C000080786

# 1 MONTH OF
# FREE
# READING

## at

## www.ForgottenBooks.com

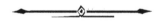

By purchasing this book you are eligible for one month membership to ForgottenBooks.com, giving you unlimited access to our entire collection of over 1,000,000 titles via our web site and mobile apps.

To claim your free month visit:

www.forgottenbooks.com/free981912

* Offer is valid for 45 days from date of purchase. Terms and conditions apply.

ISBN 978-0-260-88871-6
PIBN 10981912

This book is a reproduction of an important historical work. Forgotten Books uses
state-of-the-art technology to digitally reconstruct the work, preserving the original format
whilst repairing imperfections present in the aged copy. In rare cases, an imperfection in
the original, such as a blemish or missing page, may be replicated in our edition. We do,
however, repair the vast majority of imperfections successfully; any imperfections that
remain are intentionally left to preserve the state of such historical works.

Forgotten Books is a registered trademark of FB &c Ltd.
Copyright © 2018 FB &c Ltd.
FB &c Ltd, Dalton House, 60 Windsor Avenue, London, SW19 2RR.
Company number 08720141. Registered in England and Wales.

For support please visit www.forgottenbooks.com

# ology, Rhinology and Laryngolo

FOUNDED BY JAMES PLEASANT PARKER

INCORPORATING

THE INDEX OF OTOLARYNGOLOGY

---

H. W. LOEB, M. D., Editor-in-Chief

537 North Grand Ave., St. Louis

---

EDITORIAL BOARD

J. C. BECK, M. D., Chicago, Associate Editor

T. MELVILLE HARDIE, M. D., Chicago; G. L. RICHARDS, M. D., Fall River; THOS. J. HARRIS, M. D., New York; J. L. GOODALE, M. D., Boston; CLEMENT F. THEISEN, M. D., Albany; GEO. B. WOOD, M. D., Philadelphia; WYATT WINGRAVE, M. D., London; JOHN SENDZIAK, M. D., Warsaw; W. POSTHUMUS MEYJES, M. D., Amsterdam; N. RH. BLEGVAD, M. D., Copenhagen; VICTOR F. LUCCHETTI, M. D., San Francisco; EMIL MAYER, M. D., New York; A. J. BRADY, M. D., Sydney; S. CITELLI, M. D., Catania; H. J. B. DAVIS, M. D., London; L. W. DEAN, M. D., Iowa City; ALBERT GRAY, M. D., Glasgow; HAROLD HAYS, M. D., New York; J. D. HEITGER, M. D., Louisville; H. B. HITZ, M. D., Milwaukee; IRA FRANK, M. D., Chicago; ALBERT MILLER, M. D., St. Louis; ARTHUR I. WEIL, New Orleans; R. H. SKILLERN, M. D., Philadelphia; J. A. STUCKY, M. D., Lexington, Ky.; T. HOSHINO, M. D., Chicago.

PUBLISHED QUARTERLY
By JONES H. PARKER
TIMES BUILDING
ST. LOUIS, MO., U. S. A.

370616
25.8.39

SUBSCRIPTION PRICE, $6.00 PER ANNUM, IN ADVANCE.

Subscriptions in other countries of the Postal Union, £1 7s.

RF
A64
V. 30

# TABLE OF CONTENTS.

# ANNALS

OF

# OTOLOGY, RHINOLOGY

AND

# LARYNGOLOGY

INCORPORATING THE INDEX OF OTOLARYNGOLOGY.

| VOL. XXX. | MARCH, 1921. | No. 1. |

I.

## THE ETIOLOGY OF ACUTE INFLAMMATIONS OF THE NOSE, PHARYNX AND TONSILS.*

BY STUART MUDD, M. D., SAMUEL B. GRANT, M. D., AND ALFRED GOLDMAN, M. D.,

FROM THE DEPARTMENT OF PATHOLOGY, WASHINGTON UNIVER-
SITY SCHOOL OF MEDICINE, ST. LOUIS, MO., AND THE
LABORATORY OF BIOPHYSICS OF THE CANCER
COMMISSION OF HARVARD UNIVERSITY, BOSTON.

*The original experiments described in this paper were chiefly performed at Washington University, St. Louis, by the above authors. The paper itself is a revision of a dissertation submitted by Stuart Mudd and awarded for 1920 the Boylston Medical Prize of Harvard University, which is open to public competition. By an order adopted in 1826, the Secretary of the Boylston Medical Committee was directed to publish annually the following votes:

1. That the Board does not consider itself as approving the doctrines in any of the dissertations to which premiums may be adjudged.

2. That, in case of publication of a successful dissertation, the author be considered as bound to print the above vote in connection therewith.

SU M M ARY.

Micrococcus of Hüter.
Diplococcus coryzæ.
B. septus.
Micrococcus catarrhalis.
B. diphtheriæ.
Pneumococcus.
Bacillus of Friedländer.
B. rhinitis, Tunnicliff.
Streptococci.
B. influenzæ.
Filterable virus of influenza (?).
Filterable virus of Kruse and Foster.
Coolidge's Clinical Differentiation.

Reflex effects.
Positions of the Authorities.
Statistical Evidence.
Lowering of General Resistance by Lowering Blood Temperature.
Congestion Theory.

Methods.
Apparatus Used.
Application of the Thermopile Terminals.
Arrangement of the Subject.
Factors Determining Superficial Temperature Changes.
Control Experiments:
    (a) Respiration and Chilling.
    (b) Blood Pressure and Chilling.
    (c) Blood Temperature and Chilling.
Vasomotor Reactions to Chilling:
    Composite Graph of Temperatures of Skin and Mucous Membrane of Oropharynx and Soft Palate.
    Curve of Skin and Soft Palate.

## I.—INTRODUCTORY.

That a state of confusion exists as to the etiology of the acute inflammations of the upper respiratory tract is evident upon casual excursion into the literature. A more patient search, however, reveals certain material, notably in the form of recent laboratory work, from which definite conclusions can be drawn, and in whose light the discussions of the "common cold" in the current texts is clearly seen to be obsolete. The present dissertation is concerned with the etiology of the acute inflammations of the nose, pharynx, and fauces, particularly with reference to recent laboratory inquiries. The question of the excitation of sporadic infections by exposure of the body surface to cold is dwelt upon in considerable detail— much more at length than its relative importance deserves, indeed—simply because the newer data here presented are the contribution of the present authors.

Since the early days of bacteriology, attempt has been made by the several proponents and opponents of the infectious theory to refer the "common cold" on the one hand to the action of a specific microorganism, and on the other to various environmental and constitutional causes, such as exposure to changes of temperature, the "lithemic diathesis," and what not. Although perhaps laudable as philosophic ideals, such efforts to explain the many phenomena involved by a single cause are less deserving scientifically, and have met with just failure. The "common cold" is, as a matter of fact, in most instances the result of a local infection, but there are many types of "cold" and many infectious agents responsible for them; and the effect of various constitutional and environmental factors in determining infection is often of great importance. Furthermore there are many acute inflammations of the upper respiratory tract not primarily due to the local action of microorganisms, but rather the local expression of chemical or mechanical irritation, of nervous reflexes, of drug intoxications, of constitutional disease, or of anaphylaxis.

## II.—BACTERIOLOGY OF THE COMMON COLD.

The studies of a number of investigators have shown that, although the entrance of the nose is swarming with bacteria, the flora of the nasal cavities proper in health are kept exceedingly sparse by the action of the ciliated epithelium, the trickling of the lacrimal and mucous secretions, the inhibitory action of the mucus, and by phagocytosis. (Thomson, 1913, p. 7.) The folds of the pharyngeal mucosa and especially the crypts of the tonsils are, on the other hand, known to maintain even in health an abundant flora, including often potentially pathogenic organisms (e. g., see Davis, 1920). Bacteriologic studies of the nose and throat in the course of acute "colds" have usually shown the presence of microorganisms in unwontedly large numbers, often with one form so predominating as to suggest for it an etiologic relationship with the cold. In a number of instances immunologic and inoculation data have supported the bacteriologic evidence and would seem to warrant assumption of a causal relationship between the bacteria and the colds in question.

In 1873, Hüter described a micrococcus as a cause of coryza (cited by Benham, 1906).

Hajek (1888) described a large diplococcus, the Diplococcus coryzæ, in the early stages of acute colds. He advances no other evidence in support of his bacteriologic findings, however. Certainly in the light of recent experience with influenza, the mere presence of bacteria in large numbers during an inflammation cannot be regarded as valid ground for considering them its cause. (For a discussion of bacteriologic methods in estimating the relationship of microorganisms to respiratory disease, see Allen, 1913.)

Paulsen (1890), examining twenty-four cases of cold, of diverse clinical types, some with history of exposure to other persons with colds, and others following exposure to chilling, found various cocci and bacilli as the predominating organisms.

Cautley (1894-95) found an aerobic diphtheroid bacillus, oval, with a tendency to polar segregation of the protoplasm, in seven of eight cases of acute cold of various types. The infection started in the trachea, pharynx or nose. Cautley, believing the organism responsible for coryza, called it B. coryzæ segmentosus. Gordon (quoted by Benham, 1906) found Cautley's bacillus in all of seven cases of cold. Gordon injected two guinea pigs with the organism and noted they were sick a few days, but recovered. R. Prosser White (quoted by Benham, 1906) found Cautley's bacillus in seventeen of twenty-one cases. Inoculation experiments upon the noses and genital tracts of guinea pigs, rabbits and monkeys were negative.

Benham (1906) found a diphtheroid organism he regards as identical with Cautley's bacillus in twenty of twenty-one cases of cold. Micrococcus catarrhalis was also present in many cases. He concludes: "in view of the fact that nasal discharge was not a prominent feature of my series of cases, it seems likely that the diphtheroid organisms are rather a cause of a painful sore throat with headache, malaise and muscular pains, irritable cough and scanty, viscid expectoration. Whether they cause coryza—a cold in the head—is at · least open to question, especially in view of the presence of M. catarrhalis in nearly half my cases." Benham therefore gives Cautley's B. coryzæ segmentosus the less committal name of Bacillus septus.

Micrococcus catarrhalis was found by R. Pfeiffer (quoted by Neisser in Kolle and Wassermann's "Pathogenen Mikroorganismen," 1913) in enormous numbers in the sputum of an epidemic of mildly febrile cases of bronchitis. Gohn and H. Pfeiffer (1902) found this diplococcus in eighty-one of one hundred and forty cases of respiratory tract infection. They regarded it as a saprophyte which can under appropriate circumstances give rise to acute or subacute infection. Bezançon and de Jong (1905) found this organism very frequently in an influenza-like epidemic in Paris. Along with M. catarrhalis they found micrococcus paratetragenus, pneumococcus, Friedländer's bacillus, staphylococcus, streptococcus and diphtheroids. Dunn and Gordon (1905) believed the micrococcus catarrhalis to be the chief organism in a severe epidemic in Hertfordshire with clinical manifestations in different cases simulating cerebrospinal fever, influenza and scarlatina. Allen (1906) made claim to have isolated M. catarrhalis with ease from each case examined in a severe local epidemic of colds in England.

Neumann (1902), as a result of a considerably more extensive and thorough bacteriologic study than the foregoing, concluded that virulent diphtheria bacilli and the pneumococcus at least, perhaps other organisms, could produce the ordinary cold.

He summarizes as follows the results of his study of the flora of the noses of 111 normal persons and of 95 suffering from nasal affections of various sorts:

"The total number of bacterial species found was 19. Nevertheless in most cases there are relatively few different species found present together. Most frequently are found diphtheroid bacilli and white micrococci. Less frequently orange, gray and yellow micrococci, pneumococci, streptococci, Friedländer's bacilli, diphtheria bacilli, isolated colon bacilli, yeast, molds mixed bacilli, sarcinæ and still a few other organisms.

"Micrococcus pyogenes albus is present in 86 to 90 per cent, diphtheroids in 98 per cent of the cases, so that one can justly assert that the latter occur in every sound and pathologic nose. The more delicate form (B. xerosis) is much more frequent than the more luxuriantly growing form (Hoffman's bacillus).

"In colds the pathogenic organisms, pneumococcus, Friedländer's bacillus, streptococcus pyogenes and diphtheria bacillus are more prominent than in normal noses.

"The diphtheroid bacillus is not virulent. Seventy-eight strains cultivated from different noses in no case killed guinea pigs. In a few cases only weak infiltrations appeared at the site of injection. The organism cannot be brought into relationship with the origination of the cold and is only to be considered as a harmless saprophyte.

"Certainly it is demonstrated that virulent diphtheroid bacilli and Fränkel's pneumococcus can cause the clinical picture of the common cold. Whether and in what way other pathogenic germs are concerned in it, is still to be answered.

"A specific cause of the cold has not been found in the investigations."

Claims for the bacillus of Friedländer as a cause of "cold" are advanced, with immunilogic support, by Allen (1906). Allen asserts that in each of two epidemics of a severely infective character, in every case examined within the first 24 hours, and in some later, the bacillus was found. "It was of a very virulent stamp, being pathogenic not only for mice and guinea pigs but even for rabbits; it also clotted milk and fermented broth with ease."

Claims for an etiologic relationship are based upon the following statements, which, if true, would seem to establish the point:

"The appearance of the bacilli in the nasal passages of the people affected synchronized with the onset of the attack.

"The organism and colds disappeared together.

"The opsonic index of the patient's blood, which was particularly studied, to the bacillus of Friedländer was affected by a cold precisely in the way that would be expected in the case of an infection by that organism—that is, it rose steadily to a maximum, remained there for some time, then steadily fell to about unity during a period of perfect freedom from cold.    Second and third attacks had precisely similar results.

"The appearance in the house of a person whose nasal passages were known to be infected by the bacillus of Friedländer sufficed to start an epidemic of colds on several occasions ; and from the noses of such as were examined the bacillus of Friedländer was also isolated."

Work somewhat more convincing than any of the foregoing has been reported by Tunnicliff (1913, 1915) and Howell (1915).    The organism is an anaerobic curved bacillus.    B. rhinitis, Tunnicliff.

Miss Tunnicliff, working in Chicago, found her bacillus present in 6 per cent of some 86 normal noses examined, in 98 per cent of 82 cases of acute coryza, and in 90 per cent of twenty-odd cases of chronic rhinitis with mucoid discharge.

A slight rhinitis was produced three times in human subjects by swabbing a nose free from B. rhinitis with a pure culture.    The infection began from six to eight hours after the inoculation and lasted about 48 hours.    The organisms were present in fairly large numbers in the nose and pharynx (in the cases with pharyngitis), 18 hours after the inoculation, and persisted for three days in two of the cases.    Cultures were made twice, and the organisms isolated in pure culture both times.    The opsonic index was taken during two of the infections.    Both times it fell below normal, rising high above normal as the infection disappeared.

Vaccination of two patients with B. rhinitis produced a primary depression of the opsonic index followed by a rise above normal.

Miss Howell found that, using B. rhinitis as antigen, fixation of complement is obtained with the sera of persons with acute rhinitis and of persons injected with the bacillus after it is killed by heat.    The fixation is most marked a few days after the onset of the infection and lasts only a short time.    Sera of normal persons and of patients with various infectious diseases do not give complement fixation with the bacillus rhinitis.

It is difficult to escape the conclusion that B. rhinitis was causally related to these cases of acute coryza about Chicago.

That streptococci may be responsible for infections of the nose, and more especially the pharynx and tonsils, has been shown by many authors (vide Lingelsheim, 1912, and Barnes, 1914, p. 67).

Mathers (1917) made a careful bacteriologic study, using aerobic, anaerobic and filtration methods, of an epidemic of acute respiratory infection in Chicago, which resembled the influenza of 1889-92. He concluded that a virulent hemolytic streptococcus was the probable cause. .

Floyd (1920), as a result of bacteriologic study and vaccine therapy of the winter colds occurring in and around Boston, concluded that in acute rhinitis the organism commonly found belongs to the staphylococcus group, and that somewhat less frequently the hemolytic streptococcus has appeared. In acute pharyngitis "almost invariably the initial infection is produced by the member of the streptococcus group."

Pneumococcus has also frequently been recognized as concerned with infections of the upper respiratory tract (v. Abel, 1892; Neufeld u. Händel, 1912; Floyd, 1920).

Discussion of B. influenzæ has purposely been left out of this paper. Under this caption, however, may be quoted the conclusions of R. W. Allen (1913), based upon some ten years of bacteriologic study of the respiratory diseases, in England.

"To summarize," he writes, "it would appear that any of the seven organisms, B. influenzæ, pneumococcus, streptococcus, M. catarrhalis, M. paratetragenus, B. septus, and bacillus of Friedländer, alone or in varying combinations, may be responsible for a catarrhal condition of the upper respiratory passages. In perhaps 40 per cent of cases one organism so predominates as to justify the conclusion that it is the cause of the attack; more often two or more organisms are associated together, the B. influenzæ with the pneumococcus or M. paratetragenus, the B. septus with the M. catarrhalis or M. paratetragenus, so that it becomes very difficult to decide which organisms stand in a directly causal relationship to the attack. My own belief is that mixed infections from the beginning are fairly common.

"In uncomplicated purulent nasal catarrh the streptococcus is the most frequent cause, next to it the staphylocccus aureus. When sinus complications coexist the B. influenzæ and pneumococcus are by far the most frequent bacteria concerned."

Blake and Cecil (1920) have also reported successful infection of monkeys with B. influenzæ introduced both into the nose and intratracheally.

Cecil and Steffen (1921) have more recently produced by human inoculation with a freshly isolated virulent strain of B. influenzæ an acute self limited upper respiratory infection with local and constitutional symptoms like those of a mild endemic influenza or severe coryza.

Although any attempt at adequate discussion of the etiology of epidemic influenza is outside the scope of the present paper, its virus must be included among those capable of giving rise to acute inflammation of the upper respiratory tract. We would express our own opinion, too, that the attributes of a specific, labile and elusive virus, to which so many converging lines of evidence have pointed, are extraordinarily well filled by the filterable virus which has been the object of the past two years of careful study by Olitsky and Gates at the Rockefeller Institute (Olitsky and Gates, 1920, 1921), and which has been isolated independently by Loewe and Zeman (1921). For a bibliography and brief review of "The Epidemiology and Etiology of Influenza" reference is made to A. J. McLaughlin (1920).

A filterable virus seems without question to be the causative agent in the coryza of one fairly well defined type. Kruse (1914) diluted the secretion from the nose of an assistant with coryza, passed it through a small Berkefeld filter, and dropped a few drops of the filtrate on the nasal mucosa·of each of twelve men. Four of them developed colds in from one to four days. In a second experiment 42 per cent of thirty-six subjects so inoculated developed coryza within from one to four days. Kruse could find no living organisms in his filtrates by bacteriologic methods.

Foster (1916) in repeating and extending this work, passed through a small Berkefeld N filter, with aseptic precautions, the nasal secretion of persons suffering from acute colds. This filtrate he proved to be free from ordinary bacteria, both by ·

aerobic and anaerobic methods. From three to six drops of the filtrate was placed in each nostril of each of ten soldiers. Nine of the ten men developed the usual symptoms of acute coryza in from eight to thirty hours. Inoculated into tubes of tissue broth or tissue ascitic fluid under petrolatum, after the method of Noguchi and Flexner with rabies and poliomyelitis virus, this filtrate produced a growth which could be subcultured apparently indefinitely. Specimens of these subcultures were again diluted, passed through a Berkefeld filter, and a few drops allowed to run into the noses of eleven healthy soldiers, every one of whom developed, after an incubation period of eight to forty-eight hours, acute colds. Cultures from these individuals' nasal secretions gave the same appearance as the original cultures. They contained an abundant growth of a pleomorphic virus varying from minute globoid bodies to coccoid forms larger than staphylococci, the latter apparently in some instances with small globoid buds. (Foster, 1917.)

The clinical picture described by Foster, both for his original patients and for the subjects of the inoculation experiments, is worth giving by a typical case. The patient "complained of lassitude, chilly sensations, sneezing, unilateral nasal stuffiness, dull frontal headache with a feeling of oppression over the eyes, impairment of smell and moderate aching pain in the extremities. There was the usual lacrimation, a copious, thin, mucoid nasal discharge, which excoriated the upper lip and the alæ of the nose, and a very red, moist, swollen and boggy mucosa. The temperature was normal."

The contention of Prof. M. J. Rosenau, in whose laboratory Foster's work was done, that this type of acute coryza deserves to be considered a clinical entity, would appear to be well founded. It is extremely interesting that a symptom complex has been separated on purely clinical grounds from the remaining congeries of nose and throat affections. Coolidge (1918, p. 92) writes: "But there is one form of 'symptom complex' so common and constant that it might well be classed as a distinct and definite disease, and it is to this disease that the word 'cold' is most frequently applied." His description of it closely corresponds to Foster's.

A survey of the literature then would seem to warrant the following conclusions:

1. A common and fairly well defined clinical entity, an acute coryza, exists, probably with the filterable virus of Kruse and Foster as its causative agent. This affection is readily communicable and probably does not depend to any great extent upon the action of exciting factors in depressing the resistance of the subject. 2. A heterogeneous group of pure and mixed infections of the nose, pharynx and tonsils exists with various clinical pictures—some closely approaching that of Foster, others mere circumscribed inflammations—and with any one of a considerable number of bacteria capable, under appropriate circumstances, of acting as causative agents.

The microorganisms whose etiologic rôles seem to the writer to be best established are pneumococcus, streptococcus, B. diphtheriæ, B. rhinitis, Friedländer's bacillus, and B. influenzæ. Strong bacteriologic evidence, unsupported, however, so far as the writer knows, by immunologic or experimental data, has been advanced for M. catarrhalis, B. septus, M. paratetragenus, and S. aureus. The possibility that still other organisms may be primarily or secondarily involved is of course not excluded. Wide variations in virulence exist, both between different organisms and probably from time to time in the same bacterial strain (see Allen, 1913); some organisms are doubtless capable of causing infections in epidemic proportions, nearly or quite independent of accessory exciting factors; others may exist as harmless saprophytes upon the mucous membranes, causing infection only when the resistance of their host, local or general, is lowered by some exciting factor.

### III.—EXCESSIVE CHILLING AS AN EXCITANT OF INFECTION.

It is not the purpose of the present dissertation to attempt a sifting of the large amount of evidence, collected chiefly by ordinary and by clinical observation, which bears upon the question of the predisposing and exciting factors of upper respiratory infections. Suffice it to say that anything which lowers resistance, general or local, may disturb the equilibrium between host and parasite in the direction of exciting infection. The present section of this dissertation will concern itself with one particular factor only—namely, exposure to cold.

In the consideration of cold as an excitant of mucous membrane infection the issue has been somewhat confused by certain other effects of chilling. One of the immediate results of exposure, for instance, may be a transient rhinorrhea having no necessary relation to "catching cold." Again, a very slight draft of cool air may, in the stage of onset of a cold, be accompanied by a feeling of chilliness or even a rigor—this is obviously an effect and not, as it is sometimes wrongly considered, an antecedent of the infection.

But, in addition, it would seem to be a fact attested by long and general experience that excessive exposure to cold may be an actual excitant of rhinitis, pharyngitis or tonsillitis. For history of observation and thought on the subject, see the extensive monograph by Sticker (1916) on "Erkältungskrankheiten und Kälteschäden."

Certainly the weight of authority is in support of this thesis. Of the laryngologic texts, the following recognize chilling as an efficient factor in exciting infection: Grayson (1902), Ballenger (1908), Coakley (1914), Kyle (1914), Wright and Smith (1914), Phillips (1919), and Tilley (1919). However, Thomson (1913) and Coolidge (1918) are skeptical. In support of the affirmative are Marchand, in Krehl u. Marchand's. Handbuch d. Allgemeinen Pathologie (1908), Lingelsheim in Kolle u. Wassermann's Handbuch d. pathogenen Mikroörganismen (1912), Packard in Osler and McRae's Modern Medicine (1914), Barnes, "The Tonsils" (1914), Barker, Monographic Medicine (1916), Sticker (1916), in the Enzyklopödie der Klinischen Medizin, MacCallum's Pathology (1920), and Rosenau (1920). . The experiments of Miller and Noble (1916), who have shown that the liability of rabbits to respiratory infection by B. bovisepticus is heightened by exposure to cold after overheating or by overheating after chilling are extremely suggestive in this connection. We, too, have obtained some experimental evidence (Mudd and Grant, 1919; Grant, Mudd and Goldman, 1920), as will be shown later, which would seem to afford support to the thesis that mucous membrane infection may be excited by chilling the body surface.

What would seem to be conclusive evidence in establishing excessive exposure to cold as an efficient excitant of acute upper respiratory affections has recently come from Germany in the form of statistics for large bodies of troops during and before the war (Schade, 1919). The data in brief are as follows:

(a) Comparison of the incidence of disease during the mild winter of 1915-16 and during the very severe winter of 1916-17. The increase of disease incidence rose to almost twice the total in 1916-17; the largest single factor in this increase was the heightened incidence of respiratory affections, which in February, 1917, rose to 7.6 times the usual summer rate.

(b) Comparison of sickness among 8,000 infantry troops of whom one part (2,700 men) were subjected for three days and nights to conditions of severe cold and wet, while the rest stayed behind during the same weather in village quarters. In spite of hardening by the three previous years of trench warfare, the incidence of acute respiratory diseases, "rheumatic diseases" and acute urinary affections, chiefly acute bladder irritation with diurnal and noctural enuresis, was four times as great among the exposed as among the sheltered troops.

(c) Comparison of sickness among 8,000 infantrymen of whom one part (4,500 men) were exposed three days and nights to extreme cold (—9° to —12° C. midday temperature), accompanied by a sharp, gusty wind, while the remaining 3,500 men were in sheltered quarters. The exposed troops comprised 160 cases of "exposure disease"—i. e., 128 acute respiratory cases, 28 of rheumatism, 4 of severe bladder irritation, and 4 of freezing. Reckoned on a basis of equal numbers of men, the sheltered troops had only 40 cases of "exposure disease" and 1 of freezing.

(d) Comparison of daily incidence during three months of diseases of the respiratory tract with that of "rheumatic" affections among 8,000 troops. The curves are clearly parallel. On the same days in which the number of cases of respiratory tract catarrh increased the cases of rheumatic pain became more numerous also.

(e) Comparison of incidence of "diseases of exposure" (see above) with that of cases of freezing. Daily curves for 8,000 troops show parallelism.

The sanitary reports of the Prussian war ministry, comprising all detected diseases among all the men of Prussia, Saxony and Würtemberg in compulsory military service (more than a half million annually) have been analyzed and plotted for monthly intervals over twelve years. Of upper respiratory diseases, excluding tonsillitis, 428,714 cases are included; of "acute muscular rheumatism," 72,179 cases, and of "frost bite," 12,898 cases. Always the upper respiratory diseases show in January and February their steep winter rise; year by year the incidence of "muscular rheumatism" and of frost-bite follow in astonishing parallelism.

The curves of incidence by month for the whole twelve years combined are also given. The curve for frost bite rises from the base line in October steadily to a crest in February and returns to the base line in May. It is nearly symmetrical and of the form of the familiar frequency polygon. The curve for tonsillitis (271,852 cases) rises closely parallel to the frost bite curve from December to its peak, almost identically placed in February, and descends again almost parallel until April. The tonsillitis curve is distinguished, however, by a small secondary peak in November and by its slope becoming less steep during the spring and summer so that the base line is not approached before the October rise begins. The curve for upper respiratory diseases, exclusive of tonsillitis, runs nearly parallel to that of tonsillitis, including the secondary mode in November, but reaches its summit in January.

Such close parallelism, as Schade also gives curves to show, is not to be found between the incidence of diseases of exposure and air temperature; it is apparently with the cooling power of the air, as determined by temperature, humidity and air movement, and expressed in the frequency of frost bites, that the parallelism exists.

It is difficult to see how one could study the curves and yet escape the conclusion of the author that "chilling by the weather and the occurrence of respiratory tract catarrh stand certainly in the closest correlation."

Incidentally, to digress for a moment, the efficacy of the common respiratory affections in lowering resistance and preparing the way for the specific infections of mumps, scarlet fever and measles is shown in other curves in this most illuminating paper.

In all fairness it should be said, however, that Schade's military statistics cannot be used without some reservation in interpreting conditions of ordinary civilian life. It seems quite probable that actual lowering of body temperature may have played a much more important rôle in the incidence of respiratory disease in his statistics than most students of the subject believe it does in ordinary life.

It is probable, too, that in the general population, where the physical condition does not average so high as among the young men studied by Schade, and where exposure is not so severe, the element of contagion would play a much larger and weather a much smaller part in determining incidence of respiratory affections. However, even here, excluding the great epidemics, influenza and pneumonia begin with the frost, became severe when the temperature averages below freezing, reach a maximum when the temperature is lowest and then decline. (J. Am. M. Ass., editorial, 1920, lxxv. 1500.)

As to the mechanism of excitation of infection by chilling the skin, current opinion has gone curiously astray. Since the classic studies of Pasteur with anthrax and fowls with wet feet many authors have shown that animals whose blood temperature has been lowered may show decreased resistance to bacterial infection (Marchand, 1908). Trommsdorf (1906) further believed he showed in such animals a decreased motility and phagocytic activity of the leucocytes and a diminished capacity for regeneration of alexine and for elaboration of specific antibodies. (For literature on this subject, see Foord, 1918.) But, as Marchand himself says, and as our experiments would indicate (see below), no such considerable lowering of body temperature occurs in the majority of instances of exposure responsible for excitation of the common upper respiratory infections. Conditions in the existing animal experiments are not properly comparable to the conditions of "catching cold" in man; we must look elsewhere for an explanation.

The theory commonly advanced has been that cutaneous chilling, driving the blood inward, produces, by mechanical or reflex means, or both, congestion of the internal organs. Indeed such congestion has been demonstrated in animal experiments by a number of authors: Lassar (1880) sectioned the lungs, livers and hearts of animals after immersion in ice water, and found their vessels greatly dilated. Schüller (1881) was shown congestion of the arteries and veins of the pia mater in animals chilled by application of cold compresses. Rossbach (1901), Kisskalt (1901) and others have made similar observations upon the epithelium of the exposed trachea. Winternitz (1881) has demonstrated an increase in the volume of the arm of a human subject immersed in a cold sitz-bath, a decrease in the arm's volume when the bath water was warm.

Many authors have assumed that such findings apply equally well to the human nose and throat. The common observation that chilling may in a few minutes be followed by a feeling of stuffiness in the nose, has seemed to lend plausibility to such an assumption. That it is nevertheless absolutely at variance with what actually occurs in the nasal cavity, nasopharynx, oropharynx, tonsils and palate is shown by the experiments to be described below.

EXPERIMENTAL STUDIES OF VASOMOTOR REACTIONS OF HUMAN
SUBJECTS TO CHILLING OF THE BODY SURFACE.

Inquiry as to how the human upper respiratory mucous membranes are affected by chilling of the body surface has been undertaken by the present authors. (Mudd and Grant, 1919; Grant, Mudd and Goldman, 1920). The mucous membranes of the palate, faucial tonsils, oropharynx and nasopharynx and of the nasal cavity have been studied, primarily with regard to the vasomotor changes reflexly effected in them by chilling; and in the more recent work the changes in the bacterial flora occurring during the chilling experiments have also been considered.

Methods.—The experiments were performed upon human subjects, for the most part third and fourth year medical students and recent graduates.

Of the several criteria of vascular condition, heat seemed most readily susceptible of quantitative study. Estimation by inspection of the redness of the mucosæ was used as a check.

To follow superficial temperature changes in the sites under consideration by the direct application of thermometers was-quite impracticable.    Thermogalvanometry was of necessity employed therefore.

Apparatus used: Two similar three-element thermopiles were made up of German silver and of copper wire. In making each thermopile, three lengths of the German silver wire about a yard long were soldered alternately to three pieces of copper wire of the same length. The wires were then folded together to make a single bundle of six strands with three German silver-copper junctions at one end for application to the surface of unknown temperature, and two junctions and a loose end of copper and another of German silver at the other end of the bundle, which was to be kept at a known temperature. To each of the loose ends was soldered a copper wire leading to a rocking key. The known-temperature end of the thermopile was packed in cotton with a sensitive thermometer in a test tube suspended in the room by a clamp about its neck, or packed in a thermos bottle containing ice water.

A second three-element thermopile was similarly arranged and connected to the rocking key. From this key copper wires were led to a D'Arsonval galvanometer. Thus, by pushing down, successively, the two ends of the rocking key, each of the thermopiles could be brought successively and separately into circuit with the galvanometer.

The unknown-temperature end of the mucous membrane thermopile, when applied, was continuously bathed in mucus, containing electrolytes. Its terminals had therefore to be insulated from each other; this was accomplished by dipping them repeatedly into an alcoholic solution of shellac. The skin thermopile was similarly protected against short circuiting by sweat. The adequacy of the insulation was proved by calibrating the thermopile both in salt solution and in distilled water.

The sensitivity of the apparatus above described was such that one millimeter deflection on the galvanometer scale indicated a temperature difference of about one-tenth degree centigrade between the two ends of the thermopile in the circuit.

For calibration, the unknown temperature terminals of the thermopile were bound with elastic about the bulb of a sensitive thermometer, and this was immersed in a suspended test tube of distilled water or salt solution.

This test tube was again suspended in a beaker of water containing a stirrer. The temperature of the outer beaker was slightly raised at intervals, the water in the beaker and test tube stirred until a constant temperature had been reached, and the thermometer and galvanometer readings then taken. The calibration curves constructed from the data thus obtained were found to deviate appreciably, though very slightly, from straight lines. Temperatures were therefore taken from the curves directly.

Application of the thermopile terminals. The phase of the thermogalvanometric study of the skin and mucous surfaces which presented a new problem was that of applying the unknown temperature ends of the thermopiles. They had to be so fixed upon the site to be studied that they would remain in unchanged position, under constant and light pressure, and in such a way as not to interfere with the rise and fall of temperature in the surfaces under them in response to changing vasomotor conditions. The first two requirements were met by fastening the thermopile wires upon stiff carriers which we may designate as "applicators," and then, in the early work, fastening the latter to the appropriate surfaces by strips of adhesive plaster. Various applicators of carved wood and of wood padded with cotton covered with adhesive plaster were tried and rejected because they interfered with the normal loss of heat from the surfaces under them. Applicators satisfactory in all respects were finally made from galvanized iron wire. A medium size was used, such that it could be twisted and hammered into the required shapes, yet would bear considerable pressure without deformation. No. 13 wire proved most satisfactory.

. The several applicators used in the experiments to be considered below are shown in Fig. 1 and Fig. 2. Each consists of a body along which the thermopile wires are strung and supports placed, and a tip just large enough to allow the three terminals of the thermopile to be twisted around it. The tip is so shaped as to conform to the contour of the surface against which it is to hold the thermopile terminals. The terminals, although insulated with shellac as described above, are sepa-

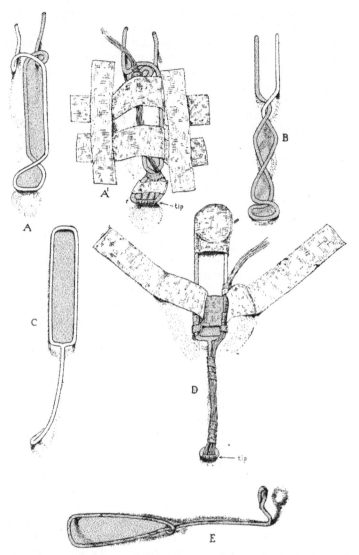

Fig. 1. Applicators: A, for skin; A', same, applied; B, for soft palate; C, for faucial tonsils; D, for oropharynx, ready for application; E, for nasopharynx.

rated from the metal tip by a single strip of adhesive plaster as a further safeguard against short circuiting. (See Fig. 1, A' and D, and Fig. 2, F.)

The skin applicators (Fig. 1, A and A') are so shaped as to form a bridge, resting stably on a support at either end, one of which is the tip, bearing the terminals. Across this raised bridge are placed the adhesive straps which hold the device in position on the skin. The tip rested usually either in the subject's supraclavicular fossa or on the forehead.

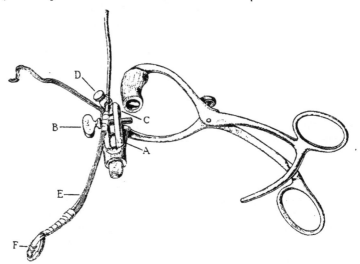

Fig. 2. Tonsillar applicator and holder: **A** and **C**, ball and socket joints made by metal spheroids and blades of head mirror; **B**, set screw for tightening joints at **A** and **C**; **D**, set screw for fastening applicator in holder; **E**, applicator; **T**, tip bearing thermopile terminals.

The mucous membrane applicators (Fig. 1, B, C, D and E) were slung in the subject's open mouth by a long adhesive strip (Fig. 1, D), which supported the body of the applicator, then passed up just in front of the corners of the mouth and was fastened on the subject's two cheeks. The tip of the applicator held the thermopile terminals against the particular site on the palate, tonsil or pharynx whose temperature changes were studied. The other end of the applicator projected out of the subject's mouth and bore a small weight.  Thus the whole device when in position constituted a lever whose fulcrum was the supporting adhesive strip, whose short arm was weighted and the tip of whose long arm held the thermopile end against the mucous surface.

In the experiments upon the faucial tonsils this method was much improved upon.  Into one arm of a Doyen mouth gag (Fig. 2) a small brass sphere, A, was screwed.  A second brass sphere bearing a groove closed by a set screw, D, was made. The two spheres were connected by means of the blades of an ordinary head mirror, C.  The blades could be clamped stably upon the spheres by means of a second set screw, B.  The applicator, E, so shaped as to have its tip fit against the tonsil, was held in place in its groove by the set screw, D.  By varying the shape and position of the applicator and arranging properly the two joints at A and C, any desired application could be made.  The subject's teeth were protected from the metal gag by rubber as shown in the drawing.

The applicator holder for the nasal cavity experiments consisted of a plate of strong but slightly flexible fiber board, about 1.5 mm. in thickness, so shaped that it could be firmly held between the subject's teeth, and cross hatched with a fine saw to prevent slipping, into which was screwed a metal sphere like that of Fig. 2, A, connected through metal blades to a second spheroid with groove and set screw, as in Fig. 2.  The arrangement of the applicator and thermopile wires was like that of Fig. 2, except that the applicator was straight and its terminal loop for the thermopile tips was very small.  The subject held his lips tight closed over the fiber board plate.

Arrangement of the subject:  The experiments were performed in a constant-temperature room, kept, on the average, between eighteen and nineteen degrees centigrade.  The subject entered the room undressed save for shoes and socks, but warmly wrapped in loose garments.  Throughout an experiment he sat in unchanging position, tongue held flat on the floor of his mouth, and applicator in position.  The sites on which the applicators were placed were of course never wrapped and were protected from direct chilling.  The experimenter removed and reapplied the wraps without disturbing the subject.  Chilling was effected by (a) removing the wraps: or (b) unwrapping and applying cold wet towels to the subject's back; or (c) unwrapping and turning an electric fan upon the subject's back. The third method was found to be by far the most efficacious.

In the earlier experiments very considerable difficulty was experienced because of the necessity for swallowing the saliva and mucus secreted in excessive amounts under these circumstances. This difficulty was subsequently minimized by continuously evacuating the liquids in the mouth through a glass tube—the ordinary saliva ejector tube of the dentists—connected through rubber tubing with a suction pump on a water faucet.

Factors determining superficial temperature changes: The factors determining the temperature changes in the skin and mucous surfaces during the course of an experiment may now readily be understood. The skin is a surface constantly being heated from below by the circulating blood in the cutaneous vessels (and to a less extent by direct conduction of heat from the deeper tissues), and constantly losing heat by evaporation of moisture, and by radiation, conduction and convection to the cold air of the room to which it is exposed. Since the temperature of the room (and of the deeper body tissues) remains virtually constant throughout the experiment, the skin temperature depends primarily upon two variable factors, viz., (a) the blood temperature and (b) the amount of blood per unit of time which circulates through the cutaneous vessels. Of these the latter is incomparably the more important. For although a rise or fall in blood temperature would of course tend to effect a corresponding change in skin temperature, yet such blood temperature changes under the conditions of our experiments were found to take place only to a relatively slight degree. It is a fact of much greater moment that, as more blood circulates through the skin, the superficial temperature must rise, that as the cutaneous vessels are constricted the superficial temperature must fall.

For theoretical completeness, alterations in rate of evaporation of sweat must also be considered. However, with the sudden changes from warmth to chilling and vice versa used in our experiments, sweat evaporation changes must have played a small part; and whatever part they did play must have been simply to make less striking the primarily important effects of vasoconstriction and vasodilation. For example, chilling the body surface was found experimentally to cause a sharp fall in superficial temperature due to reflex cutaneous vasoconstriction. But this same chilling would decrease the production of sweat and the rate of sweat evaporation and hence tend to prevent the fall in temperature incident to vasoconstriction; and similarly for warming the body, mutatis mutandis.

Also. in the mucous membranes the factor of prime importance in effecting temperature changes is that of vasomotor tone. Blood temperature, because of its relative constancy, is of minor interest. Room temperature, rate of evaporation of liquids and conduction of heat to the surface from deeper tissues are all virtually constant throughout the experiment, and so require no consideration. A third factor of consequence operating here must, however, be considered, namely, changes in rate and volume of respiration. We may assume the mucous membrane, warmed by the circulating blood, to be losing heat in three ways: (a) by direct radiation through the open mouth, (b) by inhalation of cool air and exhalation of warm air in respiration, and (c) by conduction down a thermal gradient established through the air in the mouth, and especially along the metal applicator, to the cold room outside. From what has been said above, it is evident that the rate of heat loss by (a) radiation, and (c) conduction, was kept virtually constant throughout each experiment. In all the experiments cited below (b) respiration was carefully controlled—rate of breathing in time with a metronome, and depth by the use of a thoracic and abdominal pneumograph writing on a smoked drum in sight of the subject.

Finally, the effects of air currents and eddies in the experimental room must be considered. Although the sites of application of the thermopiles were protected from the direct draft of the fan, minor currents and eddies were necessarily set up in the small closed room, and the direct cooling effect of these upon the exposed skin could not be eliminated. This direct cooling, as closely as we have been able to estimate it, probably amounted usually to between one-third and one-half of the observed skin temperature fall. The curves should be studied with this correction in mind. On the other hand, it is obvious that in experiments in which the mouth was closed and the applicator upon the pharyngeal wall, currents in the room could not have entered at all into the depression of mucous membrane temperature. Similarly with the applicator in the nasal cavity and nose breathing, or on the palate or pharyngeal wall, even with the mouth open, direct cooling by air currents in the room have entered but slightly or not at all into the observed mucous membrane temperature fall. The effect of the air currents, then, has been to make appear less striking in comparison with those of the skin the vasoconstrictor reflexes of the mucous membranes with chilling of the body surface.

The thermopiles when applied to such surfaces under the conditions described do not record precisely the absolute temperatures of the surfaces as they would in the absence of the thermopiles. However, we believe that this method does afford an accurate and sensitive means of recording superficial temperature changes, and, through these, states of vasomotor tone, and it is with these that we are concerned. Measurement of the absolute mucous membrane temperature, if desired, could be effected by a modification of the method used for the skin by Benedict, Miles and Johnson (1919).

Control Experiments.—In order to determine the validity of mucous membrane temperature as a criterion of vasomotor tone it was necessary to study changes effected in respiration, blood pressure and blood temperature by the conditions of our experiments. Without going into detail, the results of these control observations may be briefly summarized.

Chilling the body surface has, both in our controls and in animal experiments (Ansiaux, 1889, p. 569) increased the volume of respiratory change, and this in turn often depressed mucous membrane temperature. It was for this reason that control of respiration by metronome and pneumographs was necessary.

Blood pressure was not, in the two trials made, significantly altered by chilling. Animal experiments have shown an initial rise, followed, in instances of extreme chilling with depression of blood temperature, by a progressive fall (Marchand, 1908, p. 125, and Ansiaux, 1889). The depression of superficial temperature observed with cutaneous chilling was therefore not the result of lowered blood pressure.

Blood temperature, as has been said, underwent only slight alterations during the course of our experiments. So efficient is the heat regulating mechanism in man, indeed, that during chilling the blood temperature rose very slightly, to undergo a slight fall on cessation of chilling. (Fig. 3.) Liebermeister (1860) found essentially similar changes in axillary temperature with chilling of the skin.

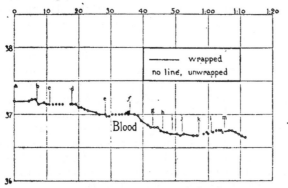

Fig. 3. Blood-temperature control: (a) electric light is reflected on thermometer; (b) light removed; (c) unwrapped; (d) wrapped; (e) unwrapped, fan on; (f) fan off, wrapped; (g) muscles of subject under tension; (h) subject feels warm; (i) subject sits comfortably, skin seems flushed; (j) subject feels cold; (k) unwrapped, cold towels to back; (l) fresh cold wet towels to back; (m) dried and wrapped.

*Vasomotor Reactions to Chilling.*—Temperature changes in the skin and exposed mucous membranes were thus established as valid criteria, under the conditions of our experiments, of vasomotor tone. The graphs to follow actually show surface temperature changes; their significance is of alterations in blood supply. Obviously, fall in temperature means reflex vasoconstriction, a rise, vasodilation.

The vasomotor responses to chilling of a distant area of the body surface exhibited in the exposed skin of the forehead and of the mucous membrane of the soft palate and oropharynx, respiration and other conditions being carefully controlled as described above, may readily be made out from Fig. 4.

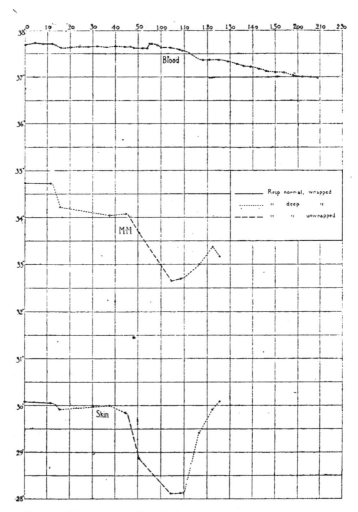

Fig. 4. Effects of chilling body surface, respiration controlled. Composite graphs of four experiments (temperatures of skin and mucous membranes of oropharynx and soft palate), and two experiments (blood temperature). Subject chilled by unwrapping, with draft of electric fan on back.

The two lower curves of this figure are composite graphs of four experiments of similar pattern. The points chosen for plotting are: The first and last readings of each experiment, the readings immediately before and after each change in experimental conditions, and the first point of maximum response of the mucous membrane to changed conditions; each point graphed is the average value of the corresponding point of the four experiments. Time is plotted on the horizontal axis, temperature on the vertical; the space between the ruled lines represents ten minutes on the abscissa, one-half degree centigrade on the ordinate. The character of the lines connecting the points gives the nature of the experimental conditions, as indicated in the legend.

While respiration is quiet and the subject wrapped, mucous membrane and skin temperatures remain constant. Deepening of respiration affects only inconsiderably the skin temperature, but causes a depression of mucous membrane temperature amounting to .68° C.; which reaches its maximum after 25.4 minutes, and then, during the remaining 8.5 minutes before chilling begins, remains virtually constant.

The subject was chilled by unwrapping him and directing the draft of an electric fan against the lower thoracic region of his back. With the start of this process, a marked depression both of mucous membrane and of skin temperature begins. The maximum fall of mucous membrane temperature is 1.42° C., reached in 18.4 minutes. The synchronous point on the skin curve represents a drop of 1.73° C. The skin curve falls away a little more sharply than the mucous membrane curve. However, even if the vasoconstriction in skin and mucous membrane were to follow an identical course, we should expect, on mechanical grounds, this difference in the curves; for the more exposed forehead would of course lose heat more readily than the mucosa of the palate and pharynx.

When it was seen the mucous membrane temperature had ceased to fall, the fan was turned off and the subject again wrapped. Here a disparity in the behavior of skin and mucous membrane vessels appears. The skin temperature climbs steeply and surmounts the level at which chilling began. The skin "reacts," as is commonly said. But the mucous membrane temperature rises only .73° C. Its maximum recovery is reached after 12.7 minutes and is .69° C. below the last point before chilling.   During the remaining 3.5 minutes of observation it falls .21° C.

No explanation in mere physics is to be found for the mucous membrane temperature remaining depressed; if its vessels returned to the same tone as before chilling, the temperature curve should return to control level.   Yet this same incomplete recovery after chilling was noted in all the crucial experiments upon soft palate and pharynx, alike in the early determinations with respiration uncontrolled and the final ones with respiration controlled.   Measurement of the respiration records for the four experiments graphed in Fig. 4 was made, and the mean figure arrived at for respiratory amplitude before chilling differed from that after chilling by only a fraction of 1 per cent.   In those experiments in which respiration was slightly deeper before as well as in those in which it was a few per cent deeper after chilling, the failure of the mucous membrane temperature to regain its former level is usually evident.   We are forced to conclude, therefore, that the vasoconstriction and ischemia reflexly produced in the palatine and pharyngeal mucous membrane by chilling the body surface persist in part for some time at least.   The skin in our experiments has tended more completely to regain its blood supply.   The tonsils have tended to regain their blood supply even more completely than the skin, in some instances actually becoming hyperemic on rewarming (Grant, Mudd and Goldman, 1920).

The uppermost curve in Fig. 4 is a composite of two blood temperature control experiments which followed the same pattern as the two lower curves.   For discussion, see above.

A few experiments, illustrating typical reactions in the several regions of the nose and throat, may now be briefly considered:

Experiment A: M. M. thermopile on anterior half of soft palate.   Skin thermopile on forehead.   Respiration, 18 per minute.   Mouth open, nose breathing.   Thoracic and abdominal pneumographs.   Room temperature, 17.9° to 18.8° C.; time, 3.55 to 5:16 p. m.

Experiment A from 0:00 to 0:50, shows the typical picture described for the composite graph above, save that the an-

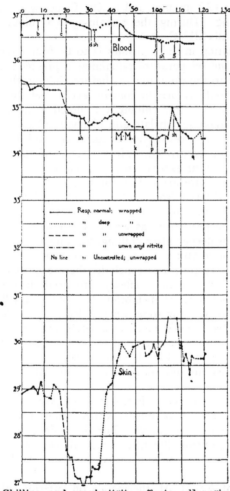

Fig. 5. Chilling and amyl-nitrite effects. Experiment A (temperatures of skin and mucous membrane of soft palate), and experiment K (blood temperature): (a) wrapped; (b) unwrapped; (c) wrapped; (d) unwrapped, fan on back; (sh) shivering begins; (e) fan off, wrapped, shivering stops; (f) unwrapped, cold, wet towel to back; (sh) is shivering; (g) dried and wrapped; (k) cold, wet towels to feet, fan on feet; (p) more cold water poured on towels around feet; (r) respiration is exaggerated; (q) fan off, feet dried and wrapped.

terior palatine mucous membrane is not affected by deepening respiration. At 0:50 the subject's feet were exposed,
wrapped in cold wet towels, and the electric fan turned on
them. This seems to have been without effect upon the forehead, but was followed apparently by a slight depression, .29°
C. of mucous membrane temperature. This effect was not
sufficiently definite to warrant much emphasis, but is at least
suggestive in view of the possible efficacy of wet feet in exciting colds.

Administration of amyl nitrite at 1:03, while the feet were
still being chilled, was followed by a steep rise in mucous and
skin temperatures with quick return to normal. The break
in the skin curve is meant to indicate that it may have risen
about 30.5° C. in the interval, 1:02 to 1:08, during which no
skin readings were made.

The uppermost curve in Fig. 5 is a blood temperature control.

Experiment B: M. M. thermopile on posterior wall of oropharynx. Skin thermopile on forehead. Respiration, 18 per
minute. Nostrils plugged with cotton, mouth breathing. Thoracic and abdominal pneumographs. Room temperature, 19.0°
to 20.6° C.; time, 10:11 p. m. to 12:33 a. m.

The curve of Experiment B (Fig. 6) shows the pharyngeal
mucous membrane reacting in essentially the manner indicated
in the composite graph, and shown also for the palatine membrane in Experiment A. The difficulties in technic are considerably greater with the thermophile applied to the pharynx
than to the palate, however, and the curve is never so smooth.
The effects of moving the pharyngeal wall against the thermopile terminals by coughing, swallowing or clearing the
throat, is shown at 0:27, 0:50.5 and 1:41. Presumably two
factors play a part in the sudden rise in temperature produced; the momentarily increased pressure between terminals
and mucous membrane slightly increased, mechanically, the
temperature of the former; the painful mechanical irritation
of the mucosa by the metal terminals and applicator probably
caused a transient blush. The rises in temperature, which
took place before chilling, although apparently elicited by less
movement, were much more marked than that which occurred

during the active vasoconstriction with chilling—1.77° and 2.69° C., as compared with .98° C.

The effect upon skin temperature of inhaling amyl nitrite is shown (2:17). A rise of .5 C. is again produced.

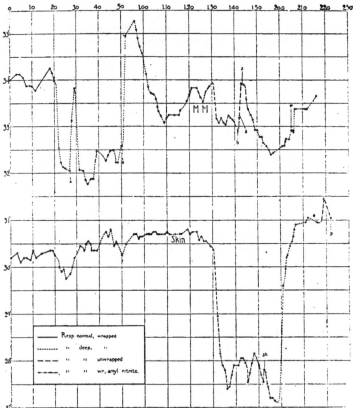

Fig. 6. Effects of chilling, mechanical irritation and amyl nitrite. Experiment B (temperatures of skin and mucous membrane of oropharynx): (a) coughs and clears the throat; (b) clears throat and swallows; (s) swallows; (sh) begins shivering; (r) misses several respirations; (p) exact time of point (p) not known; (d) coughs and clears throat.

It is to be remembered that, since the mucous membrane and skin curves of each experiment are synchronous, the annotations, although drawn in as though applying only to one curve, apply equally to both.

Experiment C: M. M. thermopile on posterior wall of naso-pharynx. Skin applicator on forehead. At first, nostrils

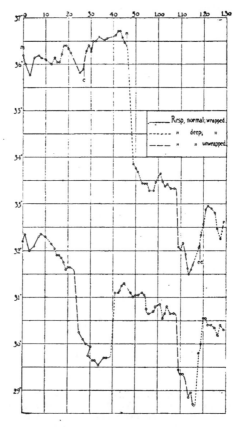

Fig. 7. Chilling effect. Experiment C (temperatures of skin and mucous membranes of nasopharynx): (m) nostrils plugged, breathing through mouth; (c) coughs; (n) plugs removed from nostrils, breathes through nose; (cc) coughs three times.

plugged, breathing through mouth; later, breathing through nose, mouth open. Respiration, 18 per minute. Thoracic and

abdominal pneumographs.  Room temperature, 15.7° to 16.9°
C.; time, 4:15 to 5:45 p. m.

With the anterior nares plugged and the soft palate raised
in mouth breathing, the nasal chamber was virtually a closed
cavity, whose temperature did not vary with the rate of blood
flow through its walls.  Correspondingly, the mucous mem-

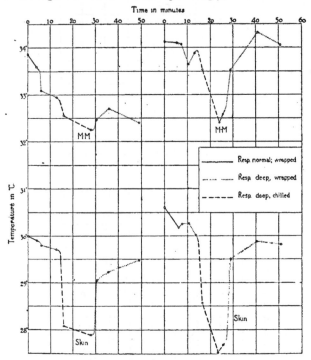

Fig. 8.  Reactions to chilling and to rewarming.  On left, composite of three experiments.  (Temperatures of skin and mucous
membrane of soft palate and oropharynx.  On right, composite of
four experiments.  Temperatures of skin and mucous membrane
of faucial tonsils.)

brane curve (Fig. 7) showed no certain change when, at
0:08.5, respiration was deepened, nor at 0:22, when the sub-.
ject was unwrapped and chilled with the electric fan.  The
skin curve, on the other hand, dropped off characteristically,
to recover when the subject was rewrapped.

At 0.46 the nostrils were unplugged and nose breathing began. The nasopharynx at once came into free communication with the outer air, and was cooled by each respiration, and became dependent upon its blood supply for maintenance of its temperature. When equilibrium had been reached, the subject was again, at 1:07.5, unwrapped and chilled with the fan. Mucous membrane and skin temperatures fell together, the former reaching a maximum depression of 1.83° C. in six minutes, the latter of 1.95° C. in eight minutes. After rewrapping at 1:16, the mucous membrane temperature rose in six minutes to a maximum point .38° below the control level, then fell slightly; the skin temperature mounted in four minutes to a maximum only .10° below control level.

In the experiments of the first series a single exception to the rule that mucous membrane temperature, upon wrapping after chilling, does not regain its original level, was found in the experiment performed upon a faucial tonsil. In this case mucous membrane temperature rose well above control level. With this idea of determining whether or not this behavior was characteristic, and because of the peculiar importance of the tonsils as a site of infection, a second series of experiments was performed with especial reference to the tonsillar reactions. These confirmed the earlier observation.

The curves on the right of Fig. 8 are a composite of four experiments upon tonsil and skin; on the left are shown for comparison composites of two experiments with the soft palate and one with the oropharynx as mucous membrane site of application.

In the tonsillar curves chilling begins at 0:15; mucous membrane and skin temperature fall away steeply together. Upon rewrapping at 0:27 skin temperature returns not quite to control level, tonsillar temperature considerably above it. In the palatine pharyngeal curve, on the other hand, the characteristic failure to regain normal relaxation of vasomotor tone after chilling is again evinced.

Experiment D: M. M. thermopile on left faucial tonsil. Skin application on forehead. Nostrils plugged, breathing through mouth. Respiration, 14 per minute. Thoracic and abdominal pneumographs. Room temperature, 17.3° to 19.45° C.; time, 11 a. m. to 12 m.

Experiment D illustrates the same reactions as the composite. With the beginning of chilling at 0:12 skin and mu-

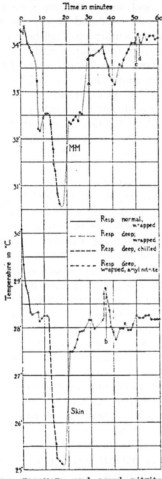

Fig. 9. Chilling, recovery and amyl nitrite reactions. Experiment D (temperatures of skin and mucous membrane of faucial tonsil): (a) applicator seen to be all right; (b) flush fading; (c) respiration shallow; (d) breathes deeper.

cosa lose heat together, to regain it on rewrapping at 0:17.5. By 0:34.5 the mucous membrane temperature had risen to

33.85° C., 1:32° above the level at which chilling began. At
0:35 an ampule of amyl nitrite is inhaled. The vasodilation
in the already hyperemic tonsillar mucous membrane was evidently insufficient to counterbalance the effect of lowered gen-

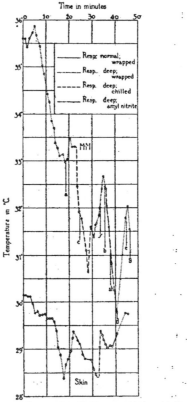

Fig. 10. Chilling and amyl nitrite reactions. Experiment E
(temperature of skin and mucous membrane of faucial tonsil):
(a) clears throat; (c) coughed; (f) face flushed; (b) flush passing,
amyl nitrite taken away; (sh) shivering; (d) clears throat; (e)
respiration too shallow, deepened; (g) subject fainted.

eral blood pressure, so that a fall in temperature resulted. The
skin temperature on the other hand, rose characteristically
with the amyl nitrite. As the flush passed, skin temperature
fell and mucosal temperature rose to their former levels.

Experiment E: M. M. thermopile on left faucial tonsil. Skin applicator on forehead. Nostrils plugged; mouth breathing. Respiration, 14 per minute. Thoracic and abdominal pneumographs. Room temperature, 17.5° to 18.55° C.; time, 10:56 to 11:43 a. m.

Figure 10 with the beginning of chilling shows the usual temperature fall; the recovery curve was terminated prematurely by the subject unfortunately fainting. Amyl nitrite was administered during chilling at 0:32.5. Vasodilation here evidently more than counterbalanced blood pressure fall, for the skin and mucous membrane temperatures each rose steeply.

The reactions of the nasal cavity have recently been found to be similar in quality to those of the oropharynx and nasopharynx, but quantitatively much more striking. Twelve experiments have been performed on seven different subjects of Aryan, Semitic and Mongolian stock. The sites tested are the nasal septum, inferior and middle turbinates, and inferior and middle meati, all, because of difficulty in application farther back, in the anterior half of the nasal cavity.

In every case chilling of the body surface has resulted in reflex vasoconstriction in the nasal mucous membrane, rewarming in vasodilation. Striking vasodilation occurs on inhaling amyl nitrite.

The reflex to the nasal mucous membrane showed a lower threshold than the corresponding reflex to the skin of the forehead. Merely unwrapping the subject in a room of 14.0° to 18.0° C. in a number of instances resulted in no change or a very slight fall in skin temperature and a fall in mucous membrane temperature of 1.5° to 2.0° C., or even more. A similar though smaller fall in mucous membrane temperature, unaccompanied by a skin temperature depression, has been observed also on unwrapping the subject with the thermopile tips on the palate, tonsil and nasopharyngeal wall.

Similarly the threshold of the chilling vasoconstrictor reflex to the forehead has been found to be higher than that to the skin of the trunk.

Application to the nasal mucosa of the thermopile terminals was extremely irritating and resulted in discharge of considerable amounts of clear mucus. The discharge was both on the side of the cavity in which application was made and on the opposite side, although more abundant on the former.

It seemed to be little if at all affected by the marked shrinkage of the mucous membrane during chilling. In three experiments the subject thought secretion was slightly

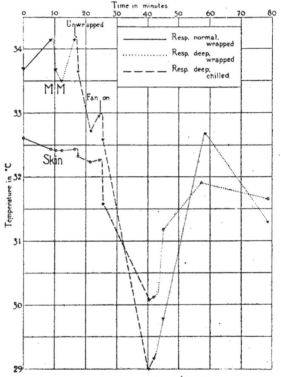

Fig. 11. Reactions of nasal cavity to chilling and rewarming of body surface. Composite graph of seven experiments. (Temperatures of skin and of mucous membrane of nasal septum, inferior turbinates and middle meatus, in anterior half of nasal cavity.)

more copious during chilling; in one he thought it slightly less. In others no change in secretion was noted. These last observations bring out two facts:

1. Discharge from the nasal cavity may be reflex and may occur in regions of the nose not directly irritated.

2. Rhinorrhea is not necessarily accompanied by vasomotor turgescence in the nasal cavity.

The nasal vasomotor reactions are illustrated by Figs. 11 and 12.*  (Footnote below.)

Figure 11 is a composite of seven experiments of similar pattern performed upon four subjects.  The sites used were the right and left sides of the nasal septum, the right and left inferior turbinates, and the left middle meatus.

A transitory fall of 0.6° C. in mucous membrane temperature followed deepened respiration.  On unwrapping the subject. mucous membrane temperature was depressed 1.4° C.; skin temperature synchronously only 0.2° C.  Turning an electric fan on the subject's lower back resulted in a further mucous membrane fall of 3.7° C. and a skin fall of 2.1° C.  Maximum recovery for mucous membrane was 3.7° C. (71 per cent); for skin the corresponding recovery was 1.8° C. (77 per cent).

Experiment F: M. M. thermopile on anterior end of left inferior turbinate.  Skin applicator on forehead.  Mouth closed; nose breathing.  Respiration, 14 per minute.  Thoracic and abdominal pneumographs.  Room temperature, 16.0° to 17.0° C.; time, 1:14 to 2:48 p. m.

Figure 12 illustrates in an individual experiment the reactions brought out in the composite.  With unwrapping at :12.0 the skin temperature is not depressed for two and a half minutes; the mucous membrane temperature in like time falls 1.6° C.  The pronounced drop in both mucous membrane and skin curves with fan on is interrupted by a sharp rise following amyl nitrite administration at 0:23.25, amounting, in the case of the mucosa, to 3.9° C., in that of the skin to 1.1° C.  After unwrapping, the mucous membrane temperature in this experiment slightly more than regained its level of before chilling (in most of the experiments it remained depressed).  Inhalation of amyl nitrite in this flushed condition of the mucous membrane resulted in a momentary depression of 0.2° C., followed by a rise of 0.6° C.  Skin temperature rose 1.0° C. approximately as before.  The experiment ends with a pro-

---

*For detailed account, see Mudd, Grant and Goldman (1921).

found vasoconstriction of mucous membrane and skin vessels incident on a second chilling with the fan.

Checking of quantitative results by qualitative observations of redness. The experimental analysis outlined above ade-

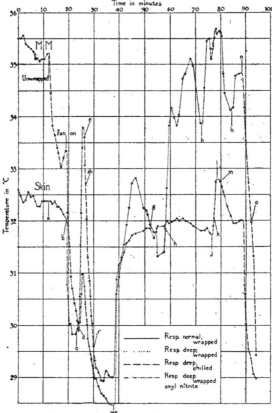

Fig. 12. Chilling, rewarming and amyl nitrite reactions. Experiment F (temperatures of skin and mucous membrane of left inferior turbinate, anterior end). (a) Subject unwrapped; (b) fan on; (c) amyl nitrite inhalation begins; (d) face has begun to flush; (e) flush fading, stops inhaling; (sh) shivers; (f) is shivering; (wr) fan off, warmly wrapped; (g) m. m. applicator feels to subject to be in correct position; (h) m, m. applicator readjusted so that subject can feel pressing against turbinate; (j) amyl nitrite administered; (k) face flushed; (l) stops inhaling amyl nitrite; (m) flush fading; (n) unwrapped, fan; (o) is shivering hard.

quately proves, it seems to us, that chilling of the body surface reflexly produces vasoconstriction in the vessels supply-
ing the normal mucous membranes of the palate, tonsils, oropharynx and nasopharynx, and of the nasal cavity. However, in order to secure still further corroboration, observations of the appearance of the mucous membranes and their
blood vessels were made.

Twelve experiments were performed. Of the five observers who noted the appearance of the buccal and oropharyngeal
membranes before and after direct exposure of those membranes to cold air, all were of the opinion that, with the direct
chilling, blanching occurred. Of the six observers who noted
the appearance of the soft palate and the seven who studied
the normal oropharynx before and after chilling of the body
surface, all said that the membranes paled while the skin was
being chilled. Only one observer specifically studied the reaction of the tonsils. He said that they blanched during the
skin's chilling. Of the three observers who watched the
changes following rewrapping, one simply said that reddening occurred; two said that reddening occurred only to a slight
extent.

The first point, i. e., the response of the mucous membranes to direct chilling, was not suitable to thermogalvanometric study. The observation that blanching occurred is,
however, in harmony with observations upon direct cooling
of the nasal mucous membrane made by Cocks (1915). (For
bibliography on effect of cold on circulation of immediate
region to which it is applied, see Nägelsbach, 1920). The
other points observed are wholly in accord with the quantitative studies.

Results in harmony with our own have been published by Tschalussow (1913), who used the nose with
posterior nares packed, as a plethysmographic chamber and studied the results of chilling the feet and lower legs
and of other sensory stimulation, and by Galeotti (1920), who
studied the effect upon the temperature of the expired air of
cutaneous chilling and warming. Tschalussow found that in
a human subject emersion of the feet and lower legs in water
at 18° C. caused a marked decrease in the volume of the nasal
cavity; electrical stimulation, needle pricks and scratching the

skin caused vasoconstriction also, but to a less degree. Galeotti (1914) found that the temperature of the expired air is depressed 1° to 2° C. by cutaneous chilling, raised correspondingly by warming. In explanation of this, he advanced the somewhat improbable hypothesis of pulmonary vasoconstriction.

Vasomotor reactions of abnormal tissues: (a) Reactions in chronic inflammatory throats: One new point of great interest was brought out by the observation experiments in which the pillars and tonsils were seen to blanch with the cutaneous chilling. The pharynx of this same subject was much injected. He gave a history of having noticed a sore throat about a week before, which he thought had cleared up; the night before the experiment he had driven an open machine without an overcoat, and his sore throat had returned. The diagnosis was chronic catarrhal pharyngitis with pustules. This inflamed throat did not pale with the rest of the mucous membrane, but, if anything, its injection was intensified by chilling the body surface.

In a thermogalvanometric experiment upon a case of chronic pharyngitis of two years' standing, a similar reaction resulted (Fig. 13).

History.—Began smoking in 1915; used about four cigarettes daily. In 1916, began smoking fifteen to twenty cigarettes daily; about this time pharyngitis began. Since has smoked eight to ten cigarettes daily. Treated April, May and June, 1917, Johns Hopkins dispensary, with argyrol, etc. No improvement. Treated twice a week with argyrol and silver nitrate, November and December, 1918, in St. Louis. No improvement. Told smoking was probable cause, and if would stop smoking throat would get well. Conditions unchanged August 2, 1918, when experiment performed.

Experiment G: M. M. thermopile on inflamed posterior wall of oropharynx. Skin thermopile on forehead. Respiration, 13 per minute. Nostrils plugged; mouth breathing. Thoracic and abdominal pneumographs. Room temperature, 18.7° to 19.5° C.; time, 10:10 to 11:35 p. m.

The skin curve in Fig. 13 is typical. The mucous membrane temperature shows the fall with deepened respiration which of necessity would follow inhalation into the pharynx through the open mouth of increased volume of cold air. However, with chilling, 0:18.5 to 0:42, the mucous membrane temperature, instead of dropping with the skin temperature, shows a slight transient rise. The shape of the curve, reaching its height in the middle of the period of chilling and then slowly sinking, apparently uninfluenced by the cessation of chilling, suggests that it records some slight changes in local vaso_motor tone quite independent of the cutaneous chilling, or

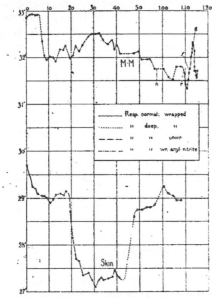

Fig. 13. Chilling and amyl nitrite effects upon chronically in-flamed oropharynx. Experiment G (temperature of skin and mucous membrane of oropharynx): (n) plugs pulled from subject's nose, begins nose breathing; (r) respiration suddenly deepened; (f) face flushed; (g) flush passing, respiration still exaggerated.

alterations in general blood pressure, or some slight accidental change in experimental conditions. At all events, there is no questioning the fact that the normal reflex vasoconstriction is absent.

Inhalation of an ampule of amyl nitrite (1:08 to 1:09.5) was followed by characteristic vasodilation. Measurement of the respiration record shows breathing to have been suddenly deepened at 1:09 (Fig. 13, r) and to have maintained itself abnormally deep until 1:14.5, when the subject could no longer maintain the slow rhythm, and respiration became quick and shallow. The preliminary fall of mucous membrane temperature from 1:09 to 1:10.5 was doubtless due, therefore, to deepened respiration and a fall in general blood pressure; the rise from 1:10.5 to 1:13.25 was unquestionably due to local vasodilation and occurred in spite of deepened respiration and lowered blood pressure.

Amyl nitrite causes vasodilation by direct action upon the smooth muscle of the blood vessel walls. This typical dilator response of the inflamed throat to amyl nitrite shows, therefore, that the vessel walls are capable of reacting normally. The typical skin curve would indicate proper functioning on the part of the afferent and association elements of the reflex arc. This failure of normal reaction to cutaneous chilling, in so far as conclusions can be drawn from a single experiment, must then be referred to the motor elements of the reflex arc, and probably has its seat in or near the inflamed mucous membrane.*

Reaction to amyl nitrite of an acute inflammatory palate: Experiment H: M. M. thermopile upon the intensely injected soft palate. Acute pharyngitis and tonsillitis. Respiration uncontrolled. Mouth breathing (except 0:00 to 0:23).

At 0:10.5 (Fig. 14) subject inhaled by mouth an ampule of amyl nitrite. A steep fall of mucous membrane temperature, amounting to 2.69° C. followed. The minimum temperature was reached in 13.5 minutes, and was followed by a rise of 2.56° C., attained in four minutes.

Evidently the vessels of the inflamed membrane were practically maximally dilated. The temperature change observed was therefore the result of the increase in depth of respiration and the depression of general blood pressure.

---

*This experiment is included as suggestive merely, not conclusive; for in later work it was found that a normal throat which ordinarily responded to chilling by reflex vasoconstriction would occasionally fail to exhibit that response. The explanation seemed to be usually or always that excessive swallowing and resultant traumatization of the pharynx occurred during the period of chilling, with consequent dilation of the vessels, as shown in Fig. 6. Such may possibly have been the case in this experiment.

Reflex reactions of scar tissue to chilling:

Experiment I: Keloid removed from chest wall August 24, 1918. Experiment performed September 25, 1918. Scar at that time 2.5 by 1 cm.; red; covered with epithelium. First thermophile on normal skin of chest near scar. Second thermopile on scar. Room temperature, 21.35° to 21.6° C. (See Fig 15, curves on left.)

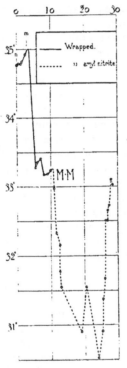

Fig. 14. Effect of amyl nitrite upon acutely inflamed soft palate. Experiment H (temperature of mucous membrane of soft palate): (n) breathing through nose; (m) changes to mouth breathing.

The subject sat wrapped from 0:00 to 0:11.5; the sites of application of the thermopiles were of course freely exposed. At 0:11.5, the subject was bared from the waist up, and chilled with ice bags to her back. Skin and scar temperatures both fell sharply. The scar temperature reached a maximum depression of .90° C. in 1.0 minute, the skin of 1.12° C. in 4.5 minutes. At 0:17.5, the subject gasped and heaved her chest. Possibly as a result of mechanical irritation, the scar temperature at once rose, although skin temperature was not affected. At 0:20.75 the subject stood up to wrap herself, and may have disturbed the position of the scar applicator, al-

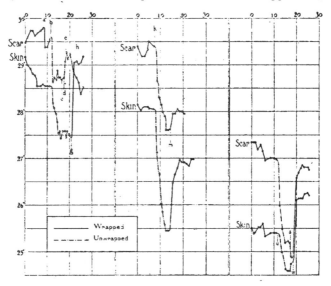

Fig. 15. Reflex effects of chilling on scar tissue. Experiments I, J and K (temperatures of scar and contiguous skin). Experiment I: (a) subject moves, sighs, etc.; (b) subject bared from waist up; ice bags to back; (c) gasps; (d) gasps, heaves chest; (g) wrapped (subject stood up to wrap self; when she sat down again the skin applicator was found to have tilted; the scar applicator seemed all right, but it also had probably moved somewhat): (h) heaves sigh. Experiment J: (k) body bared from waist up. no fan or icebag used; (m) wrapped. Experiment K: (u) body bared from waist up, fan on back, hairs on forehead not disturbed at all by draft; (s) shivers; (w) fan off, wrapped.

though no displacement was visible. After wrapping, the skin temperature rose typically, the scar temperature fell.

This experiment on new scar tissue shows, certainly, reflex vasoconstriction in response to chilling. To what degree the later atypical behavior of the scar temperature actually represents its vasomotor reactions and to what the failure of the subject to cooperate, it is difficult to say.

Experiment J: Radical operation June 7, 1918, for carcinoma of breast. Experiment performed September 23, 1918. First thermopile on normal skin near scar. Second thermopile on red scar, covered with epithelium, circular, about 2 cm. in diameter, over site of amputated breast. Sites of application exposed throughout experiment. Room temperature, 15.65° to 16.35° C. (See Fig. 15, middle curves.)

The subject was chilled at 0:07.5 merely by unwrapping in the cold room. Scar temperature dropped 1.80°C. within 5.0 minutes; skin temperature, 2.63° C. within 5.0 minutes. Upon rewrapping at 0:14.5, scar temperature rose .45° C. in 3.0 minutes; skin temperature, 1.54° C. in 4.0 minutes.

Experiment K: Admitted to hospital, February 1, 1918, with history of having ulcer on forehead for a year. Diagnosis: Syphilitic ulcer. Slow improvement under specific treatment. June 21, 1819, skin graft to ulcer from leg. Favorable. Discharged July 7, 1918. Experiment performed September 12, 1918. Scar about 5 cm. in diameter, red, covered with thin epithelium. First thermopile on normal skin near scar. Second thermopile on scar. Room temperature, 17.8° to 17.95° C. (See Fig. 15, curves on right.)

At 0:11.5 the subject was bared from the waist up, and an electric fan turned on her back. Hairs over her forehead were not disturbed; thus the sites of application were not seriously cooled by draft. The scar temperature fell 2.09° C. in 6.0 minutes, the skin 0.82° in 4.5 minutes. Upon wrapping at 0:18.5, scar temperature rose 1.96° C. in 4.0 minutes; skin, 1.55° C. in 6.5 minutes.

These reactions would seem to explain the cyanosis of fresh scars during cutaneous chilling. The arteriolar constriction doubtless renders the flow of blood through the wide capillary network scant and sluggish, thus allowing unusually complete absorption of oxygen from the oxyhemoglobin.

AFTER-EFFECTS OF CHILLING EXPERIMENTS OF SERIES OF 1918

Subject S. B. G., after being chilled as subject for fourteen experiments over a period of twenty-two days in midsummer, developed severe rhinitis, followed quickly by pharyngitis, ton-

sillitis, and injection of uvula and soft palate.   Subject retained an abnormal susceptibility to colds throughout fall and
early winter.

Subject S. M., after being chilled as subject for fifteen experiments over a period of twenty-four days in midsummer,
developed a slight neuralgia in left shoulder.   Next day was
again subject.   The day thereafter pleurisy developed in left
chest.   Neuralgia yielded to local treatment.   Pleuritic symptoms lasted two weeks.   Mucous membranes remained normal.

Chilled again in November without ill effect.   Chilled December 4; experiment 4:00 to 6:00 p. m.   By following morning slight congestion in nasopharynx had developed, which persisted three or four days.   Chilled January 2 without after-
effect other than nausea, vomiting and headache.

This subject noticed that entering the cold room from the
hot outside air of summer was frequently followed by violent
intestinal peristalsis and defecation.   This subject irrigated
his nose and throat after each exposure with a weakly alkaline
salt solution, used hot, with the idea both of cleansing and of
producing hyperemia.   Following irrigation a spray of 0.5 per
cent phenol in liquid albolene was used after the winter exposures.

Subject A. G., on August 1, chilled.   After exposure, low
grade pharyngitis developed and persisted some days.

Subject J. D. R., with chronic pharyngitis; chilled twice;
subject thought after second exposure was exacerbation of
pharyngitis.

Subject G. A. suffered after single exposure no ill effects
other than headache.

Subject B. J. F., no symptoms after an observation experiment.

CONCURRENT BACTERIOLOGIC STUDIES—SUMMER OF 1919.

Several instances during the experiments of 1918 seemed at
least suggestive of experimental excitation of infection.   The
case of S. M. in particular seemed to point to chilling as the
exciting factor.   The experiment was a blood temperature
control in which he sat from 4 to 6:09 p. m., December 4,
1918, with closed mouth, the bulb of a thermometer beneath
his tongue.   He forced respiration from 4:12 to 6:09 p. m.,

and was chilled by a fan from 4:47 to 5:09 p. m.   Shivering began at 4:48 p. m., and had become very severe by 4:52 p. m. The subject had not been aware of other recent exposure to cold or infection.   By the morning of December 5, nasopharyngeal stuffiness had developed sufficiently to cause the remark by a friend that he had a cold.   The symptoms persisted three or four days.

Similarly we have noted what we believe to be an excitation of infection after, and presumably due to chilling in a number of carefully observed instances in our everyday experience.

A study of the flora of the nose and throat during the experiments of the summer of 1919 seemed, then, to be well worth while.

Material and Method—The medium employed was a 5 per cent rabbit blood meat infusion agar.   Baked blood agar was also used in each instance as a special medium for bacillus influenzæ.   Sputum from each subject was injected into a mouse for typing pneumococcus.   Cultures were taken from the nose through the anterior nares, from the tonsil, and from the posterior pharyngeal wall by means of separate swabs. Each swab was immersed in sterile broth and then applied both to a red and baked blood agar plate; the remaining area of the plate was inoculated by means of a platinum loop.   Films were made directly from the same swab.

The cultures were incubated for 36 hours.   The plates were then divided into eight segments, and every colony in two to four segments of the plate was counted and its nature determined.   An attempt was made to detect any marked changes in the flora and particularly in the relative proportions of the bacteria present.   On account of the difficulty of differentiating pneumococcus from streptococcus viridans by morphology these two were put in the same group.

Results.—Four different subjects were used in this study. Two developed clinical sore throats; a third had some symptoms of malaise and headache; a fourth was unaffected.   The results obtained with the nose cultures were entirely negative. Subjects A. G. and S. M showed staphylococcus aureus; subjects W. G. E. and S. B. G., staphylococcus albus.   No attempt was made to sterilize the vestibule of the nose before swabbing.   The flora obtained from the nose, as has been found by other investigators (Thomson, 1913) was at all times exceedingly sparse, but the above organisms were always found to be present.   They showed no changes with exposure.   The results obtained from pharynx and tonsil in each instance are given in Tables 1 to 3.

From the pharynx and tonsil of Subject S. M. before the experiment there were cultured streptococcus viridans, pneumococcus, Type 11, atypical, and Bacillus influenzæ.   He was then subject of Experiment 7.   Within 24 hours he had a clinical sore throat; coincident with this, there was a sudden appearance of streptococcus hemolyticus in the cultures from both tonsil and pharynx.   During the days following, with the disappearance of the sore throat, the number of colonies of streptococcus hemolyticus fell off rapidly.   The remaining bacteria showed no evident change.

TABLE I.

Subject P. M. Bacteriology of Tonsil and Pharynx.

| Date | Place cultured | S. viridans and Pn. II. | | S. haemolyticus. | | B. influenzae. | | Undetermined. | | Remarks. |
|---|---|---|---|---|---|---|---|---|---|---|
| | | No. of colonies counted | Per cent of all colonies | No. of colonies counted | Per cent of all colonies | No. of colonies counted | Per cent of all colonies | No. of colonies counted | Per cent of all colonies | |
| 1919 June 4 | Left tonsil. | 28 | 93 | 0 | 0 | 2 | 7 | 0 | 0 | |
| | Pharynx. | 36 | 100 | 0 | 0 | 0 | 0 | 0 | 0 | |
| " 5 | Left tonsil. | 43 | 100 | 0 | 0 | Present in baked blood. | " | 0 | 0 | |
| | Pharynx. | 31 | 94 | 0 | 0 | " | " | 4 | 6 | |
| " 6 | Left tonsil. | 35 | 100 | 0 | 0 | 3 | 6 | 0 | 0 | |
| | Pharynx. | 24 | 86 | 0 | 0 | 4 | 13 | 4 | 14 | |
| " 7* | Left tonsil. | 52 | 94 | 0 | 0 | 7 | 8 | 0 | 0 | Subject of experiment. Application on left tonsil. Cultures after experiment. |
| | Pharynx. | 40 | 87 | 0 | 0 | 6 | 13 | 0 | 0 | |
| " 8 | Left tonsil. | 57 | 65 | 13 | 15 | | | 11 | 12 | Subjective sore throat. Pharynx shows injection with white exudate; tonsillar ring injected. |
| | Pharynx. | 26 | 56 | 14 | 31 | | | 0 | 0 | |
| " 9 | Left tonsil. | 35 | 76 | 6 | 13 | 1 | 2 | 4 | 8 | Very slight soreness. Throat no longer injected. |
| | Pharynx. | 34 | 79 | 9 | 21 | Present in baked blood. | | 0 | 0 | |
| " 11 | Left tonsil. | 34 | 94 | 1 | 3 | 1 | 3 | 0 | 0 | Throat normal. |
| | Pharynx. | 30 | 91 | 3 | 9 | Present in baked blood. | | 0 | 0 | |

* Experiment 7.

## TABLE II.

### Subject W. G. E. Bacteriology of Tonsil and Pharynx.

| Date. | Place cultured. | S. viridans. | | S. haemolyticus. | | B. influenzae. | | S. albus. | | Remarks. |
|---|---|---|---|---|---|---|---|---|---|---|
| | | No. of colonies counted | Per cent of all colonies | No. of colonies counted | Per cent of all colonies | No. of colonies counted | Per cent of all counted. | No. of colonies counted. | Per cent of all colonies | |
| *1919* June 10 | Left tonsil | 18 | 42 | 4 | 9 | 9 | 21 | 12 | 28 | |
| | Pharynx | 13 | 52 | 0 | 0 | 12 | 48 | 0 | 0 | |
| " 11* | Left tonsil | 28 | 68 | 3 | 8 | 8 | 20 | 2 | 4 | Subject of experiment. Application on left tonsil. Cultures after experiment. |
| | Pharynx | 24 | 72 | 0 | 0 | 6 | 18 | 3 | 9 | |
| " 12 | Left tonsil | 31 | 55 | 3 | 5 | 5 | 9 | 17 | 31 | No after effects. |
| | Pharynx | 18 | 54 | 0 | 0 | 12 | 36 | 4 | 9 | |
| " 16† | Left tonsil | 26 | 53 | 0 | 0 | 6 | 12 | 18 | 35 | Subject of experiment. Application on soft palate. Cultures taken before experiment. |
| | Pharynx | 32 | 60 | 0 | 0 | 9 | 17 | 12 | 23 | |
| " 17 | Left tonsil | 14 | 45 | 2 | 7 | 8 | 26 | 7 | 22 | Subject complains of general malaise; slight headache; no sore throat. Film from swab shows mostly Gram-negative bacilli with a few cocci. |
| | Red blood | 0 | 0 | 0 | 0 | | 100 | 0 | 0 | |
| | Baked blood | 0 | 0 | 0 | 0 | | 100 | 0 | 0 | |
| " 19 | Left tonsil | 19 | 56 | 2 | 6 | 5 | 15 | 8 | 24 | |
| | Pharynx | 21 | 60 | 0 | 0 | 14 | 40 | 0 | 0 | |
| " 20 | Left tonsil | 21 | 50 | 3 | 7 | 7 | 17 | 11 | 26 | |
| | Pharynx | 19 | 58 | 0 | 0 | 11 | 33 | 3 | 9 | |

* F
R

## TABLE III.

### Subject A. G. Bacteriology of Tonsil and Pharynx.

| Date. | Place cultured. | S. viridans. No. of colonies counted | Per cent of all colonies | M. catarrhalis. No. of colonies counted | Per cent of all colonies | S. aureus. No. of colonies counted | Per cent of all colonies | S. albus. No. of colonies counted | Per cent of all colonies | Remarks. |
|---|---|---|---|---|---|---|---|---|---|---|
| *1919* June 7 | Left tonsil | 29 | 85 | 0 | 0 | 0 | 0 | 5 | 15 | |
| | Pharynx | 21 | 91 | 0 | 0 | 0 | 0 | 2 | 9 | |
| " 8* | Left tonsil | 49 | 90 | 0 | 0 | 0 | 0 | 5 | 10 | Subject of experiment. Application on left tonsil. Cultures after experiment. |
| | Pharynx | 27 | 75 | 0 | 0 | 2 | 6 | 7 | 19 | No symptoms. |
| " 9 | Left tonsil | 21 | 60 | 3 | 9 | 0 | 0 | 11 | 31 | |
| | Pharynx | 31 | 57 | 15 | 27 | 1 | 2 | 7 | 14 | |
| " 10† | Left tonsil | 27 | 52 | 4 | 8 | 2 | 4 | 19 | 36 | Subject of experiment. Application on right tonsil. Cultures after experiment. |
| | Pharynx | 34 | 81 | 0 | 0 | 3 | 7 | 5 | 12 | |
| " 11 | Left tonsil | 34 | 85 | 1 | 2 | 0 | 0 | 5 | 13 | |
| | Pharynx | 39 | 93 | 0 | 0 | 0 | 0 | 3 | 7 | |
| " 12 | Right tonsil | 30 | 73 | 0 | 0 | 4 | 10 | 7 | 17 | |
| | Pharynx | 34 | 87 | 2 | 5 | 1 | 3 | 2 | 5 | |
| " 13‡ | Right tonsil | 40 | 88 | 2 | 5 | 0 | 0 | 3 | 7 | Subject of experiment. Application on pharynx. Cultures after experiment. |
| | Pharynx | 27 | 70 | 7 | 19 | 0 | 0 | 4 | 11 | |
| " 14 | Right tonsil | 21 | 58 | 12 | 34 | 0 | 0 | 3 | 8 | |
| | Pharynx | 15 | 45 | 4 | 11 | 11 | 39 | 2 | 5 | |

| | | | | | | | | | | Remarks |
|---|---|---|---|---|---|---|---|---|---|---|
| June 16§ | Right tonsil | 21 | 52 | 11 | 27 | 0 | 0 | 8 | 20 | Subject of experiment. Application on pharynx. Marked congestion of tonsillar ring and pharynx. |
| | Pharynx | 29 | 60 | 15 | 31 | 0 | 0 | 4 | 9 | |
| " 17 | Right tonsil | 34 | 72 | 3 | 7 | 8 | 17 | 2 | 4 | Throat injection milder. No soreness on swallowing. |
| | Pharynx | 27 | 75 | 6 | 16 | 3 | 8 | 0 | 0 | |
| " 18|| | Right tonsil | 25 | 59 | 2 | 5 | 15 | 36 | 0 | 0 | Subject of experiment. Application on soft palate. Cultures after experiment. |
| | Pharynx | 31 | 77 | 4 | 10 | 5 | 13 | 0 | 0 | |
| " 19 | Right tonsil | 28 | 54 | 15 | 28 | 9 | 18 | 0 | 0 | Soreness on swallowing. Injection of tonsillar ring. |
| | Pharynx | 32 | 64 | 11 | 22 | 7 | 14 | 0 | 0 | |
| " 20 | | | | | | | | | | No cultures. Sore throat disappeared. |
| " 21 | Right tonsil | 35 | 83 | 0 | 0 | 4 | 10 | 3 | 7 | No soreness. No injection. |
| | Pharynx | 31 | 93 | 1 | 3 | 0 | 0 | 1 | 3 | |
| " 23 | Right onsil | 31 | 81 | 2 | 5 | 1 | 2 | 4 | 11 | No soreness. No injection. |
| | Pharynx | 27 | 81 | 1 | 3 | 2 | 6 | 3 | 9 | |

* Experiment 9.
† Experiment 6.
‡ Experiment 10.
§ Experiment 11.
|| Experiment 12.

Experiment 7.—Subject S. M., June 7, 1919, 3:45 to 6 p. m. Mucous membrane thermopile on left tonsil. Respirations, 14 per minute. Mouth open; nostrils plugged. Room temperature, 18.10—19.60° C., 0:00 to 0:31.5. Wrapped; normal breathing; swallowed many times. 0:31.5 to 0:44. Wrapped; deep breathing. 0:44 to 0:55.5. Unwrapped; fan on back; deep breathing. 0:53. Shivers. 0:55.5. Coughs, chokes, applicator removed; blood flecks seen about terminals. 4:57 p. m., experiment started again. 0:00 to 0:06. Wrapped; deep breathing. 0:06 to 0:13.5. Unwrapped; fan on; deep breathing; shivering; swallows many times. 0:13.5 to 0:33.5. Wrapped; deep breathing. 0:33.5. Conditions the same; amyl nitrite inhaled. 0:35 to 0:44. Wrapped; deep breathing, some coughing and swallowing. 0:44 to 0:53. Hot water bag around subject; wrapped; deep breathing.

On the following morning the feeling of soreness had practically left the traumatized tonsil, but the posterior wall of the oropharynx felt sore. On inspection a localized area of injection bearing a whitish exudate was seen on the posterior wall of the oropharynx. In culturing, the contact of the swab on this area was a little painful, and the culture yielded streptococci, as explained above. The tonsillar ring was injected, but the feeling of soreness on the tonsil entirely passed off during the day and contact of the swab in culturing was hardly felt. Thus the traumatized tonsil showed less evidence of being the site of an active infection than the posterior pharyngeal wall, which was thought not to have been directly traumatized, but of course we cannot exclude the possibility that the oropharynx was infected by hemolytic streptococci from the tonsillar crypts—so commonly a habitat for them—which were missed in the earlier cultures and were disseminated by the experimental trauma and swallowing.

In subject W. G. E., there were present streptococcus viridans, bacillus influenzæ, streptococcus hemolyticus, and staphylococcus albus. Following Experiment D there were no noteworthy changes. The plate inoculated from the pharynx about 26 hours after Experiment 8, however, showed a pure culture of bacillus influenzæ; the tonsillar plate showed also a slight relative increase. The film from the pharynx showed practically all Gram negative bacilli with an occasional coccus. The subject had no sore throat, but complained of general malaise, slight headache, and some chilly sensations. (Compare the effect of infecting monkeys with bacillus influenzæ (Blake and Cecil, 1920).)

The pharynx culture made 96 hours after Experiment 8 was practically the same as before the experiment, streptococcus viridans and staphylococcus albus appearing as before.

Experiment 8 (for Experiment D, see page — above).— Subject W. G. E., June 16, 1919, 3:20 to 4:07 p. m. Mucous membrane thermopile on anterior half of soft palate, left side. Respirations, 16 per minute. Mouth open; nostrils plugged. Room temperature, 20.22—20.90° C. 0:00 to 0:05.5. Wrapped: normal breathing. 0:05.5 to 0:11. Wrapped; deep breathing. 0:11 to 0:32. Unwrapped; fan on back; deep breathing. 0:32 to 0:47. Wrapped; deep breathing.

With the applicator resting against the anterior soft palate there is no reason for supposing trauma to the tonsils and pharynx. Organisms could hardly have been introduced from outside by the applicator, for this, with the thermopile terminals attached, was freshly coated with shellac in alcoholic solution before being adjusted for an experiment.

Subject A. G. was the subject of five experiments, June 8, 10, 13, 16 and 18. On June 15 he noted a soreness on swallowing, and on June 16 the entire posterior pharynx and tonsillar ring were distinctly injected. The experiment of June 16 produced no sudden increase in symptoms; on June 17 the sore throat had practically disappeared. On June 19, 36 hours following an experiment, the subject again developed a soreness on swallowing, with congestion of the posterior pharynx and tonsillar ring. On June 20 the symptoms had subsided. On June 21 there was no longer any injection or soreness.

This subject had present in his throat streptococcus viridans, staphylococcus aureus, and staphylococcus albus. Twenty-four hours following the first experiment there was noted for the first time the appearance of micrococcus catarrhalis. Subsequently there appeared to be a certain degree of correlation between the appearances of sore throat and the rises in relative numbers of micrococcus catarrhalis colonies. No other change in the bacterial flora was apparent.

Experiment 9.—Subject A. G.  June 8, 1919, 3:38 to 5:06 p. m.  Mucous membrane applicator on left tonsil.  Respirations, 10 per minute.  Mouth open; nostrils plugged.  Room temperature, 18.1—19.45° C.  0:00 to 0:06.  Wrapped; normal breathing.  0:06 to 0:15.  Wrapped; deep breathing.  0:15 to 0:43.  Unwrapped; fan on .back; deep breathing; some swallowing, coughing, and clearing of throat; after 0:17. shivering.  0:43 to 1:20.  Wrapped; deep respiration.  1:07.  Inhales amyl nitrite.  1:20 to 1:28.  Hot water pad to back; deep respiration.

The possibility that trauma to the tonsil was responsible for the appearance of micrococcus catarrhalis after this experiment cannot be excluded.

Experiment 6.—Subject A. G.  June 10, 1919, 11:30 a. m. to 12:17 p. m.  Mucous membrane thermopile on right tonsil.  Skin thermopile·on forehead.  Respirations, 16 per minute.  Mouth open; nostrils plugged.  Room temperature, 16.9° —17.8° C.  0:00 to 0:06.5.  Wrapped, normal breathing.  0:06.5 to 0:18.5.  Wrapped, deep breathing.  0:18.5 to 0:32.  Unwrapped; fan on back; deep breathing; after 0:23.5 shivering.  0:32 to 0:47.  Wrapped; deep breathing; contraction of pharyngeal muscles.

Experiment 10.—Subject A. G.  June 13. 1919, 3 to 3:46 p. m.  Mucous membrane applicator on posterior wall of oropharynx.  Respirations, 16 per minute.  Mouth open; nostrils plugged.  Room temperature, 18.45—19.05° C.  0:00 to 0:04.5.  Wrapped; normal breathing.  0:04.5 to 0:15.  Wrapped; deep breathing.  0:15 to 0:26.  Unwrapped; fan on back; deep breathing; coughed; cleared throat; contraction of pharyngeal muscles; after 0:22, shivers.  0:26 to 0:46.  Wrapped; deep breathing; coughed and cleared throat several times; pharynx appeared normal.

Experiment 11.—Subject A. G.  June 16, 1919, 10:30 to 11:30 a. m.  Mucous membrane applicator on posterior pharyngeal wall.  Respirations, 14 per minute.  Mouth open; nostrils plugged.  Room temperature, 18.90—19.80° C.  0:00 to 0:04.5.  Wrapped; normal breathing; contractions of pharyngeal muscles.  0:04.5 to 0:23.5.  Wrapped; deep breathing.  0:23.5 to 0:32.  Unwrapped; fan on back; deep breathing.

0:32 to 1:00.  Wrapped; deep breathing; contractions of pharyngeal muscles.

Experiment 12.—Subject A. G.  June 18, 1919, 10:20 to 11:12 a. m.  Mucous membrane applicator on soft palate, middle part.  Respirations, 14 per minute.  Mouth open; nostrils plugged.  Room temperature, 18.75—19.55° C.  0:00 to 0:05.5. Wrapped; normal breathing.  0:05.5 to 0:15.5.  Wrapped; deep breathing.  0:15.5 to 0:27.  Unwrapped; fan on back; deep breathing.  0:27 to 0:52.  Wrapped; deep breathing.

In subject S. B. G., there were present in the throat streptococcus viridans, pneumococcus type IV, and staphylococcus albus.  Cultures were made daily from June 4 to 19; he was the subject of an experiment on June 6, 9, 14, and 17.  There was practically no change in the bacterial flora of this subject throughout the entire period studied.  Neither did subjective or objective signs of sore throat or cold develop.  Frequently the cultures from the pharynx were almost sterile, there being from three to ten colonies over the entire plate.

### DISCUSSION OF BACTERIOLOGIC RESULTS.

Streptococcus viridans was found in all four of the individuals studied, bacillus influenzæ in two, pneumococcus in two, and micrococcus catarrhalis in one subject.

In subject S. M., the increased number of streptococcus hemolyticus was definitely synchronous with the presence of a sore throat.  There appears to have been a correlation between the high micrococcus catarrhalis counts and the presence of sore throats in subject A. G.  The pure culture of bacillus influenzæ in the pharynx of subject W. G. E. was not coincident with sore throat, but with malaise, slight chilliness and headache.

These results in no sense prove, however, that the sore throats were caused by the increased number of bacteria cultured from the mucous membranes, or that the apparent increase of microorganisms was caused by the ischemia of the mucous membranes incident upon chilling of the body surface.  The method is subject to so many sources of error, and the amount of data thus far obtained is so small that we do not feel justified in drawing any conclusions.  To attribute the apparent proliferation of pathogenic microorganisms to the effect of chilling would seem to be in harmony with the great wealth of clinical and common. observation which points to excessive chilling, under proper circumstances, as an efficient excitant of infection of the mucous membranes by their indigenous pathogenic bacteria. Although it is possible that the apparent proliferation was due to the local ischemia incident upon chilling, the inaccuracy of the bacteriologic method and the insufficient data make it impossible to assume that this is so. The effect of trauma by the thermopiles, the possibility of transient changes in the flora of the mucous membranes caused by swallowing, gagging, or other muscular activity in the pharynx pressing a plug of bacteria from the tonsillar crypts, the . fact that the subject's mouth was held open throughout the experiments, with the accompanying accumulation of mucus on the membranes, the errors necessarily introduced in each stage of making the cultures, and the inaccuracy of any method depending upon swab cultures, all tend to confuse the results. We present the data given above as a contribution to the etiology of upper respiratory infections, and not with the idea that the study is in any sense complete in itself.

CONCURRENT BACTERIOLOGIC STUDIES—SUMMER OF 1920.*

The bacteriologic methods of 1920 were essentially those of 1919, save that the baked blood plates for bacillus influenzæ were omitted and that the vestibule of the nose was in each case washed out before the nasal culture with cotton wet with tap water.

Results: Four subjects were used in this study. Cultures were made daily (with a few omissions) from June 21 to July 19, from the right and left nasal cavities, the right faucial tonsil and the posterior pharyngeal wall of two subjects, S. M. and A. G. The third, S. B. G., was similarly cultured from June 21 to June 30. The fourth, F. J. C., was cultured only once. S. M., A. G., and F. J. C. each developed a mild coryza. S. B. G. was unaffected.

Subject S. M. showed in the nose from the outset staphylococcus albus. On June 24 and thereafter staphylococcus aureus also was found. Diphtheroids appeared in cultures from each

---

*For detailed account see Goldman, Mudd and Grant (1921).

nasal cavity made four hours after his third intranasal experiment. Streptococcus albus remained throughout all the experiments. Streptococcus aureus was present occasionally, but, except on the days following its first appearance, in smaller numbers than streptococcus albus. The diphtheroids fluctuated in numbers and were sometimes absent. There was no apparent relation between their numbers and the chilling.

The tonsil contained at the outset nonhemolytic streptococci, pneumococci. and S. albus. Streptococcus hemolyticus appeared in the tonsil culture taken 24 hours after the first experiment on June 22; the applicator in this experiment was on the nasal septum and the subject's mouth was closed. Forty-eight hours after the experiment, a pure culture of S. hemolyticus appeared in the tonsil culture. The number diminished on the following day to 11 per cent of all colonies, and subsequently remained present in numbers from 1 to 12 per cent of all colonies counted, through July 12. Nose and throat remained clinically normal throughout this time. Further experiments were performed upon this subject July 12, 15 and 17, with the thermopile tips respectively on the nasopharyngeal and oropharyngeal wall and in the air of the postnasal space. The proportion of hemolytic streptococci in the tonsil cultures slowly rose during this time—July 12, 12 per cent; July 14, 16 per cent; July 16 and 17, numerous, not counted; July 19, 25 per cent; July 20, 36 per cent. July 17, this subject began to develop symptoms of coryza. By July 19 he had cough, nasal stuffiness and rhinorrhea and malaise. Symptoms present but abated the following day. This subject's mother had had a severe cold from about July 12; his symptoms may or may not have been connected with the experiments.

The pharynx showed nonhemolytic streptococci and pneumococcus and occasionally S. albus and S. aureus. June 27, S. hemolyticus appeared, and subsequently it was obtained in four cultures, each time associated with tonsil cultures containing a like organism. S. hemolyticus is so usual an inhabitant of the tonsils (Davis, 1920) that its incidence here may or may not have been connected with the experiments.

Subject A. G. showed in the nasal cavity initially S. aureus; subsequently S. albus appeared on each side. The right side showed usually a preponderance of S. albus, the left of S.

aureus. No other organisms appeared in the nasal cultures.
The right tonsil showed nonhemolytic streptococci
throughout, i. e., from June 21 to July 19. A. G. was subject
of an experiment June 21, 23 and 24; application was made
on the anterior end of the right nasal septum, the anterior
end of the left lower turbinate and in the left middle meatus,
respectively. The symptoms of a slight rhinitis—nasal stuffiness, slight headache and slight mucopurulent discharge—
developed June 24. The secretion and stuffiness persisted until
June 29. June 24 two colonies of M. catarrhalis appeared on
the tonsil plate, and June 26 one on the tonsil and three on
the pharynx plate. June 28, S. albus began to be present in the
right nostril. Otherwise no change in bacteriology was noted,
the nose showing S. aureus and the tonsil and pharynx nonhemolytic streptococci as before. A. G. was again subject
July 7 and 17, with the applicator on the right middle turbinate
in the first case and with no mucous membrane application at
all in the second. July 17, twenty colonies (44 per cent) of
M. catarrhalis appeared on the tonsil plate. There were no
accompanying clinical symptoms. Streptococcus hemolyticus
appeared after the experiment of July 7, four colonies on the
tonsil and one on the pharynx plate July 7, one on the tonsil
plate July 8 and one on the tonsil plate July 12. These were
the only appearances of hemolytic streptococci in this subject,
either in the series of 1919 or 1920.

In Subject S. B. G. there were present in the nose S. aureus
and S. albus. On the right tonsil there were S. nonhemolyticus,
pneumococcus, S. aureus and S. albus. The pharynx showed
S. nonhemolyticus and pneumococcus. There was practically
no change in the bacterial flora throughout the period studied
nor were there any signs of a cold. The cultures from the
pharynx were frequently sterile and always showed relatively
few bacteria, as was the case in this subject in 1919.

F. J. C., whose pharyngeal culture showed abundant hemolytic streptococci, developed a mild cold the day following his
first experiment (applicator on left nasal septum). Unfortunately, a contagious origin cannot be ruled out, however, for
his baby brother developed a cold about the same time.

Discussion: Nonhemolytic streptococci were found in all
four individuals studied, pneumococci in two, S. hemo-

lyticus in three, and M. catarrhalis in one. In S. M., on one occasion there was an abundance of S. hemolyticus in the tonsil cultures before and during the symptoms of cold and sore throat. In F. J. C. a cold followed a single exposure of an individual with abundant hemolytic streptococci in his postpharynx. The appearance of M. catarrhalis in A. G. after experimentation was paralleled by a like occurrence in 1919.

### INTERPRETATION OF REACTIONS TO CHILLING.

It is a fact beyond question that potentially pathogenic bacteria may lead a saprophytic existence upon the pharyngeal and tonsillar mucous membranes of healthy subjects (e. g., see Davis, 1920). It is equally indisputable that those bacteria may under appropriate circumstances become the active agents of infection, local or generalized. We believe that exposure to cold may be one such exciting factor of infection. We have shown also that chilling of the body surface causes a reflex vasoconstriction and ischemia in the mucous membranes of the nasal cavity, postnasal space, oropharynx, palate and tonsils. That the latter is the mechanism by which local resistance is lowered and infection excited we have not proved. However, there would seem to be justification for advancing, tentatively at least, the hypothesis that the ischemia may mediate the infection. Jonathan Wright in the course of a discussion of the etiology of acute upper respiratory infection (1914), page 295), says:

"It may well be, as has been admitted, that certain bacteria are at once pathogenic when they reach the mucous membrane. Indeed, this seems very probable when they reach the mucous membranes of certain individuals. It may well be that such individuals always present, owing to systemic states, conditions of the mucosa which offer an ever open avenue to infection; but granting all this, which indeed is in reality a part of our conception of the mechanism of the process, it seems extremely likely that local biochemical change, dependent upon molecular activities acting through the sympathetic nervous system, is the antecedent in the majority of cases of bacterial infection. This molecular disturbance of the normal activities of the sympathetic nerves may be set up by external or internal agencies, by the chilling of the body surfaces, or by derangements in the activities of the internal organs. Owing to the fact that wet feet and the chilling of distant regions of the surface of the body are, at least in clinical experience, quite as frequently followed by coryzas and sore throats as the direct impact of such external influences upon the head and neck, we have the right to infer that the shock at the surface must be transferred to internal nerve ganglia and there translated into impulses which are carried to the surfaces of the mucosa of the upper air passages. There they give rise to the chain of biophysical and biochemical changes which may simply result in a mild coryza or a catarrhal pharyngitis, the resolution of which terminates the chain, or these conditions may be in themselves the starting point of bacterial invasion."

In the insufficient light of present knowledge, it would seem not improbable that the ischemia incident on cutaneous chilling, by decreasing cell respiration, or by retarding removal of the products of cell metabolism, or by increasing the permeability of the epithelial cell surfaces to the bacterial products, or by decreasing the local supply of specific antibodies, or by altering the media in the tonsillar crypts and folds of the pharyngeal mucosa in which the bacteria are living, or, especially when accompanied by direct chilling of the mucous membrane, by altering the state of aggregation of the colloids of the protoplasm (Schade, 1920), or by a combination of these factors, might effect the local change postulated by Wright and thus so disturb the equilibrium between host and parasite as to excite infection. We here use the term "infection" as denoting a process separable from that of invasion or penetration of the bacteria into or through the mucosa. For study of tonsils in the early stages of infection has usually shown the crypts swarming with bacteria with none demonstrable beneath the mucosa surface (Wright and Smith, 1914, p. 291; Wright, 1907; Goodale, 1899). There is much collateral evidence to support the hypothesis of Wright that a factor other than any of those suggested above—namely, the surface-tension relations of bacteria and mucosa cell surfaces (1909), enters into the determination of penetration or nonpenetration of bacteria through the mucosa. This hypothesis certainly deserves experimental investigation.

The demonstration that cutaneous chilling causes reflex vasoconstriction and ischemia in the nasal cavity, nasopharynx, oropharynx, tonsils and palate at least furnishes a new and correct point of departure for future investigation, to replace the former false assumption of congestion.

That the mechanism we have elucidated is the only one concerned in exciting the acute cold it would be obvious folly to believe. The conditions determining the equilibrium between host and parasite in the tonsillar crypts and folds of the pharyngeal mucosa must be so extremely complex that many different factors are capable of disturbing it, either in the direction of proliferation of the parasites and infection or of their annihilation.

A mechanism perhaps more often responsible than ours for the acute "cold" has been elucidated by Leonard Hill and F. F. Muecke (1913). These workers found that in hot, moist, crowded rooms, such as ill ventilated theaters or meeting halls, the mucous membranes over the turbinate bones and nasal septum swell, become turgid with blood and tissue lymph, and covered with a thick secretion. In such crowded places massive droplet infection is likely to occur. On going out into cold, moist, outer air, the blood vessels constrict and the nasal mucous membrane is chilled but remains swollen with tissue lymph. These authors believe—and certainly with apparent justification—that this latter condition of the nasal mucous membrane affords a suitable condition for bacterial proliferation. They find that the dangerous primary passive congestion is much less if the air in the room is kept circulating and is not overheated.

The monograph of Leonard Hill (1919) especially urges the importance in causing colds of contagion and of the unnatural conditions of indoor life, where bodily vigor is not maintained by adequate outdoor exercise, crowding favors massive infection from those already actively infected and from carriers, and overheating of the atmosphere at head level causes passive congestion of the nasal mucous membrane and predisposes to infection. In Hill's monograph is to be found detailed discussion also of the effects on the respiratory membrane of altered respiration and of changes in temperature of the inspired air, as distinguished from the phenomena we have been especially studying, namely, the reflex effects on the mucous membrane circulation of chilling the body surface without altering the quality of the inspired air. The effect of physical exertion (without excessive fatigue, of course) in increasing respiration and hence transudation of liquid through the respiratory membrane, is emphasized by Hill as a valuable factor in the prevention of initiation of infection of the respiratory membrane.

It should be clearly borne in mind that the factors of contagion and of general bodily health are probably of considerably greater importance to preventive medicine and the welfare of the ` community than the effects of chilling of the body surface.

We would reiterate also in order to minimize any possibility of misunderstanding. We are concerned in our experiments with excessive chilling of the body surface, which, like overdosage of a useful drug, we believe may have ill effects. Certainly we would not encourage the unreasoning fear of drafts and exposure so often encountered. Good ventilation and circulating air in buildings, cold weather, and out-of-door living are needed for vigorous health; many people are unquestionably benefited by cold bathing. Bnt excesses in this direction should also be avoided.

Individual differences in susceptibility should also be borne in mind. (See Sticker, 1916.) Thin, anemic and delicate persons can in general stand less exposure than stocky, "full-blooded" ones. There is evidence also that peculiar susceptibility to catching cold may exist as an individual idiosyncrasy.

We are now in a position to outline an explanation for the annual cold weather increase in incidence of upper respiratory diseases, which, although admittedly incomplete and in part speculative, would yet seem to fit well the known facts. With the beginning of cold weather, cessation of summer and autumnal out-of-door life, and beginning of hot air and steam heating, conditions of living for the average American and European become less favorable to general health and resistance. Opportunity for excitation of autoinfection by prolonged or excessive chilling become more frequent, as do those for cross-infection in crowded cars and meeting places, w¹
cous membranes are rendered more susceptible to infection by the close, hot atmosphere (Hill and Muecke, 1913). As the bacteria gain foothold and multiply on one after another

susceptible mucous membrane it is in harmony with known immunologic facts to suppose that they tend to increase in virulence and so add another factor to the general tendency to increased prevalence of respiratory infection. With moderation of the weather and return to out-of-door life in the spring, aided possibly by some as yet unknown cyclic or other change in the bacterial invaders (Journ. Am. Med. Assn., 1920, LXXV. 1500), we would expect the annual decline in prevalence.

How practically to escape respiratory infection in so far as possible? Lead a vigorous and healthful life with adequate sleep, food, exercise and fresh air. Bathe daily. Keep the houses sufficiently warm to be comfortable, but not, as most American houses are in winter, overhot and overdry. Avoid contagion from infected persons, remembering that respiratory diseases are communicated chiefly through droplets of mucous sprayed into the air through coughing, sneezing or speaking. Avoid excessive irritation of the mucous membranes by tobacco of the body surface. Avoid crowding in hot atmospheres. Obstructions to breathing or foci of infection, if present, should of course be removed. Some degree of "hardening" to exposure, graded and adapted to the needs of the individual, we believe is possible, and of the greatest service. As one valuable factor in this process, one of us at least, after some eight years' trial, is convinced of the efficacy in his own case of a daily morning shower bath with warm water, concluded with a few minutes of very cold water.

## IV.—ANAPHYLACTIC "COLDS."

The discussions of vasomotor rhinitis and of asthma in the majority of the current texts will have to be entirely rewritten. The rescue of these affections from the nebulous province of diatheses and neuroses, their establishment upon a definite and sound, if not wholly complete, etiologic and therapeutic basis, makes up one of the chapters of modern experimental medicine upon which one's imagination lingers with most satisfaction. Since, however, thoroughly modern and adequate treatments of this subject are available (v. Goodale, 1918, and Walker, 1919), they will not be further discussed here beyond pointing out a subgroup of cases recently come within the

experience of workers in the field, which simulate recurrent
common acute colds.

I cannot do better than quote briefly from Dr. Walker
(1919, p. 146):

"It is not at all uncommon for some patients to complain
of what they call hay fever symptoms or very frequent head
colds throughout the year. Since this kind of case seeks aid
from the nose specialist, who terms the condition vasomotor
rhinitis, the internist sees little of the condition, and even when
the internist does see the case first he immediately refers the
case to the nose specialist. In the future, however, such cases
should be tested for sensitization to proteins. Not infrequently are the emanations of animals the cause of these all the year
hay fever symptoms. Horse hair dandruff and cat hair are
frequently the cause of these spasmodic attacks of hay fever,
which last a few minutes to a few hours or even a day or two,
and in such instances the patient gives a positive skin test
with the proteins of the hair. Less often the injection of various foods causes spasmodic attacks of short duration simulating hay fever. True seasonal pollen cases frequently complain of frequent head colds throughout the year, and these
head colds closely simulate short attacks of hay fever. In
some of these pollen cases the sensitization serves to permanently render the mucous membranes extremely sensitive and
irritable, so that sudden temperature changes, drafts, odors
and dust particles are sufficient to produce symptoms; in other
pollen cases bacteria seem to be the cause." See also Goodale
(1916), Floyd (1920), and Walker (1920). The important
point here for the laryngologist, internist and pediatrist to remember is that frequently recurring "colds" may have protein
sensitization as their basis and to be in readiness to do the skin
tests when indicated.

V.—ACUTE INFLAMMATION DUE TO SYSTEMIC, TOXIC AND NEU-
ROTIC FACTORS, TO MECHANICAL AND CHEMICAL IRRITATION,
TO EXTREME LOW TEMPERATURE AND TO NASAL
OBSTRUCTION.

A discussion of the etiology of acute inflammation of the
nose, throat and tonsils should at least give passing mention

to various inflammatory conditions of the upper respiratory tract associated with more general affections. Acute rhinitis occurs as a local prodromal symptom of influenza, measles, scarlatina, whooping cough, enteric, typhus, smallpox, chickenpox, secondary or congenital syphilis and glanders. (Thomson, 1913, p. 113). Similarly for acute pharyngitis. Diphtheritic and gonorrheal rhinitis occur; also that of erysipelas.

Acute upper respiratory inflammations may be set up in those exposed to local irritants, as millers, furriers, sawyers, tobacco workers, ivory and steel turners, and decorators, or (Schade, 1920) when the mucous membranes are exposed to extreme low temperatures. Locally the vapors of formalin, the halogens, ammonia and the fuming mineral acids and dust and coal and tobacco smoke may give rise to them. A destructive form of rhinitis may occur in workers in bichromate of potash, mercury, arsenic or osmic acid. Acute pharyngitis not infrequently follows traumatism, as the swallowing of hot fluids, corrosives, hot condiments, raw spirits, and the impaction of foreign bodies. It may be induced by operations on the pharynx with much sponging or traction on the tissues, e. g., enucleation or morcellement of the tonsils. Secondary infection may of course aggravate any such primary condition.

Acute mucous membrane inflammation may occur in connection with the administration of certain drugs, as potassium iodid, arsenic, mercury and antimony.

Acute rhinitis "is predisposed to by all obstructive affections of the nose and postnasal space. Chronic hypertrophic rhinitis, deformities of the septum, polypi and chronic empyemata conduce to the contraction and exacerbation of acute nasal catarrh: and frequent and persistent rhinitis in children is generally due to nasopharyngeal adenoids. Indeed, a large majority of children who are reported to be always catching a 'cold in the head' will be found to possess inflamed or overgrown pharyngeal tonsils." (Thomson ibid.)

A vasomotor turgescence of the nasal mucous membrane may originate in certain individuals from some reflex, such as chilling of the feet, sudden exposure to bright light or damp air, inhalation of vitiated air, gastric disorder, or sexual irritation.

### VI.—CONCLUSIONS.

The following causes of acute inflammation of the pharynx, tonsils and nose are recognized in the present dissertation:

1. The filterable virus of Kruse and Foster, inducing apparently a clinical entity, a type of acute coryza. According to the experiments of its discoverers, this is of relatively high virulence and may cause infection practically independently of the action of exciting factors.

2. Various bacteria, including the pneumococcus, streptococci, B. rhinitis, B. diphtheriæ, Friedländer's bacillus, B. influenzæ, and probably also M. catarrhalis, B. septus, M. paratetragenus, S. aureus, the meningococcus, Vincent's spirillum and fusiform bacillus, and possibly others, seem to be capable of inducing infection of variable extent, duration and symptomatology. The relative virulence of the microorganisms also varies within wide limits—both between themselves and from time to time in the same organism—in some instances high, infections of epidemic proportions, largely independent of exciting factors, may be produced; in other instances low, sporadic infection may occur only when some factor or factors serve to depress resistance, general or local, to the point of vulnerability.

3. Protein sensitization, the basis of vasomotor rhinitis and of true bronchial asthma, the underlying cause also of a relatively infrequent subgroup of acute recurrent "colds."

4. Various systemic diseases, drugs, mechanical, thermal and chemical trauma, chronic nasal affections and reflex neuroses.

One factor by which resistance to bacterial infection may be lowered is excessive chilling.

Experiments by many workers have shown that animals whose blood temperature is lowered may have decreased resistance to infection. This, however, we believe, is not the mechanism by which chilling excites the common upper respiratory infections in man.

Experiments have shown that chilling of the body surface of animals causes congestion of many internal organs. Reasoning from a faulty analogy, the theory has been evolved and made widely current that similar congestion occurs in the upper respiratory mucous membranes of man when chilled and is responsible for the local lowering of resistance. However, the work of the present authors has shown that the opposite is true, namely, that chilling of the body surface causes reflex vasoconstriction and ischemia in the mucous membranes of the nasal cavity and postnasal space, palate, oropharynx, nasopharynx and palatine tonsils. It seems not improbable that the ischemia may be the means of lowering local resistance. In other instances the mechanism of Hill and Muecke, i. e., crowding in overheated places followed by emergence into a cold atmosphere, is doubtless responsible for colds.

During the course of the experiments by which the vasoconstrictor reaction to chilling has been demonstrated, some ten cases of cold or sore throat, usually mild, have appeared among the subjects. In a number of instances the clinical symptoms were accompanied by interesting bacterial changes.

It is a pleasure to thank the friends, without whose generous aid as subjects much of the present work would not have been possible.

A paper describing repetition, corroboration and extension of our studies upon the tonsils has come from Italy too late to be included above (Azzi, 1921). Azzi used also more circumscribed stimuli, such as a draft of cold air on one exposed foot or immersion of one of the subject's hands in cold water. Such local applications of cold elicited reflex vasoconstriction in the tonsillar mucous membrane just as more extensive chilling does, although quantitatively somewhat less. Warming the body surface generally or locally without previous chilling Azzi found to result in reflex vasodilation in the tonsils, just as with rewarming after chilling. When the subject was chilled subsequently to such heat application, however, the tonsil vessels usually remained dilated. During the experiments on himself Azzi fell sick with a febrile rheumatic affection and mild tonsillitis. His inflamed tonsils did not exhibit vasomotor response either to cutaneous chilling or warming.

Attention is also called to a late paper by E. O. Jordan and W. P. Sharp (1921), showing negative results in prophylactic vaccination against colds with W. H. Parks' Pfeiffer bacillus-streptococcus-pneumococcus vaccine, despite belief of many of the inoculated to the contrary. "'Satisfied patient' conclusions differ widely from those of controlled statistics."

## BIBLIOGRAPHY.

Abel, 1892: Centralblatt f. Bak., xii, 841.

Allen, 1906: Brit. Med. Journ., i, 1131.

Allen, 1913: Bacterial Diseases of Respiration and Vaccines in Their Treatment, London.

Ansiaux, 1889: Bull. de l'Academie Royale des Sciences, etc., de Belgique, xvii, 581.

Azzi, 1921: La riforma med., xxxvii, 175.

Ballenger, 1908: Diseases of the Nose and Throat, 109, 132, 334.

Barker, 1916: Monographic Medicine, ii, 550.

Barnes, 1914: The Tonsils, 79.

Benedict, Miles and Johnson, 1919: Proc. Nat. Acad. Sci., v, 218.

Penham, 1906: Brit. Med. Jour., i, 1023.

Bezancon et de Jong, 1905; Bull. de la Soc. Méd. des Hôp. de Paris, xxii, 165.

Blake and Cecil, 1920: Jour. Am. Med. Assoc., lxxiv, 170; Jour. Exp. Med. xxxii, 691.

Cautley, 1894-5: Report of the Local Govt. Board, Great Britain. Supplement, p. 455.

Cecil and Steffen, 1921: Jour. Infect. Dis., xxviii, 201.

Coakley, 1914: Diseases of the Nose and Throat, 79, 287.

Cocks, 1915: Tr. Amer. Laryng. Rhin. and Otol. Soc., 138.

Coolidge, 1918: Diseases of the Nose and Throat, 95.

Davis, 1920: Journ. Am. Med. Assoc., lxxiv, 317.

Dunn and Gordon, 1905: Brit. Med. Jour., ii, 421.

Floyd, 1920: Boston Med. and Surg. Journ., clxxxii, 389.

Foord, 1918: Jour. Infect. Dis., xxiii, 159.

Foster, 1916: Jour. A. M. A., lxvi, 1180.

Foster, 1917: Jour. Infect. Diseases, xxi, 451.

Galeotti, 1920: Riforma Med., xxxvi, 205; abstracted in J. Am. Med. Assoc., 1920: lxxiv, 1491.

Galeotti, 1914: Archiv. f. d. ges. Physiol., clx, 27; Galeotti, Scaftidi and Barkan, Reports of the R. Accad. Dei Lincei, 1914, xxiii, serie 5a 2o sem. fasc. 7e, Rome.

Gohn u. Pfeiffer, H., 1902: Zeitschr. f. Klin. Med., xliv, 262.

Goldman, Mudd and Grant, 1921: Jour. Infect. Dis., to be published.

Goodale, 1899: Journ. Boston Soc. Med. Sciences, iii, 68.

Goodale, 1916: Annals of Otology, Rhinology and Laryngology, 25, 527.

Goodale, 1918: Boston Med. and Surg. Journ., clxxix, 293.

Gordon, quoted by Benham, loc. cit.

Grant, Mudd and Goldman, 1920: Journ. Exp. Med., xxxii, 87.

Grayson, 1902: Diseases of the Nose, Throat and Ear, 82, 231.

Hajek, 1888: Berlin, Klin. Wochenschr., 33, 659.

Hill, 1919: Gt. Britain Med. Research Coun., Special Rep. Series Part 1, No. 32.

Hill and Muecke, 1913: Lancet, i, 1291.

Howell, 1915: Journ. Infect. Dis., xvi, 456.
Hüter, quoted by Benham, loc. cit.
Jordan and Sharp: 1921. J. Infect. Dis., xxviii, 367.
Kisskalt, 1901: Arch. f. Hygiene, xxxix, 165.
Kruse, 1914: Münch. Med. Wochenschr., lxi, 1547.
Kyle, 1914: Diseases of Nose and Throat, 73, 75, 422, 472, 521.
Lassar, 1880: Virchow's Archiv., lxxix, 168.
Liebermeister, 1860: Archiv. f. Anat., Physiol., u. Wissensch. Med., 523.
Lingelsheim, 1912: Kolle u. Wassermann's Handb. d. Pathogenen Mikroörgan, iv, 481.
Loewe and Zeman, 1921: Jour. Am. Med. Assoc., lxxvi, 986.
MacCallum, 1920: Textbook of Pathology, 386.
Marchand, 1908: Krehl u. Marchand's Handb. d. allgemeinen Path., i, 130.
Mathers, 1917: Journ. Inf. Dis., xxx, 1.
McLaughlin, 1920: Boston Med. and Surg. Jour., clxxxiii, 1.
Miller and Noble, 1916: Journ. Exp. Med., xxiv, 223.
Mudd and Grant, 1919: Journ. Med. Research, xl 53-101.
Mudd, Goldman and Grant, 1921: Jour. Exp. Med. xxxiv, July number.
Nagelsbach, 1920: Deut. Zeitschr. f. Chir., 1920, clx, 205.
Neufe'd u. Händel, 1912: Kolle u. Wassermann's Handb. d. Pathogen Mikroörgan., iv, 508.
Neumann, 1902: Zeitsch. f. Hygiene, xl, 33.
Olitsky and Gates, 1920: Jour. Am. Med. Assoc., lxxiv, 1497.
Olitsky and Gates, 1921: Jour. Exp. Med. xxxiii, 125, 361,373; Jour. Am. Med. Assoc., lxxvi, 640.
Packard, 1914: Osler and McRae's Modern Medicine, ii, 843.
Paulsen, 1890: Centra'bl. f. Bak. u. Parasit., viii, 344.
Pfeiffer, R., 1913: Cit. by Neisser in Kolle u. Wassermann's Handh. d. Pathogenen Mikroörgan, iii, 146.
Phillips, 1919: Diseases of Ear, Nose and Throat, 492.
Rosenau, 1920: Preventative Medicine and Hygiene. 195.
Rossbach u. Aschenbrandt: Cit. by Kisskalt, loc. cit.
Schade, 1919: München Med. Wochenschr., lxvi, 1021.
Schade, 1920: München Med. Wochenschr., lxvii, 449.
Schüller, 1881: Cit. by Winternitz, Die Hydrotherapie, 113.
Sticker, 1916: "Erkältungskrankheiten u. Kälteschäden in the Enzyklopädie d. Klin. Med., Berlin.
Thomson, 1913: Diseases of the Nose and Throat. 91.
Tilley, 1919: Diseases of the Nose and Throat, 26, 341.
Trommsdorf, 1906: Arch. f. Hygiene, lix, 1.
Tschalussow, 1913: Archiv. f. d. gesammte Physiol., cli, 541.
Tunnic'iff, 1913: Jour. Infect. Dis., xiii, 283.
Tunnicliff, 1915: Jour. Infect. Dis., xvi, 493.
Walker, 1919: Oxford Medicine, ii, Part 1, 115, 143.
Walker, 1920: Journ. Am. Med. Assoc., lxxv, 782.
Winternitz, 1881: Die Hydrotherapie, 113.
White, quoted by Benham, loc. cit.
Wright, 1907: New York Medical Journal. lxxxv, 437.
Wright, 1909: The Laryngoscope, xix, 321.
Wright and Smith, 1914: Diseases of the Nose and Throat. 295.

# II

# THE BORDERLAND OF OTOLARYNGOLOGY AND OPHTHALMOLOGY.

By Hanau W. Loeb, M. D., and Meyer Wiener, M. D.,

St. Louis.

Our own experience and a careful survey of the literature have forced upon us the following conclusions which it is the purpose of this paper to elucidate and to defend:

1. Lesions of the eye and its adnexa occur far more frequently from pathologic processes involving the nose and paranasal sinuses than is generally accepted.

2. A study of the minor processes would result in a more fruitful yield than that which has followed the interest in the exceptional and striking cases manifest up to the present time.

3. It is necessary to examine and to study in detail the nose and para nasal sinuses in all eye conditions for which they may be responsible, including conjunctivitis, lacrimal sac conditions, orbital cellulitis and abscess, corneal ulceration, iritis and its associates, maturing cataract, retinal hemorrhage, retinal detachment, optic neuritis, ocular and retrobulbar, optic atrophy, glaucoma, reduction of vision, diminution of the field and functional disturbances not otherwise explained.

4. It is most important to examine for and to record any changes in the orbital or ocular tissues in all cases of acute or chronic suppurative processes involving the paranasal sinuses.

5. Persistent and intelligent study along these lines must bring about a solution of many of the vexing problems which have been uncovered by the casual study of the relation between the eye and the upper respiratory tract.

## I.—THE ANATOMIC RELATIONS.

Grossly the eyes lie one on each side of the nasal cavities which, however, come into closer relation by the extension of the paranasal sinuses, below, behind, above and internal to the orbital cavity. In other words, the sinuses form a pneumatic boundary internally, superiorly and inferiorly, which, however, continues subject to nasal influences by reason of the extension of the nasal mucosa throughout each sinus.

A clear view of the intimacy of this anatomic association is shown in the illustrations herewith presented. Fig. 1* shows the bone relations of the sinuses to the orbit, the thin bone of the orbital wall of the sinuses being removed. Fig. 2 shows the bone relations of the frontal sinus to the orbits. In Fig. 3 the bone has been cut away, leaving the mucosa intact, showing how extensive and intimate is its relation to the orbital contents. The frontal, ethmoid, sphenoid and maxillary sinuses are readily recognized. Figs. 4 and 5 show this relation in coronal section, the first at the opening of the maxillary sinus into the nose, the second just anterior to the sphenoid sinus.

Of the dissections of the optic nerve and paranasal sinuses made by Loeb, that shown in Fig. 6 is presented as exhibiting the course of the nerve along the sinuses whose mucosa has been left intact.

The mere propinquity of the eye to these sinuses with their extensive mucosal covering would speak for an association of pathologic conditions both frequent and important, even if specific details were not at hand. The extension of this mucosa by continuity to the conjunctiva through the lacrimal passages adds another concrete factor to this association.

Dehiscences in bone walls, as pointed out by Zuckerkandl, Onodi and others, bring the pathologic process closer to the seat of complications. This is still further manifest in the unusual relations sometimes present between the optic nerve and the sphenoid and the ethmoid, as shown by the same authors, and the fact brought out by Loeb, that sometimes the orifice of the sphenoid sinus lies at or above the level of the optic nerve and that, in two out of thirty instances of heads studied, the course of the nerve was along the outer wall of the posterior ethmoid cell which had replaced the sphenoid. Under usual circumstances, the nearest and only point of relation to the optic nerve is the superior posteroexternal angle

---

*This and the succeeding illustrations are reproduced, by permission, from Loeb's "Operative Surgery of the Nose, Throat and Ear."

of the last posterior ethmoid cell. Compare Fig. 7 and Fig. 8.

But there are other relations quite as important if not as intimate from the standpoint of contiguity. This pertains more especially to the nerves and vessels.

The ophthalmic artery gives off the ethmoid arteries which supply the ethmoid cells and a large portion of the upper part of the nasal cavity. Still more important are the ethmoid veins which empty into superior and inferior ophthalmic veins.

In addition, the extensive anastomosis still further accentuates the vascular influence. Of the nasal and ocular lymphatics, little so far has been determined, but there is manifestly quite as intimate an association as exists in the vascular supply.

The nerve distribution is no less convincing. There are two factors in this connection. In the first place, two branches of the supraorbital supply a large portion of the nasal mucosa, the branches of the posterior ethmoidal being distributed to the sphenoid sinus and posterior ethmoidal cells, those of the anterior ethmoidal to the septum, roof, middle turbinate and anterior portion of the inferior turbinate. Anastomotic branches add to the connection between the oculoorbital and the nasal nerve supply.

In the second place, the nerve relations of the sphenoid sinus, as studied by Sluder, constitute the means by which ocular symptoms may follow disease of this sinus.

Of the anatomic relations of the ear and eye, there is little to be said. The sixth nerve, however, may become affected by pressure at the apex of the petrous pyramid through a localized leptomeningitis incident to an acute suppurative otitis media.

The pharynx and larynx have no close anatomic relations with the eye except perhaps through Meckel's ganglion, which sends branches to the pharynx as well as the eye and nose.

## II.—PATHOGENESIS.

Autopsy evidence of the pathologic relation between the ear, nose and throat and the eye is unfortunately slight. Where autopsies have been performed the process was found so extensive that little could be ascertained as to the origin of the trouble. Autopsies upon those dying of intercurrent disease in the presence of one of these conditions are rare, and when they have been performed little evidence has been uncovered.

However, we are not altogether without knowledge in this regard, as operative procedures have given some information, and inference and comparison with allied processes are of some value.

Except in malignant disease, tuberculosis, syphilis, etc., the nose, throat and ear are the original seat of the pathogenic process which brings them into relation with the eye. A malignant disease may extend from the orbit to the nose or vice versa. Tuberculosis, syphilis and diphtheria may appear either simultaneously in the eye and nose, or they may appear first in either organ.

So far little has been developed to show that any special bacterial invasion of the nose or accessory sinuses has any predilection for the eye, other than that acute virulent processes affecting the sinuses are more prone to result in orbital abscess. At any rate, with the possible exception of the work of Dewatripont upon the bacterial causes of disease of the nasolacrimal passageways, investigations have not been successful in differentiating the various types of bacteria with reference to their influence on any special oculoorbital disease of nasal and paranasal origin.

The means by which the disease process may extend from the nose, throat and ear to the eye may be summarized as follows:

1. By extension along the mucosa. This applies more especially to processes involving the nasolacrimal tract and the conjunctiva.

2. By pressure, as when the orbital wall is invaded by a mucocele or other process which bulges out the sinus wall.

3. By extension through dehiscences, mainly in the production of orbital cellulitis and abscess.

4. By destruction or necrosis of the boundary walls. Autopsies have shown that orbital abscess may originate in this way.

5. By periostitis of the sinus wall, by direct invasion or through the bone vascular system.

6. By the vascular and lymphatic systems. This group includes three divisions:

a. Cases of frank thrombophlebitis of the cavernous sinus, the ophthalmic vein and other vessels.

b. Those due to obstruction of the circulation, such as edema of the eyelids, chemosis, exophthalmus, etc. Conditions such as swelling of the papilla and optic neuritis associated with blindness almost miraculously and instantly relieved by intranasal operation are probably of vascular origin, comparable to edema glottidis occurring in connection with a severe infection of near-by tissues.

c. Those in which the vessels are merely the transmitting agent. The first two divisions of this interesting group of cases have been pathogenically faily well established. The third has the same basis as that which pertains to the origin of polyarthritis, endocarditis and nephritis from remote foci. Iritis comes under this class. For years it has been known that iritis is usually associated with syphilis or rheumatism, but only recently has the tonsil relation of polyarthritis been applied to iritis.

The lymphatic system has been included with the vascular system in spite of our lack of knoweldge of the lymphatics of the eye and nose, for the reason that the lymph flow is so closely associated with the vascular circulation and because of the behavior of lymphatic absorption elsewhere in the body.

7. By the nervous system. Of these we have two classes:

a. Cases due to pressure, extraneous or from inflammation within the nerve sheath and trophic disturbances. These include optic neuritis, with its sequelæ, optic atrophy, paralysis of the ocular muscles, blepharospasm, paralysis of accommodation. Paralysis of the abducens may result from a localized meningitis occurring in connection with a suppurative otitis media.

b. Cases in which the nervous relation is more or less indefinite or obscure. This has reference to those which for want of better pathogenic understanding are termed functional, reflex, etc. With the increase of our knowledge of pathology, this group is likely to shrink more and more by its replacement to other groups.

### III.—THE NOSE, THROAT AND EAR RELATIONS.

The paranasal sinuses are the dominating influence in the more serious oculoorbital conditions of nasal origin, yet a deflected septum or a hypertrophied middle turbinate which obstructs any of the sinus orifices may be of etiologic significance. These conditions may be responsible for a number of minor affections such as conjunctivitis of various types, inflammatory and obstructive conditions of the lacrimal passageways, and slight deficiencies in vision. Dewatripont, who has made an extensive study of the diseases of the nasolacrimal passageways, agrees with the statement made by Kuhnt that 95 per cent of the cases have a nasal origin. Magitot studied 100 cases of keratoconjunctivitis in an ophthalmic center and found 95 per cent suffering from nasal lesions as follows:

1. Acute rhinitis, followed by coryza with or without hypertrophy, 30 per cent.

2. Atrophic rhinitis with or without ozena, 5 per cent.

3. Tertiary syphilis of the nose, 7 per cent.

4. Maxillary or frontal sinusitis, acute or chronic, 13 per cent.

5. Mucous polypi often compressing the nasolacrimal canal, 3 per cent.

6. Septum deviations with large spurs, comprising the inferior meatus, 25 per cent.

7. Stenosis of the inferior meatus by approximation of the inferior against the lateral wall of the nasal fossa, 15 per cent.

8. Cicatricial lesions of the inferior meatus resulting from resection of the anterior portion of the internal wall of the maxillary sinus in the course of a radical cure of the disease.

Most of the eye complications connected with the nose result from acute or chronic suppuration of the paranasal sinuses. but some of the more interesting ones may follow acute inflammatory processes with little or no pus. The more serious complications usually occur in connection with a closed empyema. And yet, there does not seem to be a clear line of demarcation between the effects of any of these lesions on the variety, severity or duration of the resulting complications.

While most of the sequelae may result from lesions of any

of the sinuses, each sinus seems to have a fairly well established adherence to certain of these complications.

They are as follows:

1. Ethmoid Cells: Swelling of the inner angle of the upper eyelid, orbital cellulitis and abscess, exophthalmus, diplopia, visual deficiencies, disease of the nasolacrimal passageways, iritis, vitreous opacities, papilledema, optic neuritis, optic atrophy.

2. Sphenoid Sinus: Thrombosis of the cavernous sinus, optic neuritis, optic atrophy, paralysis of the third, fourth and sixth nerves.

3. Frontal Sinus: Proptosis from mucocele and suppuration, orbital cellulitis and abscess, edema of the lids, diplopia, conjunctivitis, iritis, corneal ulceration, vitreous opacities, optic neuritis and atrophy.

4. Maxillary Sinus: Edema of the lower lid, conjunctivitis, orbital cellulitis and abscess, optic neuritis and atrophy.

The ear influence is limited practically to abducens paralysis. However, no account is here taken of the interesting oculovestibular manifestations of nystagmus and of the retinal changes in the intracranial sequelæ of otitis media suppurativa, which form no part of this paper.

The tonsils have been found the focus of origin in iritis, iridokeratitis and iridocyclitis, which have heretofore been known to be associated with rheumatism. It will not be strange if other inflammatory conditions about the eye are found to be due to tonsil infection or to toxic processes originating in the tonsil.

The relation of phlyctenular keratitis to adenoids seems to be generally accepted.

There are those who consider that the thickened patches in trachoma and in follicular pharyngitis bring tnem into association, but this is quite doubtful.

#### IV.—THE EYE RELATIONS.

The eye conditions due to nose and throat lesions reported in the literature are astonishingly large, both in number and variety, in spite of the fact that the reporters have heretofore been mainly interested in the unusual and startling types. An analysis of these cases shows that the nose and throat are common factors, even making allowance for the enthusiasm of the observers. We are convinced, however, that this enthusiasm is fully warranted by the facts.

The following summarizes our observations:

1. Pain. Generally speaking, the nose or the paranasal sinuses may be held accountable for pain in the eye or eyes, in the absence of any external ocular inflammatory signs, especially when it begins in the morning or upon awakening. The pain may be described as an eyeache, a pain between the eyes or in the temple. (Usually one side.) This pain almost always disappears after the patient has been up for a while, or at least it is greatly alleviated, in contradistinction with eye pain produced by eye strain or intraocular disease, which always increases towards evening. The pain is also relievable by cocain applications to the nasal mucosa. It is often accompanied by a general redness of the bulbar conjunctiva, epiphora and more or less photophobia and dizziness.

2. Epiphora, Dacryocystitis, Stenosis of Duct, Fistula, Etc.: These long recognized and familiar signs of a nasal lesion are most frequently associated with a common cold or coryza. They may, however, be caused by a mechanical obstruction in the nasal cavity; by extension of the infection directly into the nasal duct; by extension of the infection indirectly from an infected nose and by reflex irritation in the nose.

Mechanical obstruction of tears may be due to hyperplasia of the inferior turbinate or even the middle turbinate or of the mucosa immediately surrounding the valve of Hasner.

A case has been described by Wiener in which the cause was a membrane stretched across the nasal opening of the nasal duct, the mere splitting of which relieved the tearing.

Inflammation of the nasolacrimal passageways may result from ethmoid or frontal lesions by direct pressure or contact infection, and this may sometimes occur in maxillary suppuration. Elschnig attributes 50 per cent of the cases of dacryocystitis to an extension of an ethmoiditis.

3. Lids and Orbit. Redness of the lid margins, acute or chronic blepharitis marginalis, slight edema or puffiness of the lids, dark circles under the eyes are common sequelæ of nasal obstruction or of inflammation of the nose or paranasal sinuses.

Orbital cellulitis, phlegmon and abscess have long been understood to be generally of sinus origin. Even in children and infants this has been substantiated, although the small size and seemingly slight importance of the sinuses in children has been assumed sufficient to exclude them from consideration.

Birch-Hirschfeld cites statistics of 684 cases of orbital inflammation; he found 409, or 59.8 per cent, due to sinus infection. He believes this should be much higher, as in many cases the nose and sinuses were not taken into consideration. Furthermore, as Axenfeld has pointed out, the sinusitis may subside as the cellulitis progresses, particularly in cases following influenza.

Most of the orbital complications are due to frontal sinus inflammation; the ethmoid follows, then the sphenoid, and finally the maxillary is occasionally the cause. A frontal involvement is indicated in swelling limited to the upper lid with the eyeball pushed down and towards the temple with crossed diplopia and vertical deviation; ethmoiditis, in swelling at the inner canthus evenly divided between the two lids, with the globe pushed towards the temple, and crossed diplopia with no vertical deviation; and a sphenoid empyema, in swelling of the lower lid, a predisposition to chemosis in the lower quadrant of conjunctiva.

Emphysema of orbit or lids may be due to fracture of a portion of the nasal wall of the orbit, usually the ethmoid. It also occurs from inflammatory conditions. Collections of fetid gas with pus in the orbit have been found by Grandclemont and Guyot to be of ethmoid origin.

Cases of blepharospasm have been reported in which relief was secured only when some accompanying nasal irritation was removed.

Exophthalmic goiter with complete subsidence of the exophthalmos has been cured by nasal operation. On the other hand, the exophthalmus has also been reported as having immediately followed a nasal operation. The tonsil relations of goiter are now being studied by a number of investigators.

Thrombophlebitis of the ophthalmic plexus has been found as a complication in inflammation of the posterior ethmoid or the sphenoid. Embolism of the arteria centralis retinæ and thrombosis of the central vein have been reported following sinusitis operations and paraffin injections for correcting nasal deformities. Wiener has seen a case of the embolism of the central artery of the retina occur immediately after injection of hard paraffin for cure of saddleback nose.

Paraffinomata of the lids have also occurred after injection of hard paraffin into the nose, causing partial or complete closure of the lids with more or less permanent defects.

4. Muscles. Abducens paralysis in connection with suppurative otitis media has already been considered.

Paralysis or paresis of the fourth, or one or more branches of the third nerve, is a common complication of orbital abscess or. cellulitis due to sinusitis, and paralysis of the fourth frequently results from a Killian operation. These muscle paralyses have often been permanent, although they may be merely transitory. The asthenopia often observed in patients suffering from nasal affections can be ascribed to a fatigue of the accommodation branch of the third, without producing an actual paralysis of accommodation.

5. Conjunctiva and Cornea. Inflammation of the conjunctiva or cornea must not necessarily be set down as due to nasal inflammation merely because of concommitance, for they may both be complications of measles, pemphigus, tuberculosis or syphilis.

Various forms of conjunctivitis and keratoconjunctivitis, especially the phlyctenular variety, have been reported as being caused by nasal and sinus disease. Corneal ulcer and herpes of the cornea and lids have been relieved by treatment of the nose and sinus and the removal of tonsils and adenoids. We have found that stubborn forms of dendritic keratitis, such as are not generally recognized as being of nasal origin, are relieved promptly by appropriate treatment of the nose.

Keratitis lisceformis has been reported by Elschnig as caused by sinusitis. He does not venture to ascribe the manner in which the sinus causes the condition.

6. Uveal Tract. Ophthalmologists have only in recent years awakened to the importance of looking to focal infection as a cause of iritis and uveitis. Diseased sinuses and tonsils have been found largely responsible for a great number of cases of anterior and posterior uveitis. Startling cures of acute,

chronic and recurrent cases have been recorded after removal of diesased tonsils, whereas all previous efforts at effecting a cure had failed. We have had a marked case of this type.

Increased intraocular tension may have a nasal origin. We have under observation at the present time two cases of glaucoma, one a woman, 45 years of age, who had been operated upon for cataract in the left eye and now has cataract with glaucoma in the right eye, was immediately relieved of pain with a temporary reduction of intraocular tension to normal by shrinking the middle meatus with cocain. She is already greatly improved since clearing out the diseased ethmoid cells on her right side, and we are watching with interest the ultimate outcome. The second patient, a case of glaucoma, with recurrent large blebs upon the cornea, has just been operated upon for a deflected septum. The ethmoid cells on that side were found to be diseased, but will be taken care of later. This patient also had been greatly improved temporarily by shrinking the mucous membrane of the nose.

While the contention of Ziem that cataract can be caused or at least influenced by sphenoid or ethmoid sinus disease leaves some room for doubt, Pauntz and others have unquestionably demonstrated the influence of sinusitis on postoperative cataract infection.

Hyalitis and muscae volitantes are among the conditions that have disappeared upon relieving the nasal lesion.

With sympathetic ophthalmia there is a recognized thickening of the nasal mucosa. Some authorities have held the sinuses to be the cause in a number of cases. Two are cited by Elschnig of sympathetic irritation occurring three months after enucleation, entirely cured with restored vision following treatment of the sinuses. Two reported by Moulton at the last meeting of the American Medical Association seem to be due to similar cause.

7. Optic Nerve and Retina. This is of the most vital importance, as often the question of sight or blindness rests with prompt diagnosis. Most of the cases of blindness relieved by nasal operation come within this group. Retinal hemorrhages and inflammations, retinal detachment and neuroretinitis have all been found to be due to sinus disease and infected tonsils.

We are mostly concerned, however, with optic neuritis and retrobulbar neuritis.

Evans and Fish tabulated 36 consecutive cases of optic neuritis. Sinus disease was present 26 times. Elschnig found sinus involvement in 15 per cent of all optic nerve affections.

Only a small percentage of these cases give a history of nasal trouble. There is nothing significant about the appearance of the nerve, as there may be any condition present, from a normal nerve head in retrobulbar neuritis to a choked disc, either due to sinusitis or other causes. The diagnosis is particularly difficult when sinusitis is present with some other (nerve) disease. The mere presence of tabes in a case of atrophy, or active syphilis in a case of optic neuritis, should not exclude the sinuses as having an important bearing on the neuritis. On the other hand, the association of sinusitis with optic neuritis should not deter the physician from going through the routine in an effort to discover all possible determining causes.

Van der Hoeve believes that enlargement of the blind spot, first for colors and later for white, is the first sign of retrobulbar neuritis of nasal origin. He believes that this always is the precursor of a central scotoma and could be found often if a careful and early search were made.

Elschnig does not attach much significance to enlargement of the blind spot, as it is an accompanying sign of toxic amblyopia. However, the latter can usually be eliminated by a history of the case. He believes with Fuchs that central scotoma for colors and then white is one of the earliest signs. de Kleinj, however, has verified the work of Van der Hoeve and thinks that we have in this a most valuable means for an early diagnosis, even though it may not be constant.

Ziem considers a peripheral contraction of the fields of vision common, but has received little support. Other scotomata besides the natural blind spot are sometimes found in the field. Bitemporal hemianopsia is a rare accompaniment.

Retrobulbar neuritis with resulting atrophy of the optic nerve has often been seen following fracture by blow on the orbital edge extending along the nasal wall of the orbit to the canalus opticus, and has even been reported following operation on the septum or removal of a spur or turbinate bone, causing fracture extending to the optic canal.

Optic atrophy following retrobulbar neuritis in "tower skull" has been discussed by Posey and Berger, who believe it to be due to the encroachment of bone on the optic canal and sphenoid fissure the result of enlargement of the sphenoid bone with advancing years.

It must not be forgotten that in optic nerve atrophy with bitemporal hemianopsia due to tumor of the hypophysis, the growth sometimes reaches downward into the sphenoid and may be mistaken for primary sphenoidal growth. In such a case which was under observation (Wiener) a craniectomy was unsuccessfully made, and on postmortem examination it was found that the growth extended deeply into the sphenoid. If the sinuses had been previously examined in this case, much valuable information would have been available.

Numerous cases of blindness from optic neuritis relieved by nasal operation reported by Risley, Onodi, Holmes, Evans, Fish, Elschnig, Hansell, Van der Hoeve, de Schweinitz, Sluder, Knapp, Loeb, Ring, and many others leave no doubt that there are many minor defects of vision which are dependent on nasal lesions and for which no relief is possible, except through proper attention to the nose and paranasal sinuses.

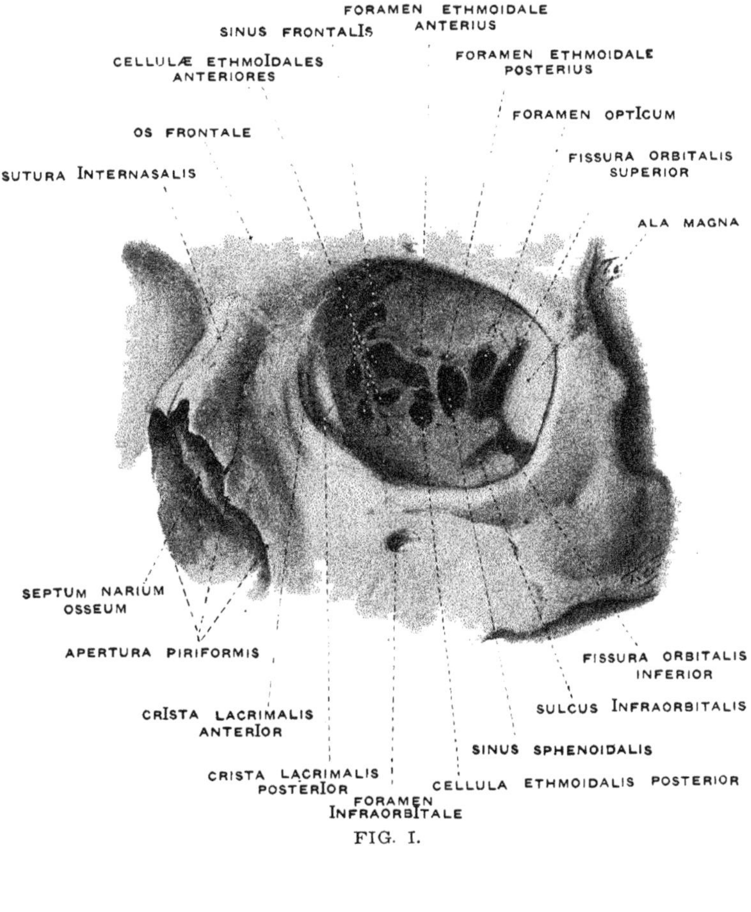

FORAMEN ETHMOIDALE
ANTERIUS

SINUS FRONTALIS

CELLULÆ ETHMOIDALES
ANTERIORES

FORAMEN ETHMOIDALE
POSTERIUS

OS FRONTALE

FORAMEN OPTICUM

SUTURA INTERNASALIS

FISSURA ORBITALIS
SUPERIOR

ALA MAGNA

SEPTUM NARIUM
OSSEUM

APERTURA PIRIFORMIS

FISSURA ORBITALIS
INFERIOR

CRISTA LACRIMALIS
ANTERIOR

SULCUS INFRAORBITALIS

CRISTA LACRIMALIS
POSTERIOR

SINUS SPHENOIDALIS

CELLULA ETHMOIDALIS POSTERIOR

FORAMEN
INFRAORBITALE

FIG. I.

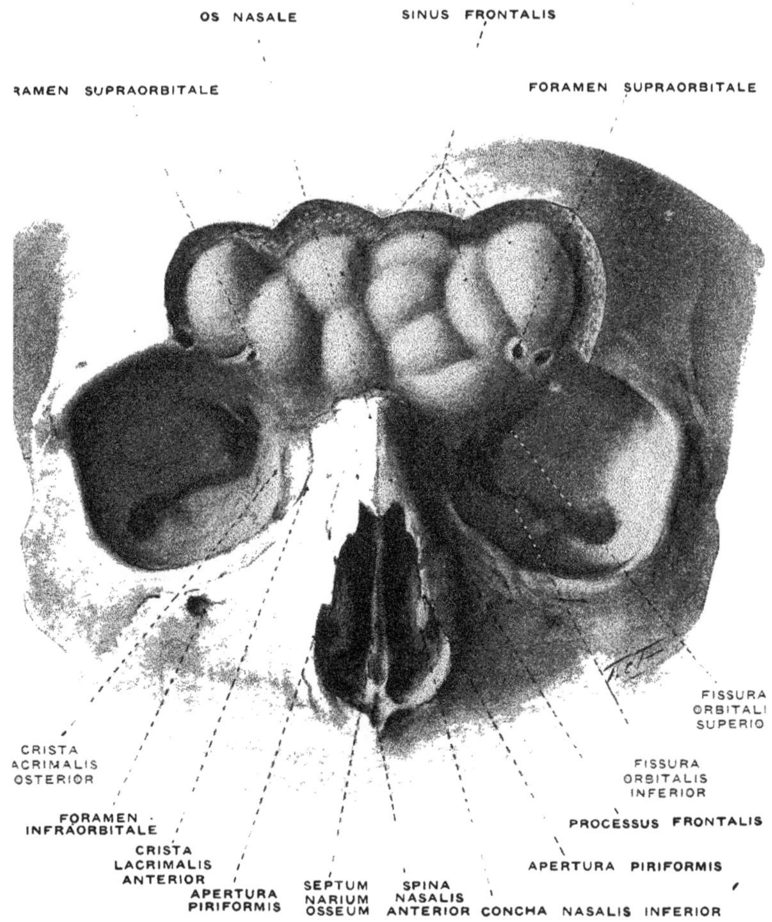

OS NASALE      SINUS FRONTALIS

RAMEN SUPRAORBITALE      FORAMEN SUPRAORBITALE

FISSURA
ORBITALI
SUPERIO

CRISTA
ACRIMALIS
OSTERIOR

FISSURA
ORBITALIS
INFERIOR

FORAMEN
INFRAORBITALE

PROCESSUS FRONTALIS

CRISTA
LACRIMALIS
ANTERIOR

APERTURA PIRIFORMIS

APERTURA  SEPTUM  SPINA
PIRIFORMIS  NARIUM  NASALIS
          OSSEUM ANTERIOR  CONCHA NASALIS INFERIOR

Fig. II.

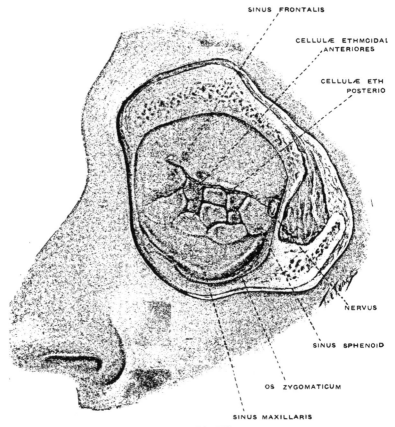

SINUS FRONTALIS

CELLULÆ ETHMOIDAL
ANTERIORES

CELLULÆ ETH
POSTERIO

NERVUS

SINUS SPHENOID

OS ZYGOMATICUM

SINUS MAXILLARIS

FIG. III.

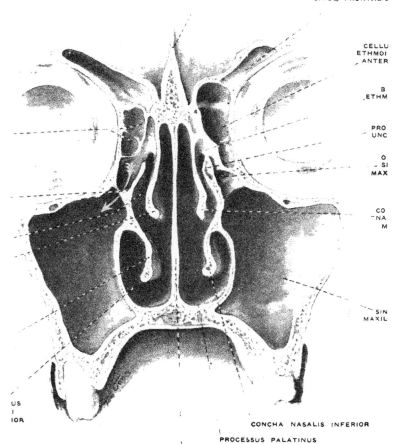

SINUS, FRONTALIS

CELLU
ETHMOI
ANTER

B
ETHM

PRO
UNC

O
SI
MAX

CO
NA
M

SIN
MAXIL

US
I
IOR

CONCHA NASALIS INFERIOR

PROCESSUS PALATINUS

SEPTUM NASI

FIG. IV.

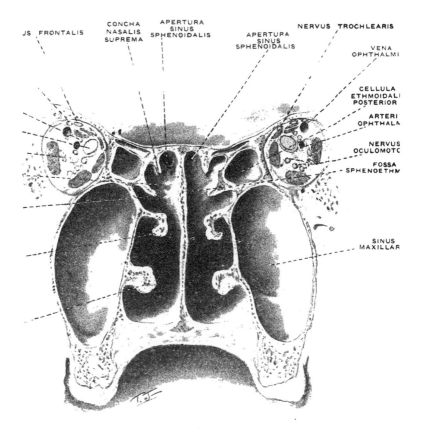

JS FRONTALIS

CONCHA
NASALIS
SUPREMA

APERTURA
SINUS
SPHENOIDALIS

APERTURA
SINUS
SPHENOIDALIS

NERVUS TROCHLEARIS

VENA
OPHTHALMI

CELLULA
ETHMOIDALI
POSTERIOR

ARTERI
OPHTHALN

NERVUS
OCULOMOTC

FOSSA
SPHENOETHM

SINUS
MAXILLAR

FIG. V.

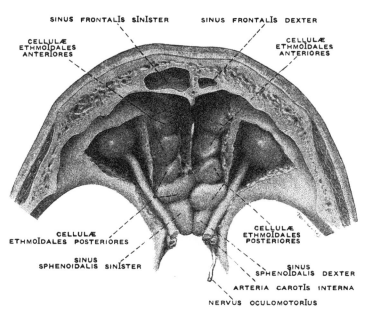

SINUS FRONTALIS SINISTER     SINUS FRONTALIS DEXTER

CELLULÆ
ETHMOIDALES
ANTERIORES

CELLULÆ
ETHMOIDALES
ANTERIORES

CELLULÆ
ETHMOIDALES POSTERIORES

CELLULÆ
ETHMOIDALES
POSTERIORES

SINUS
SPHENOIDALIS SINISTER

SINUS
SPHENOIDALIS DEXTER

ARTERIA CAROTIS INTERNA

NERVUS OCULOMOTORIUS

FIG. VI.

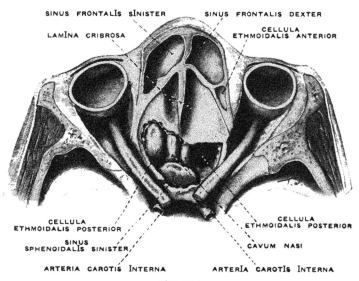

SINUS FRONTALIS SINISTER      SINUS FRONTALIS DEXTER

LAMINA CRIBROSA         CELLULA
                       ETHMOIDALIS ANTERIOR

CELLULA                          CELLULA
ETHMOIDALIS POSTERIOR            ETHMOIDALIS POSTERIOR
     SINUS
SPHENOIDALIS SINISTER           CAVUM NASI

ARTERIA CAROTIS INTERNA      ARTERIA CAROTIS INTERNA

FIG. VII.

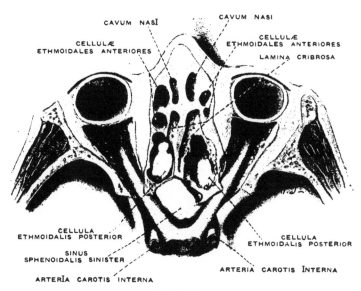

CAVUM NASI      CAVUM NASI

CELLULÆ ETHMOIDALES ANTERIORES      CELLULÆ ETHMOIDALES ANTERIORES

LAMINA CRIBROSA

CELLULA ETHMOIDALIS POSTERIOR      CELLULA ETHMOIDALIS POSTERIOR

SINUS SPHENOIDALIS SINISTER

ARTERIA CAROTIS INTERNA      ARTERIA CAROTIS INTERNA

FIG. VIII.

# III.

## OBSERVATIONS ON THE DEVELOPMENTAL ANATOMY OF THE TEMPORAL BONE.*

### By Lee Rogers, M. D.,

FROM THE INSTITUTE OF ANATOMY AND THE DEPARTMENT OF OPHTHALMOLOGY AND OTOLARYNGOLOGY.

The purpose of this paper is to record a series of observations on the development of the temporal bone in later fetal life and childhood, and to consider the varying relations of its several parts at different ages, with particular reference to their surgical significance.

The study has been limited, in the main, to those phases of the subject concerning which our information is obviously incomplete or upon which there exists a decided difference of opinion.

### MATERIAL AND METHODS.

A considerable amount of material was available for this study, including 294 temporal bones, some dried and some fresh and in situ, as well as a series of 32 skulls in various stages of development. Of the temporal bones, 14 were of fetal stages, 32 of newborn children, 18 of children of different ages (2 to 15 years, inclusive) and 230 of adults.

Of the skulls 14 were fetal, 14 were newborn, and 4 were of children. There was also available a large series of adult skulls for comparison with those of earlier stages.

To insure exactitude of measurements, and to determine accurately the relations of the various parts of the organ of hearing, the subject has been attacked with a variety of methods.

First, a series of casts in Wood's metal were prepared, reproducing the cavities of the external, middle and internal ear, together with the nerves, air cells, osseus auditory tube, tensor tympani muscle, carotid artery, aqueducts, etc. In all, 40 such

---

*Graduate thesis for Master's Degree in Ophthalmology and Otolaryngology Graduate School, University of Minnesota.

casts were prepared. Fifteen of these were of adult ears, 5 of children, 10 of newborn infants, and 10 of fetuses. Drawings of some of these preparations are shown in Figs. 1 to 14, inclusive.

Second, the antra of a series of temporal bones were filled with bismuth paste and radiographed to show their position at different ages. As a check on this procedure, the antra were later transilluminated by introducing the small electric light of a bronchoscope tube in the cavity of each bone and tracing the outline on the surface. In older children and adults an opening was drilled through the tegmen tympani into the antrum to admit the light. In the fetus and infant the antrum could be reached through the external meatus.

The size and position of the antra were determined by radiography and transillumination in 40 bones (10 adults, 7 children, 8 newborn infants and 15 fetuses). Drawings of these specimens are shown in Figs. 15 to 24, inclusive.

Third, to determine the relations of the inner structures of the ear to surface landmarks, a series of casts in Wood's metal was prepared and the bone in these specimens was later rendered transparent by the Spalteholz clearing method so that the cochlea, antrum, nerves, air cells, etc., could be observed in situ. Three of these preparations were made. Of these, one was of an adult, one of a child, three years old, and one of a newborn infant (Figs. 25 and 26).

Fourth, to further determine the relations of the antrum, facial nerve and other structures to the surface landmarks, regional dissections were made on the cadaver. Of these 8 were of the adult, 2 of children, and 8 of newborn infants. The angle of inclination of the tympanic membrane was also determined in 55 ear drums. Of these 6 were adult, 4 children, 24 newborn and 24 fetuses. As a check on measurements and relations, 32 temporal bones were sectioned in various planes. Of these 20 were adult, 2 children and 10 newborn infants.

The value of the study of the middle and inner ear by means of casts has long been recognized. As the pneumatic cavities of the ear are rather complicated in shape, it is only by representing these spaces as solids that one can obtain a clear concept of their precise form and extent, and of their relations to one another and to the neighboring nerves, vessels and other structures.   Only by a clear knowledge of the intimate topographical relations of the middle ear to the surrounding cavities is the significance of the frequent inflammations of the former fully understood.

A variety of materials have been used to replace the air spaces in making casts.   Benzold used a mixture of wax and resin, Von Stein employed a rubber and chloroform solution, and then vulcanized the mass.   Bruhl cleared the bone and injected mercury.   James Brown[1] injected dental rubber and vulcanized.   Wood's metal seems to give the most satisfactory results for this type of preparation, and certain refinements of the method introduced here have been found of considerable value in securing more perfect and complete specimens.

### TECHNIC OF MAKING CASTS OF THE TEMPORAL BONE WITH WOOD'S METAL.

To make casts of the middle and inner ear, it is best to secure well dried temporal bones in which the nerves and mucous membrane of the cavities have disintegrated and disappeared, so that the canals will be clear.   If any of these dessicated tissues remain, they should be removed with the air blast.   The canals and nerve openings are then covered with adhesive tape, with the exception of the external auditory meatus, which is left open.   After heating the encased bone at about 100 degrees centigrade for twenty-four hours in a sand bath, it is ready to receive the molten Wood's metal* which is poured into it to the level of the suprameatal (Henley's) spine.   As the bone is heated above the melting point of the metal, the latter will not solidify, and the specimen can be agitated to remove air bubbles. It is a good plan to drop a little water on the metal at the meatus to solidify it, and then the bone can be picked up, and rotated to remove the air and get the metal into all parts. After cooling, the plaster of Paris casing is removed and the specimen is placed in 30 per cent hydrochloric acid to dissolve the bone.

---

*Wood's metal is composed of tin, 4 parts, lead 8 parts, bismuth 16 parts, and cadmium 3 parts.   It has a very low melting point, about 62 degrees centigrade.

TECHNIC OF PREPARING TRANSPARENT BONE SPECIMENS.

The method used to render the injected specimens of bone transparent, as shown in Figs. 25 and 26, is that developed by Spalteholz of Leipzig in 1906.[37]

After the temporal bone is filled with Wood's metal, it is decalcified by placing it in a two per cent solution of hydrochloric acid which is changed daily for one month. It is then transferred to a one per cent solution of hydrochloric acid which is also changed daily for two weeks. The purpose of this procedure is to secure complete decalcification of the bone without destroying the specimen with the acid. The bone is then washed in running water for two weeks, or until it gives a neutral reaction to blue litmus, after which it is bleached for two hours in hydrogen peroxid and again washed. After bleaching the specimen is again washed, and is then dehydrated by passing it through a series of graded alcohols of 60, 75, 95 and 98 per cent. It should be left in each mixture about 24 hours. After dehydration, the specimen is cleared by placing it in benzol for four days, changing the solution at the end of 48 hours. The final preserving fluid in which the specimen is to remain consists of methyl salicylate 5 parts, and isosafrol 3 parts. As these fluids have the same refractive index as the prepared bone the latter becomes translucent. Sometimes it may be made more transparent by adding a little more isosafrol. Air bubbles may be removed by placing the specimen under a bell jar and exhausting the air with a suction pump.

OBSERVATIONS—THE MEMBRANA TYMPANI.

Upon examination of the literature on the tympanic membrane, one is confronted with a great variance of opinion regarding the inclination of this structure. Observers seem to be about equally divided as to whether the inclination in the newborn is equal to, or less than that of the adult, and several maintain that the ear drum is almost horizontal at birth.

The angle given by Lucian for the adult is 55 degrees. Howell[27] 130, Flint[27] 45, Kirk[27] 45, Piersol[27] 60, Gray[27] 55, Morris[27] 50, Freiligh[11] 50, Symington[20] 45, and Pollak[25] 45. Shaw,[18] Gray,[27] Henle,[24] von Troltsch, Trevis,[22] Gruber[26] and Cheatle[7] state that the tympanic membrane is nearly horizontal at birth, while Symington,[20] Pollak,[25] Cavanaugh[6] and Freiligh[11] maintain that the angle in the adult and newborn is about the same. The data obtained by the measurement of individual ear drums in this study is shown in the following table. (Table No. 1.) The figures indicate the degree of inclination from the perpendicular. The measurements as given in Table No. 1 show that a large individual variation is frequent in both newborn and adult drums. The averages show the membrane approaches a little more closely the horizontal in the fetus and that it gradually becomes more erect in later fetal life. There seems to be no constant change in the angle afterbirth.

The angles given in the following tables were determined with the Stangen goniometer of Martin and Ranke.

TABLE No. 1.

Inclination of the Tympanic Membrane.

| Age | Individual Cases | Ave. Deg. of Inclina'n |
|---|---|---|
| Four months fetus—61, 63 | | 62 |
| Five months fetus—55, 57, 60, 62, 72, 80 | | 64.4 |
| Six months fetus—58, 59, 60, 64, 64, 65 | | 61.5 |
| Seven months fetus—55, 60, 61, 62, 63 | | 60.2 |
| Eight months fetus—58, 59, 60, 65, 65 | | 61.4 |
| Nine months fetus—55, 57, 57, 61, 62, 63, 63, 68 | | 60.8 |
| Newborn—54, 55, 56, 57, 58, 58, 60, 60, 65 | | 57 |
| Child of three years—55, 60 | | 57.5 |
| Adult—45, 55, 57, 60, 60, 69 | | 57.5 |

TABLE No. 2.

Dimensions of the Tympanic Membrane.

| Age | Diameters (mm.) | Ave. Diam. (mm.) |
|---|---|---|
| Fourth fetal month—Max. 6.8, 6.8 | | 6.8 |
| Min. 5.5, 5.5 | | 5.5 |
| Fifth fetal month—Max. 7.1, 7.5, 7.5 | | 7.4 |
| Min. 6, 6, 6.5 | | 6.2 |
| Sixth fetal month—Max. 7.2, 7.3, 7.8, 8.1 | | 7.6 |
| Min. 6.3, 6.6, 6.6, 7.5 | | 6.7 |
| Seventh fetal month—Max. 7.8, 8, 9 | | 8.3 |
| Min. 7.6, 7.7, 7.8 | | 7.7 |
| Eighth fetal month—Max. 8, 9, 9.6 | | 8.9 |
| Min. 8, 8, 8.3 | | 7.8 |

Ninth fetal month—Max. 9, 9, 9.2, 9.7, 10...............    9.3
    Min. 7.5, 8, 8, 8.5, 8.5, 9.........................    8.2
Newborn—Max. 9, 9, 9.3, 9.5, 9.5, 9.8, 10, 10, 10,
        10, 10, 10.2, 10.3, 10.3.........................    9.8
    Min. 7.8, 8, 8, 8, 8, 8, 8, 8.2, 8.3, 8.4, 8.4,
        8.6, 8.8.........................    8.2
Seventh month child—Max.........................   11.
    Min. .........................    8.5
One year child—Max. .........................   11.
    Min. .........................    9.
Two year child—Max. .........................   11.
    Min. .........................    9.
Adult—Max. .........................   11.
    Min. .........................    9.

As these measurements were taken to the extreme edge of
the sulcus tympanicus they will be found to be slightly larger
than the drum membrane proper.

It is generally stated that the dimensions of the tympanic
membranes at birth are almost identical with those of the
adult, there being little or no increase in the postnatal period
of development. The figures quoted in Table No. 2 show that
the tympanic membrane increases steadily in size in the last
half of fetal life and that also there is a distinct increase in
its diameter in the first year after birth, at the end of which
period the adult dimensions are attained.

### THE ANTRUM.

The "mastoid" antrum should be called the tympanic antrum because, considered from any point of view, it is a part
of the tympanic cavity. The antrum appears in the fetus at
the same time as the tympanic cavity, and at the time of birth
is developed to about adult dimensions, but the mastoid cells
do not appear until the second year, and they are generally
diploetic till the fifth. Definite air cells first appear at the
seventh or eighth year, and are first seen as well developed
spaces after the ninth year. The antrum must also be considered at all stages as continuous with the tympanic cavity
and as lying entirely within the petrous bone. It is covered by
the tegmen tympani, which also is the roof of the tympanic
cavity and the auditory tube.

The relations of the antrum to its adjacent structures varies considerably at different ages. Up to the time of birth it is directly over the meatus, its upper part lying above the zygomatic process and its anterior margin extending forward beyond that of the meatus.

In the fetus and newborn the incus lies in the aditus and its long process projects into the antrum. As shown in Figs. 15 to 24 inclusive, as the child grows older the antrum gradually shifts from its location above the meatus to a more posterior and inferior position, and in the adult it is directly posterior to it. Its position in the child materially aids drainage in acute infections.

The lateral (external) canal of the bony labyrinth forms the inner boundary between the antrum and epitympanic recess. Its bony covering is easily recognized as a thin white ridge of dense bone. In the young child its wall is only about one-fifth of a millimeter in thickness, and a probe or curette introduced into the middle ear could easily rupture into the canal.

The thickness of the bone separating the antrum and lateral canal at different ages is approximately as follows:

Newborn, 0.2 mm.; three years old, 0.3 to 0.5 mm.; five years old, 0.5 mm.; adult, 1 mm.

As the mastoid develops, the antrum becomes farther and farther removed from the external surface of the temporal bone. The thickness of the bony wall bounding the lateral surface of the antrum at different ages is approximately as follows:

Newborn, 1 to 2 mm.; five years old, 6 mm.; ten years old, 10 mm.; adult, 15 mm.

The above figures are about the same as those given by Symington (20). The dimensions of the antrum in the newborn are about 10 by 11 mm., which is approximately the same as in the adult.

### THE FACIAL NERVE.

The general course and relations of the facial nerve in the temporal bone are much the same in the infant and adult, and there seems to be a consistent and uniform growth of its parts. The distance from the nerve's entrance into the internal auditory meatus to the central point of the geniculate ganglion is shown in the following:

Five month fetus, 8 mm.: seven month fetus, 9 mm.; newborn (average of ten cases), 10 mm.; three year child, 12 mm.; adult (average of ten cases), 13 mm.

The distance from the center of the ganglion to the point where the nerve turns sharply downward is 10 mm. in the newborn, 11 mm. at three years, and an average of 12 mm. in the adult. This portion of the nerve lies within the tympanic cavity, and in its course over the promontory around the fenestra rotundum it is protected only by a thin shell of bone in the adult, and in the child up to the fourth year it is often covered only by a thin membrane of connective tissue. This exposed condition accounts for the liability to facial paralysis in the child following acute otitis media. As the nerve runs directly beneath the anterior part of the external (horizontal) canal, a roughly used probe or Staeke's director for locating the epitympanic recess may easily injure it. As Cheatle[7] aptly says, "Such an instrument is safe only in experienced hands, and then it is not needed."

The course and relations of the facial nerve can be best seen in the superior views of the various casts. The distance from the posterior rim of the tympanic membrane to the nearest point of the facial nerve is from 3 to 5 mm., both in the fetus and the adult.

The exposed condition of the nerve, in early life, after its exit from the stylomastoid foramen, is of importance both to the obstetrician and the surgeon. In the fetus and young infant it emerges about 3 mm. behind and a little below the most posterior part of the margin of the tympanic membrane. As there is no mastoid process at this time, the nerve runs downward over the petrous portion of the bone. This condition accounts for some of the facial paralyses produced by pressure from instruments at this point during delivery. It is also to be noted that this external portion of the nerve lies in the path of an incision such as is made in operation for mastoiditis in the adult. If such an incision were made in the infant, the nerve would be cut and a facial paralysis would result; but as the antrum in the young child is much higher, and as there is no mastoid containing air cells, there is little need for such an incision. The relations of the exit of the facial nerve, the antrum, the tympanic membrane, and the developing mastoid process, are shown in Figs. 15 to 24 inclusive.

After the first year the vertical portion of the facial nerve is gradually covered by the deposit of the layers of bone forming the mastoid process, and by the outward growth of the posterior portion of the tympanic ring, which forms the external osseous meatus. The thickness of the bone over this portion of the nerve is shown by the following measurements: One year: 0 mm.; three years, 6 to 10 mm.; five years, 11 mm.; adult, 13 to 15 mm.

In all fetal and infant specimens examined the nerve came straight to the surface, but, as Freiligh[11] states, in some cases the nerve bends downward before emerging, and in these cases the exit would be two or three millimeters lower.

### THE INNER EAR.

If lines were projected through each posterior canal, they would meet a little posterior to the hypophysis and form approximately a right angle. Likewise, lines through the superior semicircular canals would meet above the posterior rim of the foramen magnum and be about at right angles to each other. It can be seen that the canals of one side are at right angles, and that either canal of one side is at right angles to its mate on the other side. This makes the posterior canal of one side parallel to the superior canal of the other and vice versa. This is shown in Figs. 29 to 30.

Upon measurement it will be found that in only about a third of the cases will these angles be exactly 90 degrees. Other cases will vary 10 degrees above or below.

The lines projected through the superior canal of the newborn meet within the foramen magnum, while in the adult they meet well back of it. This is partly due to the fact that the foramen magnum is farther posterior in the infant skull and partly because the superior canal lies more nearly in the transverse plane. The lines running forward through the posterior canals of the newborn meet in the region of the clivus, while in the adult they meet farther forward in the region of the sella turcica. This is also due to the fact that the posterior canal of the newborn lies more nearly in the transverse plane than that of the adult.

Alexander[1] and Shaw[18] found the adult inner ear larger than that of the newborn. Booth[3] found the postembryonic growth to be about 18 per cent. Hyrtle found the inner ear of the adult and child about the same size, but that there is an increase in size in old age. The diameters at different ages is shown in Tables Nos. 3 and 4.

The inner ear changes but little in size after the fifth fetal month, as is shown in the following tables (Nos. 3 and 4) :

Maximum Length of Inner Ear, Including Cochlea, Vestibule and Posterior Canal. .

### TABLE No. 3.

| | Present series mm. | Alexander[1] mm. | Seihenmann[17] mm. | Shaw[18] mm. |
|---|---|---|---|---|
| Five month fetus.... | 18 | | | |
| Seven month fetus.. | 18 | | | |
| Newborn ............ | 17 | 15 | 19 | 18 |
| Three year old........ | 18 | | | |
| Five year old.......... .. | 16 | | | |
| Adult .......... ............ | 18 | 18 | 18.5 | 20 |

### TABLE No. 4.

Diameters of the Inner Ear Parts at Different Ages.

| | Vertical diam. of cochlea mm. | Horizl. diam. of sup. canal mm. | Ant. post. diam. of ext. can. mm. | Vertical diam. of post. canal mm. |
|---|---|---|---|---|
| Five month fetus...... | 7.5 | 8. | 7. | 8. |
| Seven month fetus.... | 7. | 7.5 | 7. | |
| Newborn .................... | 7. | 8.5 | 7. | 7.25 |
| Three year old........... | 7.5 | 8.25 | 7. | |
| Five year old... .......... | 7.5 | 8.5 | 7. | 8. |
| Adult ................ | 7.5 | 8.5 | 7. | 8. |
| Seibenmann[17] Newb'n | 7.7 | 8.8 | 8.1 | 7.2 |
| Adult ........................ | 7.5 | 8.6 | 7.2 | 7.2 |
| Shaw[18] Newborn ...... | | 5. | | |
| Adult ........................... | | 6. | | |

The distance of the horizontal canal from the cortex in the infant is from 4 to 6 mm., while in the adult it is from 12 to 20 mm.  The horizontal canals and the oval window are the most frequent points of entrance for infection.  The angles of the semicircular canals to each other and their positions in relation to the rest of the skull are shown in Figs. 29 and 30.

The relation of the semicircular canals to each other is shown in the following table.  The figures indicate the degree of the angle.  (From Siebenmann[17]):

|  | Superior to external | Superior to posterior | Posterior to external |
|---|---|---|---|
| Adult | 82 | 79 | 99* |
| Newborn | 85 | 88 | 92 |

Most grateful thanks are due Professor Scammon for many helps in securing data and criticising the text of this paper.

## REFERENCES.

1. Alexander, G.: Zur Frage des postembryonalen Wachstums des menschlichen Ohrlabrinthes. Anat. Hefte., XIX (1902), pp. 571-578.

2. Alexander, G.: Diseases of the Ear in Infancy and Childhood, translated by A. Bedell, Sec. Edit., pp. 1-46.

3. Boot, G. W.: Development and Structure of the Temporal Bone, Journ. Amer. Med. Assn., LV, pp. 563-565.

4. Brown, H. P.: The Infant Temporal Bone in Its Relation to the Mastoid Operation. Bull. Lying-In Hosp., City of New York; Vol. IX (1913), p. 11.

5. Brown, J.: Bull of Med. Dept. of Wash. Univ., Vol. IV, No. 1, Aug. (1905).

6. Cavanaugh, J. A.: Topography of the Tympanic Cavity, Annals of Otol., Rhin. and Laryng. (1913), Vol. XXII, pp. 699-716.

7. Cheatle, A. H.: Some Points in the Surgical Anatomy of the Temporal Bone From Birth to Adult Life; London, 1907.

8. Cheatle, A. H.: The Report of An Examination of Both Temporal Bones from One Hundred and Twenty Individuals in Reference to the Question of Symmetry in Health and Disease. Annals of Otol., Rhin. and Laryng., Vol. XXII, pp. 19-125.

9. Clark, J. J.: Some Observations on the Temporal Bone, Chiefly in Childhood. Journ. Anat. Physiol., VII N. S. (1893), pp. 411-414.

10. Courtade, A.: Anatomie topographique comparée de l'oreille moyenne chez le nouveau-né et chez l'adulte. Ann. d Mal de l'Oreille et du Larynz., XIX (1893), pp. 682-688.

*One of the angles taken in this series of four cases was of 105 degrees, which accounts for this large angle.

11. Freiligh, C. A.: The Temporal Bone and Its Anomalies at Birth in One Hundred Fifty Cases. Bull. Lying-In Hosp.. City ot New York, Vol. IX (1913), p. 3.

12. Guthierie, T.: The Development of the Mastoid, British Med. Journ.. Vol. II, Oct., 1907, p. 986.

13. Metheny, D. G.: Some Points on the Applied Anatomy of the Temporal Bone. (Reprint) Penn. Med. Journ., Dec., 1915.

14. Politzer, A.: The Anatomical and Histological Dissection of the Human Ear in Its Normal and Diseased Condition. (English translation of G. Stone.) London, 1892.

15. Prinz, H.: The Spalteholz Method of Clearing Animal Bodies. Journ. of Missouri State Med. Assn., March, 1913; pp. 295-299.

16. Rouviere, H.: Sur le developpement de IV antre mastoidien et des cellules mastoidennes. Bibliogr. Anat.; XX (1910), pp. 24-34.

17. Siebennann, F.: Die Korrosion-Anatomie des menschlichen Ohres. Wiesbaden, 1890.

18. Shaw, A. J.: A Few Anatomical and Clinical Points in the Ear of the New-Born Infant. Amer. Gyn. and Pediat., XIII, pp. 127-142.

19. Stewart, W. H.: Radiograph Findings Illustrating the Anatomical Development of the Mastoid Bone. Annals of Otol., Rhin. and Laryn., Vol. XXII (1913), pp. 677 and 833.

20. Symington, J.: The Mastoid Portion of the Temporal Bone. Edinburg Med. Jour., 1886; pp. 293-298.

21. Trait. d Anatomie Top., 3rd Edit.

22. Trevis, F.: Surgical Applied Anatomy, 7th Edit.; pp. 91-102.

23. Spalteholz, D. W.: Über das Durchsichtigmachen con menschlichen und tiereschen Präparatin; Leipzig, 1911.

24. Henle, J.: Allgemeine Anatomie Lehre con des Menscheng und Farmbestandthei'en des menschlichen Körpers; Leipzig. 1841.
Henle, J.: Handburch der Eingeweidelehre des Menscen; 1866.

25. Pollak: Diseases of the Ear; p. 20; 1883.

26. Gruber, Jos.: Diseases of the Ear; p. 51; Sec. Amer. Edit.

27. Texts on Anatomy and Physiology:
Luciani: P. 198, Vol. IV, 1917.
Howell: P. 380, Fifth Edit.
Flint: P. 715, 1905.
Kirk: P. 739, Twentieth Edit.
Piersol: P. 1494, 1907.
Gray: P. 1125, Seventeenth Edit.
Morris: P. 1052. Fourth Edit.

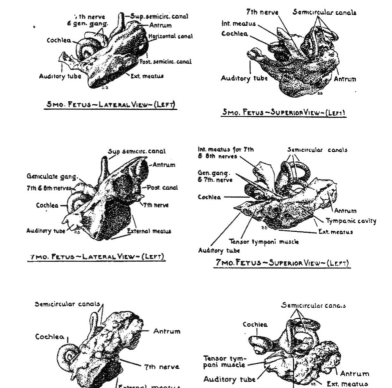

Wood's metal casts of internal and middle ear of fetus and newborn.
X—Natural size.

PLATE No. 2.

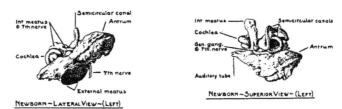

NEWBORN ~ LATERAL VIEW ~ (LEFT)

NEWBORN ~ SUPERIOR VIEW ~ (LEFT)

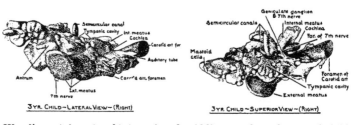

3 YR. CHILD ~ LATERAL VIEW ~ (RIGHT)

3 YR. CHILD ~ SUPERIOR VIEW ~ (RIGHT)

Wood's metal casts of internal and middle ear of newborn and child.
X—Natural size.

PLATE No. 3.

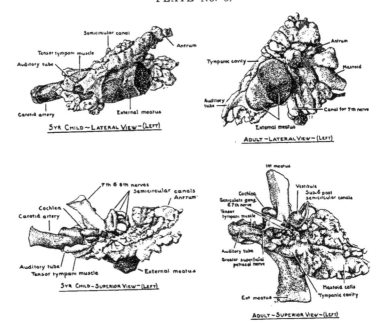

Wood's metal casts of internal and middle ear of child and adult.
X—Natural size.

PLATE XLII

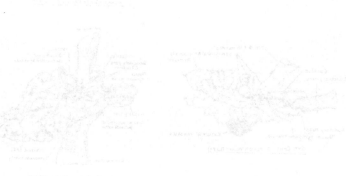

Floral parts of Gaultheria and Rubus species.—Ericaceae.

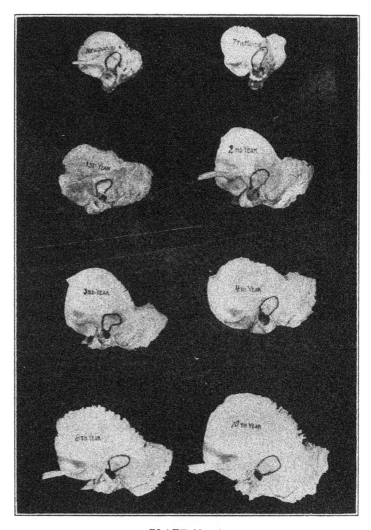

PLATE No. 4.

A series of temporal bones showing the position of the antrum as determined by X-ray and transillumination.

| | |
|---|---|
| Fig. 15. Newborn | Fig. 19. Three years old |
| Fig. 16. Seven months child | Fig. 20. Four years old |
| Fig. 17. One year old | Fig. 21. Five years old |
| Fig. 18. Two years old | Fig. 22. Ten years old |

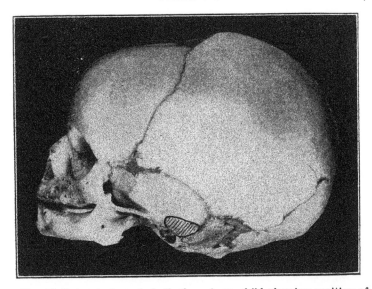

Fig. 23. Lateral view of skull of newborn child showing position of tympanic antrum as determined by X-ray and transillumination.

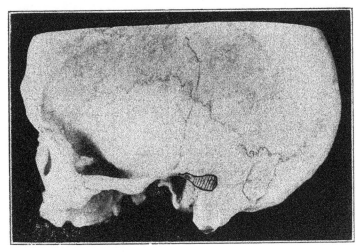

Fig. 24. Lateral view of adult skull showing position of tympanic antrum as determined by X-ray and transillumination.

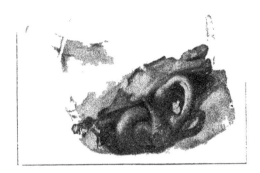

Fig. 25. Lateral view of temporal bone of newborn child which has been injected with Wood's metal and cleared with Spalteholz's method. X—1½.

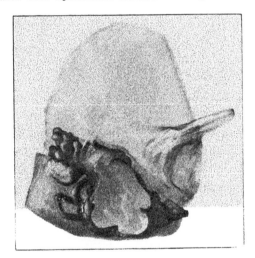

Fig. 26. Medial view of same specimen as Fig. 25. X—1½.

Fig. 5 ...

Fig. 6 ...

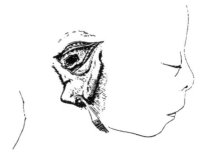

Fig. 27. Dissection showing position of antrum in relation to external osseous meatus in newborn child.

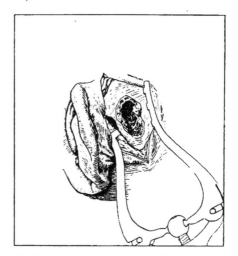

Fig. 28. Dissection showing position of antrum in relation to the external osseous meatus in the adult.

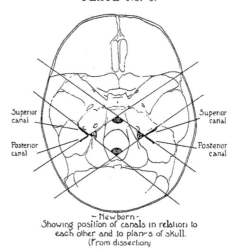

Fig. 29. Drawing of the base of the skull showing the positions and angles of the superior and posterior semicircular canals in newborn child.  X—½.

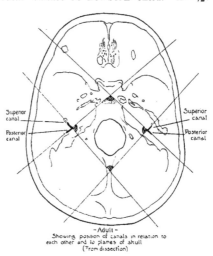

Fig. 30. Same as Fig. 29 of adult skull.  X—½.

# A RADICAL TREATMENT FOR CHRONIC SUPPURA-
## TION OF THE ANTRUM WITH MODIFICA-
### TION OF THE CANFIELD TECHNIC.*

By Walter H. Theobald, M. D.,
Chicago.

Infection of the maxillary sinus may be cured in several ways. First of all, by conservative methods: namely, irrigation of the antrum through the natural ostium or by means of the antrum trocar when the natural opening is inaccessible, and this often in chronic cases where the condition has been present for years. It is true that in most cases of chronic antrum disease a lasting cure is not effected by either of these methods. The tendency is for a mucopurulent discharge to recur intermittently or continue indefinitely in spite of frequent or daily irrigation with antiseptic solutions. The acute infections, as a rule, yield to the conservative method of irrigation, the time for recovery varying anywhere from one to five weeks. But in most cases of chronic disease a permanent opening into the sinus is necessary. In order to establish the latter an operation must be performed which will enable us to examine the interior of the antral cavity, watch the process of healing, remove the diseased or polypoid mucosa and maintain an opening that will not close within a few months or even a year's time. By means of such an artificial opening the patient may wash out his own antrum with ease and without discomfort.

Dr. Sturmann in his original paper published in Berlin, states that Berthe, Dehmer and others in their operations merely opened the lateral nasal wall for free drainage without affording a view of the changes in the mucous membrane. Such cases, however, in many instances, were not cured, but Sturmann by his improved intranasal operation, which gives a complete view of the antrum, was able to effect a perma-

*Read before the Chicago Laryngological and Otological Society, December 5, 1920.

nent cure.  The necessity of extranasal operation on the antrum was formerly advocated where examination of the cavity
for polypi, etc., was desirable, and with the publication of
Canfield's and Sturmann's intranasal operations which appeared about the same time in 1908—such methods may be
and have been abandoned since the intranasal route has proved
so eminently satisfactory in all except some rather rare instances, such as malignant growths.  This has been my experience in a series of some forty cases in which the Canfield
operation was done with some slight modifications and with
gratifying results.

Permit me now to review briefly the steps in the development of the various operations on the maxillary sinus.  In
1889 Küster published an article on operative exposure of the
antrum.  This was the first operation which gave unobstructed vision during the operation and also during the after-
treatment.  With this method many cases which resisted conservative treatment were cured, with closure of the oral opening.  Many cases, however, did not heal, even after years of
treatment, and little change was observed in results, even with
Jansen's improved method, because of the communication between the maxillary sinus and the oral cavity.  Observing
this difficulty, the intranasal operation was succeeded by the
method of Mikulicz.  Later the same idea was carried out in
the methods used by Caldwell and Luc.  Briefly, in this operation a mucous membrane incision above the alveolar margin
is made and the soft parts retracted.  The anterior antral wall
is removed, the cavity curetted, a counter opening made into
the nose, and the sinus is packed with gauze, extending into
the nasal chamber and the oral mucosa sutured for primary
union.  Many cases recovered satisfactorily by this method,
while others failed, due to the character of the chronically diseased mucosa which could not be kept under visual control.

Friedrich in 1905 departed from the methods of that time
and made a skin incision around the ala.  Through this he
removed the anterior antral wall, lateral wall of the nose, and
the pyriform process as well as the anterior half of the
inferior turbinate.  The danger of his method was the possibility of wound infection or scar contraction producing deformity.

Kretschman improved upon the Caldwell-Luc operation. He made the usual alveolar incision and also removed the lateral wall of the nose as far as the pyriform process, sparing the latter in order to avoid all deformity.

Later Denker combined these advantages by adding the removal of the lateral wall of the nose, including the lateral wall of the pyriform process—thereby converting the nose and the antrum roughly into one cavity. His results were promising and showed the importance of excluding the oral cavity. He reports three cases not successful because of complication involving the frontal sinus.

The advantages of the Canfield intranasal operation are several. First, a complete view of the antrum may be had at the time of the operation, and it can be made as radical as necessary through the nose—or comparatively conservative if the condition of the antrum renders an extensive operation unnecessary. Second, a satisfactory view of the antrum through the nose may be had during after-treatment for the control of the healing process. Third, the after-treatment is painless. Fourth, irrigation may be carried on by the patient.

Canfield's first step in the operation is the amputation of the anterior half of the inferior turbinate, and this he believes should precede the operation by about two weeks. I have found this unnecessary and in most cases have preserved the inferior turbinate entirely. In a few cases, however, it has been necessary to remove the anterior head where it was large and projected downward, covering most of the inferior meatus. In doing this, I have never removed the turbinate until the operation was completed, thereby obviating the danger of injuring the nasolacrimal duct. But in some of these cases we have been able to spare the turbinate by merely infracting it and pushing it upwards out of the field of operation, thus giving a clear held to work in. At the close of the operation it is restored to its normal position.

The technic of this procedure as suggested by Dr. Pierce and used by myself, is as follows: The operation is performed under local anesthesia, using 10 per cent cocain for the mucous membrane and 1 per cent novocain, to each dram of which three drops of the 1/1,000 adrenalin chlorid solution is added. Two or three drams is the amount usually necessary for com-

plete anesthesia. It is most important that the infiltration
be properly performed in order to have not only a painless
operation but a bloodless field to work in. For this purpose
a metal syringe with extension armed with hypodermic needle
is used. The injection is first made along the pyriform crest,
then the lateral wall and floor of the nose are infiltrated.
Lastly, the needle is introduced beneath the periostium of the
external surface of the pyriform crest and the anterior surface
of the maxilla. The finger placed over the cheek at this point
permits one to judge the extent of the infiltration. Several
injections over this area are necessary to block the nerves
completely.

Next by inserting the little or index finger into the antrium
nares, the exact location of the pyriform process is ascertained. It is a guide for the initial incision, which is made
directly over it. The incision begins above, anterior to the
point of attachment of the inferior turbinate body, and is
extended well down onto the floor of the nose, bringing into
view the sharp pyriform crest. The mucous membrane and
periosteum are then elevated on the lateral wall of the nose
from the floor up to the attachment of the inferior turbinate
and backwards about one-third its distance. On the anterior
or buccal wall it is elevated as far back as desirable. By
means of a sharp knife or scissors a longitudinal incision is
made from the upper end of the vertical incision immediately
beneath the inferior turbinate attachment backwards to the
point of periosteal elevation. From here it is carried down to
the floor of the nose parallel to the first incision by means of
a right angled knife. This makes a wide inverted U-shaped
incision with the base down, and furnishes the flap which is
laid down on the floor of the nose for the remainder of the
operation. The next step is the removal of the bone over an
area corresponding to that part from which the mucous membrane has been elevated. This is best accomplished by a Rongeur forceps, recently made by Pierce, and it is much simpler
and superior to the trephine drill which I formerly used and
with which one is apt to tear the flap. A Killian No. 1 speculum may be used to give a free view of the bony crest that is
to be first removed, and it also aids in retracting the soft parts
for examination of the cavity. After taking several bites of

bone from the pyriform process the antrum is entered without difficulty and the opening gradually enlarged in all directions so as to allow complete inspection of the sinus. At this time the antral cavity should be anesthetized. This may be done by applying ten per cent cocain with a cotton applicator or by injecting a few drops of 5 per cent cocain into the sinus with a syringe. The lateral nasal wall is removed with an antrum rasp and a biting forceps. Here the bony wall is very thin and breaks easily, while that toward the nasal floor is thick and hard to remove. But it is important that no bony projections separate the antrum from the nasal chamber—in fact, the floor of the antrum and nose must be flush or as nearly so as possible. Upon this depends much of the success of the operation. In order to remove this bone the chisel is frequently necessary. In some cases, it has been impossible to have the antral floor and nose level, because I have found that of the antrum lower than that of the nose. With an opening thus made, a comprehensive view of the interior of the antrum can be secured and its condition noted. Polypi and degenerated mucous membranes are removed with the curette and forceps, care being taken not to remove healthy or merely swollen mucous membrane. Attention should be directed to the region of the natural opening, for this is a common seat for the origin of polypi. It is well to sponge out the antrum by packing with gauze moistened in adrenalin solution. This renders the cavity bloodless for a thorough inspection, and remnants of the diseased tissue may be removed. A final irrigation with normal salt solution removes blood and secretions. This completes the operation, and the preserved flap is turned up and placed into the antrum. It is held in place by packing the cavity with xeroform gauze.

The packing is removed after forty-eight hours, the antrum irrigated and the cavity repacked for twenty-four hours longer. Rarely do I find it necessary to tampon after removing the second packing. Sturmann repacks every other day for a period of two weeks. This causes considerable discomfort to the patient and I believe is unnecessary; furthermore, the air ventilation promotes rapid healing. The subsequent treatment consists of control of granulation tissue with silver nitrate or trichloracetic acid and irrigations until secretions

stop. An excellent astringent solution is cupric sulphate, one
to six thousand, for irrigation. The usual duration until complete healing occurs is from three to five weeks.

The hole gradually becomes smaller, but the flap prevents
it from closing entirely and in no case has this occurred. I
have been able with perfect ease to wash out the antrum with
a canula in cases operated on over three years ago. All the
normal anatomic structures are preserved, and one cannot
detect evidence of operation or disease except where the
anterior head of the inferior turbinate has been sacrificed. I
have examined cases in which a pharyngoscope could be introduced into the antrum and the cavity examined through the
artificial opening two years after operation, showing that the
hole remained permanently and permitted ample room for
drainage in case of reinfection.

Necrosis is rarely found in the maxillary sinus, but when
present it is no contraindiction to the intranasal operation.
I have found necrosis of the lateral nasal wall present in two
cases, and have also noted it around the root of a diseased
tooth which penetrated the antrum. If the diseased tooth has
not been removed previous to the operation, it should be
extracted at once and the root canal curetted. In such cases
the operation can be made more radical by the removal of
as much bone as is deemed necessary by the operator.

It seems unnecessary to report the details of each of the
forty cases operated by this method, but with your permission
I will read the histories of a few typical ones:

Case 1.—Mr. J. E. B.: When first seen on April 24, 1918,
he complained of having had a foul discharge from both
sides of his nose for several years. Transillumination gave
a bilateral shadow. Pus was flowing from both middle meati
in abundance. Bilateral ethmoid disease was evidenced by
polypi in the middle meati. Irrigation of the antra through
natural opening showed a large amount of free pus present,
pea soup in character. Daily irrigation for two months did
not diminish the amount nor change the character of the pus.
On June 28th the left antrum was opened by the method described. A good view of the cavity was obtained and found
to be practically filled with polypoid growths. These were
removed with the curette and forceps, and the cavity packed

with xeroform gauze. The ethmoids were exenterated on both sides. The right antrum was not operated at this time. Cultures of pus from the left antrum showed staphylococci, streptococci, and a gram negative bacillus resembling the bacillus mucosus. Three weeks later, at which time the left, or first operated side had entirely cleared up, the right antrum was opened by the same procedure. Polypi also filled this cavity. On the third day the patient left the hospital. He was seen every day for one week; granulations were controlled with trichloracetic acid, but the antrum was irrigated only on alternate days. The discharge was scanty and mucoid in character. During the second week the sinus was irrigated twice, and during the third week once, but there was no sign of any discharge at these times. He had perfect healing in two weeks and was completely cured in twenty-one days. I have seen him at intervals since then, and there has been no recurrence of the antrum or ethmoid infection.

Case 2.—Miss B. S.: Age 31 years. When first seen on August 19, 1918, complained of pain in left side of face and a foul nasal discharge and tenderness in the region of the left maxillary sinus. Three weeks previously the left antrum had been operated upon through the canine fossa, but this opening had not entirely closed. Repeated irrigation of the sinus resulted in no improvement. The discharge was putrid and pea soup in character. On September 9, 1918, the antrum was opened in the manner above described. A large mass which filled the cavity was removed and proved to be a strip of gauze about one yard long which had inadvertently been left in the antrum at the previous operation. Bacteriologic examination showed a predominance of streptococci and a few colonies of staphylococci. The granulations were curetted and a sequestrum found at the site of the opening, originally made through the alveolar process, was removed. The patient then made an uneventful recovery within twenty-one days.

Case 3.—Miss S. St. A.: Age 21 years. Was first examined March 9, 1918, and gave a history of recurrent pain over the right maxillary sinus together with purulent discharge from the right nares. On March 21, 1918, the right antrum was operated by the procedure employed in our other cases. This was one of the cases in which the electrically driven trephine was used. Although suppuration in this instance had been a very profuse one, the patient rapidly made a complete recovery. When last examined about two years after the operation, the antrum was found perfectly dry.

### SUMMARY OF THE ADVANTAGES OF THIS PROCEDURE.

1. Operation is performed under local anesthesia with little reaction.

. 2. Operation may be radical or conservative, as judged by the pathologic condition at the time of operation.

3 A view of the antrum cavity is secured and may be maintained during after-treatment.

4. No oral incision is necessary.

5. No suturing is needed.

6. A fairly simple form of antrum operation with all the results obtained by any of the other methods.

### BIBLIOGRAPHY.

Canfield, R. B.: Tr. Am. Laryngol., Rhin. and Otol. Soc., 1907; pp. 384-393.

Watson-Williams: Jour. Laryng., London, 1914, XXIV, p. 113.

McKenzie, D.: Proc. Roy. Soc. Med., London, 1912, VI, Laryngol., Section 9.

Sturman (Berlin): Archiv. f. Laryngologie, XXIII, p. 143.

Deuber: Med. Bl., Wien, 1907, XXX, p. 601.

Andrews: Journal of Ophth. and Otolaryngology, Chicago, 1914, VIII, p. 185.

Sluder: Weekly Bull. of St. Louis Med. Soc., 1909, III, p. 461.

Denker: Jour. Laryngol., London, 1910, XXV, p. 420.

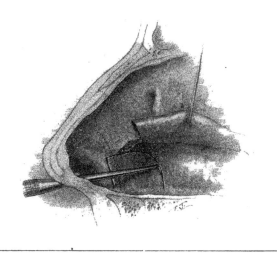

Fig. 1. Infracted turbinate showing initial incision through
mucous membrane.  Pyriform crest illustrated by dotted line.

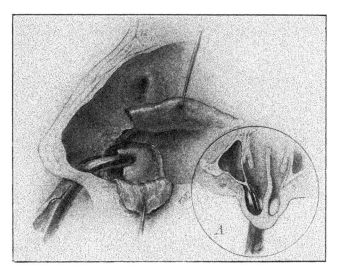

Fig. 2. Mucous membrane flap retracted. A—bone forceps in position.

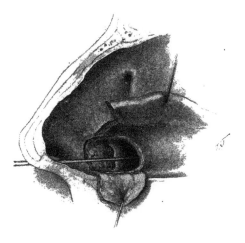

Fig. 3. Direct view into antrum through antrium nares.

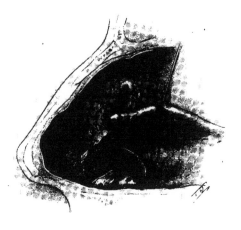

Fig. 4. Flap of mucous membrane in place; ready for packing.

# SUBMUCOUS REPLACEMENT FOR EXTERNAL DEVIATION.*

## DR. T. E. OERTEL, M. D.,

### AUGUSTA, GA.

It is with some degree of hesitancy that I come before this body to present for its consideration the procedure about to be described.

Perhaps it is seldom that any operator follows absolutely the textbook technic of an operation. More usually he fits the operation to the needs of the case and thus literally "makes the punishment fit the crime," or he may even habitually vary the operation in minor details to conform to his own notions. Such variations should not be warrant for imposing on his suffering fellows a lengthy dissertation heralding a new operation. As I have only made some minor modifications in the submucous operation, perhaps I fall within the above category. In addition to this, the cases in which I have employed the technic have not numbered more than a dozen, nor was it possible to follow these up for any considerable length of time.

Also some of them were failures. In spite of all this, I have ventured to risk taxing your patience; perhaps even my failures may be of some service in preventing their repetition by another.

The submucous resection of the nasal septum is one of the most satisfactory operations that has been devised. In any form of deviation which begins well within the vestibule one has but to have a care that the mucous membrane is preserved and that the deviating bone and cartilage is sufficiently removed to allow the two walls to fall together in the median

*Read before the American Laryngological, Rhinological and Otological Society, Boston, Mass., June 3rd, 1920.

line and form a straight partition where formerly there was a crooked one. But when, in addition to a posterior deflection the tip of the triangular cartilage is distorted and out of place, we are confronted by another and more difficult problem.

Removal of the entire cartilage results in a straight septum but a flabby one. All authors caution against removing too much of this structure on account of the deformity that will result. If, coupled with an anterior deformity of the septum there is a deviation of the external parts, the situation is still more complex.

During my service at Camp Logan I was consulted by a number of soldiers in which both conditions were present. There was obstruction to respiration on account of a deflection of the septum involving the tip of the triangular cartilage, and there was a marked deviation of the external nose.

The usual operation fails to provide for such a condition. In some of the cases the tip of the cartilage was not only displaced but was bent upon itself so that it was cupped. All of the cases gave a history of trauma. I regert that I have no more accurate records than the casts which our dentists were good enough to make for me, as these do not show the true relations, there being always more or less flattening of the tip due to pressure of the plaster. We had no means of securing photographs. I have made two models of the septum to represent the two most common forms of deviation with which I had to deal.

These models are, of course, not exact reproductions, but they will serve to show the type of deflection in which the operation may be of benefit.

In casting about for some means of reducing both the internal and external deflection it occurred to me that it might be possible to use some form of splint between the mucous surfaces—in other words, to replace the crooked cartilage and bone with some substance which would help hold the parts in proper relation and at the same time act as a support to the bridge of the nose as well as the tip and so avoid the flabby tuberosity which is an unpleasant end result. Thin plates of celluloid were used for this purpose in five cases. All of them had to be removed. Either there was infection or the irritation was so great that it was deemed best to extract them. The longest time that one was in place was three weeks. In this case there was no pus present, but the mucous membrane was swollen and thickened to several times its normal diameter, and nasal baerthing was impossible. The only service the splint rendered was in retaining the replaced tip in its proper situation. This it did, and in so far the result was good. After the failure of the celluloid splints was demonstrated I employed in several cases a splint from the perpendicular plate of the ethmoid. This was taken as the last step of the operation and served admirably, as in no case was there reaction or suppuration. Of course this result is what one would expect in an autogenous graft.

The only difficulty experienced was in obtaining a piece of bone long enough to meet the indications.

With care this may be done, as in the anterior deflections the perpendicular plate is usually little changed except at its more anterior part. Here it is often thick and spongy, and so much of it must be cut off with the biting forceps and discarded, the splint being taken from the thin portion remaining. It was found possible thus to secure a piece large enough to serve to hold in place the parts at the tip after mobilization by incisions as indicated in the individual case.

### OPERATION.

The site of the incision must depend upon the character of the deflection. Where there is a pronounced angle the cut should be made through the mucous membrane and perichondrium along the crest of this angle and well into the underlying cartilage. The deflections of this nature are always due to trauma, and the cartilage will be found to have been broken and bent upon itself at the crest of the ridge.

Usually this point is well within the vestibule. The incision, therefore, will be at least fifteen millimeters posterior to the tip of the cartilage, and it should extend from the top of the ridge along its edge to the floor of the nose, where this is possible.

The mucous membrane and perichondrium are now elevated toward the tip, so as to form a pocket in this direction and give free access to the underlying cartilage. This is accomplished with a narrow elevator, the tip of which is bent upon itself. Having nothing better at hand, I made one from a spoon handle. Fig. 1.

The mucous membrane on the opposite side being very thin, it is safer to separate the cartilage by the use of a dull elevator following the line of primary incision. This is usually easy if the original cut has been made deep enough.

The cartilage of the tip is now freed at its base, either with a knife or by elevating it from the bone with a dull dissector. It now swings free, being only attached above and to the mucous membrane of the opposite side.

The next step is to elevate the mucous membrane at both sides as in the ordinary operation and to remove the cartilage and bone posteriorly as far as may be demanded.

The mucous membrane having been elevated to the junction of the nasal bones with the cartilages, an angular knife is employed to sever the connection of these structures. External force with the finger completes the section.

The nose is now freely movable from this point forward and may be placed in the median line.

If the cartilage left at the tip is cupped it must be freely incised in such directions as to flatten it. This is accomplished by the use of a small knife with the shank bent upon itself in order to permit of its use in the anterior pocket of mucous membrane, as with a knife of the usual form it is not possible to reach this area. I devised two such knives with which cuts may be made in any direction desired, the blades being short in order that the cut may extend only through the cartilage and not wound the mucous membrane of the opposite side.

The knives are crude, as I had only two broken tonsil knives from which to fashion them, and my only tools were pliers and a three cornered file, and my forge an ordinary spirit lamp. Fig. 1.

The strip of bone from the perpendicular plate of the ethmoid is now secured and placed alongside the mobilized cartilage of the tip in the pocket of mucous membrane extending back along the line of the septum between the two mucous surfaces. The primary incision is closed with two sutures of black silk and a light pack of borated vaselin gauze placed in the size of the incision. Another useful dressing in all forms of this operation is made by packing into a rubber finger cot a thin strip of gauze with an ordinary packing instrument. The outer end is tied with a string and cut off close to the nose. To remove the pack the end is cut off, the gauze extracted and the finger cot slips out easily without giving pain to the patient or causing hemorrhage which so often follows removal of any other form of dressing.

To hold the external nose in place I have used various methods with more or less success.

That which gave the best result was dental modeling material. This is placed in hot water until pliable and moulded to fit the nose and face, a good bearing being secured on each side to avoid pressure upon the nose. After it has hardened it may be fastened with adhesive strips and should remain in place for several days.

It is best to overcorrect slightly the deviation, as there is always a tendency towards resumption of the original position. A copper splint would doubtless serve the same purpose, and has the advantage of lightness, which the dental composition has not. If, however, it is rolled out thin, not more than an eighth of an inch in thickness, it is well borne.

One must here, as in many other instances, "follow the nose." I believe the operation to be of service in the special forms of deflection for which it was devised, and it may also serve in those cases where there is a pronounced deflection of the tip of the triangular cartilage without external deviation, as a more stable tip is secured by it than if the cartilage is removed.

It would seem that in any event a replacement of structures out of place is better than a removal of them. This has been recognized by operators who have replaced the piece of cartilage removed with the Ballenger knife in the usual operation.

By this means the normal thickness of the septum is preserved. I considered using cartilage thus removed as the splint for the tip, but rejected the idea for the reason that it would be less stable than the bone and would be more bulky and narrow the vestibule.

A thin piece of rib might be employed, but this entails the rather serious operation for its removal.

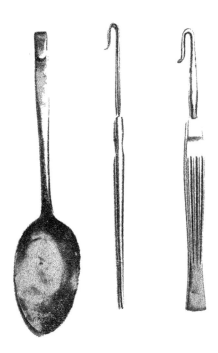

FIGURE 1.

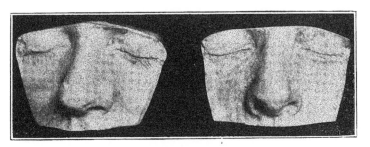

FIGURE 2.

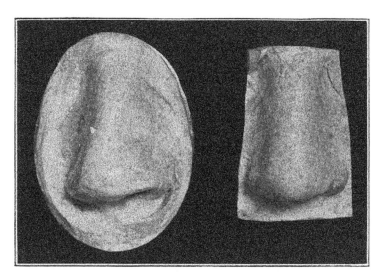

FIGURE 3.

# VI

# A CASE OF A FOREIGN BODY IN THE ESOPHAGUS REMOVED BY EXTERNAL ESOPHAGOTOMY; CURE.*

## By J. N. Roy, M. D.,

PHYSICIAN TO THE HÔTEL-DIEU, MONTREAL; LAUREATE OF THE ACADEMY OF MEDICINE OF FRANCE.

The case of a child, four years of age, having had in his esophagus, for nearly fourteen months, a foreign body which had become wedged there by one of its sharp points, and which had resisted two attempts at removal by the ordinary direct methods, presents, it seems to me, a subject sufficiently interesting to justify the following observation:

Case Report.—On April 10, 1919, H. S., four years of age, was brought to the Hôtel-Dieu Hospital, suffering with a foreign body which had lodged in the child's esophagus. The mother stated that on March 4, 1918, her child swallowed an iron washer, and as he complained of a pain in the throat, his grandmother, in attempting to remove the cause of the trouble, put her finger into the child's mouth and only succeeded in pushing this foreign body further down.

The patient's breathing continued to be normal.

The following days the child was able to swallow liquids and semiliquids, but solid food was rejected. A physician who was consulted prescribed a purgative.

During the ensuing nine months nothing special was noted in the condition of the boy, except a little constipation and a growing difficulty in swallowing. The patient never complained of pain.

Towards the end of December a medical student, relative of the family, insisted that a serious examination should be made of the child, in a hospital, and it was brought to Montreal.

---

*Read before the Canadian Medical Association, Quebec, June, 1919.

The consulting surgeon requested an examination with X-rays, and by this means the foreign body was located above the clavicules. After having administered chloroform the surgeon introduced the Kirmisson hook into the esophagus, but as all attempts at extraction were fruitless, he declared that the instrument did not even touch the foreign body.

In the presence of this failure esophagoscopy was advised. However, as New Year's Day was approaching, the mother decided to take the child back home, promising to return later. In the interval there is nothing particular to note.

On April 10th, the child began to swallow liquids with difficulty, and he was brought to the Hôtel-Dieu Hospital, where I saw him for the first time. A second radiograph, taken the previous day, showed that the foreign body was still in the clavicular region. I proposed that an esophagoscopic examination should be made, and this being accepted it was done the next morning.

Chloroform was administered and the tube was easily passed down the throat to the affected region. At that point I came in contact with an accumulation of granular tissue which commenced to bleed at the least contact.

A few touches of adrenalin diminished the hemorrhage. These granulations were so numerous that it was impossible to see the foreign body. As the wall of the esophageal canal, which had been in contact with the iron washer for more than thirteen months, seemed to be very diseased, I did not judge it proper to clean it. A pair of forceps was introduced into the tube, and by slight movements, feeling my way as it were, I was able to touch the foreign body which was lodged there. It was then not difficult to take a firm grip of it, and I slowly withdrew the esophagoscope and the forceps. After having displaced the washer and moved it over a short distance, it became wedged again, and offered marked resistance to all further efforts at removal. In order to avoid tearing the esophagus, already badly diseased, I decided to make no further attempts, and withdrew the instruments.

The child's mother was then informed of the exact situation, and external esophagotomy was proposed and accepted. However, for reasons which could not be controlled, the operation was not performed until April 24th.

There is nothing special to be noted during the intervening period.

Operation.—The patient was again put under chloroform, and his head, held in extension by means of a bolster placed under his shoulders, was slightly turned to the right. On account of the well known anatomic fact that the esophagus extends a little on the left aspect of the trachea, I operated on that side, and by the lateral way, which is the most rational. The incision practiced on the inward edge of the sternocleido-mastoid, went from the sternum to the cricoid cartilage. The vascular nervous bundle was exposed and drawn out by means of a retractor. By dissecting deeply I came across the omo-hyoid muscle and slightly raised it. The left lobe of the thyroid gland was not in the way. In order to facilitate the finding of the esophagus, the caliber of which was rather small, seeing the tender age of the little patient, a bougie was introduced into the mouth and gently passed down the esophagus. After having found the recurrent laryngeal, I made, behind that nerve, an incision of about 22 mm. and opened the esophagus near its posterior aspect. The bougie being removed, the foreign body was sought at the spot located by the X-rays. I could plainly see the granulations which bled at the slightest contact, even with the use of adrenalin, but I could not find anything more. The left index finger was then inserted in the esophagus through the vertical incision, and it immediately felt the iron washer which was pushed back into the mouth, to be seized and removed with the right hand. After disinfection of the hands, I inserted into the left nostril, for feeding purposes, a Nelaton tube which reached to the stomach and which was firmly attached to the back of the head with a point of support at the ears. Contrary to the views of a majority of surgeons, whose counsel is not to suture the esophageal wound but to let it heal of granulation, I preferred to close it with a continuous suture of catgut, after making sure that the place corresponding with the incision was not diseased. To this suture, I added three deep stitches to support the esophagus, in isolating the recurrent laryngeal nerve, and I closed the wound with silkworm gut, after having placed a drain at the point of greatest declivity. Slightly compressive dressing.

As a matter of prudence, I bound the hands of the little patient.

The foreign body measured 23 mm. in diameter and weighed 5 grams. It was not symmetrically round, and at the point where it was soldered there was a cavity whose edges were bound by a sharp point, about which I shall have more to say later on.

The outcome of this operation, which I succeeded in performing entirely with a knife, and without applying a ligature to any of the blood vessels, was very successful. The child was nourished on liquids by the Nelaton tube, and was kept in bed in a horizontal position. The first dressing, changed at the end of forty-eight hours, was hardly soiled. However, during the following days, the secretion came a little more abundant and thick from the esophageal wound. There was never any fever, and by the beginning of the second week the secretion had diminished, and I removed the drain. As during two days it seemed to be thoroughly drained, the nasal probe was withdrawn in its turn, two weeks after the operation. There remained now only to heal but a small superficial wound corresponding to the place where the drain was. The dressings were accordingly continued until June 3rd, when the child was completely cured and was able to return to his home. He now eats solid food without the slightest difficulty.

In a previous article* I have had occasion to discuss at some length the diseases of the esophagus and their treatment, so that I need not say anything further on this subject at present. I shall merely be satisfied with drawing attention to the interesting points which are contained in this observation. It is well known that the mortality, as the result of external esophagotomy, is very high, and it has gone beyond 40 per cent when intervention has been delayed for a long time after the accident.

The age of the little patient in the present case is the first thing that is striking—he was only four years old—and next is the fact that the foreign body he had swallowed had been in the esophagus for nearly fourteen months.

*J. N. Roy.—De la nécessité de l'oesophagoscopie pour le diagnostic et le traitement des affections de l'oesophage. L'Union Médicale du Canada, février, 1919.

The uncontrolled attempts made by the surgeon to extract the washer with a Kirmisson hook, while being imprudent, might have become disastrous, for, handled a little roughly, that instrument would have perforated the esophageal wall and caused a secondary suppurative mediastinitis.

In making the esophagoscopy, I did not at first wish to remove the granular tissue, in order to enable me to see the foreign body, for fear of increasing the existing injuries. and after having taken hold of the washer and moved it on a course of about 4 cm., the movement was arrested as soon as I felt it was again wedged. This wedging was easily explained when I came to examine the points of the iron washer, and its condition made it manifest that I surely would have torn the esophagus had I persisted in my efforts to extract the body.

The technic employed in this external esophagotomy followed very closely that recommended by the majority of authors, and if in this instance I have achieved success I attribute it:

1. To the great care I have exercised in my dissection:

2. To the very small incision made in the esophageal wall and to its immediate closing;

3. And finally, to the Nelaton tube passed through the nostril, which permitted me to feed the patient in reducing to a minimum the dangers of infection from the cervical wound and its possible complications.

# VII

# BORDERLINE DISEASES OF THE ESOPHAGUS.*

### By Henry Lowndes Lynah, M. D.,

### New York City.

For diagnosis and treatment of the diseases of the esophagus, the use of the esophagoscope, which enables one to study and treat the field seen by its aid, is undoubtedly a great advance in this line of work.

In the writer's opinion, it will be only a matter of a short time when all of the other methods of treatment applied to diseases of the esophagus in the dark, so to speak, will be superseded by esophagoscopy.

The chief symptom for which patients come to seek relief is difficulty in swallowing. This may be brought about by a spasm or a mechanical obstruction.

Spasm.—Normal spasm of the esophagus is a condition producing a temporary stenosis at the upper and lower ends, the cricopharyngeus and the hiatal opening of the diaphragm. This is present in all cases examined esophagoscopically without anesthesia. When this normal spasm becomes excessively irritable it is then termed esophagismus. It would, however, be well to call it a neurotic esophagismus, for it is most often encountered in neurotic subjects. Many of these patients suffer from some thyroid derangement and are extremely nervous. They also complain of a constant lump in their throat and come into the office labeled hysteria. The socalled "globus hystericus" from which patients complain of a feeling of a lump in the throat is due to this neurotic spasm element which is frequently associated with difficulty in swallowing. An ulceration may be present in some of the cases, but usually the esophagus is found to be contracted but otherwise normal. Air swallowing is a frequent accompaniment in this type of patient and they belch large quantities of gas. They also complain that certain kinds of food taken aggravate their condi-

---

*Read as part of a symposium on borderline diseases before the annual meeting of the American Laryngological, Rhinological and Otological Society, Boston, Mass., June 2-4, 1920.

tion. They recite the foods which they cannot swallow and rebel against making any attempt to even try to swallow them. They are pale and anemic, and look half starved.

A patient referred by Dr. Joseph Abraham, who had been unable to swallow for a long time on account of a persistent lump in her throat, complained that she had difficulty in swallowing at certain intervals during the day, and also that she could never swallow cake without great difficulty. She was, however, able to swallow cereals and eat bread, but with each attempt to eat cake it would stick in her throat and she would have a violent choking spell, as she described it. She had been examined by two neurologists, who pronounced her a typical case of hysteria with marked "globus hystericus." Bougies had been introduced blindly and two attempts were made to pass the esophagoscope before admission to the hospital, but were unsuccessful. The patient had a complete set of radiographic plates with her, which showed only the thoracic esophagus which appeared normal. Unfortunately, the pictures were taken not sufficiently high to show the trouble, which was in the cervical esophagus, involving the cricopharyngeus constrictor. A new set of plates made of the cervical esophagus by Dr. Charles Gottleib showed a very definite contraction which looked not unlike an esophageal stricture.

The writer has esophagoscoped several of these subjects. Some of them were apparently cured after the introduction of the esophagoscope without anesthesia. Three of the cases, however, were not cured and only temporarily relieved after the introduction of the esophagoscope, and another required esophageal dilatation at intervals for two years before she could swallow all foods with ease. The case cited had difficulty in swallowing cake, even after the large adult esophagoscope could be introduced with ease, and after ten treatments. As afore stated, spasm of the cricopharyngeus always occurs on the introduction of the esophagoscope without anesthesia, but this can be readily overcome by gentle lifting of the cricoid cartilage. However, on the other hand, there may be a marked spasticity of the cricopharyngeus in patients suffering from malignant disease of the esophagus, even when the malignancy is well below the cricopharyngeus constrictor or even at the cardiac orifice.

Spasm of the Hiatus.—The degree of contraction of the normal hiatal orifice of the esophagus is nothing in comparison to the contraction of the pharyngeus constrictor on the introduction of the tube. In the spastic stenosis at this level we all must admit that Jackson is correct in his assertion that the spasm commences at the hiatus, for such is certainly the case when viewed through the large esophagoscope. However, on the other hand, in all cases of hiatal esophagismus there is seen radiographically some of the bismuth mixture trickling through the hiatal constrictor and abdominal esophagus as a thin streak, to suddenly open as a large mass as the bismuth or barium mixture enters the stomach. While there is difficulty in observing under ocular guidance the relative amount of contraction of the abdominal esophagus and the cardia, at the same time radiographic studies seem to show that there is a complete contraction, or better, a cardio-narrowing from the entrance of the esophagus into the diaphragm to its exit at the cardiac orifice of the stomach. Jackson believes that a spasm of the cardia alone is extremely rare. He quotes Liebault and Roget on their anatomic studies that the hiatal orifice in the diaphragm is the chief factor in the production of the socalled cardiospasm. Mosher, on the other hand, in exhaustive anatomic studies of the esophagus and who knows more about the anatomy of the esophagus than any living man today, still maintains that there is a definite sphincter action of the cardia owing to demonstrable circular muscular fibers which promote a sphincter like action. The writer feels that both Jackson and Mosher are correct. The former having made all of his observations under direct ocular guidance, while Mosher, a finished anatomist, has been able to prove his findings, both by ocular guidance and extensive anatomic studies. The writer not being an anatomist and having a limited experience in this field, can only rely on visual studies and agrees with Jackson that the first definite contraction encountered is at the narrow slit like opening in the esophagus known as the hiatus. It must not be forgotten, however, that a carcinoma of the cardiac end of the esophagus may give all of the symptoms of hiatal esophagismus, cardiospasm or cardiocontraction. Cardiocontraction or cardionarrowing is certainly what is encountered, and I doubt if the spasticity is solely confined to the hiatus alone. From radiographic studies the subphrenic portion contributes to the entire contraction.

To distinguish cardioesophagismus from malignant disease of the esophagus is one of the borderline problems in diagnosis. The differential diagnosis is best accomplished by means of ocular guidance, gastric analysis and a careful study of the symptomatology and the radiographic plates.

Cicatricial Stenosis of the Esophagus.—The most frequent source of cicatricial stenosis is in the swallowing of caustic alkalies. When there is a history of a child having drunk from a cup which was used for some washing powder, and is admitted to the hospital in profound shock and suffering from acute esophagitis, it is best to wait until the acute symptoms have subsided before bouginage is attempted. Gastrostomy should be performed early as soon as it is definitely shown that the child is suffering from water and food starvation. For a long time it has interested the writer as to the final locality of the cicatricial stenosis after the subsidence of the acute attack. Guisez states that the most frequent site of the resultant stricture is at the cardia. Jackson differs with him and states that the stricture may occur in any portion of the esophagus, and that he has never seen a stricture at the cardia. In seven cases studied by the writer in children, the stenosis was at the upper orifice in three and below the bronchial crossing in all of the others. In adults the strictures encountered were usually high, but one occurred in the middle third of the esophagus. Why is it that the diluted corrosive has a predilection for attacking one portion of the mucous membrane and not the entire esophagus as in strong solutions, such as carbolic acid and ammonia, etc.? Is it because the child has been a previous sufferer from chronic esophagitis, or is it due to an anatomic peculiarity of the esophageal mucosa which is more susceptible to ulceration than other parts? It would seem that the strictures should occur at the narrowest portion and that part susceptible to narrowing, but such is not the case.

The borderline conditions resembling stricture of the esophagus in children other than impactions of food and foreign bodies resulting in strictures, are comparatively few. On the other hand, in adults there may be a good history of having accidentally swallowed some caustic alkali in childhood for which they were never treated, and have been able to swallow fairly well until recently when there had been much difficulty in swallowing. When such a case presents itself, it should be studied with great care, both fluoroscopically and radiographically, before esophagoscopy is attempted. Esophagoscopy should then be performed with great care, bearing in mind that the stricture shown in the radiographic plate may be due to a stenotic web or a malignant growth at the site of the former ulceration. Bouginage should be practiced with great care, for if it prove to be a stenosis due to malignancy the esophagus may be ruptured in the attempt to relieve the condition.

A case of this type was referred to the writer with a history of having swallowed accidentally some caustic alkali in childhood. He had never been examined, though at times he had some difficulty in swallowing. He also gave a history of having been a constant sufferer from indigestion, heartburn and belching of gas. These were looked upon by the family doctor as being more or less due to nervousness. Radiographic plates showed a narrowing in the region of the hiatus and cardia. By esophagoscopy the esophagus was found to be normal down to the hiatus and no stricture could be seen. At the hiatus there was a small mass of fungating tissue which was resistant and bled easily. A section taken showed it to be an epithelioma. Gastrostomy was performed two days later and revealed the mass involving the whole of the cardia. Whether this had been the previous site of the original caustic stricture I was unable to state. However, the contraction at the hiatus was much more resistant than a malignant stricture usually is, and no doubt the resultant ulcerative cicatrix had been the starting point for the development of the cancer.

As a rule the endoscopic picture of a cicatricial stricture is readily recognized. Cicatricial strictures usually present a whitish appearance with surrounding normal mucosa. The difference between an esophageal stricture due to a cicatrix and a neoplasm, is that the former is very firm and the surrounding esophagus does not give as it does in a malignant stricture. A cicatrix is very firm to the touch and the opening often very difficult to locate, while the malignant stricture is seldom impermeable, unless the mass has been ingrafted on a cicatricial stenosis. The cancerous mass is usually fungating and readily recognized. However, there may be a cicatricial ulceration at the site of the malignancy, and both may be present and cause complete stenosis.

Paralysis.—When there is a paralysis of the esophagus, there usually are found palsies existing in other localities. They most frequently follow the acute infectious diseases, such as diphtheria, poliomyelitis, etc. Difficulty in swallowing may occur early or late in these diseases. Sensory paralysis of the larynx as well frequently accompanies this. Often in these patients direct laryngoscopy and bronchoscopy can be performed without discomfort to the patient, for they complain of no sensation and are apparently cocainized. The writer called attention to this loss of sensation a few years ago in a treatise on diphtheria. In examining these patients with a mirror retention of secretion is seen in both pyriform sinuses. The sinuses gradually fill to overflowing, and as the secretion cannot flow into the esophagus it trickles over between the arytenoid cartilages and flows downward into the lungs. If there is complete loss of sensation and the cough reflex is impaired, these patients are unable to cough up the secretion and the lung becomes "sponge soaked," and they succumb to a terminal pneumonia. Bronchoscopic evacuation will, of course, relieve the condition, but this cannot be kept up indefinitely and the patient should be placed in a position to establish postural drainage. The best way to overcome this pouring of secretion into the lung is to insert a rubber intubation tube into the esophagus so that the secretion can flow into the esophagus and allow the lungs to act.

Case Report.—A very interesting example of what I supposed to be a bulbar paralysis came under my observation. Mrs. J. S., an old lady of seventy-two years, had a slight stroke of paralysis with involvement of the facial muscles two years previously. At that time she had a very high blood pressure, but this had fallen and she had gradually regained her health. She had been able to eat breakfast and luncheon with ease on the day of the second stroke, but when she sat down to eat dinner she was unable to swallow. She stated

that she felt peculiar before dinner, and when she sat at the
table and attempted to eat she was unable to do so. She then
drank some water and had a violent choking spell. I saw her
the same evening with Dr. Theodore H. Allen, who gave me
the foregoing history. On indirect inspection the larynx was
seen to be normal. The vocal cords moved freely; there was
no loss of sensation at this time in the pharynx or larynx. The
pyriform sinuses were filled with secretion which would pour
over between the mouthlike arytenoids into the larynx. With
inspiration the excessive tenacious salivary secretion would
flow in and then there would be a violent coughing spell, and
at this time she had some difficulty in getting it out. There
was no loss of voice or impairment of speech. She was put
in postural drainage which greatly improved the condition.
Her blood pressure at this time Dr. Allen reported as being
high, but not as high as it had been during her slight paralytic
stroke two years previously. There was slight drooping of
the corner of her mouth on the right side, but no other paralysis could be noted. The tongue protruded straight and there
was no loss of sensory reflex or cough reflex. The following
day she was admitted to St. Luke's Hospital and esophagoscoped. Before esophagoscopy was performed Dr. Le Wald
gave her some bismuth subcarbonate in an aqueous solution
to swallow to see if there had been any relaxation of the
cricopharyngeus constrictor at the upper end of the esophagus.
Watching her through the fluoroscope a teaspoonful of bismuth mixture was given, and it promptly trickled downward,
but too far forward to be in the esophagus. We watched it
carefully, and when it reached the bifurcation of the trachea
it made a turn to the left and entered the left main bronchus
and passed downward to the lower lobe branches. Having
had previous experience with the injection of bismuth mixtures into the bronchi of the living, we felt that the mixture
would do no harm. While she had an irritable cough the day
previously when secretion trickled into the trachea and bronchi, there was noted at this time that there was no attempt
to cough as the bismuth mixture entered the tracheobronchial
tree. The cough reflex was lost. It is extremely interesting
to note that the bismuth mixture was spat up by the patient
and the lung drained of the bismuth mixture even without any

sign of an expulsive cough. Of course some of it came from the reservoirs of the pyriform sinuses, but the lung was drained of the mixture before the cough reflex returned. The patient was esophagoscoped. There was a marked spasticity of the cricopharyngeus such as I had never encountered before on the introduction of the esophagoscope without anesthesia. This certainly was not a case of cricoesophagismus with which we had to deal, for the patient was not of the hysterical type and had never complained of her throat before. After the introduction of the esophagoscope and its passage through the cricopharyngeus the esophagus was found to be relaxed, but otherwise normal. On gently removing the tube the lip was violently grasped as it started to emerge through the cricopharyngeus. The esophagoscope was again pushed down and the spasm once more relaxed. Again this was tried with the same result. Finally, a stomach tube was introduced through the esophagoscope and the instrument withdrawn. The patient was fed in this manner and by having the tube in the esophagus the normal secretions were able to leak past the constriction. The trachea and larynx were covered with the bismuth mixture. The bismuth was coming out while she was in the recumbent position, but she had made little effort to cough. Bronchoscopy was not performed. The patient was fed by the stomach tube for more than six weeks before she was again able to swallow normally. In the meantime Dr. Allen had reduced her blood pressure, and I am happy to state that at the present time she is in good health.

This extremely interesting case was at first glance taken to be one of hysterical spastic esophagitis, but on further study it proved to be due to some involvement of the glossopharyngeal nerve supply, and therefore should be classified as a peculiar type of bulbar paralysis caused by a central lesion.

Another extremley interesting case I had the good fortune to see with Dr. F. J. Bevan. This young lady of twenty-two years had been in fairly good health, but was anemic and lacked outdoor life, being confined to an office all day. One evening on returning from work she had some difficulty in swallowing her dinner and choked several times. She was put to bed and the family physician notified. On his arrival at the home he found her very hysterical and attributed her

general rundown state and poor general health as the probable
cause of the condition. After a small dose of morphia the
patient quieted down and seemed to be improved. A further
test to swallow, however, proved unsuccessful. I saw the patient the same evening. At this time there was ptosis of the
left eye and a divergent squint. The pupil was widely dilated
and she complained of seeing double.

She also had difficulty with respiration but was able to
speak. She complained of pain in the region of her heart.
The larynx was examined with a mirror and the vocal cords
were found in good working order. There was no paralysis
to be seen and they moved freely. Both pyriform sinuses were
filled with secretion which would pour over into the larynx.
The cough reflex was partially lost and with each endeavor
to expel the secretion the sound produced was similar to the
paralytic nasal grunting cough so often heard in diphtheritic
paralysis. Later there was complete loss of sensation. The
patient's difficulty in breathing was due to phrenic paralysis.
The diaphragm did not move with inspiration and the epigas-
trium remained flat. An esophageal spatula was rapidly introduced and a rubber feeding tube inserted. A diagnosis
of polioencephalomyelitis was made and the spinal cord tapped.
Dr. Edward D. Fisher, the neurologist who was called to see
the patient, did not arrive in time to find her alive. The temperature remained normal throughout the attack which covered a period of fifteen hours from the time I saw her.

Pouches.—Diverticula of the esophagus are classified into
two groups according to their etiology: Traction diverticula
and pulsion diverticula. Traction diverticula are extremely
rare conditions. Jackson has reported one case. Arrowsmith
had a very remarkable case of this type which the writer had
the privilege of assisting him with at the esophagoscopic examination. Arrowsmith's case seemed to be a combination of
a traction and a pulsion diverticulum. As a rule, the traction
diverticula are seldom seen, as they are small and readily
overlooked. They usually open upwards so that the bismuth
mixture does not enter them. This was what Arrowsmith
demonstrated in his case. The traction and pulsion diverticulum occurred in a patient suffering from pulmonary tuberculosis, who also had tuberculosis of the esophagus. There

were more fungations in the esophagus which looked not unlike malignancy. The case was diagnosed by Arrowsmith from the radiographic plate and demonstrated by Mosher's ballooning esophagoscope.

Pulsion diverticula are hernial sacs which most frequently occur in the cervical esophagus. They may have a sudden onset, especially in the aged, after an attack of coughing, and produce marked dysphagia and simulate paralysis in the suddenness of the attack. Usually, however, they come on more slowly, and may give no symptoms and are only found on the introduction of the esophagoscope. This occurs when they are extremely small.

Killian was first to recognize the anatomic weak point in the production of diverticula of the cervical esophagus. The etiology of the adherent traction type has already been mentioned.

At times there may be a cicatricial stenosis of the subdiverticula orifice and also the subdiverticula esophagus, especially in large pouches which continually cause pressure by overdistention with food. In one of the writer's cases there was a complete cicatricial stenosis of the whole of the subdiverticula portion of the esophagus and the man was suffering from starvation. Gastrostomy was performed by Dr. Bodine, but unfortunately the patient did not survive. In another case there was a malignancy of the upper esophagus which simulated a pulsion diverticulum.

In a third case in an old lady of seventy-eight years the onset of the diverticulum was extremely sudden. She had never had difficulty in swallowing that she could recall. She contracted a severe cold, and it was after an attack of violent coughing that she first noticed that she was unable to swallow. The family physician was notified and pronounced the difficulty to be due to a paralysis on account of her age, high blood pressure and suddenness of the attack. No one thought of having an esophageal examination and no radiographic plates were made. She continued to suffer in this condition for seven years. She was referred to the writer on account of such difficulty in swallowing that she was beginning to suffer from starvation. By mirror inspection the larynx was seen to be normal. The pyriform sinuses were filled with secretion. An esophageal pouch was suspected from the history. which was confirmed by radiographic plates made by Dr. Charles Gottleib. Dr. Gottleib reported as follows: "There is a diverticula present in the cervical esophagus about twice the size of a hen's egg. There is a small trickle of bismuth to the left of the pouch which passes down through the sub-diverticula esophagus."

The patient was prepared for esophagoscopy. The laryngeal speculum was introduced, for from the radiographic plates the opening into the subdiverticula esophagus was extremely high. The laryngeal spatula was introduced its full length and search made on the left side for the orifice. By pulling the cricoid cartilage well forward I noticed a small dark spot on the anterolateral wall. A small bougie was readily inserted and passed through into the stomach. A 7 mm. esophagoscope was now introduced, using the bougie as a guide. but it would not enter the lumen of subdiverticula esophagus. Then a series of bougies were introduced and the orifice dilated. There was a cicatricial fold hanging over the slit of the esophageal opening. This pouch seemed to spring from the esophagus very high up, and in fact the whole of the pharynx seemed to be included in the pouch and continuous with it. After sufficient dilatation was accomplished the patient was able to swallow better. The writer had Mosher's operation in view after he had sufficiently dilated the subdiverticula esophagus.

The writer also had in mind the dangers of opening into the mediastinum. With a long pair of alligator forceps one blade was introduced into the subdiverticula esophagus and the other blade into the pouch. By this means the common wall was held firmly in between the blades of the forceps and squeezed together. The purpose of this procedure was to set up adhesions between the wall of the pouch and the esophageal wall and shut off the mediastinum before cutting the common wall, and thereby lessening danger of mediastinal infection. Perhaps this is not at all necessary, for Mosher in his series of cases does not mention clamping the common wall before cutting, and so far by opening directly into the mediastinum he has had no bad results. Perhaps these adhesions which I was trying to produce by the clamping method before cutting are already present. To the writer's great surprise the squeezing together of the subdiverticula wall and the pouch wall made the subdiverticula opening into the esophagus increase in size and the patient has been able to swallow much more comfortably ever since. She swallows semisolid food and even solid food when it is finely cut.

So far the writer has not cut the common wall, but he feels at this time that it is a perfectly safe procedure, and the danger of mediastinitis produced by cutting the common wall would be averted.

This method of treatment seems applicable to diverticula in the. aged. It relieves their suffering: adds only a minimum amount of danger, and effects a cure as far as their condition is concerned.

In younger subjects the resection operation performed by the surgeon seems to give the best results and permanent relief. A very unique operation was devised for this purpose by Gaub and Jackson, when the external operation was performed in such cases. It consisted of the esophagoscopist introducing the esophagoscope as a guide so that the redundant pouch would be removed and not the lumen of the esophagus which would result in a stricture or contraction later. This operation may be performed in one stage: but it seems best to perform all operations which are apt to involve the mediastinum in two stages to avoid fatal mediastinitis. Cryle is an advocate of the two stage operation for esophageal diverticula, and had recorded by this method gratifying results. In the cutting of the common wall, as advised by Mosher. the writer has attempted to make this a two stage operation by clamping the two sides of the common wall together to produce adhesions before any attempt is made to sever it. It was also found that by carrying out this procedure the opening into the subdiverticula esophagus may be kept open and allow sufficient food to pass. Of course a stricture of this subdiverticular portion of the esophagus must necessarily be dilated before any operation is attempted. Many of these patients refuse operations—that is, major operations proposed for relief: but on the other hand the two cases that the writer has treated by dilatation and fusing of the common wall have had relief and have improved in health.

Malignant Disease of the Esophagus.—Many cases suffering from malignant disease of the esophagus may have borderline relations to neurotic esophagismus and be mistaken for "pure neurotics," and treated as such.

In one of the writer's cases a woman of sixty-two years had been treated by six different specialists for different conditions, and after twelve months referred to the writer as a case of probable foreign body in the bronchus. All of them, however, agreed that she was suffering from some neurosis which was producing the symptoms. The history of difficulty in swallowing and constantly choking on taking food or water pointed strongly to esophageal obstruction.

On indirect examination there was seen a paralysis of the left vocal cord. Both pyriform sinuses were filled with secretion which would pour over into the larynx and produce the cough. After having seen the paralyzed left cord I naturally suspected a large aneurism to be at the bottom of the trouble, but such had not been reported by any of the physicians. On swallowing the bismuth mixture, there was plainly seen fluoroscopically a stenosis of the thoracic portion of the esophagus about the bronchial crossing. Radiographs showed no aneurism present. The following day the patient was esophagoscoped and an ulcerative fungating mass was seen and recognized as malignant. A section was taken and examined by Dr. J. G. Callison, who reported it to be an epithelioma. Gastrostomy was advised but the family refused permission. They did not object to having her treated by the tubes. Radium was applied and she was able to swallow better for one week. Then she started to completely close, so much so that a 4 mm. soft rubber intubation tube was introduced. The patient was now able to swallow liquids and was greatly encouraged. An esophageal tube may be left in for one week and then changed and cleansed and reintroduced. As a rule the smallest intubation tube has to be discontinued in time, for the malignancy as it increases will gradually close the lumen and the size of the tube used will have to be smaller and smaller until it cannot be introduced at all.

It is not difficult to introduce an esophageal intubation tube. The esophageal spatula is best for introduction and the tube is introduced through or along the side of the spatula.

Esophageal intubation has prolonged the lives of three hopeless cases of esophageal malignancy, and gastrostomy was performed just prior to the time of demise.

In removing an esophageal intubation tube the same rule applies as in removing a tube from the larynx or a tracheal cannula. There must be in readiness another tube which is immediately reintroduced, for contraction of the esophagus within a short time will render reintubation impossible. The writer has had palliative success with soft rubber esophageal intubation tubes. The writer has also made applications of radium to the esophageal lesion, but aside from the slight improvement in swallowing, there is little gained over esophageal intubation. In one instance the esophagus perforated after radium and the patient succumbed to bronchopneumonia. This, however, is frequently the termination of most of the cancerous growths of the esophagus of long duration. So far little has been accomplished by any form of treatment in esophageal cancer and the endoscopic treatment is in most cases purely palliative. Of the surgical procedure the transthoracic method as advised by Willy Meyer, Frans Torek, and others, seems to be on the road to success in cases diagnosed esophagoscopically early. Frans Torek has one case on whom he operated for a malignancy of the esophagus in the middle third who made a complete recovery and is still alive and well after seven years.

Luetic Stenosis of the Esophagus.—Luetic stenosis of the esophagus may be associated with luetic disease of the larynx. It may occur in the form of a mucous patch, an ulcer, a gumma or a cicatrix. The writer has studied two cases of luetic disease of the esophagus. One was in a man suffering from a gumma of the larynx as well, and the other was in a woman with cicatricial stenosis. The man was unable to swallow and was extremely dyspneic. He was sent to the hospital with the diagnosis of laryngeal diphtheria. Tracheotomy was performed shortly after admission to save his life. He was still unable to swallow after the introduction of the tracheotomy tube and the esophagus was examined and found to be gummatous. A soft rubber feeding tube was introduced and the patient fed in this manner. Mercury and salvarsan were administer after the Wassermann reaction

returned 4 plus. He readily improved under treatment and
was able to swallow fairly well two weeks later. An examination of the esophagus after two months' treatment showed
a cicatricial web stenosis of the upper esophagus. The larynx
greatly improved, but it was impossible to decannulate the
patient, for he preferred to wear the tube. He had a husky
voice. He insisted on leaving the hospital three months later
and was transferred to the Metropolitan Hospital and lost
sight of thereafter. At the time of discharge from the hospital he still had laryngeal stenosis, and a cicatricial esophageal
web.

Tuberculosis of the Esophagus.—The writer has seen many
cases of laryngeal tuberculosis who were also suffering from
esophageal involvement. He feels that much of the difficulty
in swallowing in laryngeal tuberculosis is often due to involvement of the esophagus as well. Esophageal ulcers may often
be present in tuberculous subjects when the lesion is not suspected, but only seen when performing the esophagoscopy.
At times there may be a tubercular lesion of the esophagus
which looks not unlike a fungating epithelioma. These healed
lesions at times may produce cicatrices and subsequent stenosis.

There are many other lesions of the esophagus which the
writer in a rather limited experienec has not been so fortunate
to see. They are angioneuritic edema, esophageal varix,
angioma and actinomycosis.

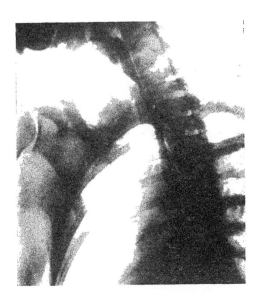

Fig. 1. Neurotic cricopharyngeal spasm. Note the narrow constriction of the bismuth mixture in the cervical esophagus. Cured after repeated introduction of the large esophagoscope.

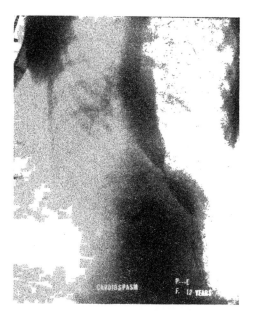

Fig. 2. Cardiocontraction and narrowing of the abdominal esophagus in a boy of twelve years. The whole of the subphrenic portion of the esophagus shows narrowing and demonstrates that the whole of the subdiaphragmatic esophagus contributes in the production of so-called cardiospasm.

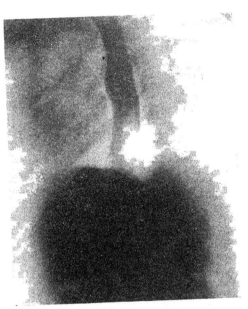

Fig. 3. Hiatal esophagismus or cardiocontraction in an adult. There is marked dilatation of the thoracic esophagus above the diaphragm.

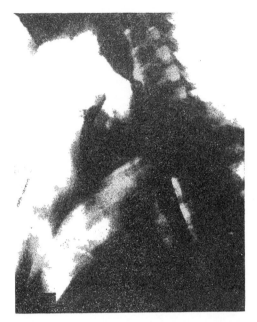

Fig. 4. Stricture of the cervical esophagus simulating neurotic cricopharyngeal spasm. The stricture was caused by the prolonged sojourn of a small spicule of bone following a submucous resection of the septum.

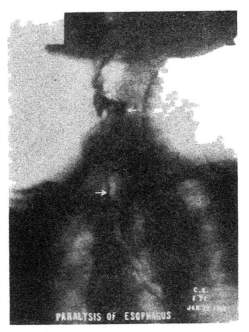

Fig. 5. Paralysis of the esophagus. The bismuth mixture was held in the reservoirs of the pyriform sinuses and poured over between the arytenoids into the larynx, trachea and bronchi. The bismuth in this instance entered the left bronchus and not the right. There was no cough reflex. It was expectorated and the lung drained of bismuth without the aid of cough.

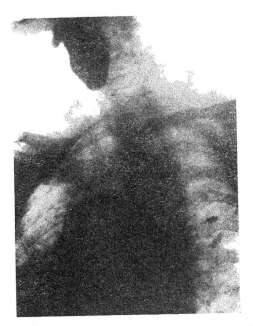

Fig. 6. Esophageal pouch in a woman of seventy-nine years.
The pouch involved the entire pharynx. There was partial stenosis
of the sub-diverticula esophagus.

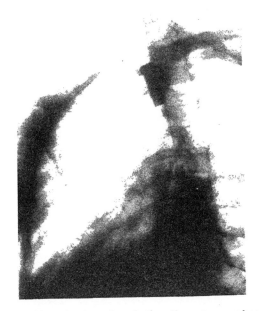

Fig. 7a. Malignant stenosis of the thoracic esophagus. The short silver intubation is covered with soft rubber and is shown as two long lines below the end of the metal tube.

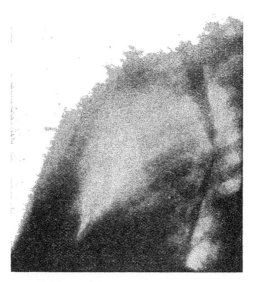

Fig. 7b. Radiograph of same patient showing the bismuth mixture passing through the tube.

# THE REMOVAL OF TONSILS IN THE PRESENCE OF A PERITONSILLAR ABSCESS.

By J. Holinger, M. D.,

Chicago.

The removal of tonsils while a peritonsillar abscess is present is not approved by physicians generally and is practiced by few. Cates in his article in the Laryngoscope of October, 1918, says: "And H. A. Barnes recommends tonsillectomy for the cure of quinsy during the attack. However, such radical forms of treatment have not received much favor as yet, not being in accord with generally accepted surgical principles." Cates does not say with which generally accepted surgical principle this procedure was not in accord, and evidently he has never tried the method himself. The objections against the procedure may concern either the clinical or the pathologic phase. Clinically, or rather clinico-historically, we may say that formerly when only parts of the tonsils were removed, the procedure may have led to sepsis, because it often did not drain all pockets of the abscess. Now with the systematic and total extirpation of the tonsil, we see the opposite. Patients who arrive in a septic condition on account of peritonsillar abscess with high fever, dry tongue, etc., make a completely different impression a few hours after the tonsils have been removed, and the writer in a comparatively large number of operations has never seen a case of sepsis following or continuing beyond the removal of the tonsils.

On the other hand, the advantages of the procedure overbalance by far all possible real or imaginary objections. We mention only a few:

1. We know that peritonsillar abscesses often recur. Therefore, sooner or later the tonsils have to be removed if the recurrences are to be prevented. Why make two operations for what can be done in one?

2. The period of recovery after the removal of tonsils in

the presence of a peritonsillar abscess is not longer than after
the removal of tonsils without abscess.

3. In peritonsillar abscesses often new abscesses are formed
next to the old ones.   In one patient we had to open a second,
a third and a fourth abscess after the first one was drained.
The duration of healing was six weeks.  Now the matter is
much simpler.  After the tonsil is out, all these pockets are
drained and heal, as said before, in the same time as the wound
after a simple tonsillectomy.

4. Patients who were in a decidedly septic condition are
relieved of their sepsis soon after the tonsils are removed.  The
pains in different parts of the body subside, and it happened
repeatedly that considerable quantities of albumin which were
found in the urine before the operation disappeared completely within the next few days after the removal.

Pathology:  The lymphatic tissue of the tonsil is arranged
in a network of connective tissue which forms its support.
This connective tissue on the outside becomes the capsule of
the tonsil and is in connection with the connective tissue of
the surrounding organs, muscles and facias.   It contains the
blood vessels, lymph vessels and nerves.  Inflammations and
especially the formation of abscesses follow the connective
tissue and leave the parenchyma comparatively free.   In a
few cases the abscess following and spreading in the capsule
practically dissected the tonsil.  As soon as the upper pole
of the tonsil was loosened from the palate and the pus removed, the tonsil was found to be quite loose in its niche, so
that it had only to be freed from the pillars.   These were the
true peritonsillar abscesses.  Several times a second and a
third gush of pus appeared during the dissection and showed
that multilocular abscesses are not so very rare.  They sometimes extend high up into the palate; sometimes they spread
between the muscles of the surroundings of the tonsils.   This
explains the stiffness and the painful mobility of the head
and neck which we usually notice in patients with peritonsillar abscesses.  This also explains why the walls of the abscess are not always smooth but often irregular.  Several times
we found that the abscess was not peritonsillar but an intra-
tonsillar abscess spreading in the connective tissue of the tonsil itself.  The tonsil in one of those cases was cut or divided
into several different parts.  At least, this is the only way

findings like the following could be explained. In dissecting the upper pole no abscess was found in the swollen and bulging soft palate. The upper pole reached far up into the soft palate, and the pus was met only in the middle or even below the middle of the tonsil. A compact or coherent mass of tonsillar tissue could not be found below the middle of the tonsil. The walls of the abscess cavity were irregular. As much of the scattered tissue as could be found was removed together with the upper pole of the tonsil. From the scattered remnants a large part of the tonsil formed again during the period of recovery. This was the only not quite satisfactory result that we have to report. It must, however, be added that the patient was unreasonable in that he smoked incessantly, even during the first days after operation.

The operation of removing the tonsils in the presence of a peritonsillar abscess has several unusual features which we will try to point out under different headings.

1. The anesthesia is general ether narcosis. In one case local cocain adrenalin anesthesia was tried, at the urgent request of the patient, but in the inflamed tissue it was very unsatisfactory to both patient and operator. The experiment will not be repeated. The ether narcosis, however, requires considerable care and experience, since often the swollen side of the pharynx and soft palate fills a large part of the pharynx and makes breathing difficult. Consequently there is often more than the usual amount of resistance till the patient is asleep. The suffocation sometimes reached very high degrees, but we never had to resort to tracheotomy or intubation. During the state of excitement the abscess broke in one case. It is a good plan to draw the attention of the anesthetist to such a possibility, that the pus may be removed before it is aspirated or swallowed.

2. At the operation the parts are often found very much distorted and the line of cleavage of the pillars is not always seen at first sight. As soon as the knife follows it, a gush of pus pours into the pharynx and is aspirated by means of the suction apparatus. Quick action is necessary, and it is evident that well trained assistants for the narcosis as well as for the operation are desirable. As soon as the pus is removed there is much more room in the pharynx. In remov-

ing the tonsil care has to be taken that no cast off lobe of the tonsil is overlooked. All the tissues are very brittle.

3. The hemorrhage is often greater than in a simple tonsillectomy. It is diffuse, but also the spurters have more caliber than under ordinary circumstances. The bleeding usually stops on compression with dry gauze or with gauze soaked in peroxide. The removal of the second tonsil is usually much easier and simpler. The after-treatment is not different from that after an ordinary tonsillectomy. A gargle of two tablespoonsful of peroxid in one glass of water will do as well as anything.

Barnes in 1915 recommended removal of tonsils during an attack of quinsy only in favorable conditions—i. e., in small abscesses. We have operated for more than seven years and have not made any distinction in small or large abscesses. We have used ether narcosis. We, too, hesitated in the beginning. but have never seen any bad results.

The following report may be of interest:

A strong young man of 19 had had several attacks of tonsillitis before. July 12, 1920, started with sore throat. July 18, was examined. The mouth could not be closed because the tongue, especially. in the base, was swollen and painful. Outside under the chin, the floor of the mouth and the sides of the jaws were bulging and very painful to touch. The glands, too, were swollen. In depressing the tongue a peritonsillar abscess was recognized. July 19th, both tonsils were removed; in the left one an abscess was met with. The swelling of the tongue improved within the next five days.

# IX

## REPORT OF CASES. 1. SIMPLE MASTOIDECTOMY ON MAN, 81 YEARS OLD. 2. INFECTIVE SIGMOID SINUS THROMBOSIS — A POSITIVE BLOOD CULTURE WITH STREPTOCOCCUS MUCOSUS CAPSULATUS PRESENT.

By J. Warren White, M. D.,

Norfolk, Va.

Case 1.—In September, 1917, I was called out of the city to see Mr. A. in consultation.

He gave a history of pain in his right ear for two weeks. On examination I found tenderness over the mastoid on pressure. The drum was very red and bulging.

A free myringotomy was done and he was removed to the Norfolk Protestant Hospital for observation. There was a profuse purulent discharge from the ear and the pain gradually became worse. On the fourth day after seeing him I decided to operate. On account of his age and general condition I attempted to operate under local anesthetic. Being unable to get any cooperation from my patient, I found it impossible, so a simple mastoidectomy was performed under ether anesthesia.

The mastoid cells were found to be pretty thoroughly destroyed. Dura was exposed in the operation.

One week after the operation he developed an infection in the left ear. A free myringotomy was done.

He made an uneventful recovery. He is living today and is enjoying comparatively good health.

Case 2.—I did a simple mastoidectomy on M. T., 10 years old, at St. Vincent's Hospital.

There was nothing unusual about the case. A culture from the mastoid showed streptococcus mucosus capsulatus. Sinus and dura were both exposed in the operation.

The child did well, and after the first week the temperature became normal and remained so until the twelfth day. On the night of the twelfth day after the operation she had a severe chill, with a rise of temperature to 105° F. The next day her temperature returned to normal. The pulse rate was 150 beats per minute, and she was completely prostrated. During the day she had another chill, with a rise of temperature to 105° F.

She was taken to the operating room. The mastoid wound was opened and the sinus freely exposed. The jugular vein was ligated and then the sinus was opened.

The report from the blood culture was positive, with streptococcus mucosus capsulatus present.

After a long illness she finally recovered.

# X

# ENCEPHALITIS LETHARGICA AS A POSTOPERATIVE COMPLICATION OF ACUTE MASTOIDITIS WITH REPORT OF A CASE.

By M. J. Siegelstein, M. D.,
New York.

The pathologic data of this form of intracranial lesion are exceeding meager, and though the records show many cases which have completely recovered following middle ear suppuration, these cases were diagnosed from their clinical findings only; and as positive diagnosis is almost impossible, the findings at operation deliver the only data to the actual conditions present in a given case, and it is with such intentions that I report the following:

Mr. O., age 37, had an attack of influenza in March, 1919, which lasted three weeks. At the end of the third week he began to have pain in the right ear with fever. Paracentesis was done, and the pain and fever relieved; the discharge from the ear was profuse and thick.

About a week later, when the discharge had almost disappeared, he began to have fever and seveer pain over the right side of the head, with rigidity of the back of the neck and twitches on the right side of the face, a temperature of 103 and pulse 120.

He was then referred to me by his physician, Dr. Bookstaber, for operation. Mastoidectomy was performed on the same day with the result that as soon as the cortex of the mastoid was removed thick white pus began to well up, and this furnished an easy guide to the antrum, which was high up under the zygomatic ridge. The antrum and cells were thoroughly cleared out down to the mastoid tip.

On the following day the temperature came down to normal and the patient remained well until the fourth day after operation, when his condition began to change and he complained of a severe diffuse headache and dizziness, and he did not sleep that night; temperature 100.

At 5 o'clock the next morning he had slight delirium, and it was with difficulty that he was restrained from getting out of bed. A few hours afterwards he began to get drowsy; temperature varied from 99 to 100; pulse, 74 to 80; conplained of general weakness as well as diplopia; answered questions slowly and incoherently; slight twitchings of face with felt facial palsy noticed. No evidence of labyrinth involvement.

He remained in stupor the entire day and had to be awakened to take nourishment, and this somnolence deepened the next day, so that he could only with difficulty be aroused, relapsing, however, into the same previous condition. Temperature 102; pulse 80 to 96. I then decided to explore the cranial cavity.

Examination revealed heart and lungs normal; no discharge from the ear or mastoid wound; accessory sinuses negative; pupils regular, dilated, reacting to light; eyegrounds normal; no local tenderness; urine negative; no Kernig, Babinski or other abnormal reflexes present; swallowing difficult; sensation markedly impaired; blood examination—white cells 12,-000, polynuclears 80 per cent; Wassermann negative; spinal fluid showed moderate pressure in the recumbent position; cell count normal; globulin negative; no bacterial growth; smear negative; Wassermann negative.

Accordingly, on the night of the sixth day following operation, the mastoid wound was again opened for revision to see if any carious bone or fistulæ were overlooked, and as it was clean, the wound was extended upwards above the zygoma for two inches, and then a horizontal incision was made from the center of the original one back to the occipital protuberance.

The bone was ronguered upwards through the zygomatic process and through the squama, starting from the tegmen antri, exposing the dura over the right temporosphenoidal lobe of the cerebrum for an area of 2 by 2 inches.

No extradural exudate was found, dura appeared to bulge, pulsated and was normal, and there was no tension of fluid between it and the cerebrum, after it was incised. Examination of the cortex showed the brain swollen and edematous, with diffuse hemorrhagic areas throughout the field.

Exploration of the temporosphenoidal lobe in various directions was done both by means of a long aspirating needle, as well as by a long narrow pointed knife for a depth of about two inches, and no abscess was discovered, but the lateral ventricle was opened, with clear fluid oozing out and not under marked tension. Working back from the lateral sinus, which was normal, the cerebellar lobe was exposed, and exploration here also proved to be negative. Dura was left unsutured for its decompressive effect and patient was returned to bed without any shock.

He reacted well and the next morning was able to open his eyes and look around him, although he still was stuporous. On arousing him, only indistinct mutterings were heard and he immediately went back to sleep.

The day following, somnolence was still present, and during the afternoon he had an attack of pulmonary edema which lasted about one hour and disappeared, leaving his lungs clear, but in a few hours the coma deepened, with Cheyne-Stokes respirations, and he made his exitus.

Autopsy in this case was unfortunately not obtained because of family objections.

Remarks.—In this case the difficulty of arriving at a differential diagnosis was obvious, and resort to exploration to give the patient the benefit of the doubt was indicated.

Brain tumor was excluded by the absence of changes in the eyegrounds as well as the presence of fever.

Meningitis (serous, suppurative, tubercular and syphilitic) were excluded by lumbar puncture, examination of spinal fluid and the exploration.

Abscesses (extradural, cerebral and cerebellar) were excluded by the exploration; sinus thrombosis by history and examination of sinus at operation.

The presence of cortical hemorrhagic areas with swollen and edematous brain substance noticed in the operative field is characteristic of encephalitis and the clinical history confirms the findings.

The onset of the encephalitis during the convalescence of the mastoid operation is confusing, when the more common complications, as abscesses, meningitis and sinus infection, are ordinarily looked for.

Körner from the report of those cases supposed to have recovered believed that the eradication of the primary lesion in the temporal bone was sufficient, or in addition the free exposure of the affected area will often result in a cure ·and that ventricular and lumbar puncture would help combat the disease. There is no doubt that those cases that have recovered would have recovered without operation, as attested to by the many reports now published, and that those who died could not have been benefited by operation. Operation is only indicated in those cases complicating mastoid operations where the exploration will exclude other complications requiring surgical treatment.

## REFERENCES.

Skversky: Lethargic Encephalitis, Am. Journ. Med. Sc., December, 1919.

Kopetzky: Surgery of the Ear.

Dench: Diseases of Ear.

British Med. Journ., February, 1919.

Wien. Klin. Wochenschr., May, 1917.

Paris Med., August, 1918.

Journ. Am. Med. Assn., January, 1919.

Journ. Am. Med. Assn., March, 1919.

Korner: Die otitische erkrankung des Hirns, 1902.

# XI

## TONSILLAR HEMORRHAGE.*

### By T. E. Fuller, M. D.,

#### Texarkana, Ark.

The factors which influence postoperative tonsillar hemorrhage are so varied that accurate statistics are difficult to obtain. In 700 consecutive cases in children in Barnes' service at the Boston Dispensary only two hemorrhages occurred that required suturing the pillars. In 140 tonsillectomies on patients over 16 years of age at the Massachusetts General Hospital there were four hemorrhages that required suturing of the faucial pillars.

The replies to a questionnaire sent out by L. G. Hill indicate that troublesome hemorrhages range from ½ to 8 per cent, the majority being from 2 to 5 per cent. Troublesome hemorrhages are 4 per cent greater in adults than in children.

Relative to dangerous hemorrhages, 10 per cent of the replies were zero, the balance ranging from 1 to 6 per cent. One prominent operator reported twelve cases of fatal hemorrhage, one reported four cases, one reported three cases, four reported two cases and others reported none. It is interesting to note that out of the 14,042 tonsillectomies done in our army there was only one death from tonsillar hemorrhage.

As to whether the number of hemorrhages was greater following local or general anesthesia, the majority stated that the percentage was greater under general. About 30 per cent, however, stated that the hemorrhage under local anesthesia was higher. Many of them accounted for this fact by the large number of adults operated upon by this method. The report of the Committee on Local Anesthetics read before the section on laryngology, rhinology and otology of the American Medical Association at New Orleans indicates that the percentage of hemorrhages, when local anesthesia is used, is not greater.

---

*Accepted as a candidate's thesis by the American Laryngological, Rhinological and Otological Society.

The above figures confirm what one from his own experience and observations knows to be true, namely, that everyone who performs the operation of tonsillectomy will sooner or later encounter hemorrhages, some of which may be severe enough to tax his skill to the utmost, and yet when we consider the methods of hemostasis used by many operators and note those advocated in certain textbooks and journals, we wonder if the reproach that the control of hemorrhage, during and following tonsillectomy, is most inexact and unsurgical, is altogether unmerited.

The tonsil receives its blood supply from the dorsalis linguæ, a branch of the lingual, which supplies the anterior pillar and sends branches into the anterior surface of the gland. From the ascending pharyngeal of the external carotid branches enter from the posterior pillar. The descending palatine from the internal maxillary sends a branch to the superior lobe. The most important arteries are the tonsillar and ascending palatine branches of the facial. These pierce the superior constrictor muscle at the lower pole of the tonsil, where they usually break up into two or more branches before entering the capsule. The arrangement of these branches is variable. Davis observes that they are most commonly found just behind and about one-quarter of an inch from the margin of the anterior faucial pillar, about midway between the top and base of the tonsil, or a little below this point. It is said that occasionally by anastomosis of the above named vessels an arterial plexus is formed just outside the capsule. The writer has not observed such an arrangement. The internal carotid artery is almost an inch behind and to the outer side of the tonsil. The external carotid is still further away, and is protected by the styloglossus and stylopharyngeus muscles. It will thus be seen that the carotids, when normally placed, are in very little danger of being wounded during a tonsil operation. Dr. Gwilym G. Davis has demonstrated a specimen in which the internal carotid could have been wounded by incision of the tonsil.

The facial artery when it makes a high loop before crossing the ramus of the jaw has only the superior constrictor muscle between it and the lower pole of the tonsil. The ascending pharyngeal and ascending palatine arteries are also separated from the tonsil by the thickness of the superior constrictor muscle alone. When very firm peritonsillar adhesions exist it is possible to wound one of the three last named vessels and have a fatal hemorrhage. As the ascending palatine frequently takes its origin from the external carotid instead of the facial, it would seem more certain to ligate the external carotid and not the facial in cases of serious tonsillar bleeding.

The ligature on the external carotid should be placed as low as possible in order to control the ascending pharyngeal, which arises close to or immediately at the origin of the external carotid. The veins terminate in the tonsillar plexus which joins the pharyngeal and pterygoid plexuses to empty into the internal jugular or facial vein. Some small veins empty into the larger vessels at the base of the tongue. A large vein frequently runs the length of the tonsillar fossa just external to the posterior pillar. When wounded, it bleeds profusely. The writer has seen one troublesome postoperative hemorrhage from this vessel.

The successful arrest of hemorrhage depends on the clotting power of the blood. No doubt the statement of Bayliss, who writes "It cannot be said that the coagulation of the blood is yet understood," is correct; nevertheless, the theories of Howell are the most generally accepted, and as the action of a number of hemostatic agents is best explained by his researches, brief reference to them will be made.

When blood clots, the circulating fibrinogen of the serum is transformed into an insoluble protein fibrin by the action of fibrin ferment or thrombin. Thrombin, as such, does not exist in the blood, but its precursor, prothrombin, does, and this is converted into thrombin. In order that this change may take place calcium salts are necessary; also an element derived from the blood platelets, or injured tissue, or from both, called by Howell "thromboplastin." Blood does not coagulate in the vessels, because this prothrombin is combined wtih an antithrombin, which prevents it from acting. When the blood is shed and flows over injured tissue, the thromboplastin, derived from the blood cells, blood platelets or tissue cells, unites with the antithrombin, liberating the prothrombin. This in turn combines with calcium salts, and thrombin is formed. The thrombin converts the fibrinogen of the plasma into fibrin and coagulation sets in. It has been shown that thromboplastin, from whatever source, gives the reaction of lipoid kephalin, the principal lipoid of the brain. This fact has been taken advantage of in the preparation of many substances used to hasten coagulation. The recent work of Mills indicates that extracts from lung tissue are even more active than those of brain tissue in inducing coagulation.

The part taken by the platelets in the process of clotting has been further studied by Tait, who believes that when a vessel is cut the labile platelets, or spindle cells, called thigmocytes, adhere to the edges of the vessel wall and build up a plug. By cytolysis these same cells produce the thrombin which causes the plasma to clot, thus taking two distinct parts in the checking of hemorrhage.

Types of Hemorrhage.—The types of hemorrhage encountered in tonsil cases are:

Primary, which occurs at the time of operation;

Early secondary, which comes on in a few hours, and is frequently the continuation of a primary hemorrhage which was not checked, and

Late secondary, which most frequently occurs at the end of four or five days or a week. As a rule it is not serious, being produced by the opening up of small vessels during the separation of the slough.

Predisposing Causes.—The conditions which render troublesome bleeding more likely to occur are certain blood dyscrasias, such as hemophilia and the purpuras, high blood pressure, arteriosclerosis, acute inflammation of the tonsils or surrounding structures and peritonsillar adhesions. Anemic and poorly nourished children have a tendency to bleed.

It is said that during and immediately following the menstrual period the clotting time of the blood is delayed. The exciting cause of tonsillar hemorrhage is, of course, the operation, during which the vessels are severed.

Prophylaxis.—The radical removal of tonsils is an important surgical procedure, and the cases are entitled to a more careful selection than many of them receive. The condition of the heart and kidneys should be ascertained, and in adults the blood pressure taken. Operation should not be done in the presence of acute inflammation of the tonsils or surrounding structures. The general condition of anemic and poorly nourished children should be improved by the use of proper food and iron tonics. In the case of females the operation should not be done during or for a week following the menstrual period.

Tonsillectomy should always be done in a hospital. If the patient is an adult, he must remain for 24 hours afterward. Children may in some instances be allowed to go out in 12 hours. In taking the case history care should be exercised to learn if any unusual tendency to bleed exists in the patient or his family.

The bleeding and coagulation time should be determined in all doubtful cases. When the coagulation time is delayed and when it cannot be shortened by measures to be discussed later, operation should be refused. In cases where the bleeding time is prolonged, a count of the platelets should be made, and not until their number has been made to approach normal should the tonsils be removed.

Treatment.—No attempt will be made to consider all the measures advised for the control of hemorrhage. Some are uncertain, and others too unsurgical to deserve a permanent place in our armamentarium.

The measures used may be grouped into:

1. Those acting on the blood to influence its clotting, or on the blood vessel walls, or on both.

2. Mechanical measures.

Remedies whose dominant action is to lower blood pressure are not included, because we believe that cases of hypertension should be under the care of an internist, and that he should have lowered the blood pressure, at least temporarily, before operation is attempted.

### AGENTS ACTING ON THE BLOOD OR BLOOD VESSELS.

Preparations of the Suprarenal Glands.—Considerable work has been done on these glands ever since the time of Addison, but it was not until 1901 that Takamine succeeded in isolating the active principle in pure and stable form. He gave to the preparation the name of adrenalin. Adrenalin stimulates the sympathetic system in general. When it enters the blood stream it causes elevation of blood pressure and increased action of the heart. The vasoconstrictor action is peripheral. When applied locally, marked contraction of the arterioles occurs. This is followed by a relaxation of the vessels. Richards and Vosburgh found that adrenalin increased the coagulability of the blood. Wiggins was unable to corroborate these findings. Conman and Gray showed that small doses intravenously and larger amounts subcutaneously shortened the coagulation time one-third or even one-half. Grabfeld finds that the prothrombin is increased by it. When added in small amounts to the solution used to induce local anesthesia, adrenalin is of value. Care must be taken, however, not to have the solutions too strong, or the vasodilatation following its use will render secondary hemorrhage very likely to occur. There is this same objection to its local use following the removal of tonsils. When it is desired to increase the coagulability of the blood there are other substances which are more certain and more desirable. The use of adrenalin then should be limited to the small amount added to the solution to be injected when local anesthesia is used in the removal of tonsils.

Emetin.—Trousseau recommended ipecacuanha as a hemostatic. Its active principle—emetin—has been used for hemorrhages of various kinds since soon after its isolation. Emetin hydrochlorid causes a short rise in blood pressure. Pelline and Wallace obtained no change or only a slight contraction of the arteries. Enous Smith and Middleton found transient vasoconstriction followed by vasodilatation. Howell has noted a deficiency in the fibrinogen in the blood as a result of which the clotting is retarded and the clot not retractile. Bostedo concludes that neither clinical results nor pharmacologic action justify its use in any internal hemorrhage.

Weinstein was the first to report the use of this drug in nasopharyngeal surgery. He found that by injecting emetin he could reduce the coagulation time by one-third. The writer was able to check the bleeding in a case of late secondary hemorrhage following removal of tonsils by the use of emetin. In view of the fact that we have agents more reliable in their action, the use of emetin seems unnecessary.

Pituitary Extract.—The functions of the pituitary gland and the pharmacology of its preparations are still being investigated. It seems from the work done, however, that it may be said that pituitrin constricts the peripheral blood vessels, probably by direct muscular action, and that it slows and strengthens the heart. The coagulation time of the blood is reduced in fifteen minutes after a hypodermic injection, according to Kahn.

This action on the blood is what makes pituitary extracts valuable in the prevention and treatment of tonsillar hemorrhage. Moore fiuds that given fifteen to thirty minutes before the removal of tonsils it reduces the loss of blood and shortens the coagulation time by one-third or one-half. Salinger reviews 87 cases in which pituitrin was administered as a prophylactic prior to operation, 52 under general and 35 under local anesthesia. In two of the cases there was severe bleeding, the pituitrin apparently exerting no influence. He is convinced, however, that the drug has a marked hemostatic action, as 62 out of the 87 cases showed only slight bleeding which required no pressure or other hemostasis. He concludes from his experience that pituitrin will, in most cases, diminish the amount of blood lost, particularly under general anesthesia, and that for the control of secondary hemorrhage its action is prompt and successful. On the other hand, Donelon's experience leads him to consider pituitrin as uncertain, its chief use being to support the heart and prevent shock.

The writer's experience agrees with that of Salinger. He has used it in a number of cases. While it is not a sure preventive, in most instances it will shorten the coagulation time and lessen the amount of blood lost. Several cases of secondary hemorrhage of moderate degree have been checked by its use alone. The dose is ½ cc. for children; for adults, 1 cc. It should be given one-half hour before the operation.

Calcium Salts.—It was believed that a lack of ionic calcium was the common cause of delayed coagulability of the blood. In order to supply this deficiency calcium lactate or chlorid was given for a variable length of time before operation. In much of the literature on tonsillar hemorrhage these remedies are given a prominent place, but later studies have shown that insufficient calcium is rarely, if ever, the cause of delayed clotting, and further, that it is difficult, if not impossible, to increase the calcium content in the blood by the ingestion of calcium salts.

Rudolf and Cole in 1911 conclude that the exhibition of calcium lactate by the mouth has no appreciable effect on the coagulation of the blood. Van Lier in 1912, after taking the coagulation time in forty persons before and after the administration of calcium lactate, has arrived at the same conclusion. Lee and Vincent draw different conclusions from the above, believing with Wright and Paramore that a distinct difference in the coagulation time can be produced by the injection of calcium. In addition to the above, clinical evidence supports the contention that the calcium salts are not worthy of confidence when it is necessary to shorten the coagulation time of the blood.

Tissue Extracts and Sera.—The knowledge that thromboplastin from whatever source obtained gives the reaction of lipoid kephalin was made use of in the preparation of various substances to increase the coagulability of the blood. The work of Hiss in this field is well known. The substance he prepared came from ox brains. E. R. Squibb and Sons manufacture it and offer it under the name of thromboplastin, which was first given it by Hiss. A thromboplastin solution is prepared by Armour & Company, who also manufacture kephalin, which they describe as "hemostatic phosphotid from spinal cord and brain tissue." Their remedies are in two forms, one for local use and the other for hypodermic administration. The former is used on gauze sponges applied directly to the bleeding area.

It is not expected that this will stop the bleeding from large vessels, but where there is a general oozing or small vessels are involved, the results are very satisfactory. The hypodermic preparation is used in cases of delayed coagulation time.

Coagulen Ciba.—Coagulen Ciba is made solely from the blood platelets. It comes in the form of powder, compressed tablets, and in sterilized ampules. It is used in the same manner as thromboplastin. Bann and de Tarnowsky in this country and many foreign observers testify to the usefulness of coagulen.

Normal Horse Serum.—Normal horse serum and, when it was not obtainable, antitoxin has long been used to check hemorrhage. The results obtained have been variable, and the danger of anaphylaxis is present. A comparison of the various physiologic hemostatics was made by Hanzlink and Weidenthal. Their results are quoted below:

"From the summary it is seen that the thromboplastins were distinctly superior to all other products tested, the Squibb product possessing a median efficiency of more than three times that of the Armour product, and seven times that of the freshest and some old kephalins."

"The freshest specimens of dry coagulen, coagulen solution in ampules, coagulose and hemostatic serum are seen to occupy the same grouping and efficiency values as normal saline. In other words, these products did not accelerate the coagulation of plasmas and blood in vitro, and accordingly are regarded as entirely inert as thromboplastic agents."

"The freshly obtained and prepared thromboplastic agents which were tested arrange themselves in descending order of the plasma and blood clotting efficiency in vitro, as follows: First, thromboplastin (Squibb); second, thromboplastin (Armour); third, kephalins (fresh and some old specimens); fourth, coagulen, coagulose, hemostatic serum and normal saline."

It would seem that because of its efficiency and because the risk of anaphylaxis is reduced to the minimum, thromboplastin is the remedy of choice when agents of this class are to be used.

Blood Transfusion.—In hemorrhage due to delayed coagulation the best remedy by far is a blood transfusion from a properly grouped donor. In cases where for lack of time or facilities the grouping is not possible, a member of the patient's family should be used as the donor. Some of the agents above enumerated are of great assistance, but their use should be limited to mild cases, or to cases where for some reason a blood transfusion is impossible.

Mechanical Measures.—Pressure, properly applied, will check capillary bleeding and bleeding from small vessels. If kept up for some time hemorrhage from vessels of considerable size can be controlled.

Pressure is made by sponges, held in clamps, or sponge forceps, suturing the pillars with a sponge between them, by the use of pillar compression forceps, such as those of Ber-

geron, and by tonsil hemostats, of which there are many kinds.
After the tonsil is removed one or two gauze sponges, held
by forceps, should be placed firmly in the fossa for a few
moments. This will stop the capillary hemorrhage and the
bleeding from the smaller vessels. When these are removed,
if one or more vessels bleed, they should be dealt with by
other means, and no further time should be consumed in an
attempt to check the hemorrhage by pressure.

To suture a sponge between the pillars increases the reaction, is painful to remove and other means are more certain.
These same objections apply to the use of tonsil hemostats,
and in the writer's opinion they should never be used unless
it be to make pressure in the fossa of the first tonsil removed
while the second is being operated. To send the patient out
of the operating room with one of these hemostats in place
or to use one in an attempt to check secondary hemorrhage
should not be done.

Ligation of Vessels.—When pressure, as described above,
does not control and one or more bleeding points are revealed
in the fossa, they should be ligated. Savage of Baltimore says:

"There is no excuse for omitting ligation on account of
imaginary difficulties, and resorting to suture of the pillars,
or using the clumsy Mikulicz instrument, or mere pressure by
gauze sponges until the hemorrhage has apparently ceased to
recur after the patient has left the operating table, and then
to call it, improperly, secondary hemorrhage."

With this view the writer is in entire accord. Boettcher
credits Cohen of Baltimore as being the first to systematically employ ligature of the tonsillar vessels in tonsillectomy.
Cohen's method of ligating the vessels is, in the writer's opinion, the simplest and best. It is well illustrated and described
in the second volume of Loeb's Surgery of the Nose. Throat
and Ear. Other good methods are those described by Parkes
and by Gross.

It is necessary to expose the fossa well by the use of a
pillar retractor. When a good exposure is obtained, there
is, as a rule, little difficulty in placing a ligature around the
bleeding point. Occasionally there is too much tissue in the
bite of the artery forceps. This will make the pedicle too
large and the ligature may slip off. When it is seen that this

is likely to occur, it is well to use a suture ligature. In the placing of these suture ligatures, the writer has found the needle holder of Baum to be the most satisfactory. In cases where it is difficult to grasp the bleeding point, one or two properly applied suture ligatures will control the hemorrhage. There have been a number of special instruments devised to render the placing of ligatures or suture ligatures more simple. Cavanaugh's is one of the best of these.

Instead of using sutures a number of operators employ Michel clips to control the bleeding points. There is no doubt that their use is simple and effective, but one had to be removed from the bronchus of a patient where it had been inspired from the tonsillar fossa. With other reliable means at our command, we should not subject our patients to this additional risk, slight though it be.

Suturing the Faucial Pillars.—Boettcher in the article referred to above states that suturing of the pillars is the most approved, present day method of controlling hemorrhage. If the bleeding vessels are ligated, as a matter of routine, very few cases which require suturing of the pillars will be seen. At times there is a general oozing from the entire bed of the tonsil. Pressure does not control it and individual bleeding points cannot be found. In these cases suture of the pillars must be done. The sutures must be placed in such a way as to include not only the pillars, but the floor of the fossa as well, so when they are tied no dead space will remain.

In this, as in the placing of suture ligatures, the needle holder of Baum has served me well.

In discussing the tonsil question at the meeting of the Southern Section of the American Laryngological, Rhinological and Otological Society, held in New Orleans, in April, 1920, Dr. J. O. McReynolds, of Dallas, Texas, stated that for some time he had been obliterating the tonsillar fossa as a part of every tonsillectomy. He compared this with the closure of wounds made by the general surgeon in other parts of the body. It not only controls hemorrhage, but is an attempt to secure primary union. In the cases where the writer has found it necessary to obliterate the fossa, the stitches have given away in a few days and the same granulating fossa has been left that we are accustomed to see following tonsillectomy.

the only difference being that there was more reaction. For that reason he believes that suture of the pillars should be done only after other measures have failed.

Ligation of the External Carotid.—The writer has not seen a case where it was necessary to ligate any of the vessels in the neck. A number of such cases, however, have been reported, and if all other measures fail one should not hesitate to ligate. Some advise ligation of the facial, and in most cases this would be sufficient, but if it happens to be the ascending palatin that is bleeding and it takes its origin from the external carotid instead of the facial, nothing would be accomplished. For this reason, where it is necessary to ligate a vessel in the neck the external carotid should be selected.

Case No. 1.—A colleague, a general surgeon, removed the tonsils of an eight year old boy, using a Beck instrument. The operation was done early in the morning. At noon the writer was called to the hospital to see the case. The child was expectorating mouthfuls of blood, and showed plainly the effects of acute anemia. The patient was sent to the operating room and gas ether given. A mouth gag was introduced, and by the use of suction and sponges it was seen that the bleeding came from the left tonsillar fossa. This was packed with two or three gauze sponges. By removing these one at a time we were able to locate the bleeding vessel. It was a large vein which ran the entire length of the fossa, just external to the posterior pillar. A section of the vein had been removed about its center, and it was bleeding from both ends. Each end was caught with a clamp, which controlled the hemorrhage perfectly. The surgeon, whose case it was, came in at that time, so the patient was given into his care. He left the clamps on a few hours. When they were removed no further bleeding occurred. The boy made an uninterrupted recovery. In this case I feel certain that the hemorrhage at the time of operation had never been checked.

Case No. 2.—A male, aged 25, was operated upon under local anesthesia. The writer follows the technic of Matthews of Minneapolis. In snaring off the pedicle of the first tonsil two or three wires were broken. The tonsil was unusually fibrous and large. When we came to remove the second tonsil we broke our entire stock of wires and the tonsil was still in place. The hospital had no wire; the only instrument they had was an old fashioned tonsillotome with a sharp blade. This was used to cut the pedicle. The hemorrhage was slight. The case was watched a few minutes. The anterior pillar was retracted and the fossa inspected. As it seemed to be dry, the patient was sent to his room. About an hour later the interne requested me to come to the hospital, as the patient was bleeding and he was unable to control the hemorrhage. Inspection showed the hemorrhage to be coming from the second tonsillar fossa. A sponge was introduced and held in place. This controlled the hemorrhage. After the sponge was removed the fossa remained dry, so no further measures were necessary. Patient made an uninterrupted recovery.

Case No. 3.—Patient, a female, aged 23, was operated upon under local anesthesia at 8 o'clock in the morning. There was nothing unusual during the operation. The tonsils came out readily and cleanly. The hemorrhage ceased spontaneously. At 9 o'clock that night the nurse asked me to see the patient, stating that she was having some hemorrhage. When seen she was having a moderate hemorrhage, but as it had kept up for some time and pituitrin had no effect on it we felt it unwise to wait longer. Inspection revealed the fact that the bleeding was from the left fossa. It was difficult to locate the exact points. There seemed to be a general oozing. Accordingly catgut sutures, two in number, were taken through the pillars and bed of the fossa. When there were tied the bleeding ceased. At the end of 24 hours the stitches were cut. The patient's recovery was uneventful.

Case No. 4.—Patient, a male, aged 20, were operated on under local anesthesia at 2 p. m. The tonsils were firmly adherent to the surrounding structures and considerable difficulty was encountered in the dissection. They were removed entirely, however, but the fossæ were rather ragged looking. There was a moderate degree of hemorrhage, but it ceased spontaneously, inspection showing dry fossæ. About 6 o'clock the house surgeon reported that the patient was having some hemorrhage, and that he had been given pituitrin hypodermically. This did no good, so normal horse serum was given. An hour later I saw the patient, but the hemorrhage had ceased, so he was not disturbed. Early the next morning I was requested to see the case, as he had been bleeding some all night. The patient's throat was very sensitive, but we managed to introduce catgut sutures into the pillars on the right side, the one that was bleeding. This, however, did not control the hemorrhage. The patient was anesthetized and the sutures removed. The fossa was again found to be filled with clot from around the edges from which the blood oozed. This clot was thoroughly removed, and as there was a general bleeding from the fossa the pillars were sutured with silk. This controlled the hemorrhage. The patient's recovery was uneventful.

Case No. 5.—Patient, a male, aged 30, was operated on under local anesthesia. The tonsils were easily removed, and the hemorrhage ceased spontaneously. Five days later we were requested to see the case because of hemorrhage. There was a moderate but continuous oozing from under the edges of the slough in the left fossa. Pressure was made with gauze sponges and a hypodermic of emetin given. The hemorrhage was soon controlled and did not recur.

### CONCLUSIONS.

1. Everyone who undertakes the operation of tonsillectomy should have in mind definite methods of controlling hemorrhage.

2. Each case should be thoroughly examined. Any tendency to bleed must be overcome by transfusion or injections of thromboplastin or, except in cases of extreme urgency, the operation refused.

3. During tonsillectomy every vessel that bleeds after a moderate amount of pressure has been made should be tied as a matter of routine. In exceptional cases it may be necessary to suture the pillars because of generalized oozing.

4. Postoperative hemorrhage is to be controlled in the same way. The clot must be removed from the fossa. In many instances it is necessary to reanesthetize the patient.

### BIBLIOGRAPHY.

Barnes, Harry A.: The Tonsils.

Hill, L. G.: Hemorrhage Following Tonsillectomies. Journal Lancet, Minneapolis, 1919.

Mosher, Harris P.: Observations on Otolaryngology in the War. Annals of Otology, Rhinology and Laryngology, September, 1919.

Wood, George B.: Loeb's Operative Surgery of the Ear, Nose and Throat, Volume 1.

Davis, J. Leslie: Tonsillectomy, Why, When and How. Pennsylvania Medical Journal, November, 1911.

Piersol, George O.: Human Anatomy.

Gray, Henry: Anatomy Descriptive and Surgical, edited by John Chambers Da Costa.

Bayless, Wm. Maddock: Principles of General Physiology. .

Howell, Wm. H.: Text Book of Physiology.

Mills, C. A.: The Activity of Lung Extract as Compared to Extracts of Other Tissues in Inducing Coagulation of the Blood. Journal Biological Chemistry, December, 1919.

Tait, J.: Natural Arrest of Hemorrhage From a Wound. Journal of Physiology, September 5th, 1919.

Moore, Irwin: Hemorrhage Following Removal of the Tonsils and Its Treatment. Practitioner, London, 100; pp. 334-361, 1918.

Oppenheimer, Seymour, and Gotlieb, Mark J.: Blood Examinations in the Surgery of the Nose and Throat. The Laryngoscope, July, 1919.

Oppenheimer, Seymour, and Spencer, Henry James: The Value of Laboratory Examinations in Diagnosis and Prognosis in Otolaryngology. Transactions of the American Academy of Ophthalmology and Otolaryngology, 1919.

Bastedo. Walter A.: Materia Medica, Pharmacology and Therapeutics.

Wood, Horatio C.: Therapeutics, Its Principles and Practice.

Weinstein, Joseph: A Clinical Report of the Successful Use of Emetin in the Control of Hemorrhage Following Nasopharyngeal Operations. Medical Record, January 16th, 1915.

Weinstein, Joseph: Nature and Control of Hemorrhage in Nasopharyngeal Operations. The Laryngoscope, March, 1917.

Wiggins, Carl J.: The Physiology of the Pituitary Glands and the Action of Its Extracts. American Journal of Medical Sciences, April, 1911.

Salinger, Samuel: Pituitrin in Tonsillar and Nasal Hemorrhage. Therapeutic Gazette, January 15th, 1918.

Donelon, James: Critical Notes on the Value of Pituitrin Preparations in Reducing Operative or Post-Operative Hemorrhage. Journal of Laryngology, Rhinology and Otology, Vol. 28, p. 353, 1913.

Dennis, W., and Minot, A. S.: Effects of Feeding With Calcium Salts on the Calcium Content of the Blood. Journal Biological Chemistry, March, 1920.

Hiss, A. F.: Thromboplastin (Tissue Extract), as a Hemostatic. Journal of the American Medical Association, April 24th, 1915.

Bonm, H. K.: Further Clinical Studies of Coagulen Ciba (Kocher-Fonio). Indianapolis Medical Journal, March, 1919.

DeTarnowsky, Geo.: Surgery, Gynecology and Obstetrics, May, 1914.

Hanzlink, P. J., and Weidenthal, C. M.: Study of the Coagulation Efficiency of Various Thromboplastic Agents. Journal of Pharmocology and Experimental Therapeutics, October, 1919.

Bergeron, J. Z.: Pillar Compression Forceps for Controlling Hemorrhage Following Tonsillectomy. Journal of the American Medical Association, February, 1916.

Savage, M. M.: Control of Tonsillar Hemorrhage. Journal of the American Medical Association, 53, p. 698, 1909.

Boettcher, Henry R.: Ligature of the Vessels to Arrest Hemorrhage After Tonsillectomy. Illinois Medical Journal, 34, pp. 212-216, 1918.

Parkes, William B.: Control of Hemorrhage in Tonsillectomies. Surgery, Gynecology and Obstetrics, November, 1919.

Gross, William A.: New Forceps for the Control of Hemorrhage After the Removal of Tonsils. Surgery, Gynecology and Obstetrics, March, 1919.

Baum, Harry L.: Complications and Sequelae of Tonsil and Adenoid Operations, Their Prevention and Management. Transactions of the American Academy of Ophthalmology and Otolaryngology, 1919.

Cavanaugh, John A.: A New Instrument for Ligating Bleeding Blood Vessels After the Removal of Tonsils. Journal of the American Medical Association, May 1st, 1920.

Matthews, Justus: Technique of Tonsillectomy. The Journal Lancet, Minneapolis, March 15th, 1917.

# XII

# PATHOLOGIC NASAL ACCESSORY SINUSES IN CHILDREN.*

By Francis W. White, M. D.,

New York.

Never before has the adage "The child is father of the man" been brought to the attention of the economist, statesman, publicist, and medical fraternity as it has since a short time after the beginning of the Great War. The slaughter of the physically fit, the biologic crises brought about by the radical changes in dietary due to the blockades and shortage of crops in belligerent countries has brought home the necessity of not only conserving the life of the infant and child, but also the best means of making it possible for them to become 100 per cent men and women, both mentally and physically. The reduction of child mortality is being considered from all angles, as are the best methods, not only of curing ailments of later years, but of preventing them entirely if possible. Every specialty is, so to speak, vying with the other in this respect. To quote Kugelmass,[2] "The time is here, the place everywhere and the obligation everyone's to serve in the cause of national upbuilding through child welfare, for the child is the embryo of the nation's progress, and the parent of the future generation, the potential citizen." From birth to 17 or 18 years of age the human economy undergoes its most rapid growth and physiologic changes, and naturally if predisposing causes for chronic or semichronic diseases or conditions can be eliminated during this period, what a vast amount of good may be accomplished. To do this a coordination of all branches of medicine and science must be consummated. In our particular line of endeavor monumental work had been done in eliminating foci of infection by the removal of the adenoids and tonsils. Are these the only preadult enemies we have to deal with? Are our little adenoid and tonsil patients getting their

*Candidate's thesis, American Laryngological, Rhinological and Otological Society.

full due when these offending members are removed without
further endeavor being made to ascertain whether other remaining parts are not potential or undermining factors?  In
one large special hospital about 5,000 tonsil and adenoid operations have been performed in a year.  How many of these
patients were actual patients for the future, or even at that
time should have been retained as patients?  The familiar
history of a child breathing through the mouth and incapable
of blowing the nose—certainly the removal of the adenoids
in the majority of these instances will greatly benefit this class
of individuals.  The mere fact that for a definite length of
time there has been more or less complete stoppage of the
nasal passages and consequently a lessened ventilation of these
and neighboring parts strikes one as being far from physiologic.  The normal secretions of the body soon become pathologic secretions when denied their normal flow.  This is particularly so when secretions which have undergone such
changes are located in positions to act in a dual rôle—first
by the absorption of their toxins directly; secondly, by the
disturbance of the digestion, due to their being taken into the
alimentary tract.  Children are notoriously more inclined to
swallow nasopharyngeal discharges than to expectorate them.
It demands but very low mentality to appreciate the train of
disaster that may follow continued interference with the
digestion, particularly in a child who requires sustenance not
only for the repair which is great, due to their activities, but
also to keep pace with the increase in glandular and bodily
growth.

As noted by Mayer,[3] the first recorded case of sinusitis in
an infant was reported by G. A. Rees.[4]  In this instance, as
in so many cases that have been reported since, there were
signs and symptoms so definite that no mistake could be made
regarding the condition present.  The patient was two weeks
old, there was swelling in the left cheek and all the signs of
an active inflammation were present.  Protrusion of the eyeball with the swelling of the eyelids and pointing below the
eye, also sagging of the hard palate of the same side.  Numerous cases have been reported since in infants, from the newborn to several months of age—all, however, with a very
definite symptomatology.  Arvellis[5] in 1898 took up the sub-

ject, and in a very strong and scathing article denied there was
such a condition as maxillary sinus empyema.  He claimed it
to be a tuberculous infection of the bone and offers a case
history in support of his view.  With the advent of the roentgen ray there has been progressive advancement in the early
diagnosis of sinusitis in children, but unfortunately it has
not been impressed upon the minds of rhinologists and others
sufficiently enough that sinusitis is so prevalent in children.
Coffin,[6] one of the earliest if not the earliest, to bring to the
attention of the rhinologist the prevalence of sinusitis in children, carried out an extensive series of roentgen ray examinations of children suffering from eye and ear infections, prov-
ing the association of, if not the actual cause of the above
mentioned conditions.  Dean[7] in a much larger number of
patients comes to the conclusion that in his series about 15
per cent had sinusitis, and that as one single means of diagnosis the roentgen ray examination was the most important,
although he calls attention to the fact that in the antrum of
Highmore a necrosis of the floor may exist with so little discharge that a negative report is rendered, and yet be a cause
of systemic reaction.  The necrosis is found only upon exploring the sinus.

Being impressed with the radiographic reports so frequently
stating "thickened membrane or granulations" in this or that
sinus, it seemed that if roentgen ray examinations of young
patients taken at random from a group of patients about to
be operated upon for adenoid and tonsils (the patients having
been admitted for the sole purpose of adenoid and tonsil
removal), it might throw some light upon these vague reports
in older subjects, therefore in this series on one operative day
a week, five patients were taken from a group of children
awaiting operation.  The first set of five were anesthetized as
for operation and then were radiographed.  This proved very
tedious and required much help and great care, especially as
the X-ray department was on a different floor from the operating room.  These things delayed the operations considerably
and kept the patients under ether an inordinate length of
time for an adenoid and tonsil operation.  Besides these annoying conditions, the inevitable sighing or sobbing respiration was a very difficult problem to handle, from the stand-

point of radiography technic. There was also a great tendency for the nose of the patient to be flattened on the plate
when in frontal position. The hands and other exposed parts
of the person holding the patient's head in position were also
prone to be affected by the rays after one or two exposures.
The remaining 45 were radiographed without anesthesia, and
out of a possible 45 only 3 refused, for upon the least sign
of hesitancy they were quickly separated from the group, as
an old, age long element was being used namely, "mob physiology." First, a general invitation was extended to a group
of waiting patients to visit the "moving picture" room, and
from the volunteers five were selected. Each patient was
asked his or her favorite "movie" star and was designated
as such. The most eager to be "pictured" was allowed to
mount the table first, and from that time on a hearty cooperation of the others was, to say the least, highly amusing. In
this way there was no delay whatever, and the personal interest of each patient was such as to endeavor to make his or
her "picture" the best. Due to this factor excellent plates
were obtainable. Neither punctures of the antra nor any other
line of procedure or treatment as carried out in Dean's[7] series
of cases were attempted. The enormous amount of operative
work and the congested conditions of all wards precluded such
a lengthy routine. (The main reason for such congestion was
the holding in abeyance of all surgical work as far as possible
during the influenza epidemic.) In taking the history of the
50 patients it was impressive to note that 32, or 64 per cent,
had suffered from measles; next was whooping cough, 29
cases, or 58 per cent. Both of these diseases being a highly
catarrhal nature is significant. Next in order of frequency
came a history of colds, ordinary and severe, giving a percentage of 36, and then mumps, 16 per cent. A tubotympanic
catarrh of varying intensity was observed in nearly all patients, but neither from the history nor by examination was
any case of suppurative otitis media listed. Practically all
had some degree of nasopharyngitis with discharge of varying
amount from their noses. The youngest radiographed was
3½ and the eldest 9.

There is some diversity of opinion regarding sinusitis as
an entity, Skillern[8] pointing out that it is a purulent infection

of the antrum, ethmoids and surrounding and intervening bone, and that in children over five years of age it is usually the termination of a socalled cold in the head, when not a sequel to scarlet fever or diphtheria, but he places great stress upon roentgen ray findings. Kerley,[9] discussing Oppenheimer's[9] paper upon sinusitis in children, said that he thought the rhinologist often overlooked cases of sinusitis in children and related how in one instance the rhinologist had cut out everything in sight and out of sight, and still the patient had a profuse discharge from the nose—the sinusitis, according to the inference, having been overlooked entirely. Much laudable work has been done, but there is still much to be accomplished in order to bring to the attention of medical men in general that this condition in children is prevalent. In this series of fifty patients the roentgen ray examinations are of intense interest, for while, as stated previously, detailed and routine examinations of the sinuses were not carried out, the report of the roentgenologist gives an affected sinus as being pathologic, minus or plus, as compared to a sinus being clear. While working out the details of these cases several patients have come under observation, suffering from a suppurative sinusitis, in whom an adenoid and tonsil operation had been performed from one to five or six years previously, but without a curative effect upon the bronchial or discharging nasal condition. All of these patients gave a history of one or more attacks of the diseases of childhood or of catching colds.

A detailed tabulation of the X-ray reports is submitted, and it may not be amiss to call attention to the fact that there is quite a difference in the findings concerning the frontal sinus and the postmortem findings of Davis.[10] Referring to the five different sources of the origin of the frontal sinus he sums up by stating that in any event this sinus has its origin from the ethmoid area. The statement is also made that as an average the frontal sinus is about 3.8 mm. above the nasion at three years of age, and advances at an average of about 1.5 mm. a year until the fifteenth year of age. This would naturally seem at variance with the X-ray findings in which so many absent frontal sinuses were noted. However, one report is an actual findings and the other is on interpretation of shadows, a diametrically opposite starting point. Assuming that the above measurements are correct, in the youngest of the cases tabulated herewith, namely 3½ years, the upper limit of the frontal sinus should be about 4.55 mm. above the nasion, and in the eldest in which the frontal sinus is reported absent, 9 years, it should be about 12.8 mm. Considering the small amount of space involved, it is within the realm of possibility that a frontal sinus may be charted as an ethmoid cell, thereby increasing the number of frontals tabulated as absent.

It is hoped that, due to the interest of a few, children presenting themselves for adenoid and tonsil operation, upon inquiring into the past medical history revealing their having passed through an attack of one or more of the infectious diseases of childhood or of catching colds, a general interest may be aroused to undertake a searching investigation for the presence of a pathologic sinus, and if present to care for such a condition at that time. In other words, to become an expert adenotonsillectomist is not the zenith to be sought by constant application to this operation.

### REFERENCES.

1. Rubner: The Military Surgeon, September, 1919.
2. Kugelmass: The Scientific Monthly, October, 1919.
3. Mayer: The Medical Record, August 10, 1901.
4. Reese: Medical Gazette, N. S., Vol. 45, 1898.
5. Arvellis: Muench Med. Wochensch., No. 45, 1898.
6. Coffin: Trans. Amer. Laryn. Assn., 1914.
7. Dean: Annals Otol., Rhin. and Laryn., June, 1918.
8. Skillern, R. H.: Jour. A. M. A., Vol. 69, No. 11.
9. Oppenheimer: Jour. A. M. A., August 30, 1919.
10. Davis: Sec. Laryn., Otol. and Rhin., Jour. A. M. A., 1918.

| | AGE. | FRONTALS. | ANTRUM. | ETHMOID. | INFECTIOUS DISEASES. |
|---|---|---|---|---|---|
| 1. | 5 | ab. | .......................... | .......................... | meas., whoopg.-cough, colds. |
| 2. | 3½ | ab. | .......................... | .......................... | measles, whooping-cough. |
| 3. | 5 | ab. | .......................... | .......................... | mumps, whoopg.-cough, colds. |
| 4. | 3½ | ab. | .......................... | .......................... | meas., whoopg.-cough, colds. |
| 5. | 6 | ab. | P— | .......................... | meas., mumps, whpg. c., colds. |
| 6. | 5 | ab. | .......................... | P— | meas., whoopg.-cough, colds. |
| 7. | 6 | ex. smll. | P+ | P— | measles, whooping-cough. |
| 8. | 7 | ex. smll. | P+ | .......................... | measles, whooping-cough. |
| 9. | 5 | vy. smll. | P+ | P— | measles, whooping-cough. |
| 10. | 4 | ab. | R&L. P+ | P+ | meas., whopg.-cough, colds. |
| 11. | 6 | ex. smll. | R. P— | .......................... | meas., whopg.-cough, colds. |
| 12. | 7 | ab. | .......................... | .......................... | measles, whooping-cough. |
| 13. | 6 | ab. | .......................... | P— | measles, colds frequent. |
| 14. | 7 | R. P— | .......................... | .......................... | colds frequent. |
| 15. | 7 | .......................... | .......................... | R. P— | meas., mumps, colds frequent. |
| 16. | 9 | R. ab. | R. P— | P—(sph. pr) | .......................... |
| 17. | 4½ | .......................... | L. P— | .......................... | whooping-cough, colds. |
| 18. | 6 | R. ab. | R. P— | .......................... | measles, whooping-cough. |
| 19. | 8 | L. P— | L. P—(sph. vy. lge) | .......................... | measles, whooping-cough. |
| 20. | 7 | L. ab. | R. P—, L. P— | P— | measles, whooping-cough. |
| 21. | 7 | .......................... | P—(sph. pr) | .......................... | measles. |
| 22. | 6 | ab. | .......................... | P— | measles. |
| 23. | 6 | ab. | P+ | P— | meas., mumps, whoopg.-cough. |
| 24. | 5 | ab. | R&L. P— | R&L. P— | measles, whooping-cough. |
| 25. | 7 | ab. | R. P+, L. P— | L. P— | measles, whooping-cough. |
| 26. | 5 | ab. | R&L. P+ | R. P—, L. P+ | .......................... |
| 27. | 5½ | ab. | L. P— | L. P— | measles. |
| 28. | 5 | ab. | R. P+, L. P— | R&L. P— | .......................... |
| 29. | 8 | ex. smll. | R. P—, L. P+ | R&L. P— | .......................... |
| 30. | 6 | smll. | .......................... | .......................... | .......................... |
| 31. | 4 | ab. | R&L. P— | R&L. P— | .......................... |
| 32. | 4 | ab. | R&L. P+ | R&L. P— | measles. |
| 33. | 6 | ab. | R&L. P— | .......................... | .......................... |
| 34. | 7 | ab. | R. P+, L. P— | L. P— | meas., mumps, whoopg.-cough. |
| 35. | 6 | ex. smll. | R. P— | R&L. P— | whooping-cough. |
| 36. | 5 | R. smll, L. ab. | R&L. P— | R&L. P— | measles, colds. |
| 37. | 7 | ab. | R. P— | L. P— | .......................... |
| 38. | 6 | ab. | .......................... | .......................... | meas., whoopg.-cough, colds. |
| 39. | 9 | smll. | .......................... | .......................... | meas., whoopg.-cough, colds. |
| 40. | 5 | R. smll, L. ab. | R&L. P— | R&L. P— | mumps, whooping-cough. |
| 41. | 6 | R. smll, L. ab. | R. P+, L. P— | R&L. P— | meas., mumps, whpg.-c, colds. |
| 42. | 4 | ab. | .......................... | .......................... | mumps, whpg.-cough, colds. |
| 43. | 5 | ab. | R. P—, L. P+ | R&L. P— | .......................... |
| 44. | 3 | ab. | R&L. P+ | .......................... | measles, whooping-cough. |
| 45. | 7 | smll. | L. P— | L. P—(sph. pr) | .......................... |
| 46. | 4 | ab. | .......................... | R&L. P+ | diphtheria, colds. |
| 47. | 6 | ab. | R. P— | R&L. P— | measles. |
| 48. | 8 | smll.R.P&ex.S.L. | R&L. P+ | R&L. P—(sph. pr) | measles, diphtheria. |
| 49. | 4 | ab. | R&L. P+ | R&L. P+ | meas., whpg.-c., diphth. colds. |
| 50. | 6 | ex. smll. | L. P— | R&L. P— | whooping-cough. |

10 patients gave no history of childhood diseases.
 8 patients had no pathological sinus with history of childhood diseases.
32 patients with pathological sinus had history of childhood diseases.
29 patients with pathological sinus had history of whooping-cough.
 8 patients with pathological sinus had history of mumps.
18 patients with pathological sinus had history of colds.
 3 patients with pathological sinus had history of diphtheria.
41 patients radiographically showed pathological sinuses.

# XIII

# ATYPICAL MASTOIDITIS WITH REPORT OF THREE CASES.

By Elbyrne Gill, M. D.,

Roanoke, Va.

Etiology, pathology, symptoms and signs of uncomplicated typical mastoiditis are well known to all competent otologists, and a mere narration of these conditions would be of no avail. It is the purpose of the writer to report what is to his mind three cases of atypical mastoiditis.

Case 1.—Carl D., age 11. History: March 7, 1920, left ear began discharging. March 11, swelling appeared above his zygoma. On the following day, March 12, the swelling had extended almost to the median line of the head. Also swelling extended across his face to the left eye which resembled erysipelas. On the following day, March 13, the right eyelid was swollen shut, and on March 15 the swelling had left the eyelids on both sides. The swelling above his zygoma had increased in size and was now extended to the median line of the forehead. From March 7 to March 15 the patient ran a temperature of 101 to 103. On March 15 I advised and performed a simple mastoid operation, making the regular mastoid incision, different only in that I carried the incision higher than usual. When the incision extended through the periosteum about eight ounces of pus escaped. Pus was under the periosteum. On exposing the mastoid cortex two small perforations were found, one just above and one just posterior to the spine of Henley. The mastoid cortex was opened and the antrum entered. There was no pus in the mastoid bone or antrum. The bone was in the stage of hyperemia, and there were a few granulations in the mastoid antrum. The infection from the ear and from the evacuated pus was pneumococcus. The patient left the hospital a week following the operation and made a complete and uneventful recovery. The points of interest in this case are: 1. The short aural history, which was not preceded by any systemic condition. 2. The subperiosteal swelling was above the temporal ridge and extended to the median line of the forehead.  3. Absence of any pus in the mastoid process.

Case 2.—L. T. S., age 50, was first seen March 5, 1920. Patient gave a history of having had influenza for the week previous and was now suffering with pain in the left ear. Physical examination revealed a red and bulging drum membrane, which was incised and was followed by profuse discharge.  Patient did not give history of any previous ear trouble.  The discharge continued for two weeks, during which time the patient had no mastoid tenderness and no pain but was running a temperature of 101 to 102½ each day. At the end of two weeks, on account of the profuse discharge, which showed a pneumococcus infection and considerable elevation of temperature, I decided to send the patient to the hospital, where she could have an X-ray examination of the mastoid as well as of the chest.  The X-ray examination of the mastoid showed increased density and cloudiness, but was not operative from an X-ray standpoint.  The X-ray examination of the chest revealed a resolving bronchopneumonia.  In a few days her chest condition cleared up and her temperature dropped to the normal line and remained so for an entire week, during which time the aural discharge continued to be profuse.  During this week the patient had absolutely no pain and no mastoid tenderness, and the second X-ray examination of the mastoid showed a slight increase in the density and cloudiness but was not operative from an X-ray standpoint. The physical examination of the fundus of the ear showed a distinct sagging of the posterosuperior wall.  In spite of the negative X-ray reports and the normal temperature for a week and absence of any other signs of mastoiditis a simple mastoid operation was advised for the following reasons: 1. There had been a continuous and profuse discharge for three weeks, with no sign of abatement. 2. The distinct sagging of the posterosuperior wall.  The operation was done March 26, 1920.  On opening the mastoid cortex, which was very thick, a profuse amount of pus escaped which was under pressure. The entire mastoid process was broken down throughout. There were a large number of postsinus cells.  The entire mastoid tip was broken down and was removed.  A small area of dura was exposed in the middle fossa. The sinus was not exposed. The patient left the hospital one week following the operation. On May 10, 1920, her hearing in the operative ear was practically as good as in the other. The points of interest in this case are as follows: 1. The absence of mastoid tenderness. 2. Normal temperature for one week preceding the operation. 3. Entire absence of pain. 4. The two X-ray examinations which did not indicate an operation from an X-ray standpoint.

Case 3.—D. L. R., age 56, was first seen April 20, 1920. Patient gave the following history: On April 18, patient began having pain in the right ear. Had had tonsillitis for a week previous. Physical examination on April 20 showed a marked furuncular condition of his external auditory canal. The swelling was so extensive as to prevent a satisfactory examination of the drum membrane. Patient had considerable pain and marked tenderness of the mastoid tip but not of the mastoid antrum. Pressure on the tragus caused severe pain. His temperature at this time was 103. My diagnosis at this time was furunculosis of the external auditory canal. The patient was placed on treatment for this condition, and when seen on the following day, Wednesday, April 21, was feeling more comfortable and his temperature was 101. The swelling of the external canal still prevented a satisfactory examination of the drum membrane. On Thursday morning, April 22, I received a telephone call from a member of the patient's family saying that his condition was worse than it had been and that he was suffering most excruciating pain. Examination at this date showed a small perforation in the superior quadrant of the drum membrane in the region of the vault. From it there was escaping a small amount of serosanguinous discharge. Patient was exceedingly tender over entire mastoid process. I was satisfied that the patient was suffering from suppurative mastoiditis, and upon that conviction I advised an operation. The X-ray examination revealed a marked increased density and cloudiness of the bone. The bacteriologic examination of the aural discharge showed a pneumococcus infection. On Thursday, April 22, 1920, a simple mastoid operation was performed. The entire mastoid process was very soft and broken down. Pus was present in the mastoid tip and mastoid antrum.   A number of large cells were found posterior to the lateral sinus.   Four days following the operation the patient developed erysipelas which disappeared after a week's duration.   Patient left the hospital two weeks following the operation and has made a complete recovery.   The points of interest in this case are as follows:   1. History of ear trouble which was of only four days' standing. 2. The extensive furuncular condition which to a certain extent masked the symptoms arising from the middle ear.

# XIV

# ACCIDENTS IN AURAL PARACENTESIS.

## By Jerome F. Strauss, M. D.,

### Chicago.

A severe hemorrhage from the ear, necessitating actual hemostatic measures for control, and a similar case with a less severe but continuous loss of blood for a period of several days occurred some time ago in my hospital service, following incisions in the tympanic membrane for acute purulent otitis media. These accidents, being the first of my experience and also in the larger experience of those gentlemen with whom I am associated, led me to search otologic literature with the idea of obtaining some information regarding the frequency of such cases. I have found but little to reward my search. either because accidents of the kind are rare or because professional pride places such episodes in the category of unreportable cases. I found in all less than twenty references to the subject, but sufficient, I hope, to interest you for a few moments.

When Riolanus first suggested the perforation of the tympanic membrane as a relief for deafness, in the middle of the seventeenth century, his proposal was based on the result of the accidental perforation of the drum in a deaf patient with subsequent partial restoration of hearing. His contention, and that of Plemp a few years later, that air was necessary in the tympanic cavity to permit normal hearing, was supported by Valsalva's demonstration that there was a passage of air from the mouth to the middle ear. The operation was first performed by Valsalva in 1740 without success, and again by Eli, who has something of the reputation of a charlatan, in 1760. The latter's success or failure is not on record.

In 1800, Cooper, who first published the experiments of Wm. Cheselden, cited four cases of deafness cured by perforation of the ear drum. These cases, together with a successfully operated case reported by Hymly, aroused a marked degree of enthusiasm in the profession and even among the laity; and for a short time paracentesis was hailed as a panacea for deafness. Hymly and Cooper gave as indications for the operation the closure of the eustachian tube and blood extravasation into the tympanic cavity. Saunders, of London, in 1804, was probably the first to recommend empyema of the tympanum as an indication.

These indications were not universally accepted by the profession, and a great number of the medical men of the period practiced and advised the puncture as a cure for deafness. This large group includes such names as Ribes, Itard, Dubois and Deleau in France, S. Cooper, Hunold and Wright in England, and Rust, Kawerz and Arneman in Germany. In consequence of the activity of this school and the relatively few successful results of their work, the general enthusiasm was soon dampened, and the emphasis by Hymly on the fact that the operation could be applicable in only certain selected cases brought about a temporary discarding of the operation.

The accidents in the early days of paracentesis were many and varied. The records are, of course, meager and inexact, and in the light of present day knowledge, were practically entirely due to infections and the crude instrumentation of the time. Thus, Hymly, in 1806, cited examples of grave and fatal accidents following perforation, and Fuchs, in 1810, reported many cases in which the operation was followed by headaches, convulsions, and fevers of a serious nature. It is probable, judging from the incomplete evidence now obtainable, that the fatalities which occurred were due to sinus thrombosis, meningitis and intracranial abscess. Muller, in his inaugural dissertation at Halle in 1890, stated that the operative procedure was considered relatively if not absolutely free from danger until the middle of the nineteenth century when deaths were reported by Hubert-Valleroux in France and by Butcher, an English physician.

Secondary infection of the ear cavity was a frequent occurrence in those cases in which paracentesis was performed to relieve deafness. Schwartze found it in 20 per cent of the cases operated upon at Halle, and he intimates that this percentage increased proportionately as new and more complicated intraaural operative procedures were devised.

In present day otology the one accident complicating incision of the tympanic membrane in ordinary cases of suppurative otitis media seems to be extensive hemorrhage. The first case on record is mentioned by Gruber in the 1888 edition of his textbook. The accident occurred with a patient whose drum membrane had been opened a few days previous uneventfully. Symptoms requiring a repetition of the operation developed, and an incision was made in the posterior inferior segment. The blood poured out so copiously that it appeared as if a large vein had been divided. More than ten ounces of blood were lost before the hemorrhage was controlled by tightly packing the canal with cotton wool soaked with perchlorid of iron.

In 1890 Ludwig reported the first case of such hemorrhage in periodic literature. In this case a translucent blue coloration was noticeable in the posterior inferior quadrant, but was not considered of any importance. The first incision permitted a clear serous fluid to escape, and the opening was then dilated with a needle. This maneuver brought forth a sudden stream of dark blood which filled a large pus basin before the canal was effectively packed with firm tampons. Recovery was uneventful.

Hildebrant reported a case in 1891 occurring in a rhacitic child showing well marked deformities of the joints and cranium. Paracentesis was performed on a lusterless, reddened bulging membrane in the usual manner. Immediately there escaped a stream of venous blood as large as the small finger in diameter. Because the canal was promptly packed the loss of blood was not great. It was shown later on this patient that the light reflex on the affected side changed its shape when the internal jugular vein of that side was compressed. It was also noted that all the veins of the neck and scalp were enlarged on this side.

The first fatal case was reported by Brieger in 1892. After paracentesis of the membrane in this case, the incision was enlarged with the pointed galvanocautery, and the jugular vein was perforated. The hemorrhage was readily controlled by tamponade, but pyemia and death resulted.

Seligman demonstrated a case of injury to the bulbus vena jugularis during paracentesis, in 1893, and McKernon reported the first instance of the kind in this country in 1894. The latter case McKernon claimed was arterial hemorrhage, the blood spurting out with rhythmic pressure for a distance of two feet. Firmly tamponing the canal, and pressure on the carotid artery for half an hour controlled the bleeding.

Other instances recorded are those of Max (1905), Castex (1905) and two of Lueder's (1912). Castex's patient developed a facial paralysis nine days after the injury to the bulb. In one of Lueder's cases bleeding recurred in spite of all external precautions, and it was necessary to expose the lateral sinus and pack above and below the bulb. Pyemia developed in this case and resulted fatally.

The anatomic changes necessary to produce these accidents are not many. A congenital absence or thinning of the bony capsule of the bulb may exist, or the condition may be acquired through metabolic disease in the early developing years of life. Friedlowsky, in 1868, published a report on the dissection of one thousand skulls, in only one of which the bulb protruded into the tympanic cavity. Muller found more frequent anomalies, and these occurred in skulls which showed other anatomic defects of bone formation, partly congenital and partly as a result of rhacitis. The cases of Ludwig, Hildebrandt and Max, cited above, were definitely rhacitic, the osseous changes being apparent in joints and skull. Körner in 1892 published his study of two negro heads, wherein, had paracentesis been performed, severe hemorrhage could scarcely have been avoided. Zuckerkandl, Toynbee, Von Troltsch and others have made similar observations, and I might add the unusual case of Lannois, a "venous hernia," in which the jugular fossa was dilated to an extent that it replaced the middle ear cavity and a portion of the external auditory canal.

In 1903 Hansen reported a case in which the internal carotid artery coursed through the tympanum in such a way that if the ear drum had been incised during life the vessel must have been seriously injured. A similar case was published by Max, discovered during life, attention being called to it by the rhythmic pulsation of the drum synchronous with the heart beat, and which was not apparent after firm pressure was applied to the internal carotid artery. It is very probable that McKernon's case was one of this type, in which, during violent exercise the artery or an anomalous branch ruptured within the tympanic cavity and thus produced the symptoms for which the ear drum was incised.

The following cases attracted my attention to the literature on this subject:

. Case 1.—C. S., age 8 years. After thirty-six hours of acute earache he had been taken to a physician's office, where, after otoscopy, a paracentesis was performed, following which there was an immediate gush of blood from the auditory canal, which evidently was sufficient to cause concern to the operator, who hastily inserted a firm wad of cotton and brought the patient to the hospital. When seen by us, blood was steadily oozing through the temporary packing. On removal of the cotton wad the gushing of venous blood was resumed, and the only course to pursue was immediate firm repacking of the canal. This served to control the bleeding and the patient recovered uneventfully. The patient was subsequently examined by Dr. Abt, who was able to demonstrate a Harrison's grove, some deformities of the heads of the long bones and the remnants of a rhacitic rosary.

Case 2.—B. D., age 7 months. This infant was brought to the hospital forty-eight hours after a paracentesis, during which period he had continued to ooze a slow but steady drip of blood from the ear. The little canal had been packed with gauze twice without success, and the condition was becoming serious. Pallor was marked and pulse rapid.

An adrenalin soaked tape was inserted deeply into the canal and tightly packed. This treatment evidently slowed up the hemorrhage, for though the packing was blood soaked in a few hours there was no further bleeding. Subsequent history and examination revealed the fact that the patient was a hemophiliac. The patient made a recovery after treatment with horse serum, which was in vogue at the time, and a course of calcium internally.

# XV

## ASTHENIC HYPOACOUSIS.*
### BY H. J. INGLIS, M. D.,
#### BOSTON.

Fatigue of the auditory nerve as it appears in its aggravated forms, such as occupational disease, and in certain phases of neurasthenia is commonly recognized and promptly classified by the average aurist. I doubt, however, that the loss of auditory function as an indication, or a consequence of general debility, is given the discriminating consideration and the importance which it deserves in the differentiation of nonsuppurative forms of ear disease.

Dr. Emerson and others have told us of the effects of toxins, emanating from infected tonsils and suppurating nasal sinuses, which exercise a selective action upon the auditory apparatus. The type of cases which I wish to consider are independent of toxemia, having as their etiology overwork, mental strain, prolonged anxiety, and other conditions resulting in lowered physical and nervous vitality.

The recognition of this type of disorder is most important from the standpoint of prognosis; for the outstanding features which the functional examination shows are diminished bone conduction and lowering of the upper tone limit, and we are very apt to look upon these points in a hearing test as discouraging evidence of actual degeneration of the sound perceptive apparatus.

From a rather large amount of material I have selected for study fifty cases of asthenic hypoacousis which are "pure"— that is to say, from them all possibility of confusing concurrent conditions such as middle ear dsiease, syphilis, hysteria, etc., has been eliminated. These fifty cases have been divided into three groups according to the characteristics of the hearing tests.

These groups are: 1. Those showing little loss of quantitative hearing, diminished bone conduction and lowering of the

---

*Candidate's thesis. American Laryngological, Rhinological and Otological Society.

upper tone limit. 2. Those showing noticeable loss of hearing, diminished bone conduction and no disturbance of the upper tone limit. 3. Those showing noticeable loss of hearing, diminished bone conduction and lowering of upper tone limit.

In none of these cases is the perception of low tones affected. Tinnitus and various types of discomfort about the ears are common but not characteristic.

Only a few cases fall into Group 1, chiefly because most of these were discovered by chance while the patients were being examined for some entirely different condition. Also many cases which might have been included in this group were discarded because of a possible hysterical element.

This group is typified by the story of a gentleman who had brought himself up, by hard work, from a humble position to one of great responsibility in a manufacturing concern, and who was induced by a medical friend, interested in the relation of physical fitness to business efficiency, to undergo a general physical examination.

He went about it with characteristic thoroughness, entered a private hospital for twenty-four hours and was examined by an oculist, an aurist and an internist. His urine was examined, the Wassermann test performed and an X-ray examination for abscessed teeth carried through.

The story which he told of his present condition was that he was tired and somewhat nervous, worked very hard, had occasional palpitation, and, about every ten days, had severe headache centering in his eyes, which he ascribed to overwork. He did not use alcohol or tobacco. He was 44 years old.

The positive findings on examination, as submitted by the various men were: Blood pressure, 164-120; slightest possible trace of albumen and very rare small fine granular casts in the urine; refractive error well corrected by glasses, and considerable strain of the eye muscles, due to overuse; some pyorrhea alveolaris and hemorrhoids. His hearing test showed:

| A.D. 20/20 | 40/12 | 16 | 1.00 |
|---|---|---|---|
| W.V.(Numbers) | Rinné (512) | Low limit | Upper limit |
| | | (Dench fork) | Galton |
| A.S. 20/20 | 40/15 | 16 | .9 |

The unanimous diagnosis was overwork.

In Group 2, which comprises 38 per cent of the cases, comes a professor of music in a large college, who had just finished his year's work.

Three years previously he had had tinnitus for a while, which disappeared spontaneously. There was no further trouble until one week before he presented himself for examination, when his ears began to feel stuffy and a buzzing tinnitus intruded. He had recently felt tired and nervous.

Examination of ears, nose and throat showed nothing of moment. His eustachian tubes opened easily and inflation did not affect his hearing or his tinnitus.

His hearing test showed:

| A.D. 10/20 | 60/20 | 16 | N |
|---|---|---|---|
| W.V. (Numbers) | Rinné | Low limit (Dench fork) | High tones |
| A.S. 12/20 | 50/18 | 16 | N |

Group 3 produced 50 per cent of the cases and includes a lady 47 years old, an employe of a publishing house, who had suffered great and prolonged mental distress.

Her general physical and nervous condition was deplorable. She fainted during the examination.

For about one year she had been growing deaf in her right ear. The hearing in her left ear had recently fallen off steadily and rapidly.

Her hearing test showed:

| A.D. 4/20 | 50/20 | 16 | 1.00 |
|---|---|---|---|
| W.V. (Numbers) | Rinné (512) | Low limit (Dench fork) | Upper limit Galton |
| A.S. 3/20 | 40/12 | 16 | 1.00 |

The details of the history and examination in these cases have been rather sketchily presented, but let it be understood that what has not been mentioned did not occur. Each case throughout the series was completely examined as to nose, throat, nasopharynx and eustachian tubes, and, where indicated, a general examination was obtained and the investigation completed with X-ray plates and the Wassermann reaction.

One lapse in the functional examination needs explanation. That is the use of numbers only, in estimating the perception of the whispered voice. This method is, in a measure, inaccurate; for patients with their attention fixed on certain known sounds, where combinations are. limited, will more easily interpret these sounds than they will those represented by isolated words or a series of words making up a sentence. The result is that their perception for voice is overestimated.

On the other hand, the use of numbers has an advantage in so far as high and low pitched sounds may be systematically employed at will, the result easily recorded and an adequate basis is established for comparison in future tests. In a whispered sentence we not only bring in the element of enunciation but letters and syllables of varied pitch are uncontrollably intermingled, and it is very difficult to record the results, unless the same words and sentences are employed at subsequent examination. This is particularly true in these cases where the nerve is quickly fatigued.

From the material in hand I have tried to produce a sort of composite hearing test representative of auditory asthenia, in order to form a comparison between it and the derangements produced in other disorders of the cochlear nerve. This empiric record has been produced by a general averaging of the various tests with the exception of the Rinné, which is founded on an average of the air conduction and a ratio estimation of the bone conduction. The result is as follows:

| Whispered voice | Rinné | Low limit | Upper limit |
|---|---|---|---|
| | | | Galton |
| 14/20 | 50/17 | 16 | .9 |

The Weber test is uncertain. As a rule it simply follows to the ear with the best bone conduction.

Although the above is an average of the perception for whispered voice and high pitched sounds, in some cases the former was as low as 1/20, and loss of high tones as much as 2.1 on the Galton whistle.

The condition is usually bilateral with the two ears showing a fairly uniform deterioration.

In examining this hearing test the one distinguishing feature which is apparent is the preservation of air conduction for the C2 tuning fork used in the Rinné, and in going over the whole series no case was found in which duration of perception for the C2 fork by air was below the normal limits, even where the whispered voice and perception of high tones were most affected. In other words, within the ordinary register, the defect in function is failure of the capacity for the fine discrimination required in selecting and coordinating sounds rather than the lack of response to simple tone.

Of course, where there is a defect in the peripheral portion of the sound perceptive apparatus, regardless of pathology, the functional examination must show fairly uniform results; but it is interesting to compare simple asthenia with some of the other diseases from the standpoint of the Rinné tests.

For example: In secondary degeneration of the organ of Corti following long standing middle ear disease, we find such a hearing test.

| Forced whisper | Rinné | Low limit | Galton |
|---|---|---|---|
| 8 in. | 5/0 | 512 | 2.00 |

Occupational disease in a man who worked many years in a boiler shop gives us the following:

| Whispered voice | Rinné | Low limit | Galton |
|---|---|---|---|
| 2/30 | 10/10 | 64 | 20 |

The effect of large doses of quinin is shown in this:

| Whispered voice | Rinné | Low limit | Galton |
|---|---|---|---|
| 4/20 | 20/15 | 16 | 2.00 |

Advanced otosclerosis showed:

| Forced whisper | Rinné | Low limit | Galton |
|---|---|---|---|
| 6 in. | 14/22 | 96 | 2.5 |

In all of these examples (actual ones taken from records) the proportionate falling off of the air conduction for the C2 fork is obvious.

The nearest approach to the tests found in asthenia of the auditory apparatus is shown in a case of active secondary syphilis which had not been treated. Incidentally this young man laid his difficulty to overwork and excessive outdoor speaking, for he was engaged in lecturing to soldiers on sexual hygiene and the curse of "social diseases."

He gave the following results:

| | | | | |
|---|---|---|---|---|
| A. D. | 1 foot | 30/10 | 16 | .9 |
| | Forced whisper | Rinné | Low limit | Galton |
| A. S. | 1 foot | 40/10 | 16 | 1.2 |

He had a secondary rash and a positive Wassermann.

A short time ago loss of bone conduction was given a good deal of attention as a diagnostic point in syphilis. This has recently been descredited to a large extent, and I venture to say that while a large proportion of cases that have syphilis actually involving the auditory apparatus may have reduced bone conduction, in the general run of patients, nervous debility will be found to be responsible for the loss of bone conduction much more frequently than syphilis.

Auditory neurasthenia must not be confused with hysteria. The latter is always easily detected by the variety of results obtained in repeated hearing tests. One case gave me in three hearing tests in a few days the following results for the Rinné:

$$\text{A. D.} \quad 40/10 \quad 60/28 \quad 60/10$$
$$\text{A. S.} \quad 55/20 \quad 58/23 \quad 45/15$$

In asthenic hypoacousis, then, we have patients who tell a story of general fatigue or nerve strain, a rather sudden realization that they do not hear conversation as well as formerly —perhaps of tinnitus, a sensation of stuffiness or slight shootings pains about the ears. Vertigo is not particularly common.

Upon examination there is no serious abnormality found about the nose or throat, the appearance of the tympanic membrane gives no impression of disease, and the eustachian tubes are normal patent. The functional examination shows a certain degree of loss of hearing for the whispered voice, relatively high preservation of perception by air of the C2 fork and absolute diminution of perception for the same fork by bone conduction, the apprehension of low tones unaffected and in the majority of cases a lowering of the upper tone limit.

When we have a pure case of asthenia presented the diagnosis should be fairly easy. Unfortunately, it is often confused by the coincidental existence of some other form of disease. This is most likely to be simple chronic otitis media and, as a rule, careful scrutiny of the hearing test and a shrewd estimation of the potential pathology about the nose and throat, especially if the middle ear disease be one sided, will serve to disentangle the two elements of the disorder. If, however, the complicating disease is one involving the labyrinth or auditory nerve the immediate diagnosis is difficult.

The failure to properly segregate the neurasthenic element from other complicating conditions undoubtedly explains the surprising improvement which sometimes occurs in patients whom we have considered the victims of an incurable form of deafness.

As was mentioned at the beginning, the recognition of auditory neurasthenia is of great importance from a prognostic standpoint; for in this disease the prognosis is good for the recovery of a large part of the lost hearing, whereas, in the other conditions where the functional examination gives similar results the prognosis is bad.

The recovery of the hearing is directly dependent upon the individual's capacity for recuperating his general condition. Under favorable conditions, even where the perception for voice has fallen off considerably, the restoration of function may be rapid, as is shown in the case described above to illustrate Group 3. At the end of two weeks, after a course of general treatment had been instituted, her perception for whispered voice had more than doubled.

Under rigid general treatment, in cases where the change in the upper register is slight, and the relative loss of bone conduction in the Rinné does not exceed one-third, one can promise the patient practically complete recovery. The dropping of the high tones and the loss of bone conduction are the factors which determine the measure of recovery, rather than the extent to which the perception of voice has suffered. By the time the upper tone limit has been reduced to 1.00 on the Galton and the perception for the C2 fork by bone has fallen below ten seconds the promises of recovery must be restricted.

One word must be added in regard to treatment. It does not suffice to give the patients a tonic and tell them to rest, but rather they should be entrusted to the care of a patient and careful internist who is capable of carrying out a scientific regulation of the patient's daily life.

Local treatment is of little use.

## XVI.

## PARALYSIS OF THE EXTERNAL RECTUS IN THE RIGHT EYE FOLLOWING MASTOIDITIS IN THE LEFT EAR.

By DUNBAR ROY, M. D.,

ATLANTA.

There has been reported by several observers such a fairly authentic number of cases of abducens paralysis of the eye in conjunction with diseased conditions of the middle ear and mastoid, as to make the subject one of clinical interest and to establish the fact that it is a complication by no means of infrequent. occurrence.

Practically all of the cases reported have shown the paralysis to exist on the same side as the ear involved, and it is for this reason that I present the following case where the abducens paralysis occurred on the opposite side.

In the last few years this subject has been much discussed and several cases reported under various captions. The most exhaustive article has probably been written by Dr. Chas. E. Perkins, published in the ANNALS OF OTOLOGY, RHINOLOGY AND LARYNGOLOGY, for September, 1910. All the succeeding writers have referred extensively to this article and have really made it the basis of their own conclusions. The article by Dr. John M. Wheeler in the A. M. A. Journal, November 23, 1918, and the one by Dr. T. J. Maybaum of New York deal with the report of cases and at the same time discuss the subject in a very similar manner.

Ophthalmologists recognize the fact that isolated paralysis of the abducens nerve is by no means of infrequent occurrence. Its etiology in the large majority of cases is obscure. In 1919 the writer read a paper before this society on "Malignant Diseases of the Sphenoid Sinus" in which he called attention to the fact that the paralysis of the abducens nerve was one of the first symptoms observed and gave in detail its anatomic position, showing that it was the one most easily affected from pressure of any character at the base of the brain or even a slight meningitis. For this reason it is very difficult to trace the etiology of abducens paralysis unless an unfortunate postmortem should have given this important information, as has been mentioned by Perkins in his very excellent bibliography. Isolated cases of abducens paralysis bear a strong resemblance to the isolated cases of facial nerve paralysis. The etiology of both of these conditions is quite obscure, and yet if they occur in conjunction with a middle ear involvement their etiology takes on a more definite aspect. Syphilis, rheumatic diathesis, catching cold, are all supposedly a possible cause for these isolated paralyses, but just what is the real anatomic pathology can only be conjectured.

Extension of an inflammation from the middle ear and mastoid along the various routes mentioned by Perkins would certainly be sufficiently explanatory in the large majority of cases, but where the paralysis occurs in the abducens on the opposite side from the ear involved, it is quite difficult to arrive at a satisfactory explanation. One of the triad symptoms —i. e., severe pain on the side of the face, was entirely absent in my case, which would lead us to conclude that the gasserian ganglion was not involved. The peculiar feature in this case was the opposite side paralysis showing the difficulty in tracing its pathology, and following its clinical report I have taken the liberty of compiling a report of all cases to be found in the literature where the paralysis occurred in the eye opposite to the ear involved.

L. J., white, age 10½ years, was brought to my office by his physician on July 17, 1915, with the following history:

On January 3, a month previous, the patient was suddenly seized with an earache in the right ear. Six days later it began to discharge, following which all pain and fever disappeared, and with the exception of the discharge the patient seemed thoroughly comfortable. On July 4, one month after the initial symptoms, the discharge suddenly ceased, some pain returned and a swelling developed over the mastoid. This was treated by his physician without results, hence the consultation. The writer was requested to take charge of the case. The temperature at this time was 101 F. The swelling over the mastoid was tender and fluctuating, showing every evidence of a subperiosteal abscess. The patient's appearance was cachectic.

He was immediately sent to the hospital, and next day, February 18, a complete exenteration of the mastoid was made. On making my incision no pus escaped as was expected but, on the contrary, we found the swelling due to an enlarged gland. Underneath this the cortex of the mastoid was soft and the whole tip was found to be necrotic. There was very little pus in the antrum, but the sinus was exposed when necrotic sequestra of bone were removed. The cavity was lightly packed with iodoform gauze and the lower end of the wound left open. This was removed on the fifth day. There was never any pain or rise in temperature. Patient left the hospital in one week. The next day after the operation it was noticed that the patient kept the lids of the right eye closed, although they could be voluntarily opened. Two weeks after the operation the wound was nearly healed, and for the first time the writer noticed a paralysis of the left external rectus with the consequent internal strabismus of the same eye. The patient also complained of diplopia.

Examination showed vision to be normal in both eyes and absolutely no fundus changes. Three weeks after the operation the mastoid cavity was healed, showing remarkable tissue vitality, the only complaint being the double vision. A Wassermann examination was negative, as also a tuberculin test.

The patient was placed upon gradually increasing doses of the iodid of potassium and allowed to go away in the country. Two months later he was again seen and the hearing test showed this to be normal. He had much improved in appearance, having gained ten pounds. The paralysis was gradually subsiding. On June 15th, five months after the initial symptoms of middle ear suppuration, the patient had recovered and the paralysis of the external rectus had entirely disappeared.

### CASE REPORTS AND COMMENTS.

Rimini, S.: La paralysis de l'oculomoteur externe d'origine auriculaire. Arch Internal. de Laryngol., XXI, 125, 1906.

One case in a child aged 7. Bilateral otitis after scarlatina, followed by mastoiditis on the left side; mastoid operation.

After the operation patient complained of frontal headache, pain in the left eye and diplopia. Examination showed paralysis of the external rectus of both eyes, at first more marked on the right side. As this paralysis in the right side gradually diminished, that on the left side gradually increased. In two months all eye symptoms had disappeared.

Collinet: Meningite d'origine otique avec paralysis due moteur oculàire externe. Bull. d. Laryngol., Otol. and Rhinol., X, 90, 1907.

Reports one case in a young woman age 20. In August, 1905, suppurative otitis in the left ear, the pain being alleviated when ear began to discharge. Toward the end of September, return of symptoms with severe headache, nausea and constipation. Diplopia noted at this time. In the early part of October symptoms became more severe, with evidences of meningitis, and the mastoid operation was performed. Before the operation a very decided strabismus in the right eye was observed. After the operation all symptoms improved, but the eye muscle paralysis persisted for some time, diminishing gradually. Four weeks after the operation the right eye could be normally abducted, and diplopia was noted whenever the patient was tired. These symptoms finally disappeared entirely, and the patient was in excellent general health after a rest in the country. No lumbar puncture was done in this case, but the symptoms indicated meningitis. The paralysis of the external rectus of the eye on the side opposite to the diseased ear is difficult to explain; there was evidently some lesion along the course of the nerve which healed gradually.

Quadri, A.: Otite meyenne aigue gauche; mastoidite; paralysis de la sixieme pairs du cote droit. Rev. hebd. de laryngol., II, 100, 1908.

One case, man, age 48. Acute otitis in the left ear. In spite of repeated paracentesis and thorough drainage of the ear, mastoiditis resulted, and the mastoid operation was performed; no cerebral lesion. Four weeks after the operation the patient complained of headache; a cervical swelling developed on the left side which was repeatedly drained. The patient one day complained of diplopia, and examination showed paralysis of the sixth cranial nerve on the right side. This paralysis lasted

36 days. The cervical phlegmon did not heal for several months. The author is unable to explain the eye paralysis in this case.

Furet, F.: Otite suppurée droite ancienne; mastoidite; operation. paralysie de la sixieme paire gauche; guerison. Ann. d. mal. de l'oreille, du larynx (etc.), 34, 659, 1908.

Reports one case observed in 1895. Boy, age 14; chronic suppurative on the right side. Mastoid operation. Fifteen days later, patient saw double, complained of severe headache. Examination showed paralysis of the sixth cranial nerve on the left side; nystagmus and diplopia.

General condition of the patient improved, and eye symptoms had disappeared in a month.

Commenting on the case, the author notes that this paralysis of the external rectus of the eye on the side opposite to the diseased ear is very rare. He has found in literature only two other cases—Collinet and Quadri.

Savariaud and Dutheillet de Lamothe: Un cas de meningite sereuse otogene guerie avec paralysie du moteur oculaire externe du cote oppose à la lesion auriculaire. Bull. d'oto-rhino-laryngol., XV, 206, 1912.

One case in a child aged 8½ with acute otitis and symptoms of meningitis on the right side. Operation at which an extradural abscess was found. The day after the operation, horizontal nystagmus, five days later a sudden rise in temperature and meningitis with the cerebrospinal fluid under greatly increased pressure. Condition was greatly improved by repeated lumbar punctures, but two days later, paralysis of external rectus of the eye on the left side developed with diplopia and internal strabismus. At the time of the report the child was in excellent general health, but the ocular paralysis was still present, although gradually diminishing. The mastoid operation was done on December 21, 1911: the date of the report was February 9, 1912.

Paullier, A.: Contribution a l'etude des paralysies de la vle paire cran iene survenant au cours de lesions auriculaires du cote oppose a ces lesions. Paris Thesis, 1912.

Pallier reviews the cases cited above and adds the following from the literature:

1. Bonnier (Compt. rend. soc. d. biol. ser. X, 2, 368, 1895). After the Stacke operation for a chronic otitis in the left ear patient complained of seeing double, and of incessant vertigo. The left eye was in forced adduction; this condition later extended to the right eye, probably due to paralysis of abducens extending from the left side to the right.

2. Strazza (Arch. ifal. d. d. otol., XVIII, 403, 1907). Patient age 51; otitis media on left side with mastoiditis. Previous to the mastoid operation, paralysis of the abducens nerve on the left side was noted; about one month after the operation headaches recurred, and a paralysis of the abducens on the right side developed. The symptoms gradually disappeared.

3. Blauluet (Report to societe parisienne d'tologie, 1909, original not found here). Patient 18, otitis in the right ear in March, 1908, resulting later in mastoiditis, for which the mastoid operation was performed on April 7, 1909. Previous to operation the patient saw double, and a slight strabismus was noted in the right eye. After the operation, on April 12, convergent strabismus and diplopia due to a paralysis of the external rectus of both eyes developed, but more accentuated on the left side. Lumbar puncture showed increased pressure of cerebrospinal fluid; after the puncture the eye symptoms greatly improved, and in a short time disappeared altogether.

The author in discussing these cases points out that where lumbar puncture has been performed, it has always shown increased pressure of the cerebrospinal fluid. He believes that paralysis of the abducens nerve on the side opposite to the diseased ear is due to the increased pressure of the cerebrospinal fluid acting upon a nerve which for some cause or other shows diminished resistance.

In treatment, he believes no further operation is necessary except to insure proper drainage of the diseased mastoid. Lumbar puncture, however, is indicated until the cerebrospinal hypertension is reduced.

Rousseau, F.: Les paralysies des nerfs moteurs le l'oeil au cours les otites moyennes suppurees et leurs complications. Ann. d'ocul., CLIII, 530, 1916.

Rousseau states that the paralysis of the external rectus of the eye in otitis is usually noted on the side of the affected ear, but may be observed on the opposite side and exceptionally is bilateral. In cases where the rectus paralysis occurs on the opposite side he considers that it must be due to cerebrospinal hypertension compressing the nerve trunk of the abducens. Cites no new cases.

Wheeler, J. M.: Paralysis of sixth cranial nerve associated with otitis media. J. Am. M. Ass., LXXI, 1718, 1918.

Wheeler reports one case with mastoiditis on the left side, operated upon on February 13, 1918. On examination on March 9 the patient "exhibited a most interesting condition in a double external rectus paralysis (complete on the right side and partial on the left) without any involvement of the other muscles of the eye." It is to be noted in this case that the paralysis, while bilateral, was most complete on the side opposite to the affected ear.

ADDITIONAL BIBLIOGRAPHY.

Baldenweck, L.: Les altérations du ganglion de Gasser et de la vie paire au cours des inflammations de l'oreille moyenne. Ann. d'ocul., CXXXIX, 246, 1908.

Baratoux, J.: De la paralysie du moteur oculaire externe au cours des otitis. Arch. Internal. de Laryngol., XXIII, 63, 414, 1907. Also in Pratique méd., XXI, 33, 49, 1907.

Barr, J. S.: Paralysis of the Sixth Cranial Nerve Consequent Upon Chronic Purulent Middle Ear Disease. J. Laryngol., XXIII, 553, 1908.

Downey, J. W.: One Hundred Cases of Mastoiditis and Its Complications. Ann. Otol., Rhinol. and Laryngol., XXV, 994, 1916.

Graham, H. B.: Gradenigo's Syndrome: Analysis of Published Cases. Laryngoscope, XXVIII, 1146, 1913.

Kerrison, P. P.: Abducens Paralysis Complicating Mastoiditis. Med. Rec., XCIV, 941, 1918.

Lannois and Perretiere: Paralysis du moteur oculaire externe d'origine otique. Bull. Soc. méd. d. hop. de Lyon, V, 72, 1916.

Perkins, C. E.: Abducens Paralysis and Otitis Media Purulenta.  Ann Otol., Rhinol. and Laryngol., XIX, 692, 1910.

Sauvineau: Les paralysies oculaires dans les affèctions de l'oreille.  Ann. d'ocul., XXXVIII, 321, 1907.  Notes the same case published by Fauret.

Schwarzkopf: Die otogene abducenslahmung: Sammelreferat.  Internat. Centralbl. f. Ohrenheilk., V, 215, 1907.

Sears, W. H.: Isolated Paralysis of the External Rectus in Acute Suppurative Otitis Media.  Penn. M. J., XIII, 844, 1909-10.

Grand Opera House.

# SOCIETY PROCEEDINGS.

## CHICAGO LARYNGOLOGICAL AND OTOLOGICAL SOCIETY.

*Meeting of November 3, 1920.*

THE PRESIDENT, DR. ALFRED LEWY, IN THE CHAIR.

### Sebaceous Cyst of the Mouth.

Dr. Otto Stein reported a sebaceous cyst of the mouth and exhibited the patient and the cyst. This case was first seen by Dr. Stein three or four months ago. A young woman appeared at the hospital with her mouth so full that she could scarcely talk or swallow. At that time, about the middle of July, she was beginning to have difficulty in swallowing and great interference with speech. She had very little pain, only from the inconvenience from the size of the growth. Examination showed a mass in the floor of the mouth, which was a smooth symmetrical swelling. There was no inflammation, no particular soreness, and it was cystic to the touch. The mass pushed the tongue away up to the roof of the mouth, and below the chin in the sublingual region was a similar swelling which on palpation one could readily feel was a part of the mass in the mouth. The tumor was about the size of a small orange. The speaker was not sure whether it contained fluid or not. He decided to use a local injection and make an incision in the floor of the mouth, which he did under 1 per cent procain, which gave very good anesthesia. After making the incision through the mucous membrane only, he came down upon the sac and started to dissect it, but found it was too large to remove that way unless he emptied the contents through a small incision. Opening the sac readily revealed the contents to be sebaceous material. All of it was practically scooped out before any attempt was made to remove the sac; otherwise, he would have had to enlarge the incision considerably. The dissection was very easy, and the cyst was removed through a small incision. He exhibited the mass he removed in its entirety, containing whatever sebaceous material was left. There was a narrow prolongation in the median line in the submental region. Cysts of this type may appear anywhere along the branchial cleft. The patient had had no difficulty since the operation.

Dr. Joseph C. Beck asked how many of these cases Dr. Stein had found in the literature.

Dr. J. Holinger asked whether the sublingual salivary glands were implicated, did they discharge any saliva, or were they obstructed.

Dr. Robert Sonnenschein asked whether the cyst contained any hair.

Dr. Stein, in replying to Dr. Beck, stated he had not gone into the literature of the subject. Dermoids of the mouth were not uncommon. This was the second one he had seen; the other one was not of this type. This one contained only sebaceous material and had no connection with any salivary mucous gland.

These growths belonged to the class known as teratomas. They were a well known class of tumors, in which there was a wandering of epithelial tissue from its normal source or residence. They wandered sometimes in early fetal life and became included in other tissues, as in this case. Frequently they were pinched or squeezed off in the development of the fetus, and when the cleft closed they remained as a common condition in various parts of the body, without anything happening, but when they developed, as in this case, there was tissue according to the elements present in the particular rests that had wandered or were pinched off. In this case evidently a piece of the ectoderm of the fetus was extruded or was caught within the submaxillary cleft (this being the particular cleft that made up both sides of the tongue) and here later developed. These dermoids are usually congenital growths. The epithelial tissue in this case contained sebaceous elements that developed later on and formed the sebaceous material. The cyst grew until it could not grow any further. Dr. Stein recalled seeing the picture of a case in Senn's book on tumors that contained something like two or three pints of sebaceous material. The patient was an East Indian negro with a large mass protruding from his mouth. The cyst developed in the floor of the mouth, protruded from the mouth and when operated upon contained nothing but sebaceous material. If some of the epithelial elements contained mucous glands, hair follicles or fatty tissue, or any of the elements of the skin, they were liable to develop also in this tissue until there was almost the development of normal tissue. A certain kind of dermoid could develop where all the elements were present, resulting in the formation of various degrees of monstrosities.

There are several types of this growth. One, a simple teratoma made up of the normal stratified epithelial cells. Another contains various elements of the skin, hair follicles, sweat glands, sebaceous glands, mucous glands, and some fatty tissue. In the same way the mesoderm may develop in the ectodermal or endodermal area and produce a teratoma there.

An interesting point was the matter of diagnosis. When one looked into the mouth and saw a mass of this character he thought of several things, probably a mucous cyst, a ranula, or an occlusion of a salivary duct. Usually they were one-sided, but this was absolutely in the midline, both sides of the tongue having been lifted up. In the region below the chin one could press the floor of the mouth down and the mass would protrude in the neck.

The patient felt this cyst when a child six or seven years of age. It gradually grew until last year it bothered her a great deal, was painful and became objectionable.

Dr. G. W. Boot demonstrated a case of brain abscess.

The patient was a man, aged 24 years, who fell from a high chair when nine months old and had a hemorrhage from the right ear, with continuous discharge since that time. He served in the Army for two years.

August 27, 1920, he entered the Presbyterian Hospital with an otitis externa. The abscess was opened and the patient went home the following day.  September 4th he returned complaining of headache, dizziness, nausea and vomiting, stiffness of the neck and a slight earache.  He was slightly delirious and constipated.  A spinal puncture revealed a cloudy fluid, with 6,250 cells; small diplococcus questionable.  The cultures remained sterile after seventy-two hours.  He was seen on September 5, and a diagnosis of meningitis secondary to a chronic discharge of the ear was made.  A mastoid operation was performed and a large cholesteatomatous mass was found in the left antrum.  The tegmen seemed softened; the dura was incised and clear fluid found.  The temporosphenoidal lobe was incised and a thin, grayish turbid fluid with broken down brain tissue escaped.  A drainage tube was inserted after the sinus had been exposed and found normal; the wound was tamponed. The patient had a stormy convalescence until September 19th; on the 21st, sixteen days after the first operation, a probe was passed up the path of the drainage tube and thick pus was removed, which contained colon bacilli and pneumococcus on culture.  After that the headache disappeared, the patient felt fine and only complained that he could not go home.  On September 26th he was permitted to go home, as there was no longer any drainage and the wound was granulating nicely.

The temperature before the operation was 101.8° F., at operation 100°, and most of the time was subnormal up to the time of the drainage.

The case was presented at this time because the otologists are divided as to the advisability of operating on these cases.  One group said one should not operate on meningitis, another said not to operate on a brain abscess in the initiatory stage or in the terminal stage.  This patient in the beginning stage of brain abscess had been operated.  Dr. Boot had repeatedly operated on patients in that stage and they recovered.  He felt sure the attitude taken by the men at the Mayo clinic was wrong—just like the men who said not to operate on the appendix until there was a well walled off abscess.  He had now operated upon eight temporosphenoidal abscess and had four recoveries and had operated on three cerebellar abscesses, with one recovery.

Dr. Jerome F. Strauss presented his membership thesis entitled:

### Accidents in Aural Paracentesis.*

### DISCUSSION.

Dr. Otto Stein said that the paper of Dr. Strauss was very timely, and he did not think one could lay too much stress on the possibility of a hemorrhage occurring in any case of incision of the drum membrane.  It was almost an axiom with teachers in otology to impress students.  He knew that in postgraduate teaching they impressed upon physicians who were learning otology the greater care needed in the incision of the drum membrane on account of the possibility of fiuding anomalous conditions in the floor of the middle ear.  Such cases had been reported from time to time, and those who were experienced in otology were constantly on the lookout for such a possibility.  Therefore, this paper was of extreme interest at any time, in emphasizing the care one should exercise

---

See page 232.

in performing the operation of incision of the drum membrane. This condition of the floor of the middle ear, where there was no bone proper and the jugular bulb presented prominently, was more commonly found in children in whom there was an acute condition of the middle ear.

Dr. Stein was particularly interested in the arterial type of hemorrhage. Venous hemorrhages could be readily detected and recognized on account of the character of the blood escaping, but the arterial cases were far more rare. He had presented to the society a case of an anomalous arterial vessel in the anteroinferior wall of the middle ear. The case was studied by several gentlemen and carefully gone over by the members at that time, and had been seen by the speaker frequently. He could not determine exactly from the X-ray pictures whether this was a case of anomaly of the internal carotid artery, or a branch of some large arterial vessel in the anteroinferior part of the middle ear. The patient had a suppurating ear for some time before it healed. He had some loose connective tissue which formed a fair drum, but this drum bulged forward, and there was a distinct pulsation which was controlled by the blood pressure in the neck. He applied for relief from an annoying pulsating tinnitus. All this, taken with the X-ray findings, showed it to be one of the arterial cases. He did not attempt to puncture the swelling.

There was another class of cases, that did not come under this heading, where there was a terrific hemorrhage from cutting, and this was where there was a malignant growth in behind. Of course, there was destruction of part or all of the drum at the time, but in incising or curetting this mass at the bottom through the canal alarming hemorrhage might take place from the erosion the growth had produced around the carotid artery, with severe hemorrhage following.

Dr. Joseph C. Beck stated that this paper brought to his attention the thesis he wrote on the only case on record, so far as he knew, of primary actinomycosis of the middle ear. He had observed the case in the Allgemeiner Krankenhaus in Prague from the beginning. The patient came in with the diagnosis of otitis media. Subsequently Dr. Hektoen of this city and the speaker worked on it from a pathologic point of view, examining the yellow bodies that were discharging from the mastoid wound, which proved to be actinomyces. This case progressed and terminated in a fatal hemorrhage from the ear.

The remarks made by the previous speaker with reference to erosion from growths were also applicable to his case for erosion from osteitis of actinomycotic origin followed. A postmortem examination was made, and they studied the temporal bone, which was excised and made serial sections of it, especially in the vicinity of the ruptured internal carotid artery, which was from an erosion caused by the actinomycotic process. The erosion occurred in the carotid canal and just at its relation to the eustachian tube.

The point in this case was the treatment of the hemorrhage. The patient did not die from the immediate hemorrhage that occurred from the ear. He was not able to control the hemorrhage from the eustachian tube. It was necessary to do a ligation of the carotid; then the patient lived for a little while longer, but it was the tremendous loss of blood at the time of the first hemorrhage that killed the patient.

In another case of an endothelioma, of the endovascular type, of the middle ear, one did not expect a great deal of hemorrhage on account of this tumor developing within a vessel. But Werner in his surgical pathology showed the fallacy of this thing in bleeding tumors. The speaker had a great deal of difficulty in treating the case and in dealing with the hemorrhage from the ear. It was not always possible to control this by packing, even though one had a firm canal. In this case, too, the blood went into the mouth, the lady expectorating large quantities of blood. It finally was necessary to ligate the common carotid. She was still living, although with marked facial paralysis. The endothelioma had not recurred, when he heard from her about six weeks ago.

Another point should be considered: If one accidentally opened the sinus and knew he probably had an infection pouring in from the suppurating ear, would it not be safer to shut off the general circulation, both cerebral and in the neck? In a case of that kind threatened with pyemia, Dr. Beck would rather do a ligation and pack off the lateral sinuses than to let the case go along and take chances, providing the patient was at all safe for such procedure.

Dr. J. Holinger said that he was of the impression that cases of hemorrhage after paracentesis were not quite as rare, and mentioned a case in the Chicago Eye and Ear Infirmary. It occurred in the year 1901 or 1902, when in making a paracentesis the knife of a colleague struck the jugular bulb which was protruding abnormally from below into the middle ear. Since there are usually anatomic abnormalities which give rise to hemorrhage, he called the author's attention to the fact that in 1899 at the International Otological Congress, held in London, Dr. Rohrer, of Zurich, showed a picture of a drumhead with a number of ectatic veins in the upper part, and described it as a blue drum membrane. They might have given rise to hemorrhages if an incision had been found necessary. This hemorrhage would have occurred in the upper part of the membrane, while hemorrhages from protruding bulbs of jugular vein occur in the lower part. In the normal membrane the bulb appears as a bluish cupola through the transparent gray membrane, but in inflammations, when the membrane is red and swollen, there is no possibility of recognizing the abnormality of a protruding jugular bulb in making a paracentesis in an acutely inflamed drum membrane.

Dr. George W. Boot read a paper entitled:

"Abscess of the Frontal Lobe Secondary to Sinus Infection."

### DISCUSSION.

Dr. Sonnenschein stated that about four and a half years ago he had an unfortunate experience in the case of a medical student who developed a very acute right frontal sinusitis. Within twenty-four hours from the onset of the pain he had a tremendous edema of the eyelid, and despite the use of ordinary measures for two or three days, pain and swelling did not subside, nor did the temperature.

The anterior tip of the middle turbinate was then removed and a large quantity of pus evacuated. The symptoms did not improve. He then took the patient to the Michael Reese Hospital, and Dr.

Frank and himself opened the sinus externally and found a good deal of pus which was drained. The patient recovered and reached the point where he expected to go home the following day, but on that day he had a chill and the temperature rose to almost 106° F. Spinal puncture was made twenty-four hours later and turbid fluid found. A neurologist in consultation suggested frontal lobe abscess. They then opened the wound and explored the posterior wall of the sinus, but found no dehiscence and no necrosis. They removed the posterior wall and put a trocar into the frontal lobe and a large quantity of pus escaped. The patient, unfortunately, died. Whether the infection spread through small veins he did not know, but no macroscopic lesion was present.

Dr. G. Henry Mundt stated that in conversation with Dr. Boot he had told him of the most spectacular case of frontal lobe abscess he had ever had. Five or six years ago he did an intranasal operation on a young man, seventeen years of age, for a frontal sinusitis. The case apparently cleared up. Some months afterward he presented himself and was again having symptoms. He had a roentgenogram taken at this time, and the roentgenologist stated there was some osteomyelitis in the frontal sinus. An external operation was advised but refused. The patient got into the hands of some other practitioner, and eventually, when Dr. Mundt saw the boy, in company with two general practitioners, he had paralysis of respiration. He was kept alive for two or three hours with the pulmotor until his fingers and toes got cold. This boy was walking about the street six or eight hours before had this attack. He had eaten dinner in the evening at 6 o'clock and the paralysis of respiration came on about 7 o'clock. The patient died, and immediate postmortem revealed from four to six ounces of pus in a frontal lobe abscess. There were no symptoms previously that were referable to the frontal lobe abscess.

Dr. Joseph C. Beck asked whether the ventricles were opened in the postmortem examination.

Dr. Mundt replied that he could not recall whether they were or not.

Dr. Alfred Lewy asked Dr. Boot if he had observed in the patient with frontal lobe abscess any focal symptoms or anything that could be classed as focal symptoms of the mouth, movement of the tongue, jaw or lips.

He had seen two frontal lobe abscesses, one of which had as the only socalled focal symptom a licking movement with the tongue. The tongue was constantly protruding in licking the mouth. That patient was practically comatose. He did not recall the particulars of this first case, which was seen several years ago.

The second patient was a male child, four years of age, who entered the Eye and Ear Infirmary with an orbital abscess and was transferred from the eye department to the nose and throat division, and one of the men operated by, the external route. The speaker was present at the first operation. An incision was made in the eyebrow and the orbit entered; the abscess was subperiosteal on the nasal side of the orbit. The periosteum was incised and pus lying between the lamina papyracea and the orbital periosteum was released. The lamina papyracea and for a distance behind was necrotic, so that the operator curetted out what he could find of the ethmoid cells. The child apparently made a perfect recovery. The eye went back into place, the wound healed, leaving a good looking pale scar, and for several weeks the child stayed well. Then he was brought back and entered the speaker's service complaining of headache and vomiting. There was an occasional rise of temperature. The eye grounds, when the patient first entered, were doubtful, but the next day the eye men agreed there was some beginning choked disc. The patient was gone over for several days by a neurologist, who failed to detect any focal symptoms which would locate an intracranial lesion. There were no focal symptoms except a constant chewing movement. Spinal puncture showed 52 cells, the majority of which were polynuclears. The fluid was under slight pressure. The speaker operated upon the child in the presence of Dr. Sonnenschein, who helped him with his advice. An incision was made above the eyebrow and the bone removed. A number of X-ray plates indicated there was no frontal sinus, and no frontal sinus was found at the operation. He removed the bone, exploring the orbital ridge, and found the dura bulging but pulsating and practically normal. At one part of the dura there were a few spots, pinhead in size, that looked like granulations. The dura was incised and the brain tissue began to exude. The patient had extensive encephalitis. The speaker then went in with Gifford's searcher, and it entered the tissue of its own weight to a distance of two and three-quarters inches. He struck something that offered resistance and did not know whether he was against the wall of the ventricle or abscess cavity wall, but the child was in such a desperate condition he thought he had better take a chance. He perforated the abscess wall and got thick yellow pus. A rubber tube drain was inserted, which was later changed to glass. The headaches were immediately relieved, vomiting stopped, and the patient apparently did well for about five days. On the fifth night the child tore off the dressing, pulled out the drainage tube, and when he saw him there was a marked hernia of the brain but the child was not unconscious. As nearly as he could learn, the child had complained of headaches for the first time since the operation just before he tore off the bandage. The child lived three weeks; was fully conscious and perfectly bright in every respect up to five days before operation, and even with the headache, vomiting and choked disc his mentality was not disturbed. The only symptom that might be construed as focal was the chewing motion, and he wondered whether this was of any clinical value.

Dr. Joseph C. Beck thought the report of Dr. Boot should be criticised because it was not complete. He had left out a good many things that the members would like to know more about. Very little was known thus far about the functions of the frontal lobe.

Schaefer had called attention to some of these cases in reference to the olfactory function and had pointed out that in unilateral involvement of the frontal lobe there were frequently demonstrable changes in the olfaction. There was parosmia or symptoms of disturbed function of the sense of smell. There was not a loss of the sense of smell, but rather an irritation and an abnormal interpretation of odors. This was an early symptom.

The members ought also to have been shown the X-ray picture

of the case to determine whether there was really an absence of
the frontal sinus. If he found it at the operation, Dr. Beck thought,
no matter how much it was involved in the process of necrosis or
filled up with pus, a good X-ray plate of one side of the nose or on
the other side of the sinus would show some indication of a frontal
sinus.

The blood picture given of 4,000 and some odd leukocytes without any differential count was another thing which was not clear.
Assuming the patient was in a very bad condition, septic, run
down, and had leucopenia, the differential count would have clari-
fied the point as to whether there was a deficiency in the polymorphonuclear cells, or what was the cause.

Another point: The doctor said he had incised the subperiosteal
abscess, yet there was no statement made as to an examination to
determine whether the turbinates were cut. This was an important
point to determine. While the patient was relieved after an intranasal operation, might not this patient have had an acute exacerbation if an old abscess due to a chronic condition?

The speaker's experience with cases of frontal lobe abscess was
limited to about twenty, on which he had operated, but of this number there was only one of the real brain abscess cases that survived operation.

As to the prognosis of frontal lobe abscess in contradistinction
to brain abscess from the middle ear, Dr. Beck believed the circulation had something to do with it.

In reference to the central vein that went through the foramen
cecum and the longitudinal sinus, with distribution of the circulation at this point, it was a venous circulation. This point was
never referred to very clearly by anyone in reports of frontal lobe
abscesses.

A thing that had impressed the speaker in connection with these
brain abscesses was the anatomic formation of the anterior horn
of the lateral ventricle, which was so close to the frontal lobe that
infection could readily take place in such a case as Dr. Boot had
reported. The speaker had had such an experience. A patient, who
had felt perfectly well one week previously presented symptoms
of frontal lobe abscess which soon resulted fatally. At the postmortem examination a complete section of the brain was made,
which showed perforation into the ventricle with a sudden increase
in pressure on the vital centers, and this would give the symptoms
Dr. Boot had described.

Dr. J. Holinger was impressed with the progress of the suppuration through the diploe and stated that this was not a very exceptional finding in the author's experience. It was not rare in a case
of empyema of the frontal sinus for the pus not to show itself at
the point where one might expect to find it. He observed in the
mastoid as well as in the frontal sinus that the pus may spread in
the diploe and appear in very unexpected places either below the
skin or in the skull cavity. He recalled one patient, a girl, who
complained of indefinite symptoms until one night she cried out
and in the morning was found unconscious. Before that she was
able to go out and play with other children. When he saw her,
she showed a decided reaction on pressure over the frontal sinus
on the left side. He operated from the outside at once and fol-

lowed the pus along the diploe and was led to an abscess in the temporal lobe six or seven cm. away from the frontal sinus. The spreading of pus in the diploe around the mastoid is more frequent, especially in traumatic mastoiditis. In one such patient he had to uncover in four successive operations a large part of the inner plate of the occipital bone till past the middle line, where an emissary vein led the thromboses to very near the torcular. The suppuration spread in the diploe after each operation, but finally stopped and the patient recovered.

Dr. Boot, in closing the discussion, said he would not expect in lesions of the frontal lobe to find focal symptoms except of a mental nature, and in the case he had reported he had been unable to elicit them since the patient spoke only Bohemian and because of the short time the patient was under observation.

He was in hopes some member of the society might say something about streptococcus infection. Not long ago at a meeting of this society the subject of streptococcus meningitis was brought up and the statement was made that streptococcus meningitis did not recover. Dr. Holinger had one such case at the County Hospital that Dr. Boot also saw that did recover. Sptertococci were found in the spinal fluid. The speaker also had a patient with abscess of the right temporosphenoidal lobe in which the lateral ventricle burst when the explorer was but half way through the cortex, and the cerebrospinal fluid was thrown out some eight inches. The fluid, which was of a greenish tint, was collected and smears made at once showing many short chains of streptococci. The abscess was evacuated and the patient did very well for a week or more and then became more and more sleeply, finally dying in coma. Apparently an encephalitis had developed. There were no further signs of brain abscess.

In the case reported in the paper the X-ray examination failed to show the presence of a frontal sinus, although one was found 2 cm. in diameter and .5 cm. deep, filled with pus. The skull was very thick.

In answer to Dr. Holinger's question, the pus was seen oozing through the bone when the pericranium had been elevated.

In answer to Dr. Lewy's question, there were no chewing motions or other focal signs until the tonic spasm of the left arm and hand developed.

In answer to Dr. Beck's criticism, the serious symptoms developed so rapidly when they did come that there was not time enough to get a Wassermann reaction or to do other things that one would like to do to get a complete report. It was a question of doing what was possible in time to give the patient a chance for his life by operating.

The reason why abscess of the frontal lobe secondary to sinus disease has a worse prognosis than temporosphenoidal abscess is because the diagnosis is not made early, because focal symptoms are late in developing. This case was reported to show how serious a case might become before definite localizing symptoms occurred and to urge the members of the society to operate early on cases of frontal sinus infection where things were not running smoothly, without waiting for localizing symyptoms. In other words, to do an exploratory operation.

# CHICAGO LARYNGOLOGICAL AND OTOLOGICAL SOCIETY.

*Meeting of December 5, 1920.*

THE PRESIDENT, DR. ALFRED LEWY, IN THE CHAIR.

## Multiple Brain Tumor.

Dr. Joseph C. Beck showed a specimen of a brain from a case of multiple brain tumor. Many diagnoses had been made in the case by various neurologists who had seen the patient and made careful examinations, each of them having placed the lesion in a different part of the brain. When the patient was first seen by Dr. Beck, he diagnosed a frontal lobe abscess associated with frontal sinusitis. Operation being decided upon, Dr. Beck exposed the frontal sinus and found it full of thick pus and the lining membrane markedly thickened. The nasofrontal duct appeared completely blocked. Nowhere could there be found any fistula or atrium towards the brain.

Leaving the area entirely separate and going into the aseptic area corresponding to the frontal lobe region, he found a thickened dura coming on from the posterior or cerebral surface of the frontal sinus. Upon opening this dura no abscess was found intradurally or within the brain; there was nothing but the thickened dura, a piece of which he excised for subsequent microscopic study. After some time (five and one-half months) the patient succumbed to the disease. The symptoms during this period were exceedingly variable; there were tonic and clonic contractions of the feet which disappeared. and mental and cerebellar symptoms became more evident.

Necropsy, performed by Dr. Beck, showed that each of the diagnoses based on frontal symptoms was correct. He found many encapsulated tumors, some of which dropped out when the brain was sectioned after hardening. These tumors were found in the cerebrum as well as in the cerebellum, which accounted for the great variety of symptoms. At first Dr. Beck thought that the tumors were multiple syphilomas, but histologic sections showed that they were walled off eipthelial tumors—walled off carcinoma of the brain. Dr. Beck had never before known of this as a primary growth, but in the literature he found two cases, reported by Fraser, and one man in Spain (cited by Greenwood of England) reported seven cases. It was interesting to note that Lewis Fisher of Philadelphia, who saw the man, localized the lesion exactly corresponding to one of the lesions that were found postmortem.

Dr. Beck called attention to the method by which this specimen was imbedded in a block of paraffin, which made it very easy to display, and he thought it would preserve the sections well. (Fig. 1.).

## Bezold's Abscess.

Dr. Beck also showed two cases of unusual mastoiditis. The first case was that of a man whose trouble first manifested itself in June,

1917, by earache in the right ear and dizziness. These symptoms continued for two or three weeks, the patient being unable to work; gradually the symptoms improved and the patient returned to work, but soon they returned, more marked than formerly, and he again went to bed. One morning he arose and found himself staggering to such an extent that he could not walk. A doctor was called, who applied hot water bottles to the head; this gave no relief and ice packs were then used. Later the patient was taken to DeKalb, where he consulted Dr. Smith, who, after a careful examination, including an X-ray of the head, diagnosed sinus disease. The physician who had formerly seen the patient declared that it was not a case of mastoid disease.

Two days after the diagnosis was made the patient was operated upon; after the operation he was told by the doctor that the mastoid cells were full of pus. The operation afforded no relief from the symptoms, and the wound continued to drain. In November the patient left the service of Dr. Smith and placed himself in the care of Dr. Thiele, who brought him to Dr. Beck.

Examination at that time showed a fistula behind the right auricle which was discharging pus, which proved to be of mixed culture. A probe followed the fistula down toward the neck, somewhat posteriorly. The patient complained of lack of motion of the neck, and examination revealed resistance to movements, though by persistence and patience it was found that almost all movements of the head and neck were possible. Examination of the ear revealed no evidence of any suppuration ever having existed. Tests showed the ear to be reduced to one-half of normal. The Weber was lateralized to the right and bone conduction was markedly increased The test of jumping back from the tips of the toes to strike the heels against the floor gave a suggestion of spinal caries.

The patient was kept under observation in the hospital for one week, during which time the vestibular apparatus was explored; all the reactions proved practically normal, as did also the symptoms referable to the cerebellum. X-ray pictures of the head and neck, with special reference to spondylitis, showed no evidence of any vertebral trouble. The temperature remained constantly normal; all laboratory tests proved negative. A diagnosis of osteomyelitis of the temporal bone finally was made and the patient was operated upon.

Operation revealed granulation tissue around the fistula, and upon its removal there was soft bone at the tip which appeared much like detritus. A continuous bleeding vein was encountered at the depth of the tip of the mastoid toward the neck; the bleeding was controlled by the use of surgical wax, and the incision was continued through the mastoid backwards and outwards toward the occiput, where a collection of pus was found between the occipital bone and vertebral column. The under surface of the occipital bone in the vicinity of the pus pocket was eroded, and it was scraped down almost to the dura, but the dura was not exposed. The wound was closed by bringing the flap back and sewing it in position. Drainage was established by means of a stab wound behind the incision. The drainage was continued for about two weeks, when a bismuth injection was made under considerable pressure. Immediately following this the patient felt something in the middle ear, which was assumed to be particles of bismuth escaping through aditus and antrum into the middle ear. There was a feeling of fullness in the ear about two weeks, when all symptoms began to subside. Aural inspection failed to reveal any foreign substance, and it was concluded that there was some secretion rather than bismuth in the middle ear. The wound healed and there had been no recurrence in three years, and the hearing was not affected. No spinal puncture was made, but it was concluded that the symptoms were irritative.

The second case was that of a man who had an acute otitis media, followed by a rapidly developing mastoiditis. He was first seen on May 12, 1920. A simple mastoid operation revealed no evidence of erosion or other necrosis in the region of the tip in the neck. He made an uneventful recovery, and in thirteen days was out of the hospital. The wound healed and the recovery was absolutely normal. Two or three weeks later there was slight swelling over the mastoid, which was opened and cleaned out and drainage instituted. The fistula continued and a larger exploration was made. Following down into the region of the occiput, they found destruction of bone, and upon exploring the sinus and dura at that point pus was found. The sinus had been thought of, but there were no symptoms referable to it. However, upon pushing back the tissues of the neck, pus exuded, but on pressure of the neck there was no pus. Drainage was continued for several weeks, but on pressing back the tissues of the neck small quantities of pus continued to escape. Afterward they made a still larger exploration and found that the pus ran much more forward than in the previous case, collecting close to the region of the external jugular.

Another operation was performed, going down to the neck and opening through the sinus to get at the infected area, which was cleaned out and drained. The patient made a good recovery and went along practically without temperature but the pus persisted. Later an incision was made through the clinoid muscle, which was followed down to the depths of the neck and the cavity cleaned out. This had not been done before because of fear of infection of the jugular wound. The patient had been perfectly well for four weeks.

Smears showed a mixed bacteria, diplococci predominating; cultures also showed a predominance of diplococci, both at the primary examination and subsequently. The Wassermann reaction was negative.

## DISCUSSION.

Dr. C. H. Long asked Dr. Beck if he had gone in the first time posteriorly if he would have accomplished the same results.

Dr. Beck said that on going down the same as in the first case he found that the pus went forward and he could not go posteriorly, but had to go through the mastoid foramen, sacrificing the facial nerve, or go through the sinus in the way he did. It was impossible to reach it from the back and get the necrosis which he could see and feel. It was only by going through the sinus that he was able to reach it.

Dr. Edwin McGinnis showed a patient who had had

### Double External Frontal Sinus Operations

following two intranasal operations.

The patient was a man who had a double frontal sinus infection, with an intranasal operation on both of them. The first operation was performed by Dr. Good eight years ago; at that time the anterior end of the middle turbinate was removed, and the anterior ethmoid cells were rasped forward. Dr. McGinnis had seen Dr. Good perform this operation several times, but thought he had not reached the frontal sinus in this case. The other side had been operated by the late Dr. Friedberg. In 1918 the patient entered the Presbyterian Hospital with severe frontal pain, and pain through the eye, but did not wish the intranasal operation again. All the landmarks were gone, so it was decided to do an external operation. They opened through the eyebrow and made a little peek-hole through into the frontal sinus. The front wall of the sinus was one-fourth inch thick. On the floor of the frontal wall of the sinus there were two quite large polypi, one attached to the posterior and one to the anterior wall. The sinus was filled with pus. The polypi were removed, the base curetted and on going down gently into the nose, a couple of ethmoid cells were found that had not been touched by the first operation.

The other sinus was operated in August, 1920. An incision was made through the eyebrow, the brow elevated and a small opening made in the front wall. The case was interesting because all of the sinus lining was detached and the mucosa seemed about three-sixteenths of an inch thick.

The patient made a pretty good recovery with a freely movable scar; the discharge had cleared up and the nose was in about the same shape as before the operation. The Wassermann reaction was negative with both blood and spinal fluid.

### DISCUSSION.

Dr. E. P. Norcross asked whether Dr. McGinnis operated through the peekhole or whether he enlarged the opening.

Dr. McGinnis replied that he did a modified Lothrop operation, butting up through the nose. He had never been able to use the burr successfully through the nose because it seemed to tear things so much. The septum was not removed in this case.

Dr. Walter H. Theobald presented a thesis entitled

### "A Radical Treatment for Chronic Suppuration of the Antrum with Modification of the Canfield Technic for Operation."*

### DISCUSSION.

Dr. Joseph C. Beck said he was much pleased to see an operation illustrated which he had been doing for some time. He though he got it from Pierce or Skillern, and had published it in Ochsner's book on diagnosis, both the posterior incision and turning the flap over, not taking out but raising the flap toward the septum. He

---

*See page 131.

called it the "Skillern operation" because Skillern had the opening through the pyriform fossa, but later gave it up because it was too irritating. Dr. Beck used the electric burr, doing the operation very quickly, and that gave more room to work with than the large nose instruments. It was not necessary to see, because after exposing the margin of the pyriform fossa one could bite it through. He had obtained more satisfactory results from this than from any other antrum procedure.

Dr. Beck congratulated Dr. Theobald on bringing up the subject and was glad to have heard his description, although he believed someone else had done it.

Dr. Norval H. Pierce thought that the matter of priority was always a small matter to argue about. He had been doing the operation Dr. Theobald described for over ten years. It was founded on the Denker idea, the natural suggestion that would come to one's mind—could we not do away with the buccal incision? When that thought came to his mind he made the incision through the pyriform crest, and found that by reflecting the facial soft parts and lateral wall of the nose one could get an ample view of all parts of the antrum. He thought it rather an original idea to not sacrifice the inferior turbinate. He was not sure whether it was quite the right thing to do in all cases. He believed it caused a more rapid contracture of the hole, but he had seen a number of cases that had returned after five years with an ample orifice in the inferior meatus, and the anterior fifth, which had been temporarily detached, had grown back into place. The operation certainly gave a complete view of the antrum with a minimum amount of destruction, and he considered it as corrective as any operation could be.

In regard to the tape being left in, this is most frequently due to the gauze tearing. In his opinion, it would be a good plan to measure the tape before putting it in and check it up after taking it out, as it was a very simple matter to leave a piece in, but it was a very unpleasant occurrence after the wound had practically healed and was rather small to have the discharge persist and the unpleasant odor continue. When such a thing occurred, it was pretty safe to say that the packing had been left in, and the best thing to do was to reopen the wound and remove it.

Dr. Robert Sonneschein said that he had asked Dr. Skillern about his operation some years ago and was told that he used it only in acute cases, and expected to use it only in acute cases where he wished to keep the antrum open for a few weeks. He did not make a flap. In the operation described by Dr. Theobald, a flap was made, and if it stayed in place it prevented closure of the wound.

Dr. Sonneschein had had his own antrum operated upon by the essayist some time ago, and the work was very skillfully and almost pleasantly done, except for one feature—the use of the trephine. He was very glad that had been discarded, for when one felt the vibration as it struck the roots of the teeth it was very unpleasant. He felt that the rongeur method would be much more agreeable. His operation was very successful, and while sometimes infection occurred, a few irrigations caused it to subside. The only disagreeable feature remaining was some anesthesia of the teeth most adjacent to the antrum.

Dr. Sonnenschein congratulated Dr. Theobald on his thesis and upon his entrance into the society.

Dr. E. P. Norcross said that Dr. Skillern termed this operation the "preturbinal operation." As he remembered it, he described it to him as. a modification of the Canfield operation, but said it was a much less radical procedure. Dr. Norcross had performed the operation several times and to him the most surprising thing was the thickness of the pyriform crest. In his opinion, the point that should be appreciated even more than the method of operation was the fact that all kinds of antra, having all kinds of pathology, had been cured by a comparatively simple operation. It did no harm to try this method first, and if after a time it did not cure the trouble there was no objection to doing a Caldwell-Luc or Denker operation. He had been more successful by removing the anterior tip of the turbinate, thus getting a more permanent opening. In the last year Dr. Norcross had seen a number of cases that had been operated by the Krause-Mikulicz operation, simply making a hole in the nasal wall. This had relieved the patients of all symptoms, and they had had no unpleasant symptoms following the operation, all of which went to show that too radical surgery on the antrum or any other part of the body was not always necessary to obtain the desired result.

Dr. Norcross thought the essayist was to be congratulated on having a series of forty cases that had been cured. That fact alone must bear out the practicability of the operation.

Dr. Charles M. Robertson thought this operation was a good one but that there are so many good operations for the antrum that one could not do any one in all cases.

There was one place in this operation that made trouble. When the anterior inner edge of the cavity was taken away it left a place where the cavity was covered by the soft tissues of the cheek, at which site granulations would occur, and, as the essayist said, he had to apply nitrate of silver during the first week, which showed a piling up of granulation tissue in the opening of the antrum. The soft tissues must be watched in all antral cases. Granulations in this place encroach on the opening and destroy the opening from the anterior end.

The operation Dr. Robertson had always advocated was a modified Caldwell-Luc with special features as to the meatal flap of mucous membrane. In going through on the buccal surface one could easily determine at a glance the position of the attachment of the inferior turbinate body, as it shows a bulge on the nasal wall extending from before backward and downward, corresponding to the attachment of the inferior turbinated bone. In the operation he advocated the wall of the inferior meatus was removed in its entirety down to the floor, leaving the floor of the antrum and the floor of the nose on a level so there would be no interference with drainage from the antrum.

The mucous membrane of the inferior meatus was not attacked until the bone had been completely removed and the edges of the wound smoothed. The nasal mucous membrane was then cut in the form of a letter X from before and upwards downward and backward and from below and forward, upward and backward, which created four flaps which were reflected into the antrum and held in place by the pack which was introduced into the antrum. These flaps cover the edge of the bony wound and part of the anterior antral wall and no soft tissue comes into contact with the nasal wound.

Thus the edge of the wound into the nose is covered with mucous membrane which secures a permanent opening as large as at the time of operation. Dr. Robertson thought operating through the buccal cavity gave a most beautiful result, and affords a better view of every part of the antral cavity. He had operated in this way for eight or ten years and had measured. the opening into the antral cavity afterward and found that the opening remained the same as at the completion of the operation. This operation gave the advantage of a cavity in which one could see, and if one desired to drain the sphenoid into the antrum through the posterior ethmoid cells, it could be done under direct inspection. The operation could be done just as quickly as the other, and the buccal wound was not objectionable, being at the gingivobuccal junction, which precluded gaping, and which closed in from three to four days.

Dr. Robertson considered the operation under discussion admirable, but wished to enter a protest against displacing. the turbinate or cutting any off. In his opinion, this would be sufficient cause for perverted physiologic function of the inferior turbinate.

In case the inferior turbinate extended to the floor of the nose enough might be trimmed from its lower edge to allow a ventilation space of six to eight millimeters between the lower edge of the turbinate and the nasal floor.

Dr. Frank Brawley said that he had seen Dr. Pierce and Dr. Theobald perform this operation and had since done six of them himself. He believed it was the best procedure for the chronic antrum that he had ever tried. He had experienced no difficulty in the after healing in any of the six cases. he had had. However, he had taken off the tip of the turbinate in every case, but would try refracting the turbinate in the future.

One point was important in order to get a clear field, and this was to be careful to make the incision over the pyriform crest in the mucosa. Before he had much experience he made the incision at the mucocutaneous junction and got a good deal of bleeding, which he had difficulty in controlling. It was just as easy to make the incision in the mucosa, and there was much better control. It had appealed to him particularly, because it was such a safe operation, so far as the lacrimal duct was concerned. There was no danger of injuring the lower end of the duct by this method.

Dr. Alfred Lewy stated that he had the pleasure of working in Sturmann's clinic in 1898 when he perfected his operation, and Sturmann was surprised to know that Canfield had already perfected the operation and published it. He thought Canfield beat Sturmann to the publication.

Several years ago Dr. Lewy saw Dr. Robertson perform his operation, which looked like a modification of the Caldwell-Luc. He did not remove the tip of the turbinate. He operated under general anesthesia, and Dr. Lewy thought it took exquisite skill to peel off the bone from the membrane as he did. The unusual skill required would probably prevent Dr. Robertson's technic from becoming popular.

Dr. Walter H. Theobald (closing the discussion) thanked the members for their discussion, and stated that in the first fifteen or twenty cases he used the electric driven trephine or drill, but found it to be a great discomfort to the patient. It was as disagreeable as having one's teeth drilled, so he discontinued using it.

The operation mentioned by Dr. Beck as the Skillern, the writer assumed was used only in acute cases.

Dr. Theobald believed Dr. Robertson would have some difficulty in keeping his flaps in place. The operations which the writer had reported were of the intranasal type. Canfield claimed priority for this operation in that his publication preceded Dr. Sturmann's of Berlin by two months.

As to the after-treatment, it consisted largely in controlling the granulation tissue which formed so rapidly around the first incision. After the packing was removed he irrigated the antrum through the canula until the secretion subsided, which usually took about ten days. The patient came in for irrigation a week later and perhaps two weeks later for further irrigation. For this purpose he usually used an astringent solution of cupric sulphate in dilution, about 1:6,000.

Dr. Edwin McGinnis read a paper on

### "Problems in Bronchoscopy and Esophagoscopy"

illustrated with lantern slides.

Dr. McGinnis presented graphically some of the phases of this large subject and showed examples of the place of arrest of foreign bodies in the esophagus.

Case 1.—Child, 9 months old. Open safety pin resting in the laryngopharynx with the points upward and ring wedged in the introitus esophagi. It had been in this position for two weeks and was removed by turning and extraction with direct laryngoscope.

Cases 2 to 8 were coins and telephone slugs in the esophagus either at the introitus or further down at the sternoclavicular notch. Removed by means of direct vision.

Case 8.—Ring from an alarm clock lodged in the esophagus at level of the sternoclavicular notch. Three previous attempts at removal were unsuccessful. By means of fluoroscopic esophagoscopy it was removed and the child recovered.

Case 9.—Lead horse's head, prize from popcorn package, lodged in upper end of the esophagus. Kindly referred by Dr. H. R. Boettcher. Removed under direct vision.

Case 10.—Child with dorsal Pott's disease. Penny lodged at cardia. Passage of esophagoscope set up peristalsis, and penny could be seen passing through into the stomach.

### BRONCHOSCOPIC CASES.

Case 1.—Upholsterer's tack in right bronchus of child 3 years of age, which had been in position six weeks. X-ray revealed tack. Removed fluoroscopically by means of upper bronchoscopy. Uneventful recovery.

Case 2.—Kindly referred by Dr. Harry Pollock. Six penny nail in left bronchus of child 20 months old. Nail had been in position for about six months. Fluoroscopically removed nail from bronchus, but point stuck into larynx and it was necessary to do a thyrotomy to remove nail tracheotomy. This child died one week later from a pneumonia.

Case 3.—Upholsterer's tack right bronchus of an adult aged 33. Removed fluoroscopically. Uneventful recovery.

Case 4.—Rubber in right bronchus. Child. Kindly referred by Dr. Joseph Beck. Lung on the same side appeared of greater density than the other lung on X-ray plate. Removed fluoroscopically. Recovery uneventful.

Case 5.—Patient, aged 43 years. Referred by Dr. Oliver of Chicago. Six weeks previously had had fourteen teeth extracted with nitrous oxid gas anesthesia. Was normal for about two weeks and then began to cough. One week later pain appeared in the right chest, and X-ray showed foreign body in right bronchus. Removed fluoroscopically and was found to be part of a molar tooth. On looking again another object presented itself. This proved to be an amalgam filling and was removed. Recovery was uneventful.

Case 6.—Watermelon seed in the right bronchus of an infant of 8 months. Faint shadow on the X-ray plate. Removed by upper bronchoscopy. Recovery uneventful.

Case 7.—G. J., age 5, seen November 8, 1918. In the morning the child was eating some raw carrot; with a sudden sharp intake of breath, she was seized with a violent fit of coughing which persisted for some time. She became hoarse and decidedly wheezy. On admittance to the hospital, breathing was slightly accelerated. Examination: Right lung, increased breath sounds, bronchial breathing with wheezing rales anteriorly. Left lung, absence of breath sounds, no area of dullness.

November 8, 1918, at 8 p. m., at Presbyterian Hospital, without anesthetic, upper bronchoscopy. The larynx and upper part of the trachea were clear; at bifurcation and extending into left bronchus several small yellowish objects were seen. These were removed with forceps, there being two large pieces of carrot, about the size of a small pea, with several smaller pieces in a great quantity of mucus. The patient left the operating room in good condition. At 11:05 the examination revealed air going into both lungs and considerable roughening of breath sounds. Four days afterwards the temperature went up to 103.6°, but the next day dropped to normal. She left the hospital November 13, 1918. Her mother wrote that she had pneumonia afterwards and coughed up a little piece of carrot.

Case 8.—L. H., aged 1 year, referred by Dr. A. E. Loewy. Three days before admittance, or on June 9, 1920, the baby was eating a hard boiled egg and some of the eggshell became lodged in the larynx. This produced difficulty in respiration which gradually became worse. At the time of entrance into the hospital there was marked retraction of the sternum with each respiration, as well as marked movement of the lower ribs. The feet were becoming cyanotic. The child acted like one with laryngeal diphtheria in need of intubation.

Coarse rales could be heard all over the chest in front and be-hind. On June 12, 1920, at the Presbyterian Hospital, by direct laryngeal examination could see a piece of eggshell in the larynx anteroposteriorly between the cords. This broke up into little pieces under the grasp of the forceps. Breathing was not much better after this, so a tracheotomy was performed under local an-esthesia. Upon opening the trachea, some eggshell presented in the wound and this was removed. Breathing was better with the tube in place.

Temperature at the time of the operation: 102.6 degrees; June 13, 102; June 14, 103.2; June 17, 99.6; June 18, 103.

On June 17th the tracheotomy tube was removed for cleansing and the patient had great difficulty in breathing until the tube was replaced. On June 18, 1920, at 4:25 a. m., the child died gasping for air.

Postmortem examination: Beginning just at the lower edge of the tracheotomy opening was a large fibrinous exudate almost fill-ing the lower trachea and extending down into the bronchi at the bifurcation, which was the cause of death. No diphtheria organ-isms were found.

Case 9.—H. H., aged 3 years, referred by Dr. John E. Rhodes. On September 22, 1920, the patient's parents noticed the boy playing with some acorns. A short time later they found him in a fit of coughing, and becoming quite blue, breathing rapidly and with great difficulty. In a short time breathing became better and the color became normal. When first seen by Dr. McGinnis on Sep-tember 12, 1920, he had been having asthmatic attacks for six or seven months. Upon X-ray examination, the upper lobe appeared to be more dense. No shadow of a foreign body was seen. Direct laryngoscopic examination revealed something coming into the larynx and receding with inspiration and expiration. It was grasped with a forceps but could not be extracted. Then it disappeared and a good deal of secretion was coughed out. Upon insertion of the bronchoscope some obstruction was noted, but careful search failed to reveal any foreign body in the bronchus.

An intubation tube was inserted, which was removed the next day. In one week another examination revealed a swelling of the right side of the subglottic space. The child became cyanotic and a tracheotomy was performed. The incision opened up a large peri-tracheal abscess, probably due to a broken down cervical gland. The child improved and was sent home with the tracheotomy tube in place.

In conclusion, Dr. McGinnis said that these cases now have an earlier diagnosis and are in better shape for operation. His early experience in the practice of the late Dr. Ingals was discouraging in that the foreign bodies remained so long unrecognized. There was usually abscess formation and extraction was almost im-possible.

### DISCUSSION.

Dr. George W. Boot congratulated Dr. McGinnis on his success in this very difficult kind of work. In his opinion, no work is quite so difficult as removing foreign bodies from the bronchi and esoph-agus. He was surprised to know that Dr. Ingals had not had more foreign bodies to remove than Dr. McGinnis reported. Dr. Ingals' finder was altogether different from Dr. Boot's, as his has only one turn, and the end, and Dr. Boot's was a regular corkscrew, so that by rotating it the point of the open safety pin was brought within the spiral and protected in such a way that the safety pin could be extracted without tearing the mucosa.

There was one point in which he did not agree with Dr. McGinnis: he thought no one should ever search blindly for these foreign bodies. Wherever possible, the foreign body should first be seen before attempting to grasp it. He very recently had an experience with a foreign body, which was a little different from the usual. The patient was a child of 18 months, who had inhaled a piece of carrot and the family physician had tried to extract it. The child was taken to the hospital and an interne tried to remove it and the piece of carrot turned and shut off the breathing. The intern did a hurried tracheotomy and then Dr. Boot was called. He found it impossible to use a suspension apparatus and then the bronchoscope as he ordinarily did because of the tracheotomy tube's being in place, but he finally located the foreign body and removed it.

He thought it was surprising how many of the patients swallowed coins. He once had a colored servant maid who stole her mistress' jewelry and swallowed a diamond ring. By the time he reached the patient the foreign body had passed into the stomach and out of his territory. The hospital people were going to do a gastroenterostomy, but Dr. Boot told them to wait for a while, so two policemen were kept on guard, and in two or three days the patient passed the ring.

Dr. Otto J. Stein has been interested in this subject since the inception of the work, and in the spatula which Kirstein first brought out, which he had used very persistently in his work. He then became very enthusiastic about the work with the bube, as brought out by Killian, and thought it was remarkable how much success one could obtain in patients with real pathologic lesions within the esophagus or tracheobronchial tract, as well as in finding foreign bodies if one gave a lot of time to it and allowed others to know they were doing the work.

A number of years ago there was difficulty in finding such patients to work upon. After realizing that he never would become an expert, he almost dropped the work and found that by unanimous consent this particularly difficult work of scoping really belonged in the hands of only one or two who were especially interested and who had the peculiar ability to apply their skill. It seemed to be the unanimous opinion that the work should be in the hands of Dr. Friedberg. Aside from the foreign body extraction he used the tube work quite often as a means of diagnosis and in the treatment of tracheal ulcers and some years ago used it a good deal in bronchial asthma, thinking that by dilatation of the trachea some of these cases could be relieved, and it did bring relief in many cases.

Aside from the foreign body work there was a very definite field for this work. In making applications to ulcers in the trachea, in removing sections of tumors below the glottis and in the larynx, diagnosing stenosis in the esophagus and trachea, made the application of the method much broader than one ordinarily thought.

Dr. Stein believed every laryngologist should practice tubing, and it was now being taught at the Postgraduate Hospital. In that way it was possible to teach the hand and eye to locate different parts of the trachea by demonstrating that one could work bimanually. With the probe and forceps and measuring the distance, one did not have to do this very often before becoming accustomed to the localization of the parts, and the method was often of much assistance.

Dr. Harry L. Pollock referred to a case seen recently which was very interesting along this line. The patient was a man who had a tracheotomy performed in June. The surgeon who did this died within a few days afterward, and everyone was afraid to remove the tube. The patient was sent in to him with a history of having cleaned the tube with cotton wrapped about an applicator. He was cleaning it in this way one day, when suddenly the cotton and applicator disappeared down the trachea, and the patient stated that when he was sitting up it obstructed his breathing. He came in bending away forward, for in that position there was no obstruction. Dr. Pollock took out the tube and did a lower bronchoscopy, but could see no cotton or applicator, and decided that possibly the thing had gone upward, above the tube. If it had been below the tube, he felt that it would have dropped further down. The patient was breathing fairly comfortably lying on his abdomen and the following morning they suspended him. Examination showed complete edema which closed the entire larynx. The following day the tube was again removed, and when it was replaced again the patient said he could feel the applicator at the end of the tube. The tube was pulled out again and the cotton and applicator came out with it. He thought it had gone upward and when the tube was removed it permitted it to fall down.

Dr. Pollock said they had had a good many cases of foreign body removal, and he agreed with Dr. Boot that one should never search for them blindly. He believed that all the trouble in these cases came from laryngologists going down and grasping the membrane. He was certain that every such case that had been referred to them that had died, had died as the result of having the mucous membrane torn and infected. He recalled a case seen with Dr. Friedberg, in which the patient had swallowed a tack, and they could not find it. He used the fluoroscope and directed the tube the same as Dr. McGinnis showed in the nail case, but Dr. Friedberg could not get the tack either way. They could see several times that he was immediately over it, but he was unable to get it. Dr. Pollock thought that the fluoroscope, to be of the most service, should have two tubes, a lateral and an up and down, and that it was far better to go right down and see what was being done rather than depending on the fluoroscope.

Another case which had astonished him was that of a little child 2 years old, who had swallowed a quarter. They took an X-ray picture and found the quarter in the stomach, although he had thought that a quarter would not go through a child's esophagus. A neighbor had told the mother to give the child a big dose of castor oil and that same evening the child passed the quarter.

Dr. Norval H. Pierce said that lately he removed a sandbur from the larynx of a young woman after it had been in position for almost a week. The sandbur was situated in the anterior portion of the larynx, between the vocal cords. The patient, a young lady, was walking with some friends, and in going through the grass the sandbar had attached itself to her skirt. She had on a pair of mitts, and in removing the bur from her skirt it attached itself to the mitt and she attempted to remove it with her teeth, and in doing so she inhaled the sandbur. The remarkable thing about the case was that the patient had very little discomfort. There was no edema and little pain in the larynx and the bur was removed very easily. The patient went home in a day or two.

Dr. Edwin McGinnis (closing the discussion) thanked the members for their liberal discussion. He felt that there was one serious side to the question: if anyone wished to go into bronchoscopic work thinking to get rich, he would get badly fooled. Most of the people who get foreign bodies into the trachea and bronchus are the children who are not taken care of, and the parents are unable to pay very large fees. The instruments are very expensive. Those that Dr. Ingals had used were given to Dr. Friedberg and had now passed on to Dr. McBride. The remunerative side of the work was not great, but the patients came to the office, as they had done in the days of Dr. Ingals and Dr. Friedberg, and someone had to take care of them.

# SOCIETY PROCEEDINGS.

## ABSTRACT OF THE SCIENTIFIC PROCEEDINGS OF THE FORTY-SECOND ANNUAL CONGRESS OF THE AMERICAN LARYNGOLOGICAL ASSOCIATION, HELD AT BOSTON, MASS., MAY 27-29, 1920.

Reported by Emil Mayer, M. D., Abstract Editor.

President A. Lawrence Lowell, of Harvard University, delivered an address of welcome.

Looking at American professional men and comparing them with men of the same class in Europe, one is brought to the conclusion that the American specializes more and earlier than does the European. It takes men a longer time here to fit themselves for medicine than for other subjects, because the amount of material they have to command is very much greater. One looks forward to the time when a simplification will take place; when some particular form of information will make way for the advent of general principles that simplify the processes of education and which will permit of the command of a larger variety of facts than could be available through isolated factors. These processes occur from time to time. Thus the bacterial theory of disease has simplified a great many problems which otherwise would have remained separate and complex.

The whole process of medical education is interesting to one who sees it as part of the total plan of education for a large number of professions. In the other professions men are trained to be citizens as well as professional men, as for instance in the legal profession or in engineering. In medicine it is all the other way. Medicine is a field of specialists.

If it is true that there is a time for everything; a time to be born, a time to wed, and a time to die, and it is generally conceded to be a mistake to do any of these things at the wrong time, then it is especially true that there is a time to enter a profession. There is a period when men acquire knowledge more easily and launch out with more energy and force into their career. I feel that men today are entering too late, especially in medicine. The amount of preparation required could readily be extended so as to make it impossible for men to enter at all before forty years and then it would be useless. The entrance time now is nearly thirty, much older than in other countries.

Our education begins too late. Children are sent to school much later with us than in European countries. Two years are lost and are never made up. The speaker believes that boys are capable of commencing college life at sixteen. The mind is more active at twenty than at twenty-five. The war showed us that our boys could rise to anything that occasion required of them. The speaker then extended a very cordial welcome to Harvard University to the members of the association.

### President's Address.

The President of the association, Dr. Norval H. Pierce, of Chicago, then addressed the association.

Attention was called to the history of the association and the high standard held to be requisite for membership.

If ever an esprit de corps existed among a body of men in the finest manner, it has existed in our association, but the speaker believes that we stand on the threshold of a new period in our development. In all the domains of human endeavor a great change is taking place in social, scientific and economic life. We will no longer be content with things as they were. There is a desire in the air for new and more productive effort, and that which interferes or tends to check the fulfillment of that desire will sooner or later be swept aside.

We must at all hazards widen the scope of those who practice within the confined limits of laryngology. First, by the preliminary education of specialists. (The speaker then quoted from a report by a committee composed of the heads of the departments of otolaryngology of three universities in Chicago, of which he was a member.) Second, association with other branches of medicine. Third, investigation and research.

The speaker called attention to the danger of regarding the association as an elysium where effort ceases, and to this end suggested that the method of program preparation be radically altered by the formation of a program committee who shall hold office for a term of five years. He then declared the meeting open for the reading of scientific papers.

## Retention Crypts in the Infratonsillar Nodules as Common and Extensive Harbors of Pathogenic Bacteria.

### By THOMAS R. FRENCH, M. D., Brooklyn, N. Y.

Our especial attention was drawn to the infratonsillar nodules, in tonsilloscopic studies in situ of the inferior lobes of pathologic tonsils, including a few which had been permitted to remain after tonsillectomies. The tonsilloscope must, therefore, be regarded as the responsible agent in detecting and exposing those germ-laden menaces to health, for that little instrument of precision had led us to at least the beginning of a knowledge of common and often very extensive harbors of infectious material, which of necessity must be reckoned with.

This study deals only with the chains of nodules lying on the lateral walls of the pharynx and the base of the tongue, directly beneath the faucial tonsils.

In the first actual removal of nodular tissues, which was from the throat of a girl, seven years of age, a section a quarter of an inch in length was enucleated with the tonsil, and in that short tonsillar appendage three collections of pus-like debris were found. And in conjunction with that revelation, we were cheered by what seemed to be another, of only slightly less importance, that on the under surface of the appendage there was a smooth limiting membrane which was manifestly a section of a fibrous capsule. The double display was, naturally, quite sufficient to stimulate thought for devising means to secure the removal of the whole of the structure, and when that had been accomplished and many entire nodular columns had been enucleated and their contents examined, it was made wholly apparent that here was a hidden, but probably common source of infection, which, no doubt, had been responsible for the inception and continuation of physical ills which had long baffled understanding. And it also was made clear that after we have become skilled in removing those masses of disordered tissue within the limits of safety to the patient, we will have no more right to permit such tissue to remain attached to the throat in our tonsil operations, than we now feel we have the right to perform a tonsillectomy, or even an incomplete tonsillectomy, when the tonsils are seen to be infiltrated with the products of past attacks of acute inflammation.

The pathologist reported that the removed nodules had well developed fibrous capsules and a few crypts but did not contain pus.

An examination of those specimens in the external tonsilloscope before they were sent to the laboratory, showed what we believed to be superficial abscesses, as each of the closely set collections of foreign material lying near the surface, was surrounded by a zone of hyperemia such as is always seen surrounding abscesses in other lymphoid tissues. Despite the position pronouncements of the tonsilloscope, we did not feel justified in continuing the removal of nodules until a solution of this vexing question could be found.

These examinations were made with the tonsilloscope, and also with a direct illumination of the nodules from a concentrated beam of an arc light, the field of observation meanwhile being magnified with a large warmed lens held in front of the mouth. While the nodules were glowing with the light of the tonsil lamp, or were being directly illuminated and magnified in the way just described, numerous small slits and pin-point spots, flush with the surfaces, were seen upon the tops of the lymphoid bodies. With the aid of a very thin bent probe, or searcher, those slits and spots were shown to be minute openings to crypts of varying sizes, but often relatively very large, and which at once were proved to be veritable traps to the unwary ingesta of secretions gravitating downward from the mouth and throat, for each of them was filled, and some of them were distended, with necrotic material which could easily be culled out with a curette. The constant presence of pathogenic bacteria in the crypts of the nodules has now, seemingly, been established, and those tissues, therefore, constitute still another field to which we must look for possible sources of chronic systemic infections.

## OBSERVATIONS ON THE ANATOMY, PATHOLOGY AND BACTERIOLOGY OF THE NODULES.

Except in broken chains and in minute form the nodules are not present in a state of health. Their presence in continuous lines or solid columns is an expression of a pathologic state. The four tonsils are constant structures. The nodules are constant only in minute form, but the fields, or pathways, over which they may develop, almost as if they were new growths, are definitely mapped out. The extent to which those fields, or pathways, may be occupied by the nodular tissues depends largely upon the amount of and the degree of irritation occasioned by the foreign material deposited within them.

The nodules are of a piece with the tonsils, as their underlying capsules are a continuation of the capsules of the tonsils. The mucous membrane covering the nodules is attached to the lower edges of the inferior poles of the tonsils, but the loosely attached ends of the lymphoid bodies extend upward to and occasionally slightly overlap the under surfaces of the posterior lateral halves of the inferior lobes.

It, therefore, would seem to be a fact that while in late childhood and youth, in association with diseased tonsils, there are always pharyngeal nodules which later may become branches, the lingual nodules are always branches, for they do not exist without trunks made by their junction with the pharyngeal nodules. The lingual branches are apparently developed in youth, and then only in association with extensively diseased tonsils.

Our observations lead us to the belief that the lingual tonsil is far less frequently enlarged than the nodules which connect it with the faucial tonsils, and when it is enlarged it is very much less so than the nodules. Indeed, it seems to be a fact that when the lingual tonsil is enlarged, and the associated nodules are connected with pus tonsils above, the nodules are apt to be several times larger than the lingual tonsil.

We believe that the free ends of the lingual branches are much more often the cause of pressure-cough in adults than is the lingual tonsil which is usually credited with it. This has occasionally been interestingly illustrated in the subjects of long standing irritative cough who were almost instantly relieved by the emptying of crypts in the nodular tissues which were lying in contact with the epiglottis.

Pus is not often found in the nodules. We have opened abscesses in several trunk specimens, but have not seen pus elsewhere in those structures. The necrotic tissue is practically all in the crypts, and in many of them it is so tightly locked in by the constricted mouths, that it seems almost as if it was sealed in, for in order to rupture such crypts in a fresh specimen it is necessary to apply heavy pressure to the sides of the nodules. As the lymphoid nodules described in this paper were believed to be devoid of lymph paths or crypts and also of capsules, objection has been made to their being classed as tonsils. Both of the missing links have been found to be cryptic, or in hiding, and as we now know that all the elements which characterize the faucial tonsils are, with a somewhat different arrangement and grouping, also present in the nodules, it would seem to be entirely correct to place them in the tonsil class. As they are in truth but offshoots or branches of the faucial tonsils, it may come to be a habit to speak of them as parts of the faucial tonsils, instead of separate structures. But future developments will affect their proper classification.

## DIAGNOSIS.

By depressing the tongue far back upon its base the lingual branches and the upper parts of the nodular trunks will be directly exposed. The tonsil lamp is then made to slide along behind the ridges of tissue to produce in its passage a luminous display of the pathologic conditions in every part of them. If, however, the fauces are too irritable even to permit the manipulation just described, then the condition in a nodule can, with a fair degree of accuracy, be determined by ascertaining the condition in its associated tonsil, for a situation in which the lamp cannot be quickly slipped behind a tonsil is scarcely conceivable. If the diseased condition of the tonsil is extensive enough to give a uniform bright rose-shade of color in transillumination, it is a fair assumption that in subjects above the age of six or eight years, filled retention crypts, varying in a general way in number and size according to the age of the subject and the extent of the disease in the tonsil, are present in its annexed nodule.

## ENUCLEATION OF THE NODULES, PUNCTURE AND CURETTAGE.

The key to the method of enucleating the pharyngeal nodules at any age and the nodular trunks and their pharyngeal branches in adults, lies in a block molded to fit over the angle and under the lower edge of the jaw in such a way that it will serve as a resisting wall, or outside runway, for an undercutting scoop of the arc of the Sluder guillotine.

The block duty usually falls to the anesthetist. After the block-mold is in place, the forefinger of the free hand of the operator is introduced into the fauces to press the tonsil firmly outward and downward upon the nodule to be removed. The guillotine, with the flat surface of the shaft in a horizontal position, is then introduced obliquely into the mouth and dipped gently downward over the side of the base of the tongue, close to the end of the forefinger pressing upon the tonsil, until the arc meets with the resistance of the pharyngoepiglottic fold. The edge of the shaft is then pressed forward deeply into the base of the tongue as near its outer limit as possible. The arc is now pressed outward with moderate firmness in order to sink it into the tissues below the free end of the nodule, and, while maintaining the pressure of the shaft against the tongue, the arc is drawn slowly upward along the block-supported wall toward the finger pressing upon the tonsil.

Upon reaching the inferior pole the upward movement of the arc is checked and at the same instant it is pressed hard against the ramus of the jaw to maintain its hold upon the stretched mucous membrane of the lateral wall of the pharynx. That membrane is highly elastic and is drawn under the nodule in ridges, like the wake of a moving hull, and put under considerable strain as the lower end of the nodule is doubled under itself by the arc. The finger holding the tonsil is then slipped down to the dislocated nodule overhanging the arc, to manipulate it into the grip of the blade of the guillotine—when after a half minute of compression it is cut off and the guillotine withdrawn.

A pharyngeal nodule is removed after a tonsillectomy—the block-mold being in position outside of the neck—by a scoop of the arc of the guillotine upward against a resisting finger held in the lower part of the empty tonsillar fossa, where it also may be made to assist in manipulating the dislocated tissues into the grip of the blade.

.While enucleation of the lingual branches with their capsules is most appealing to our ideas of completeness, it is possible that a less thorough removal of them will be quite as effective in obliterating the retention crypts, and also that the resulting wound will be less liable to inflammatory reaction during the healing process. An incision from the free end to the trunk made midway between the capsule and the upper surface would, in a fully developed nodule, undercut many crypts and probably convert the remainder into more or less wide-mouthed cups which could never again entrap foreign material. A very promising plan of accomplishing the midway severance of those tissues is to shave off their tops with the guillotine, for with it the alignment is more accurately made, compression can be practiced, and, if the lymphoid masses are not drawn through the fenestrum of the instrument, there is no danger of wounding the subjacent tissues or the numerous small varices which in adults often overlap the bases of the nodules. In all the subjects operated upon for the removal of infratonsillar nodules, the somewhat surprising and altogether pleasing fact has been that the blood loss from that source during operations was negligible, apparently adding little or nothing to the drain of the tonsil and adenoid procedure, and also that there has been no postoperative hemorrhage, no deterrent effect upon recovery from the enlargement of the pharyngeal wound and no added pain during the healing process. Indeed, the clinical picture following tonsil and adenoid operations including the removal of the nodules, has been the same as the familiar picture after similar operations without the removal of nodules. The above statement is based upon a "follow up" of most of the patients from whom nodules were removed, but, of course, we are not yet in a position to determine whether there are to be late postoperative effects. The operations for the removal of nodules were all performed under general anesthesia while the patients were in both recumbent and upright positions. Much of the best results were obtained in the upright position, as the gravid tongue not only permitted an easier manipulation of its base but greatly broadened the operative field. We presume the nodules can be enucleated under local anesthesia, but a consideration of that feature of the subject has not yet been reached. Where operation is not performed, nearly perfect results can be obtained by puncture through the sides of the crypts and curettage of all nodular structures.

Skilful curettage is an art which requires considerable practice to acquire, but the value of the method as a conservative measure makes it worth the while to develop, if possible, the deftness needed for the procedure. For high walled, narrow topped, jellylike lingual branches, in which the crypts are long and their openings minute, an effective method of emptying the crypts is by compressing the nodules with an oval sponge-stick and then expressing the cryptic contents.

## DISCUSSION OF DR. FRENCH'S PAPER.

Dr. D. Bryson Delavan, New York: This splendid contribution of Dr. French is the result of long continued, painstaking, exhaustive work. It is presented not as a theory, but as a series of abundantly demonstrated scientific facts. It is a valuable addition to the established knowledge of the anatomy and pathology of the lymphoid elements of the lower pharynx. In the clearness and force of the presentation, the convincing character of the pathologic specimens exhibited and the beauty of the illustrations, the association has rarely received a contribution of equal merit. I have had the privilege of following Dr. French's investigations for a long while. The practical application of his ideas has proved their truthfulness and well established their value.

Dr. Greenfield Sluder, St. Louis, Mo.: Upon the introduction of Dr. French's tonsillcscope, five or six years ago, I predicted that it had a future capable of great development. This work is the result of careful, painstaking and industrious investigation. The nodules spoken of seem to be in close proximity to the lingual mass and cross over behind the lingual fossa. In five or ten years these masses fill up and practically reproduce the entire tonsil.

Dr. Henry L. Swain, New Haven, Conn.: There are two or three points that I should like to make. The first is that we are told that all the new work is being done by the young men; but this wonderful piece of work is done by one of our oldest members. Another point is that this tissue is definitely encapsulated and mechanically loosens upon enucleation. As to the location of the nodes: I have been a little in doubt as to where they are located. It is not clear to me what the lateral column of the pharynx has to do with the situation, but we have to deal with groups of lymphoid tissue, which seems to be identical with the pharyngeal and lingual tonsil. This structure has the same ill effect upon the system as the tonsil and the importance of removal is equal in value to that of the tonsil in any other situation.

Dr. George L. Richards, Fall River, Mass.: I would like to express my personal thanks to Dr. French for this splendid contribution, coming as it does from one who has been a member of this association for forty-one years.

Dr. French, closing the discussion, expressed his appreciation of the gratifying and eloquent remarks on the paper by Dr. Delavan and Dr. Swain. He was glad to learn that the description of the nodules alone had been sufficient to enable Dr. Sluder readily to find an explanation of the recurrent tonsil or infiltrate, for, as with many other features contained in the body of the paper, that was not brought forward in the necessarily limited presentation of the subject. As to age, referred to by Dr. Richardson, the present outlook was that many more years must be added to his score before he could even begin to comprehend its existence.

### An Unusual Type of Nasal Tuberculosis.

By DR. GEORGE E. SHAMBAUGH, Chicago, Ill.

Read by title.

### A Case of Multiple Strictures of the Esophagus, Apparently Cured by Repeated Dilatation with Graduated Bougies.

By CLEMENT F. THEISEN, M. D., Albany, N. Y.

Female, aged 51, under care by the writer for eight months. She had been unable to swallow anything but liquids for the past year.

She had lost 28 pounds in weight and was markedly cachectic. She traced her difficulties to the accidental swallowing of a small amount of the fluid contained in a bottle of smelling salts, about two years ago.

The difficulty in swallowing became gradually worse until for the last year she could swallow only liquid food, and that often with difficulty.

Examination, both fluoroscopic and with X-ray plates, showed five distinct strictures, the first about the cricoid and the other four almost equal distances apart, the lowest about 2½ inches above the stomach.

After a period of rest a small, very flexible, metal bougie was passed through the first stricture. This was repeated several times before any attempt to pass through the others. She was able to take a little more liquid nourishment after the first few weeks. During the next six weeks the other strictures were successfully passed, the lowest one causing the greatest difficulty. Increasing sizes were used until an almost normal size could be introduced.

The patient gained rapidly, her weight became normal, and is able to take three full meals a day.

Dilatation was practiced every two weeks with fairly soft flexible fibre bougies.

The writer calls attention to the need of dilatation over a long period of time before it may be regarded as cured.

### Report of a Case of Syphilis, Vincent's Angina and Sarcoma of the Pharynx, Following Each Other in the Order Named.

#### By CLEMENT F. THEISEN, M. D., Albany, N. Y.

Male, aged 38, had deep ulceration almost covering the surface of both tonsils. Wassermann was positive, syphilitic history not obtained. Iodid of potash given, but the ulcerative process extended.

Vincent's angina was now apparent, being confirmed by an examination of the smears. In spite of vigorous treatment, including salvarsan, the process extended.

He then developed a large very hard mass in the left side of the neck. A piece of the very firm nodular mass from the edges of the tonsillar ulceration was removed, and upon examination proved to be a round celled sarcoma.

Serious hemorrhages from eroded blood vessels took place. The nodular mass, which broke down rapidly, extended to the base of the tongue and finally into the larynx, and the patient died soon thereafter.

This case is reported because of the unusual combination of diseases; the writer believes this occurs more frequently than the records show.

#### DISCUSSIONS OF DR. THEISEN'S PAPER.

Dr. Francis R. Packard, Philadelphia, Pa.: I had a similar case to the second one reported by Dr. Theisen. It had been diagnosed as quinsy and there was an ulcer where the incision had been made. Wassermann was strongly positive, salvarsan was injected and three weeks later the throat condition was very much worse. Removing a portion, the pathologist diagnosed it round celled sarcoma. Coley's fluid was given with beneficial results as far as the sarcoma was concerned.

Dr. James E. Logan, Kansas City, Mo.: I do not think it of any advantage to the patient to administer salvarsan without being absolutely certain of the specific nature of the lesion.

Dr. Thomas H. Halsted, Syracuse, N. Y.: A young man came to me with beginning ulcer of the throat. In spite of salvarsan and the iodids he grew steadily worse, and the ulceration extended to the soft palate, then he lost the whole roof of the mouth, nasal bone and external nose. Section removed showed round-celled sarcoma. The man denied ever having syphilis. He died within three months. I think other conditions than syphilis caused a positive Wassermann at times.

Dr. John E. Mackenty, New York: I have seen three cases in the clinic in which there was sarcoma of the neck or throat. There was a positive Wassermann, but the lesion did not clear up with specific treatment. I don't believe a positive Wassermann is to be taken absolutely seriously.

Dr. Lewis A. Coffin, New York City: I cannot but feel that the underlying cause in Dr. Theisen's case was lues; we not unfrequently have cases showing specific lesions and positive Wassermann that fail to respond to the most thorough antispecific treatment, these cases often have at some point a focal infection. If the latter be cleared up by ordinary means the specific symptoms clear up and the blood becomes negative to the Wassermann test.

Dr. Hanau W. Loeb, St. Louis, Mo.: I recall my experience with certain cases of Vincent's angina in the army, in which there was no way of differentiating from syphilis except by the course of the disease.

Dr. W. B. Chamberlin, Cleveland, Ohio: We do get cases of Vincent's angina complicating syphilis. In a recent case we made a diagnosis of Vincent's angina of the left tonsil. Microscopic examination showed spirillae and fusiform bacilli. The case cleared up under salvarsan. Subsequently the characteristic rash of syphilis developed and we found that there had been a primary sore on the tonsil. The condition was masked by the complicating Vincent's. The primary sore had been acquired during what our patient was pleased to call his vocation.

Dr. H. L. Swain, New Haven, Conn.: I think Dr. Theisen's first case should not go without mention. We have all had these cases of multiple stricture of the esophagus and work as hard over those cases as over anything we do. I had one case of complete stricture. The patient disappeared and later was seen after an operation in which someone had tried to reach the stricture through an external opening. The esophagus passed below the cricoid; lower down there was complete stricture behind the arch of the aorta. I dilated with a bougie, and the patient began to take liquid nourishment. I tried to pass a flexible tube into the stomach and the patient immediately complained of pain. The stomach tube had apparently ruptured adhesions between the posterior side of the stricture, and she developed an empyema. Resection of the ribs was done and she nearly died. Finally a complete stricture supervened. The patient is a young girl of 17, and I shall do all I can to avoid for her the fate of passing a long life of having to be fed through a gastrostomy opening.

Dr. D. Crosby Greene, Boston, Mass.: I understood in these cases Dr. Theisen say that radium never did any good. I would take exception that statement. In my experience remarkable improvement has occurred in many cases of this type.

Dr. Theisen, closing the discussion: I want to correct an error in the title of my paper. It says "cured," but I would like to change that to "apparently cured." These cases do recur. Dr. Swain's case reminds me of a procedure which you may have tried. I saw a child with complete stricture of the esophagus, after swallowing caustic potash. The child had a gastrostomy done in the hospital, by one of the surgeons, and we finally got a piece of fine whalebone through from above attached to a ligature, and we then sawed through the stricture. It was many months, however, before the gastrostomy wound could be closed. The child swallowed fairly well after a while. As regards syphilis and Vincent's angina, I think often syphilis makes a good foundation for the Vincent's angina to be grafted on. One is subsequent to the other, or they often occur together.

## SYMPOSIUM ON RADIUM.

### Treatment of Epithelioma of the Larynx by Radium.

#### By DR. H. H. JANEWAY, New York.

Read by title.

### Dosage and Methods of Treatment.

#### By PROFESSOR WILLIAM DUANE, Harvard University.

In deciding upon the details of an application of radium, or of any of the radioactive substances to a case of malignant disease, one must bear in mind the general principles underlying the methods of radiotherapy. There is no evidence that rays from radioactive substance can transform tumor cells directly into normal cells. The fundamental principle of radio treatment appears to be one of destruction. The rays from the radioactive substance destroy the tumor cells either by passing through them and exerting a direct action on them, or by cutting off their supply of nutrition; just as invading armies are destroyed either by shooting individual soldiers, or by cuttting off their food supply. In order to destroy a tumor by radiation we must fill the tumor and part of the surrounding healthy tissue with rays sufficiently intense to kill the tumor cells, but at the same time we must avoid too great destruction of the normal tissues. The problem becomes largely one of solid geometry. The source, or sources, of radiation must be placed in such positions in or near the lesion as to produce the required effects throughout the volume of the tumor.

The primary effect of the passage of radioactive rays through a substance appears to be the ejection of atoms of electricity called electrons from the atoms of ordinary matter. As a secondary effect a regrouping of the atoms takes place. For instance, if the rays pass through water, $H_2O$, they split up the water in molecules, and, as a regrouping of the atoms, we get molecules of hydrogen, H; of oxygen, $O_2$; of hydrogen peroxid, $H_2O_2$, etc. Just what regrouping of atoms take place when the rays pass through living tissue we do not know, and, in the nature of the case, are not likely to find out, until we have learned more about the actual distribution of the atoms before the rays passed through them.

Although we do not understand the mechanism of the effects produced by rays on living cells, we do know something about the gross behavior of tumors after radiation. One of the most important effects due to rays appears to be a retardation of the growth of the tumor. This retardation may last for many generation of cells after the generation that has actually received the radiation. The retardation effect is of great value in cases where the situation of a tumor does not allow its complete destruction or removal. The direct action of rays from a radioactive substance on a cell appears to be more pronounced during mitosis than at other times. For this reason prolonged radiation ought to be more effective than short radiation, for there would be more chance of catching a greater number of cells during their most vulnerable period in the former than in the latter case. Over five years ago I used a method of treating certain types of malignant disease with radioactive substances, which has the following advantages: (a) the active sources of the rays may be placed and kept in position with considerable precision, thus ensuring an accurate distribution of the radiation throughout the tumor; (b) very little effect is produced in normal tissue at a short distance from the source of the rays; and (c) the length of the treatment may be prolonged continuously for days, weeks or even months. The method consists in introducing very minute glass tubes containing a very small quantity of radium emanation (often less than one millicurie) into the tumor itself through a trocar. The tubes and emanations are left in place until most, or practically all of the emanation has disappeared. As is well known half of a given quantity of emanation disappears in slightly less than four days, so that in this way the tumor tissue may be subjected to weak radiation lasting a long time.

The emanation in the tubes transforms itself into substances called radium A, B and C, Radium B and C (not the emanation, nor radium A) produce the rays that are used in therapy. The walls of the glass tubes being very thin the radiation passes easily through them, and is absorbed in the tissues immediately surrounding them—most of it within 6 or 7 mm. of the tubes. Hence by accurately placing the tubes in position the radiation can be confined to the required volume of tissue with precision.

Owing to the fact that most of the radiation is absorbed close to the tubes, very little effect is produced at a distance from them. Normal tissue appears to be able to withstand indefinitely the weak rays that reach a distance of 10 or 15 mm. from the tubes. Thus excessive destruction of healthy tissue may be avoided, if the tubes are properly placed.

In certain types of cases, which are particularly well suited to it, the method appears to be the best procedure to follow in applying radioactive substances to malignant disease.

This method has been extensively used in our own hospital and in the Memorial Hospital, New York.

### Factors Influencing the Quantitative Effects of Radiation.

By DR. WILLIAM T. BOVIE, Harvard University.

For every treatment in radiotherapy the clinician must decide the following question:

Under a given set of conditions, what exposure must I give to produce the desired effects? The decision is frequently a mere guess, for many more factors are involved in the dosage of radiotherapy than are involved in the dosage of chemotherapy, and chemotherapeutics can scarcely be classed as an exact science.

The students of photography have very successfully solved the dosage problem for the blackening of the photographic plate. Undoubtedly there is much which the clinician may learn from them. With the speed of the plate determined and stamped on the box, formula given for making up developers and fixing solutions, full directions as to temperature control, duration of development, etc., the only thing left to the judgment of the photographer is the intensity of the light to which the plate is exposed, and even here he has been provided witht chemical devices, actinometers, for accurately measuring the power which the light has to bring the silver bromide of the photographic film into the developable condition.

It is not always convenient in clinical problems to measure the intensity of radiations at the place where they are absorbed, but when a point source is used, if the intensity of the radiation is known at any one distance from the source, it is possible by means of Lambert's "inverse square law" to calculate the intensity. This does not apply, however, to other than point sources, nor to sources of the corpuscular radiations A and B rays. By exploring with photographic paper as an actinometer I have measured the intensity of the radiation about small cylindrical sources, such as glass tubes containing radium emanation and have constructed diagrams of surfaces of equal intensity.

It is not sufficient to know only the intensity of the radiation. One of the oldest laws in photochemistry is Grotthus' law which states that "it is only that fraction of the rays which is absorbed that is effective in bringing about a photochemical change." It is necessary, therefore, to know, besides the intensity of the radiation, the fraction of the rays which will be absorbed. Again using photographic paper as an actinometer and beeswax as a typical homogeneous absorbing medium, I have constructed charts and diagrams showing radiation intensities within such an absorbing medium when it encloses a tube of radium emanation as a source for rays.

Photography would not be possible if manufacturers possessed no method of measuring and indicating the sensitiveness of their plates to light. It would undoubtedly help tremendously if we possessed a similar sensitometry for tissues. (Dr. Bovie then discussed the methods of sensitometry of the photographic plate, and showed how these methods may be applied directly to the sensitometry of tissues.)

In order to arrive at a mathematic expression giving the relationship between the exposure and the physiologic effect, it will be necessary to have a term for the intensity of the radiation, a term for the amount of energy required to produce the particular change sought in a single cell or tissue element, a term expressing the absorption index of the tissue to the particular radiation used, a term showing the concentration of the unaffected cells or elements of tissue, and a term expressing the number of cells or elements already altered by the exposure. It may be shown that an expression of this kind leads to the conclusion that the effect produced should vary with the logarithm of the exposure (intensity times the time).

It follows, therefore, that a short exposure is relatively more effective than a long exposure.

One other term must be introduced into such a mathematical expression, namely, a term which the photographer calls "the factor of development." The initial photochemical change latent image, produced by the exposure cannot be detected. It is only after a period of development, in therapy a period of physiologic change, that the effects of the radiation are manifest. Unfortunately at the present time we are quite ignorant of the nature of, and the laws which govern, the rate of these physiologic changes. It is for this reason that many of the results of radiation treatment are charged to the idiosyncrasies of the patient.

It is a step in advance to formulate a problem even if we are unable to solve it.

### The Results of Treatment of Malignant Disease of the Upper Air Tract by Radiation.

(From the Clinic of the Huntington Memorial Hospital, Boston.)

#### By D. CROSBY GREENE, M. D.

In treating carcinoma of the larynx with radium, we are confronted at the outset with the problem of making accurate applications of the desired dosage to the exact location required. Owing to the intolerance of the larynx to foreign bodies and the involuntary movements of gagging, swallowing, and coughing, even after thorough cocainization, such accurate application is not practicable by any method of surface application from within. I believe that some improved method of insertion will prove to be effective in a fair proportion of cases which are not far advanced.

This method is especially applicable to the cases of extrinsic cancer involving the tissues about the orifice of the larynx in which complete surgical removal would involve excision ot the tongue, total extirpation of the larynx, and resection of the upper esophagus.

In cases of intrinsic carcinoma, operation by window resection of the thyroid cartilage, leaving the wound open for immediate and subsequent radiation, is an effective method of treatment in some cases.

The effectiveness of any method of radiation from a clinical standpoint, depends on the extent of destruction of tumor tissue. While the tumor cells have been shown to be less resistant to the action of the rays than normal tissue, in order to furnish sufficient strength of dosage to reach those tumor cells which have invaded normal tissue beyond the limit of gross inspection, some normal tissue also must be destroyed in the process. Unfortunately, cartilage which forms the framework of the larynx although peculiarly resistant to invasion by cancer, is especially vulnerable to the rays. Therefore, as a result of radiation, perichondritis and necrosis of the cartilage is likely to take place, resulting later in permanent stenosis of the laryngeal passage.

In early intrinsic cancer, surgical treatment by thyrotomy without radiation, up to the present time has yielded such brilliant results that it is still the method of choice.

The speaker presents the following conclusions:

1. In malignant disease of the regions we have considered, the chief value of radium lies in supplementing rather than supplanting operation.

2. In cases of extensive extrinsic laryngeal carcinoma about the upper orifice, in which operative removal entails excessive operative risk, benefit may be expected in a small proportion of cases by radium treatment alone. In our hands the method of insertion of seeds under direct inspection has been the most effective in such cases.

3. In early intrinsic carcinoma of the larynx, the operation of thyrotomy and excision without radiation is still the method of choice. This conclusion is based on the untoward secondary results which have followed in certain cases caused by the destructive effects of active radiation on the cartilaginous framework of the larynx. The results from thyrotomy in early cases are too favorable to lead one to employ radium treatment under these circumstances. In moderately advanced cases, however, the use of radium to supplement operation is advisable.

4. In most cases palliative results in the way of retardation of the growth and relief of pain may be expected by radium treatment in some form.

5. In advanced upper jaw cases treatment by operation followed by radiation has given promising results.

## DISCUSSION.

Dr. D. Bryson Delavan: From personal experience as well as that of many others practically interested in the subject with whom I have conversed, and from what may be deduced from the statements of various authorities whose views upon the subject have been published, it would seem that the present situation with regard to the value of radium in malignant disease of the upper air passages may be thus summarized:

1. The histological character of a growth to which radium may be applied will have an important influence upon its effect.

2. In certain types of malignant growth under favorable conditions, the use of radium may effect a cure.

3. In cases where the prospect of a cure is not probable, under the use of radium there has often been observed a distinct temporary retrogression of the growth.

4. Even in otherwise hopeless cases radium is likely to relieve distressing symptoms of pain, discharge and their attendant sequels.

Dr. J. Payson Clark, Boston, Mass., showed a man, 33 years old, who has had a large tumor involving the right tonsil and adjacent structures, clinically diagnosed as sarcoma. Later a small piece, snipped off for examination, was pronounced by the microscopist "malignant lymphoma."

The tumor was treated by imbedding small glass tubes of radium emanation into it. The tumor was compleetly destroyed after four months' treatment, and there has been no recurrence a year and a half from the completion of the treatment.

Dr. F. E. Hopkins, Springfield, Mass., presented the history of a boy of 17, native, extraordinarily tall and slender, who stated that during the previous summer he had an acute infection of his throat, "a severe tonsillitis," with high temperature and marked prostration. A prominent symptom was difficulty in swallowing, which became serious because of interference with nutrition. .He was taken to a hospital and fed by tube, and bougies were passed to dilate the supposed stricture of the esophagus. This was continued for six weeks, the patient meanwhile becoming very weak and unable to sit up. X-ray plate showed an obstruction near the cricoid cartilage, displacing and closing the esophagus from the posterior and right side. The question of an abscess was considered, palpation showed a yielding mass but not a fluid content. It was then suggested that this growth was an accessory thyroid and the patient treated by radium and X-ray. The technic of the treatment is fully given, with illustrations of the fluoroscopic picture. There was a steady improvement following this treatment, the patient gained 30 pounds in weight and can now partake of food in a perfectly normal manner.

## DISCUSSION ON SYMPOSIUM.

Dr. C. G. Coakley, New York: It has been proven experimentally and clinically that while there is a partial destruction of the tissues of the pharynx and larynx and improvement of the patient, there is apt to occur suddenly a rapid extension and increase of the growth, such as occurs in no other way. One point observed in radium treatment of the nose and nasopharynx is the extraordinary amount of pain and burning produced which no medication will allay.

I have had eleven cases of cancer of the larynx treated by radium. In one of them the growth was limited to one-half of the cord. The man was given an improperly screened dosage, and while the growth diminished there was terrible destruction of tissue, including the trachea.

There was not a trace of epithelioma found at autopsy. There was a septic bronchopneumonia due to absorption of toxic material. In another case there was an epithelioma involving the upper part of the larynx. Tracheotomy had been performed two weeks previously. Considerable granulation tissue about the tube was radiumized, leaving a healed surface.

Five cases of fibroma of the nasopharynx did remarkably well. One of epithelioma of the palate had a recurrence after eight months. One case of constant asthma caused by nasal polyps was treated by radium with relief of the asthma and disappearance of the polyps.

Dr. H. P. Mosher, Boston, Mass.: I have had more experience with cancer of the upper jaw than with cancer of the larynx. Radium has proved to be of most use in superficial growths, and in growths like those of the upper jaw that have been made superficial by operation. In jaw cases I am strongly against opening into the mouth if it can be avoided.

Dr. Harry A. Barnes, Boston, Mass.: My results with radium alone have been uniformly discouraging. I have, however, found it an invaluable adjunct to operative measures, used, immediately after removal of the growth, on the whole operative field. In eight cases of malignant disease of the accessory sinuses, a radium tube of 35 to 40 milicuries was placed in the center of the postoperative pack and allowed to remain there throughout convalescence. Subsequent radium treatments were given through an opening in the cheek made by cutting away a triangular flap from the facial integument at the end of the operation. These radium exposures were given, not because of any recurrence, but with the idea of destroying microscopic particles of tumor impossible of removal by operation, and also to counteract the possible tendency of metastatic formation which the crushing nature of the operation might have produced. Of six cases of carcinoma, three are dead; two are alive and with no signs of recurrence after 26 and 17 months, respectively. Two cases of sarcoma are alive and without recurrence after 28 and 18 months, respectively. There was one death directly attributable to operation. Of the eighth cases, four (50 per cent) are alive and without recurrence after intervals of from 17 to 28 months.

Dr. Harmon Smith, New York: I regret exceedingly the absence of Dr. Janeway, as he had embodied in his paper the histories of a number of my cases, and their absence lessens materially the force of my remarks.

My earliest cases were far advanced, and it became often necessary to perform a tracheotomy before they could be turned over to Dr. Janeway, and all these went on to their doom in about a year and one-half.

Following this in a case of lymphosarcoma of the tonsils of a boy of 18, I had removed the right tonsil; then in about 18 months a similar involvement of the left occurred and was removed, and then radium was applied. He remained free for about two years, and there never was any recurrence in the pharynx, but there was metastasis in the chest and head, and he ultimately died.

The next case was one of lymphosarcoma of the tonsil. There was no operation; radium was applied, and though observed for two years there was no evidence of return.

The next two cases were typical nasofibroma. The first in a boy of 16. In spite of repeated removal, and the injection of monochloracetic acid the recurrence was fearfully rapid. Radium treatment at several intervals had no effect and he died of hemorrhage.

The second case was of the same character, as the first. The patient disappeared and did not return for about a year. There then was a marked improvement in his condition, and monochloracetic acid was again injected and after a few months the growth had almost entirely disappeared.

The next in the series are those of cancer in the larynx.

It occurs so frequently that patients come to us with the direct request for radium to be applied, and the question of operation is a secondary matter, that I feel the need for calling attention to the fact that the cure of cancer by radium has been unjustifiably advertised to the laity. In many cases we may lose the crucial importance that we promptly determine exactly what radium can moment by applying radium first. It is certainly of the greatest do and likewise ascertain its limitations.

Dr. J. E. Mackenty, New York, presented a larynx, which shows the effect of radium treatment. Radium gas was injected into the larynx direct and left in. Three weeks later there was an enormous edema of the larynx, tracheotomy and nasal feeding became necessary. Septic bronchitis followed and operation was done under local and general anesthesia. The larynx was the site of a large abscess cavity. The patient made a rapid recovery.

### Acute Abscess of the Lateral Wall of the Lower Pharynx.

### By DR. CHARLES W. RICHARDSON, Washington.

The speaker described an unusual type of abscess of the laryngopharynx. The origin of it was uncertain. Symptomalogic characterized by the sudden onset and the severity of the pain; tumefaction not manifest until the second or third day. Pointing takes place deep down in the lateral wall of the lower pharynx. There is little alteration of voice or interference with breathing; deglutition very painful, but not impossible. Septic temperature of moderate type. Treatment: Early evacuation.

### DISCUSSION.

Dr. Henry L. Swain, New Haven, Conn.: In 1913 I published in the Transactions of this association a report of five or six cases of a similar nature, which I called abscesses of the lateral column of the pharynx. There was marked edema of the larynx. A recent case of mine had no edema and was exactly like the one described by Dr. Richardson.

Dr. J. E. Mackenty, New York City: I had several cases of this affection last winter. In one there was danger from edema of the larynx and the neck was opened. I believe external operation is far safer, as probing for pus in the edematous tissues of the throat is a very dangerous procedure.

Dr. Richardson, closing the discussion: Dr. Swain's cases are not quite like the cases reported. His cases were those of descending infection of the lateral wall and the posterior pillar.

### Nasociliary Neuralgia.

### By GREENFIELD SLUDER, M. D., St. Louis.

Pain in the eyes, brow, and root of the nose is frequent and may be of different origins. Localization of the pain of the several origins by the patient is not precise. Pains of frontal, ethmoid and sphenoid sinuses, or nasal (sphenopalatine-Meckel's) ganglion, or supraorbital or nasociliary nerve origin may overlap in their sensations. This last pain is usually referred to the small district bounded by the supraciliary ridge above the supraorbital notch laterally and the nasal bones below. Sometimes it extends to the tip of the nose. Rarely it is referred to the eyes. Patients often complain that they cannot wear their glasses because of soreness of the nasal bones. Severe degrees, however, of whatever origin, may be referred beyond these limits. Pain of supraorbital neuralgia is more widespread. Pain of suppuration of the frontal or ethmoid sinuses under pressure is of long known recognition.

(Here follows careful anatomic description of the nasal nerve and its branches.—E. M.).

It is to be seen that the nasociliary nerve, as it enters the nose in its uppermost anterior limit, is quite near the surface of the membrane. It is more superficial than the nasal ganglion (usually). The ganglion may, however, be quite superficial (submucous). So it is easily understandable that an inflammation of the membrane in this part may irritate or inflame the nerve and produce pain. In older cases with general hyperplasia of membrane and bone, it is also easily understandable that the ethmoidal slit may be encroached upon to narrow its caliber and place the nerve in a more easily vulnerable position.

## DIFFERENTIAL DIAGNOSIS.

The nasociliary nerve is more easily cocainized than the nasal ganglion. A small applicator with 20 per cent sol. suffices. It is passed upward on the inside of the nose, being held forward in contact with the anterior limit of the nasal fossa until it reaches the roof of the fossa. By this procedure it arrives automatically in the apex of the angle formed by the cribriform plate above and the anterior limit of the nasal fossa. It is at this point that the nasociliary nerve enters the nasal fossa. When the pain in this region is of nasociliary origin, such an application of cocain will stop it in a few minutes. Should it be of the other origins mentioned above, it will not be influenced by such an application.

My observation so far has been that nasociliary neuralgia has usually been a transitory phenomenon in the course of cases which have been in observation or treatment for something else. The nasociliary neuralgia would appear from time to time in the course of other clinical conditions, and was usually not obstinate. It would yield to cocainization and applications of dilute carbolic acid, ½ per cent. Four times, however, I have seen it the only clinical phenomenon. Once I injected the nerve trunk at its entrance into the nose, with relief to the patient. The technic is that first advocated by Otto J. Stein in his alcohol injection treatment of hyperesthetic rhinitis.

A straight needle is passed upward in the nose in the same way as the applicator for cocainization described above. A few drops of 95 per cent alcohol with 5 per cent phenol are instilled into the nerve trunk at its exit from the ethmoid slit.

## DISCUSSION.

Dr. Henry L. Swain, New Haven, Conn.: Dr. Sluder gave us the sphenopalatine ganglion syndrome, and now he is teaching us the nasociliary type to be added to the neuralgias which have borne his name all over the world. I have had an interesting case of this affection, of which Dr. Sluder writes me that it is an exquisite case. The Ewing's sign was very marked. That was relieved by the application of cocain to the sphenopalatine ganglion. In this case the pain in the angle of the orbit was the troublesome feature, and treatment to the eye was of no avail, while a single application to the ganglion achieved the effect immediately.

In my hands a weak solution of nitrate of silver prolonged the beneficial effect of the cocain. I hesitate to apply carbolic and alcohol for fear of severe reaction, which occurred in this patient and lasted 24 hours, from the simple application of nitrate of silver.

Dr. Harmon Smith, New York: The excellence of Dr. Sluder's articles has been manifest to me in my official capacity, in that the copies of the Transactions of this Association containing his reports have been in unusual demand.

In one case of mine the patient, a lady from California, who had several operations upon her left maxillary sinus. These were followed by intense pain on that side.

I was to try the Sluder method, but expecting him in New York shortly, I awaited his arrival and submitted the case to him.

Local anesthetization had no effect, and Sluder was averse to have the patient return with him for further treatment. I should like to have Dr. Sluder state his reasons for that decision.

Dr. Faulkner injected the ganglion with alcohol with only temporary effect. Radium within the antrum produced excruciating pain. Dr. Sharp removed the semilunar ganglion with immediate relief.

Dr. J. E. Mackenty, New York: A patient of mine had a nasociliary neuralgia, with considerable inflammatory tissue. This was removed with the Sluder knives, with cure of her pain. In another type of case there is a sense of pressure over the distribution of the nasal nerve, a pressure from within which causes great distress and does not yield to treatment. I would like to know if Dr. Sluder would include this in the nasociliary cases?

Dr. H. W. Loeb, St. Louis: The interesting part of this report is that it makes it possible to differentiate this type of pain from other types of nasal origin. Has Dr. Sluder met any cases with pain referred to this region but with a distinct point of origin?

Dr. Norval H. Pierce, Chicago, mentioned the case of a minister who was compelled to give up his work in church on account of a phonetic spasm associated with grotesque facial contortions.

As he complained of pressure symptoms in the nose, equal parts of cocain and sugar of milk were blown up the nose, with the surprising result of the disappearance of the spasm and the return of a normal voice. After that, whenever he had to preach or talk he used a tablet of 50 per cent cocain and sugar of milk. This occurred before Dr. Sluder published his work. It is possible that the case may have been one of reflex trouble from the nose. It was remarkable that cocain relieved the pain, whether applied to right or left side of the nose, also that hypodermic injections had the same effect. Hence in these conditions I feel that we cannot eliminate the systemic effects of cocain.

Dr. James E. Logan, Kansas City: Dr. Sajous used cocain on the turbinates in his study of the reflex neuroses of the nasal cavity, but Dr. Sluder has brought out more clearly the relations of the subject from the diagnostic and remedial standpoint.

Dr. Sluder, closing the discussion: Dr. Swain's case was evidently a nasal ganglion neurosis and I suggested that he inject it. I presume, also, that she was very neurotic and difficult. In such cases the injection should be carried out under nitrous oxid anesthesia and a small amount of cocain applied to the nasal ganglion. The gas does not complicate the issue. By adding methylene blue to the alcohol it can be seen if it enters the throat. Nitrous oxid is preferable to ether, and a straight needle better than a curved one.

Dr. Harmon Smith: The case I mentioned had been operated on for maxillary sinusitis, and continued to suffer from neuralgia. Cocain did no good. Dr. Sluder advised against continuing.

Dr. Sluder: Such cases are extremely difficult. The nerve supply of the nasal ganglion may come through the sphenoid fossa. In Dr. Smith's case a Gasserian ganglionectomy was done, I presume. If the entire sensory supply is removed a cure follows in some cases but not in all. The question is what is the source of pain. My opinion is that the pain is transmitted by the sympathetic fibers that run through the nose. It is claimed by some that the sympathetic is purely a motor system and that there are no fibers of a sensory nature at all. While, on the other hand, there is sufficient at hand to show that there exists a motor and sensory supply taking in the spinal ganglion. Cushing thinks that all this work is a mistake, and I hope to argue it with him shortly, before the American Laryngological, Rhinological and Otological Society.

Dr. Pierce's case is very interesting and raises the question as to how much of this effect is due to absorption and systemic influence. This effect has been so carefully watched since 1903 and the prompt response of relief when the proper spot was touched, and only then would indicate the localization of the diseased condition and its prompt relief.

I have seen similar cases to that of Dr. Pierce, complicated with blepharospasm. Cocainization of the nasal ganglion relieved the orbicularis spasm and soft palate for 12 hours. I shall try, however, the subcutaneous injection of cocain in my next case. I have injected in the edema of hay fever when the whole nose was occluded and this was cleared up by injection.

### Esophagismus and Allied Disorders.

### By DR. THOMAS HUBBARD, Toledo.

Complete reversal of peristalsis culminates in emesis, but the interesting fact is that the important clinical manifestations are partial or abortive reversals. Globus, heartburn, erophagia and belching, regurgitation and nausea are familiar clinical examples.

We are inclined to attribute socalled biliousness and bad taste in mouth and foul breath exclusively to throat, nose and mouth conditions, and certain it is that we have met disappointments in attempts to give relief by ordinary treatment.

Recent clinical and experimental observations are convincing that reverse peristalsis can be a factor in causing any of these symptoms.

Pyloric and cardiac control are influenced by the chemical reactions, and likewise the cricoid may react against the acid of reversed peristalsis. This may produce the symptoms which we call globus.

Attention has been called to the blending of involuntary and voluntary nervous energy in this region and with true globus hystericus in mind we can appreciate what is meant by psychic interference. It is characteristic of the psychic factor that the function as a whole rather than certain nerve tracts give evidence of interference. The hypoglossal, glossopharyngeal, pneumogastric and spinal accessory, and even the phrenic, controlling salivary and mucous membrane secretions and the muscular action direct and auxiliary of food ingestion may any or all be affected.

With consciousness of dysphagia, the psychic factor of alarm may cause a reaction of hyperesthesia in areas previously anesthetic, and the tonic spasm results—a spasmogenic phenomenon. The foreign body sensation is very common in this type of throat trouble, and reversely, throat hysteria can be induced by a real foreign body.

The terminal·of the tube at the hiatal orifice, commonly called the cardia, is subject to spasmodic constriction enduring even to the degree of threatening life. (Jackson objects to the term "cardiospasm," preferring hiatal spasm, and he is correct, as usual.) It is primarily a phenomenon of partial reversal. Chronicity, in this instance, naturally follows distortion due to sacculation above the stricture, and even in fatal cases—death from starvation— there is found little or no hypertrophy of circular muscle fibers at cardia or hiatal regions.

The following conclusions are presented:

1. The pharyngeal plexus is concerned with a primitive function of such vital importance that even slight disturbance may provoke psychic interference with resulting confusion of automatic reflexes.

2. Chronic spasmogenic phenomena, esophagism and cardiospasm, may be primarily manifestations of irregular or reversed peristalsis.

3. The hysterical throat is a manifestation of paresthesia and incoordinated muscle actions with psychic fixation in neuropathic individuals.

4. It is probable that disease conditions and local irritations of the gastrointestinal tract may initiate the reverse peristalsis involving the esophagus. Abnormal reflexes and sensations are naturally referred to the beginning of the vegetative tract—the region of the pharyngeal plexus.

5. Through intimate anatomic association, the throat and larynx participate in the clinical syndrome. The gastric factor in asthma may be thus explained.

6. The more we emphasize peristalsis as a factor in digestion, the more important is it to properly interpret abnormal peristalsis as a factor in disease.

Dr. R. B. Shurley, Detroit, Mich.: We see a number of these cases in this rapid, nervous age. They can be watched through the fluoroscope and the spasm seen. Dilatation causes great relief, as also full doses of the bromides. These cases represent instability of the nervous system of the vasomotor type. Reestablishment of the nerve tone by hypodermic injections of iron and glycerophosphates and dilatation of the esophagus are beneficial. I had one patient who was unable to eat when anyone was looking, and another who could only eat while standing. Patients of this type would eat sandwiches and other foods in the office which they declared they could not eat at home.

Dr. Lewis A. Coffin, New York City: I have long laid stress on the importance of the care of the gastrointestinal tract in affections of the upper air passages. This holds specially where there isa disturbance of the vasomotor system. Rhinorrhea, sneezing, hay fever and asthma are not infrequently caused by gastrointestinal disorders, and are frequently relieved by appropriate treatment to the cause.

Dr. H. L. Swain, New Haven, Conn.: In the exhibit by Dr. Mosher, I noted that the lobe of the liver was very near the lower pole of the esophagus. Supposing this lower lobe impinged on the esophagus, a marked effect might be produced, both mechanical and obstructive, as well as inducing spasm.

Dr. Henry L. Lynah, New York City: A great many cases of malignant disease of the esophagus occur and are labeled hysteria, and they are only discovered after death. The functional spasms become organic sooner or later.

Dr. Hubbard, closing the discussion: There is no disease more difficult to cure than cardiospasm. Many cases of this affection are diagnosed as organic stricture, and the autopsy shows no lesion. Just what makes the formation of the sacculation is not determined. Dr. Coffin wrongly labels his cases granular pharyngitis. All pharyngitis is caused by chemical irritation and autointoxication, perhaps due to retarded peristalsis. Chemical digestion takes place in the gastrointestinal tract, and disturbances of rhythm upset the whole process. Organic disease is the cause of spasm. I have one case of a man who could only swallow liquids, who has a small, pendulous, nonmalignant tumor just below the cricoid which I expect to snare off. The importance of reverse peristalsis as a cause of obscure throat lesions has long been apparent to me.

## Intrinsic Carcinoma of the Larynx, with a Second Report of the Cases Operated on by Suspension and Dissection.

### By DR. R. C. LYNCH, New Orleans.

Every case has been carefully studied with a negative Wassermann and a negative clinical test against syphilis and tuberculosis, and the tumor mass removed in each instance has been carefully submitted to a pathologist of repute with the simple notation that the tissue is from the larynx.

Under suspension it is perfectly possible to palpate with a feeler with quite as much certainty as one does with his fingers upon the surface of the body, and because of the peculiar location of the lesion and the anatomic construction of the cartilaginous box in which this growth takes its origin, it seems very easy, for me at least, to make out quite definitely, the area of involvement, and thereby making due allowance for microscopic invasion, to cut sufficiently wide the growth to insure its removal, at least with as much assurance of success as one operates for this dread disease in any other part of the body, including thyrotomy and the total extirpation of the larynx.

These are a few points to be remembered:

First, after having determined that the case is suitable for intrinsic dissection, it is necessary to have the consent of the patient to do all or anything that is necessary, for while under suspension you may determine that thyrotomy or even laryngectomy is the only possible chance to save the individual from this disease and preserve his natural breathway. If you have done a few thyrotomies for intrinsic cancers diagnosed by mirror only, then I feel sure that you have been surprised at the extent of involvement—usually far beyond your expectation.

Second, that since it is determined that the case is suitable for intrinsic dissection, when once the forceps take hold of the mass they should not let go to avoid the possibility of cell implantation from this source.

Third, that the tumor circumscribed, as is possible from an anatomic standpoint, and is usually delivered upon a cartilaginous plate, not having permitted the cutting instruments to come in contact with the tumor mass again to avoid implantation.

Fourth, there must be no special desire to save tissue for subsequent functional use, for fear that in your desire to save tissue the removal will not be complete.

Fifth, all raw surfaces should be sealed with the actual cautery at a cherry red heat that this may seal the lymphatic drainage outlet from the raw surface and with the hope that the heat thus applied will kill any remaining cancer cells that may have been displaced during the operation.

The advantages of the operation are that, being especially suitable for the very early cases where there is apparently very little involvement of tissue, it can be done quickly and without external incision; that the normal breathway is not interfered with, since trachectomy is at no time necessary, and the chances of postoperative contraction are most remote; that the operation is carried on entirely within the closed box, which should offer the very best opportunity against metastasis, spread or involvement without the box; that convalescence is unusually short and the surface can easily be watched by mirror, and finally, when convalescence has been completed there is more likelihood of nature establishing a cord with which the voice function can be reestablished.

The histories of nine cases are presented. One is dead of recurrence. Two others had a recurrence; they were subjected to a laryngectomy and are still well and healthy and useful citizens. The other six are perfectly well. One, six years after the operation; one, four years after operation; one, three years after operation; two, two years after operation, and, at this time, one, six months after operation.

## DISCUSSION.

Dr. D. C. Greene, Boston, Mass.: I have no objection to any method of removing cancer provided the entire mass with a sufficient margin of healthy tissue is removed intact. I believe that Dr. Lynch's method is successful in his hands on account of his extraordinary skill, and I do not believe it can take the place of thyrotomy in general. I have, however, found the Lynch apparatus most useful as an adjunct in the thyrotomy operation.

Dr. J. E. Mackenty, New York City: Dr. Lynch's results, nine cases and eight recoveries, are far better than the external method of operation, and probably he sees them in the early stages. Seventy-five per cent of the cases I saw last year were inoperable. I did three thyrotomies, otherwise a total laryngectomy. We have but one choice, recurrence spells death. One objection is leaving the cartilaginous wall of the larynx. It leaves an indurated mass which will granulate and give trouble. Removal of the laryngeal wall with the cancer mass is of advantage in the technic of this operation.

Dr. Lynch: I removed the perichondrium but not the cartilage.

Dr. Mackenty (continuing): I believe that it is disadvantageous to leave the cartilage there with such a poor blood supply. It is difficult to judge of the extension of a cancer of the larynx looking down upon it while under suspension. I am averse to removing tissue for examination, as it disseminates morbid cells.

Dr. Norval H. Pierce, Chicago, Ill.: In operating for the removal of early malignant neoplasms of the larynx he preferred laryngofissure to suspension. While no one can question the superior operative dexterity of Dr. Lynch, still he regards laryngofissure as the preferable procedure in these cases because it gives a better view of the operative field, the removal can be accomplished with greater accuracy and the dangers are no greater. He can report a little over 50 per cent of recoveries which have remained well over a year in cases where early malignant neoplasms have been removed by laryngofissure. His greatest mortality has occurred in cases which have been left open for the purpose of applying radium.

Dr. Shurley asked if radium was used in these cases? Dr. Logan asked if any galvanocautery was used. Dr. Hubbard asked to have the technic of combined suspension and laryngectomy explained.

Dr. Lynch, closing the discussion: This report is preliminary and may be extended later on. None of the cases had radium, either before or after operation. In one case I had to do laryngectomy where radium had been used, and there was so much slough that the case ended fatally. All open surfaces were touched with the galvanocautery after operation, in the hope of destroying any scattered cells. Students watching the operation are apt to be impressed with the fact that these cases can be dealt with early. I have been seeing more early cases than formerly. The suspension is ideal for extirpation of the larynx and trachea. I always refrain from removing tissue for diagnosis, except at time of operation.

## Lung Mapping by the Injection of Bismuth Mixtures in the Living. Preliminary Report.

### By DR. HENRY LOWNDES LYNAH, New York.

The following summary is presented:

1. That bismuth substances can be injected into the bronchi and lung of a living patient without doing damage.

2 That the injection of an opaque substance into the lung of the living patient will open up an enormous field of usefulness in the study of cough the expulsion of substances from the lung and lung drainage. It will also localize bronchial strictures in the same manner as seen in the esophagus. Furthermore it will be of the greatest aid to the thoracic surgeon by mapping out the abscess cavity in the respective lobe of the lung.

3. A definite lung abscess cavity is seldom seen bronchoscopically and pus is usually seen coming from a branch bronchus. The abscess cavity may be well around the corner and not in that portion of the lung from which the pus is oozing. An injection of bismuth mixture or some other opaque mixture will close up this error.

4. Bismuth, when it enters the abscess cavity, is interpreted by its metallic luster and when it is in the lobular lung structure it is interpreted as a dull opaque spot. Pus diffuses and soaks the lobular structure, and this often makes the area involved appear many times larger than it really is.

5. The amount of bismuth injected in these patients was an 8 cc. mixture of bismuth subcarbonate on part, in pure olive oil, two to three parts. The mixture is rendered sterile before injection by boiling.

6. The injection should be made slowly and not with a squirt, for the picture may be spoiled by bismuth lung soaking.

7. There seems to be from these preliminary studies that cough and the action of cilia are not the only means of expelling secretions from the lungs.

8. While bismuth mixtures were originally injected by the author for the purposes of lung mapping of abscess cavities in their respective lobes it seems to have been of apparent benefit to the two patients upon whom it was tried. So far it has done no harm.

### DISCUSSION.

Dr. Thomas Hubbard, Toledo, Ohio: I think Dr. Lynah's technic is marvelous and the possibilities immense. Besides the diagnostic there is the therapeutic aid of the healing properties of bismuth. I had one experience of the accidental aspiration of bismuth.

Dr. Mackenty asked how much importance the speaker attributes to cleaning out the cavity and how much to bismuth.

Other speakers asked the strength of bismuth in the mixture and how much was injected.

Dr. Norval H. Pierce, Chicago: In connection with the subject of inspection of bismuth for the purpose of outlining cavities, Dr. Pierce desired to bring to the attention of the society certain work that is being done by Dr. Cavanaugh of Chicago in this direction for the purpose of ascertaining the position and extent of the sphenoid sinus. The removal of this mass after the picture has been taken may be attended with some difficulty; also, in consequence of the density of the bismuth mass usually employed it may not reach all parts of the cavity. In order to overcome these two objections Dr. Pierce suggests that it might be found feasible to make a sprayable mixture of bismuth or barium in an albumin fixing menstruum, and this, by means of a suitable spray, might be sprayed into the cavity Or the albumin fixing mixture might precede the bismuth.

Dr. Lynah, closing the discussion: I used 8 cc., the cases had improved before bismuth was injected. The bismuth was only injected for diagnostic purposes.

### Some Indications for Operation on the Nasal Sinuses in Children.

By DR. L. W. DEAN, Iowa City, Iowa.

Three cases of arthritis vastly improved as a result of sinus operation are fully recorded.

With rather a large number of cases of multiple arthritis referred to the laryngologic clinic, it has only been necessary to treat or operate the sinuses in a very few cases. When we have found nasal sinus disease present in this condition and the etiological factor is the hemolytic streptococcus we have found great difficulty in eradicating the nasal sinus disease as compared with non-complicated, sinus disease in children.

We feel that all cases of systemic infection in children that are ordinarily due to foci about the upper respiratory tract, if not checked by the removal of diseased tonsils and adenoids, should come in the hospital for study of the nasal sinuses. We have only been able to study them satisfactorily by having the patients in the wards where they are under constant supervision. If the nasal sinus disease is present we find it necessary to hospitalize these patients for six to nine months in order to get satisfactory results. This gives the best opportunity for that careful study which must precede all operative work in the sinuses.

With the cases just cited we feel that the focus of infection was in the nasal sinuses and that it could only be removed by operation on these sinuses. The removal of middle turbinate and the destruction of sinuses have been justified by the results. In these three cases if the foci had not been obliterated the result would probably have been an ankylosis of all joints utter helplessness, and a slow, painful death.

As the result of the work our patients, although cripples are well nourished, happy, free from pain, enjoy play and, with proper education, will be self-supporting. These children are our best friends, their gratitude compensates us many times over for the time and work necessary for the proper handling of their cases.

Dr. Ross Hall Skillern, Philadelphia, Pa.: We do not see these cases in Philadelphia, and there are three reasons for this: 1, we may not have them; 2, I doubt if we would recognize them, and 3, the parents would not allow us to keep the children long enough in the hospital to study them carefully. The diagnosis of these cases require long and careful study.

Dr. Harmon Smith New York: During the past winter I had an unusual number of children with sinus involvement. Most of them had bronchitis which had failed to yield to treatment. After shrinking the puffy mucosa with solution of adrenalin, 1-1600 of rosewater, I either douched their nares with a hot alkaline solution with a Douglas douche, or the postnasal douche as first suggested by Chappell. I then employed a 1 per cent argyrol solution in my sinus suction syringe, which not only sucked out the remaining pus but also introduced the argyrol solution. The majority of these cases recovered completely within from two to three weeks, both from the sinus affection and the bronchitis.

For a number of years we have employed filtered sea water, to which 1 minim of carbolic acid to the ounce has been added, for irrigating purposes. This is much more valuable than normal saline.

Dr. B. Alex. Randall, Philadelphia, Pa.: In 35 years' duty at the Children's Hospital we saw many cases of diseased sinus. In extreme cases we passed alligator forceps into the sphenoid and withdrawing them open divulsed the front wall and thus opened drainage.

Dr. Charles W. Richardson, Washington, D. C., reported a case of extreme exophthalmos, primarily an acute mastoid infection, right side, acute suppurative otitis left side, when first seen. Incision of the left ear; subsidence of ear symptoms; exophthalmos left eye gradually increased, blood, bacteriologic and other examinations seemed to show it to be a case of orbital leukemia.

Dr. Henry L. Swain, New Haven, Conn.: I had one case in which the infection of the orbit was caused by a single tooth extracted from the lower jaw. The infection passed up the ramus of the jaw out by the pterygoid fossa and pterygomaxillary fossa and into the orbit. No pus occurred in the orbit, but exophthalmos was sufficient to cause permanent blindness.

Dr. H. P. Mosher, Boston, Mass., asked at what age it was feasible to wash out the antrum of a child and how early the sphenoidal sinus was an operable cavity?

Dr. J. H. Bryan, Washington, D. C.: These are desperate operations but, nevertheless, are justified. Many think that because a child is young radical measures are cantraindicated.

Dr. J. E. Logan, Kansas City, Mo., asked if Dr. Dean used autogenous vaccine before or after operating. This has proved a potent factor in clearing up the cases before operation. He has used it as a regular procedure.

Dr. G. Sluder, St. Louis, Mo.: No matter how much bone you take out of a child's nose the activity of the bone cells is such that in three months' time the bone will be replaced. You take desperate chances in bone removal in children. Do not operate on the paranasal sinus in children except in conditions of dire distress. We may consider the sphenoid as a sinus to be dealt with at the age of five.

Dr. J. E. Mackenty, New York City: As regards the bacteriology in these cases the S. hemolyticus is one of the most difficult to deal with and eradicate. In the long chronic cases the S. aureus is the most common germ. The sphenoid sinus is the most devilish to treat. The question to settle is how much we are justified in operating on the sinus in children?

Dr. Dean, closing the discussion: I have performed extensive operations on the nasal sinuses in children only a very few times. The youngest operative sphenoid was 5 years and 4 months. A prolonged study of the case is most essential in diagnosing nasal sinus disease in infants and young children. Every possible method of examination must be used. The nasopharynogscope is of particular value. Microscopic examination as well as cultures of the contents of the sinuses give a most definite result. X-ray picture is always necessary. To secure the contents of the Highmorian antrum for microscopic examination and culturing the following procedure is used: With an X-ray plate before us a trocar is introduced into the sinus through the inferior meatus. Even if the floor of the Highmorian antrum does not extend below the inferior turbinate if the X-ray plate is carefully watched, the sinus may be readily entered without danger of complications. Through this trocar a very slender sterile needle is inserted into the sinus and its contents aspirated. Within the last few days in a boy 2 years old suffering from trophoneurosis of obscure origin such an examination gave from one Highmorian antrum thick, yellowish-white pus. The culturing of the sphenoid is not so exact as the Highmorian antrum. In this instance, after cleansing the upper nasal chambers with 50 per cent alcohol a slender German silver canula is inserted into the sphenoidal sinus and its contents aspirated. Naturally, the needle becomes contaminated with its passage through the nose and it is always questionable as to whether organisms cultured are from the sinus or from the nose. When, however, the material thus secured is found to contain pus cells or pyogenic organisms we feel certain that sphenoid sinus disease is present. In cases where we have painted the neighborhood of the ostium of the sphenoid with a solution of methylene blue, the methylene blue has not appeared in the material aspirated from the sphenoid.

I was very much interested in Dr. Richardson's report of his case. I believe it to be a case of chloroma. I feel certain that his case will come to autopsy and the characteristic greenish tumor will be found.

### A New or Hitherto Undescribed Form of Maxillary Sinusitis.

By DR. ROSS HALL SKILLERN, Philadelphia, Pa.

The history of the case of a female aged 50, single, is presented. A severe cold began some six months previous, remaining in a more or less chronic form with occasional acute exacerbations. Soon thereafter a postnasal discharge containing blood, but no pus, made its appearance. Later the blood became darker and more profuse. Still later the expectorated blood assumed the appearance of clots. The discharge always came from the posterior nares, never from the anterior. The expectoration often occurred during the night. Examination was negative, but as a routine measure both antra were punctured, the right with a negative result. On needle puncture of the left antrum, however, as soon as the air was forced into the sinus there escaped an ounce or more of apparently pure unclotted blood, the quantity of which was considerably increased on lavage with the normal, salt solution. No sign of pus either granular or en masse was present. The lining mucosa of the sinus did not appear to be greatly thickened as the lumen of the cavity was found without difficulty by the point of the needle, and the sound made by the injected air proved without question that the point was not imbedded in thickened mucosa. Irrigation was continued until the flow returned clear, after which 50 per cent alcohol with 1/2000 bichloride, sufficient to fill the sinus, was injected and the needle withdrawn. Bacteriological examination of the blood showed an abundance of streptococcus hemolyticus.

The injections were continued daily, the discharge gradually losing its hemorrhagic appearance only to assume more and more a purulent content, the total amount of secretion remaining about constant. It was therefore apparent that the irrigations were exerting little influence on the course of the disease, the character of the secretion, however, was changing from sanguineous to purulent. At the end of fifteen days, after about the same number of treatments, the blood had to all intents and purposes disappeared leaving a thin purulent, granular secretion which mixed readily with the irrigating fluid and formed with it a milky appearance.

About this time a swelling appeared upon the septum which rapidly developed into an abscess. This was incised and in a few days subsided, but was followed by a bloody discharge from the right side of the nose, the secretion hitherto had been entirely unilateral and confined to the left side. Needle puncture of the right antrum brought forth a large quantity of blood identical with that which had originally appeared from the opposite sinus. Previous to this the right side had not been affected.

The present condition of the patient is unsatisfactory in that she is fairly comfortable under bi-weekly treatments, but if un treated the disease shows a great tendency to revert to the hemorrhagic form.

This case is unique. The peculiar bloody discharge, unaccompanied by any subjective sign of inflammation with its tendency to diminish, but become purulent after irrigations, and on non-interference to revert to its original type, is puzzling, to say the least.

The advisability of a radical operation has been thoroughly discussed and finally decided upon where, it is hoped, by pathologic investigations the exact status of the infection will be determined.

### DISCUSSION.

Dr. H. P. Mosher, Boston, Mass.: I recall operating a number of cases of apparent mucocele of the frontal sinus in which the sinus was filled with a sterile blood clot. These cases I never could explain. They resemble in a measure the case of Dr. Skillern. In the three cases that I have had, the modified Killian operation gave a successful result.

### Report of a Case of Extradural and Subdural. Abscess Following Suppurating Frontal Sinusitis and Osteomyelitis of the Frontal Bone.

By DR. JOSEPH H. BRYAN, Washington, D. C.

Male, aged 15, first seen May 6, 1919, with a history of having had a distinct swelling over the left frontal sinus, with pus under the middle turbinate on that same side in January previous. There was a temperature around 100 or 101 degrees. The left frontal sinus was opened the following day. Discharge continued and an abscess of the left upper lid developed. Operated again January 31 and a sequestrum of bone was removed from the inner wall of the sinus, leaving a perforation into the cranium and exposing the dura.

Again operated April 15, owing to continuance of the discharge. The right maxillary sinus now became infected. On one occasion a canula was inserted in the wound and the sinus washed out under mild pressure with a warm boric acid solution. Following this he complained of severe headache, numbness in the right hand and thickness of speech. This would indicate intracerebral pressure.

On May 6, when first seen by the writer, the whole of the left frontal region was markedly swollen, pitting, bloody, purulent secretion with entire absence of symptoms from his condition. Operation the following day, bone curetted and thoroughly cleansed. Packing with gauze in a solution of dichloramine T. Convalescence was long and tedious, pus flowing still two months later. On one occasion a probe first passed into the cranial cavity through the opening in the posterior wall of the sinus. In the following September the patient's general condition was good. Locally there remained a fistulous opening at the inner angle of the orbit through which the secretions continued to flow freely. The probe was introduced as formerly and an X-ray examination made with the probe in situ. Another X-ray examination was made after injecting through the sinus opening a 10 per cent solution of nitrate of thorium. This revealed a large extradural abscess. Operation, September 25, with drainage. The pus from the extradural abscess showed nonhemolytic streptococci in pure culture. By December all discharge had ceased and patient felt well. An attack of influenza in January followed. In the middle of February he became seriously ill, had a marked septic appearance, temperature 103, swelling over left frontal region associated with headache. The old wound was reopened the next day and a larger segment of bone removed, as well as necrotic bone. One week later he died.

A neurologic study of this patient's condition at this time then follows.

The bacteriologic report states that the organisms here found was the enterococcus, which occasionally becomes pathogenic.

The report of the autopsy shows the conditions as indicated in the title of the paper.

The author presents the following summary:

1. This case presents many points of interest, both from the pathologic and surgical sides. The obstinate character of the original inflammation in the frontal sinus; the exposure of the dura

in the course of one of the operations through which the infection passed to produce the extradural abscess.

2. It is unfortunate there was no bacteriological examination made from the sinus secretion at the time of the original operation.

3. The value of nitrate of thorium as an aid in differentiating between an extradural and cerebral abscess during an X-ray examination.

4. The complete relief of the osteomyelitis, generally a progrossive condition.

5. The fulminating process developing so rapidly and resulting in a subdural abscess after the extradural abscess had seemed to be relieved.

## Meningitis Due to Frontal Sinus Suppuration with a Report of Three Fatal Cases.

### By RALPH BUTLER, M. D., Philadelphia.

Considering the vast number of cases of sinus suppuration that exist, the number of reports of intracranial involvement from them are relatively few. A search of the literature shows the greater number of intracranial cases of otitic as compared to those of nasal origin. That these complications of sinus inflammation are not common is borne out by statistics.

The writer then quotes from the literature as to the occurrence and relative frequency of meningitis following frontal sinus disease.

Meningitis may complicate either chronic or acute sinusitis and is more common in the male during the second and third decades.

The infection may be transmitted through a congenital or a carious defect in the posterior wall of the sinus, through the veins or lymphatics, by infection of the diploe or by the formation of an osteomyelitis.

After purulent leptomeningitis has developed the prognosis is very bad. There is considerable evidence to show that the mortality has been increased by operation on the sinuses.

As there is considerable operative risk, the cosmetic results are not always satisfactory and complete cure is uncertain, many surgeons hesitate to do a radical operation unless intracranial infection is suspected or the bone is diseased. One should not hesitate beyond this point.

As illustrating the value of late operation, the writer presents the history of a 14-year-old boy who had marked proptosis of the left eyeball; the left frontal ethmoidal and maxillary sinuses were operated upon. The dura was exposed in the ehmoidal and frontal regions with local meningitis. The roof and inner wall of the orbit were largely destroyed, and staphylococci were found in pure culture. The patient has shown no evidence of extension of the intracranial involvement.

Three fatal cases are next recorded:

Case 1. Male, aged 11, had an acute inflammation of the left frontal sinus, with swelling and tenderness for about two weeks. Three months previous had an attack of influenza.

There was neither tenderness nor swelling over other sinuses. postural tests were negative and there was no abnormal secretion in the nose or throat. The roentgenologist could not determine whether the left frontal sinus was absent or full of exudate. Blood count showed 20,000 leucocytes. The neurologist gave a negative report.

Admitted to hospital and a few hours later became unconscious, with signs of meningitis. At 2 p. m. the following day he was comatose, the neck was stiff, pupils did not react to light and accommodation, the left widely dilated, the right contracted, with hemorrhage in each fundus. A second X-ray examination showed exudate in the left frontal sinus.

The sinus was opened and found to be filled with a thick brown fluid. While the wound was being sutured the patient suddenly stopped breathing, probably from paralysis of the respiratory center. No autopsy.

Case 2. Male, aged 21. Had been kicked by a horse 14 years previously. Three months later he noticed a swelling over the inner end of the eyebrow. He had slight symptoms from this. Unilateral anosmia on that side.

Examination showed it to be a mucocele of the frontal sinus.

Removing the anterior end of the middle turbinal and opening the frontal sinus, a large cavity was found filled with thick, ropy mucus; a rubber drainage tube was inserted. On the removal of the tube the artificial duct closed and the swelling reappeared.

The wound was reopened later and a gold tube inserted, with recovery and marked improvement of his mental condition.

The patient then reappeared in four years with the tube in situ, was treated a few times, then disappeared, returning four years afterwards with a recurrence of acute symptoms. One month later he developed a typical attack of meningitis and died. No autopsy.

Case 3. Male, aged 77. The examination showed tenderness over the floor of the right frontal sinus with induration of the tissues of the upper part of the right orbit and a supraorbital fistula extending into the frontal sinus from which pus was draining. The X-ray showed marked clouding of the right frontal and roughening of its median wall with slight clouding of the right antrum and of the ethmoids on both sides.

The right middle turbinal was removed and the right antrum irrigated. Three days later an external operation was performed. The front wall containing the fistula was removed, the sinus was found filled with pulsating pus, the posterior wall was necrosed, through which the inflamed dura could be seen. At this point the operation was discontinued as the patient was doing badly. On the third day after operation the patient became irrational and had one general convulsion which was attributed to uremia. The patient died during the night.

Autopsy showed bilateral chronic suppuration of the frontal, ethmoidal and sphenoidal sinuses and of the right antrum of Highmore. Chronic suppurative meningitis with secondary atrophy of the cortical substance of the frontal lobes of the brain, estimated to be of six months' duration. Infection probably pneumococcic. Gram positive diplococci.

## DISCUSSION OF DR. BRYAN'S AND DR. BUTLER'S PAPERS.

Dr. Ross Hall Skillern, Philadelphia, Pa.: I lost two cases after the Killian operation of meningitis. One point to be considered is the route by which this infection travels to the brain. In one of my cases the man died three days after operation. At autopsy the whole brain was a mass of inflammatory reaction, but no path could be traced. The cases that die are old cases who in the years have built up for themselves a kind of resistance. Operation frequently breaks this down and then they go off very quickly.

Dr. C. W. Richardson, Washington, D. C.: I believe that a latent form of meningitis exists which is started up immediately after operation. I noticed this in two of my cases.

Dr. Henry L. Swain, New Haven, Conn.:   On one occasion I advised against operating on a patient sent to the hospital with meningitis and a discharging ear. The fluid from lumbar puncture contained pneumococcus, the ear secretion staphylococcus, the nose pneumococcus. The patient recovered {with a succession of spinal punctures when indicated. Had the usual ear operation been done the patient would in all probability have died.

Dr. B. Alex. Randall, Philadelphia, Pa., verbally reported a case of probable noma of the nose in a man of 68, suggesting malignant disease of syphilis, but justifying neither diagnosis. Typical noma of the ala nasi later developed, but did not improve under diphtheria antitoxin.

# INDEX OF THE LITERATURE.

## SECTION 1.—LARYNGOLOGY AND OTOLOGY—GENERAL AND HISTORICAL.

**Ballenger, Edgar G., and Elder, Omar F.** Orchitis from mumps: the need of conserving the testes by incision of the tunica albuginea.
J. Am. M. Ass., Chicago, 1920—LXXV—1257.

**Beck, J. C., and Deutsch, E.** Interrelation between eye, ear, nose and throat with presentation of cases.
Am. J. Ophthalmol., Chicago, 1920—III—349.

**Berens, C., and Uren, C. T.** Effect of nose and throat infections on ocular functions of aviators.
Am. J. Ophthalmol., Chicago, 1920—III—170.

**Bilancioni, G.** Illumination of the throat by transparency.
Policlin., Roma, 1920—XXVII—915.

**Bledsoe, R. W.** Influenza: management of nose, throat and ears.
Kentucky M. J., Louisville, 1920—XVIII—289.

**Brühl, G.** Otologic hints for the general practitioner.
Deutsche med Wchnschr., Berl., 1920—XLVI—861, 919.

**Burton, F. A.** Prehistoric trephining of frontal sinus.
Calif. State J. M., San Fran., 1920—XVIII—321.

**Carpenter, E. R.** Surgical problems in otologic work.
Texas State J. M., Fort Worth, 1920—XVI—121.

**Dufourmentel, L.** Otorhinolaryngology in 1920.
Paris méd., 1920—X—176.

**Finder.** Rhinolaryngologic hints for general practitioner.
Deutsche med. Wchnschr., Berl., 1920—XLVI—547, 660, 691, 717, 743, 775, 802.

**Friesell, H. F.** Progress in dental education.
J. Am. M. Ass., Chicago, 1920—LXXV—1247.

**Keyes, F. A.** Institutional dentistry; results, report No. 4.
Boston M. & S. J., 1920—CLXXXIII—464.

**Lanier, L. H.** Essential points in successful laryngologic practice.
Laryngoscope. St. Louis, 1920—XXX—530.

**Marks, H. J.** Evolution of otorhinolaryngology.
Med. J. Australia, Sydney, 1920—II—331.

**New, G. B.** Mixed tumors of the throat, mouth and face.
J. Am. M. Ass., Chicago, 1920—LXXV—732.

**Pearson, W. W.** Chloroma with special reference to ear, nose and throat manifestations, with report of two cases.
Ann. Otol., Rhinol. & Laryngol., St. Louis, 1920—XXIX—806.

**Randall, B. Alexander.** Trifles that count for efficiency.
Ann. Otol., Rhinol. & Laryngol., St. Louis, 1920—XXIX—796.

**Robertson, H. E.** Local amyloid with special reference to socalled amyloid tumors of the tongue.
Ann. Otol., Rhinol. & Laryngol., St. Louis, 1920—XXIX—773.

**Sauer, W. E.** Reactions of ear, nose and throat in syphilis.
Am. J. Syphilis, St. Louis, 1920—IV—430.

**Schulze, W.** Etiology of postoperative parotitis.
Zentralb. f. Gynäk., Leipz., 1920—XLIV—613.

**Sonnenschein, Robert.** Radium in the treatment of malignant tumors of the nose and throat: its use and possible abuse.
J. Am. M. Ass., Chicago, 1920—LXXV—860.

**Thompson, J. A.** Laryngologist and diseases of the lungs.
Ohio M. J., Columbus, 1920—XVI—655.

**Tydings, O.** Eye, ear, nose and throat in general disease.
Ark. M. Soc. J., Little Rock, 1920—XVII—74.

**Von Dworzak, Z.** Radium therapy in diseases of nose, ear and throat.
Colorado Med., Denver, 1920—XVII—238.

**Wieder, H. S.** Relationship of anatomy and physiology to pathology of nose, throat and ear.
Laryngoscope, St. Louis, 1920—XXX—543.

**Yeasley, M.** Recent work in otology.
Practitioner, Lond., 1920—CV—139.

## SECTION 2.—RESPIRATORY SYSTEM, EXCLUSIVE OF THE EAR, NOSE AND THROAT.

**Adkinson, J., and Walter, I. C.** Types of streptococci found in sputum of bronchial asthmatics.
J. Med. Research, Bost., 1920—XLI—457.

**Gottlieb, Mark J.** Results of tests in hay fever and asthma.
J. Am. M. Ass., Chicago, 1920—LXXV—814.

**Mayo, C. H.** Adenoma with hyperthyroidism.
Ann. Surg., Phila., 1920—LXXII—134.

## SECTION 3.—ACUTE GENERAL INFECTIONS, INCLUDING DIPHTHERIA, SCARLET FEVER AND MEASLES.

**Allen, E. D.** Influenza.
Iowa M. J., Des Moines, 1920—X—337.

**Baez, M. Quevedo.** Clinical studies on influenza.
Porto Rico M. Ass. Bull., San Juan, 1920—XIII—104.

**Bardes, A.** Aural aftermaths of influenza.
Med. Rec., N. Y., 1920—XCVIII—810.

**Bichel, J.** Influenza in Greenland.
Ugeskr. f. Laeger, Kjobenh., 1920—LXXXII—1163.

**Bird, R. L.** Symptoms, diagnosis and treatment of influenza.
Kentucky M. J., Louisville, 1920—XVIII—291.

**Blau, A. I.** Schick test, its control, and active immunization against diphtheria.
N. York M. J., 1920—CXII—279.

**Bleyer, A.** Concerning direct smears in diphtheria.
Am. J. Dis. Child., Chicago, 1920—445.

**Boisliniere, L. C.** Influenza as factor in activation of latent tuberculosis.
Am. Rev. of Tuberculosis, Balt., 1920—IV—534.

**Bonar, D. S.** Influenza.
Kentucky M. J., Louisville, 1920—XVIII—288.

**Bosler, A. B.** Diphtheria immunization.
Illinois M. J. Oak Park, 1920—XXXVIII—185.

**Bradbury, S.** Recurrence of influenza in a regiment.
Mil. Surgeon, 1920—XLVII—471.

**Burne, W.** Influenza.
Kentucky M. J., Louisville, 1920—XVIII—295.

**Chaney, W. C.** Treatment of fifty-one selected cases of influenza in epidemic of 1920.
Minnesota Med., St. Paul, 1920—III—436.

**Clark, F. S.** Influenza sequels.
Kentucky M. J., Louisville, 1920—XVIII—293.

**Dorn, E.** Influenza and tuberculosis.
Ztschr. f. Tuberk., Leipz., 1920—XXXI—257.

**Edington, J. W.** Causal organism of influenza.
Lancet, London, 1920—II—340.

**Falcioni D.** Immunity to influenza.
Riforma med., 1920—XXXVI—692.

**Fildes, P., and McIntosh, J.** Etiology of influenza.
Brit. J. Exper. Path., London, 1920—I—119, 159.

**Fildes, P.** New medium for growth of B. influenza.
Brit. J. Exper. Path., London, 1920—I—129.

**Fishberg, M., and Boas, E. P.** Influenza in tuberculosis.
Am. J. M. Sc., Phila., 1920—CLX—214.

**Friedemann, U.** The present influenza epidemic.
Deutsche med. Wchnschr., Berl., 1920—XLVI—283.

**Gomibuchi, T.** Use of diphtheria serum in treatment of influenza.
Japan Med. World, Tokyo, 1920—X—840.

**Granthamhill, C.** Symptomless influenzal (streptococcal) mastoiditis.
Lancet, London, 1920—II—241.

**Hammond, L. J.** Condition of chest in influenza.
N. York M. J., 1920—CXII—212.

**Kitano, T.** Results of practical application of influenza vaccine.
Japan Med. World, Tokyo, 1920—X—.

**Lambert.** Manifestations of diphtheria in nose and ears.
Arch. med. Belges, Liege, 1920—LXXIII—382.

**Lavergne, De, and Zoeller.** Schick reaction- in postdiphtheric paralysis.
Bull. soc. med. de hop., Paris, 1920—XLIV—954.

**Loewenhardt.** Bacteriologic findings in influenza.
Deutsche med. Wchnschr., Berl., 1920—XLVI—794.

**Lohrig, A.** Grave diphtheria in children.
Jahrb. f. Kinderh., Berl., 1920—XCIII—49.

**Lopez, J. A.**  Treatment of influenza.
Semana med., Buenos Aires, 1920—XXVII—535.

**Majumdar, B.**  Influenza epidemic in Calcutta.
Indian J. Med., Calcutta, 1920—I—46.

**Markel, C.**  Pulse, temperature and respiration in influenza.
Colorado Med., Denver, 1920—XVII—244.

**Marriott, W. McKim.**  Postdiphtheritic paralysis of the respiratory
muscles: Report of case treated by prolonged artificial
respiration.
J. Am. M. Ass., Chicago, 1920—LXXV—668.

**McCulloch, H.**  Effect of diphtheria on heart.
Am. J. Dis. Child, Chicago, 1920—XX—87.

**McGill, E. L.**  Intubation for laryngeal diphtheria.
Virginia M. Month., Richmond, 1920—XLVII—250.

**Menninger, Karl A.**  Influenza and hypophrenia: the interrelation
of an acute epidemic infection and a chronic endemic
(brain) affection.
J. Am. M. Ass., Chicago, 1920—LXXV—1044.

**Morquio, L.**  Diphtheria and diphtheria antitoxin in Uruguay.
Rev. med. d. Uruguay, Montevideo, 1920—XXIII—260.

**Opitz, H.**  Active immunization against diphtheria.
Jahrb. f. Kinderh., Berl., 1920—XCII—189.

**Reese, G. H.**  Management of influenza at "Old Hickory."
Virginia M. Month., Richmond, 1920—XLVII—254.

**Richardson, C. B.**  Influenza and its treatment with phenol.
Practitioner, Lond., 1920—CV—150.

**Rosenow, E. C.**  Etiology of and prophylactic inoculation in influenza.
Iowa M. J., Des Moines, 1920—X—335.

**St. Lawrence, Wm.**  Effect of tonsillectomy on the recurrence of
acute rheumatic fever and chorea: a study of ninety-four
children.
J. Am. M. Ass., Chicago, 1920—LXXV—1035.

**Salomon, H.**  Iodin prophylaxis in influenza.
Deutsche med. Wchnschr., Berl., 1920—XLVI—882.

**Sindoni, Maria.**  Bacteriologic research in influenza.
Pediatria, Naples, 1920—XXVIII—851.

**Sorenson, S. T.**  Operations for scarlatinal otitis.
Hosp.-Tid., Khenh., 1920—LXIII—457.

**Speidel.**  Late results of encephalitis after influenza.
Münchener med. Wchnschr., Munich, 1920—LXVII—630.

**Sur, T.**  Influenza epidemic in Calcutta.
Indian J. Med., Calcutta, 1920—I—57.

**Tyler, W. L.**  Diagnosis of influenza.
Kentucky M. J., Louisville, 1920—XVIII—294.

**Waters, H. G.**  Influenza in India, 1918-1920.
Brit. M. J., Loud., 1920—591.

**Wesselhoeft, C.**  Orchitis in mumps.
Boston M. & S. J., 1920—CLXXXIII—425, 458, 520.

**Wiesner, R.** Pathogenesis of influenza.
Wien. klin. Wchnschr., 1920—XXXIII—531.

**Zingher, Abraham.** Accuracy of the Schick reaction: influence of variations in diphtheria toxin content in Schick outfits.
J. Am. M. Ass., Chicago, 1920—LXXV—1333.

## SECTION 4.—SYPHILIS.

**Davidsohn, H.** Hutchinson's teeth.
Deutsche med. Wchnschr., Berl., 1920—XLVI—295.

**Kranz, P.** Hutchinson's teeth (a reply).
Deutsche med. Wchnschr., Berl., 1920—XLVI—773.

**Sauer, W. E.** Reactions of ear, nose and throat in syphilis.
Am. J. Syphilis, St. Louis, 1920—IV—430.

**Schmidt, V.** Syphilitic disease of nasal accessory cavities.
Hosp.-Tid., Khenh., 1920—LXIII—544.

## SECTION 5.—TUBERCULOSIS.

**Boisliniere, L. C.** Influenza as factor in activation of latent tuberculosis.
Am. Rev. of Tuberculosis, Balt., 1920—IV—534.

**Dorn, E.** Influenza and tuberculosis.
Ztschr. f. Tuberk., Leipz., 1920—XXXI—257.

**Fishberg, M., and Boas, E. P.** Influenza in tuberculosis.
Am. J. M. Sc., Phila., 1920—CLX—214.

**Mieres, J. F.** Exophthalmic goiter in the tuberculous.
Semana med., Buenos Aires, 1920—XXVII—507.

**Sergent, E.** Exophthalmic goiter mistaken for tuberculosis.
Paris méd., 1920—X—80.

**Sloan, E. P.** Tubercular goiter patient.
Illinois M. J., Oak Park, 1920—XXXVIII—144.

## SECTION 6.—ANATOMY, PHYSIOLOGY AND PATHOLOGY.

**Adkinson, J., and Walter, I. C.** Types of streptococci found in sputum of bronchial asthmatics.
J. Med. Research, Bost., 1920—XLI—457.

**Canelli, A. F.** Anatomy and pathology of the thymus in young children.
Pediatria, Napoli, 1920—XXVIII—573.

**Floyd, C.** Study of streptococci obtained from mouth in cases of chorea.
J. Med. Research, Bost., 1920—XLI—467.

**Kellert, E.** Pathologic histology of tonsils containing hemolytic streptococci.
J. Med. Research, Bost., 1920—XLI—387.

**Loewenhardt.** Bacteriologic findings in influenza.
Deutsche med. Wchnschr., Berl., 1920—XLVI—794.

**Meyer, Jacob.** Types of pneumococci in the throats of one hundred normal persons.
J. Am. M. Ass., Chicago, 1920—LXXV—1268.

**Marine, D.** Physiology of normal thyroid and physiology of thyroid in exophthalmic goiter.
Ohio M. J., Columbus, 1920—XVI—735.

**Sindoni, Maria.** Bacteriologic research in influenza.
Pediatria, Naples, 1920—XXVIII—851.

**Tanaka, F., and Yoshida, C.** Vital fixation of auricular órgans and staining of nerves.
Japan Med. World, Tokyo, 1920—X—.

**Wieder, H. S.** Relationship of anatomy and physiology to pathology of nose, throat and ear.
Laryngoscope, St. Louis, 1920—XXX—543.

**Wood, G. B.** Anatomy, physiology and pathology of tonsillar structures in relation to cryptogenic infections.
Med. Rec., N. Y., 1920—XCVIII—593.

## SECTION 7.—EXTERNAL NOSE.

**Carter, W. W.** Nasal deformities due to submucous operation; their prevention and treatment.
Med. Rec., N. Y., 1920—XCVIII—808.

**Chubb, G.** New method in rhinoplasty.
Lancet, London, 1920—II—354.

**Cohen, L.** Correct rhinoplasty.
Surg., Gynec. & Obst., Chicago, 1920—XXXI—412.

**Hartzell, M. B.** Lupus erythematosus and focal infection.
Arch. of dermat. and syphil., Chicago, 1920—II—441.

**Oppenheimer, S.** Condemnatory note on use of paraffin in cosmetic rhinoplasty.
Laryngoscope, St. Louis, 1920—XXX—595.

**Oppenheimer, S.** Implantation methods in cosmetic rhinoplasty.
Boston M. & S. J., 1920—CLXXXIII—329.

## SECTION 8.—NASAL CAVITIES.

**Agar, M.** Method of treating hay fever and paroxysmal rhinorrhea.
Brit. M. J., London, 1920—II—125.

**Caldera, C.** Etiology of ozena.
Ann. d'ig., Rome, 1920—XXX—168.

**Carter, W. W.** Nasal deformities due to submucous operation; their prevention and treatment.
Med. Rec., N. Y., 1920—XCVIII—808.

**Gottlieb, Mark J.** Results of tests in hay fever and asthma.
J. Am. M. Ass., Chicago, 1920—LXXV—814.

**Heermann.** Treatment of hay fever.
Deutsche med. Wchnschr., Berl., 1920—XLVI—211.

**Imperatori, C. J.** Apparatus for irrigating nasal cavities, useful in home treatment.
Laryngoscope, St. Louis, 1920—XXX—550.

**Meller.** Relation of retrobulbar neuritis to nasal cavity.
Wien. klin. Wchnschr., 1920—XXXIII—205.

**Nagel, C. S. G.** Congenital atresia of lacrimal duct.
Am. J. Ophth., Chicago, 1920—III—406.

**Patton, W. T.** Simplified technic for local anesthesia of tonsils; intranasal surgery without packing.
South. M. J., Birmingham; Ala., 1920—XIII—750.

**Potts, J. B.** Nasal infection basis of certain ocular lesions.
Am. J. Ophthalmol., Chicago, 1920—III—195.

**Walker, I. Chandler.** Frequent causes and the treatment of perennial hay fever. :
J. Am. M. Ass., Chicago, 1920—LXXV—782.

**Walter, Will.** Inoculation against hay fever.
J. Am. M. Ass., Chicago, 1920—LXXV—670.

**Wiener, Meyer and Sauer, W. E.** A new operation for the relief of dacryocystitis through the nasal route.
J. Am. M. Ass., Chicago, 1920—LXXV—868.

## SECTION 9.—ACCESSORY SINUSES.

**Burton, F. A.** Prehistoric trephining of frontal sinus.
Calif. State J. M., San Fran., 1920—XVIII—321.

**Dunning, Henry S.** Surgical treatment of chronic maxillary sinusitis of oral origin.
J. Am. M. Ass., Chicago, 1920—LXXV—1391.

**Ellett, E. C.** Optic neuritis, associated with disease of the nasal sinuses; report of two cases.
J. Am. M. Ass., Chicago, 1920—LXXV—805.

**Harter, J. H.** Diseases of ethmoid and sphenoid sinuses.
Northwest Med., Seattle, 1920—XIX—199.

**Liebault, G.** Acute frontal sinusitis and ptosis.
Bull. méd., Par., 1920—XXXIV—815.

**Loeb, H. W.** Two cases of blindness relieved by ethmoid exenteration; case of keratoiritis due to tonsil infection.
J. Missouri M. Ass., St. Louis, 1920—XVII—409.

**Meller.** Relation of retrobulbar neuritis to nasal cavity.
Wien. klin. Wchnschr., 1920—XXXIII—205.

**Novitsky, J.** Dead teeth and antral pathology.
Illinois M. J., Oak Park, 1920—XXXVIII—143.

**Patton, W. T.** Simplified technic for local anesthesia of tonsils; intranasal surgery without packing.
South. M. J., Birmingham, Ala., 1920—XIII—750.

**Potts, J. B.** Nasal infection basis of certain ocular lesions.
Am. J. Ophthalmol., Chicago, 1920—III—195.

**Schmidt, V.** Syphilitic disease of nasal accessory cavities.
Hosp.-Tid., Kbenh., 1920—LXIII—544.

**Skillern, R. H.** Ethmoid problem.
Texas State J. M., Fort Worth, 1920—XVI—116.

**Unger, M.** New instrument and method for washing and draining nasal sinuses.
Laryngoscope, St. Louis, 1920—XXX—561.

**Welty, Cullen, F.** Closure of fistulous openings through alveolar process into antrum of Highmore.
J. Am. M. Ass., Chicago, 1920—LXXV—867.

White, L. E. Diagnosis of accessory sinus disease causing loss of vision.
Laryngoscope, St. Louis, 1920—XXX—551.

## SECTION 10.—PHARYNX, INCLUDING TONSILS AND ADENOIDS.

Anderson, H. B., Mann, R. W., and Sharpe, N. C. Chronic tonsillar infections.
Med. Rec., N. Y., 1920—XCVIII—589.

Bernstein, E. J. Sluder operation.
J. Mich. M. Soc., Grand Rapids, 1920—XIX—448.

Boyd, F. D. General vs. local faucial tonsil removal.
South. M. J., Birmingham, Ala., 1920—XIII—748.

Boyd, F. Plea for more careful tonsil and adenoid operation.
Texas State J. M., Fort Worth, 1920—XVI—131.

Brüggemann, A. Plaut-Vincent angina.
München. med. Wchnschr., 1920—LXII—772.

Flores, A. Mycosis of pharynx and larynx.
Cron. med., Lima., 1920—XXXVII—225.

Frantz. C. P. Tonsils cases I have met.
Iowa M. J., Des Moines, 1920—X—309.

Ganley, J. E. Vincent's angina-stomatitis.
Boston M. & S. J., 1920—CLXXXIII—466.

Hirsch. Treatment of Plaut-Vincent angina with arsphenamin.
München. med. Wchnschr., Munich, 1920—LXVII—718.

Kellert, E. Pathologic histology of tonsils containing hemolytic streptococci.
J. Med. Research, Bost., 1920—XLI—387.

Key, S. N. Status of tonsillectomy in Texas.
Texas State J. M., Fort Worth, 1920—XVI—130.

Lapat, Wm. Catheterization of eustachian tubes through the mouth.
J. Am. M. Ass., Chicago, 1920—LXXV—1498.

Lapsley, R. M. Diseased tonsils.
Iowa M. J., Des Moines, 1920—X—308.

McReynolds, G. S. Tonsil operation, with special reference to hemorrhage control.
Texas State J. M., Fort Worth, 1920—XVI—132.

Meyer, Jacob. Types of pneumococci in the throats of one hundred normal persons.
J. Am. M. Ass., Chicago, 1920—LXXV—1268.

Neugebauer, G. Angino ludovici.
Deutsche. med. Wchnschr., Berl., 1920—XLVI—942.

Orendorff, Otis. Foreign body in nasopharynx.
J. Am. M. Ass., Chicago, 1920—LXXV—1343.

Patton, W. T. Simplified technic for local anesthesia of tonsils; intranasal surgery without packing.
South. M. J., Birmingham, Ala., 1920—XIII—750.

Quackenbos, M. Chronic peritonsillar abscess.
N. York M. J., 1920—LXII—193.

Ramós, A. Aurelio. Pneumococcus tonsillitis.
    Arch. espan. de Pediatria, Madrid, 1920—IV—273.

Rich, A. B. Innervation of tensor veli palatini and levator veli pala-
    tini muscles.
    Johns Hopkins Hosp. Bull., Balt., 1920—XXXI—305.

Richardson, Charles W. Acute abscess of the lateral wall of the
    laryngopharynx.
    Ann. Otol., Rhinol. & Laryngol., St. Louis, 1920—XXIX—804.

Rosenblatt, S. Simple bloodless tonsillectomy, with local anes-
    thesia.
    Laryngoscope, St. Louis, 1920—XXX—576.

St. Lawrence, Wm. Effect of-tonsillectomy on the recurrence of
    acute rheumatic fever and chorea: a study of ninety-four
    children.
    J. Am. M. Ass., Chicago, 1920—LXXV—1035.

Shapiro, A. F. Instrument for simplifying tonsillectomy by snare.
    N. York M. J., 1920—CXII—681.

Sparata, L. B. Tonsillectomies.
    Kansas M. Soc. J., Topeka, 1920—XX—221.

Thompson, W. R. Abortive treatment of peritonsillar infection.
    Texas State J. M., Fort Worth, 1920—XVI—129.

Trotter. W. Method of lateral pharyngotomy for exposure of large
    growths in epilaryngeal region.
    J. Laryngol., Lon., 1920—XXXV—289.

Voss, J. Vincent's angina.
    Norsk Mag. f. Laegevidensk., Kristiania, 1920—XXCI—778.

Wood, G. B. Anatomy, physiology and pathology of tonsillar
    structures in relation to cryptogenic infections.
    Med. Rec., N. Y., 1920—XCVIII—593.

Yorke, C. Anesthesia in tonsil and adenoid operations.
    British M. J., London, 1920—318.

## SECTION 11.—LARYNX.

Flores, A. Mycosis of pharynx and larynx.
    Cron. med., Lima., 1920—XXXVII—225.

Garland, J., and White, P. D. Paralysis of left recurrent laryngeal
    nerve associated with mitral stenosis.
    Arch. Int. Med., Chicago, 1920—XXVI—343.

Goodloe, A. E. Laryngo-tracheo bronchoscopy.
    Tenn. M. Ass. J., Nashville, 1920—XIII—141.

Hofer, G. Chronic stenosis of larynx and trachea.
    Kien. klin. Wchnschr. Vienna, 1920—XXXIII—515.

Jackson, C. Peroral endoscopy and laryngeal surgery.
    Laryngoscope, St. Louis, 1920—XXX—520.

MacKenzie, G. W. Motor neuroses of larynx.
    Laryngoscope, St. Louis, 1920—XXX—585.

McGill, E. L. Intubation for laryngeal diphtheria.
    Virginia M. Month., Richmond, 1920—XLVII—250.

Portmann, G. Technic and indications for biopsy of the larynx.
    Paris méd., 1920—X—185.

**Richardson, Charles W.**  Acute abscess of the lateral wall of the laryngopharynx.
Ann. Otol., Rhinol. & Laryngol., St. Louis, 1920—XXIX—804.

**Rosenthal, G.**  Technic for intercricothyroid injections.
Paris méd., 1920—X—521.

**Stern, H.**  Laryngectomy and retraining of the voice.
Wien. klin. Wchnschr., 1920—XXXIII—540.

**Symonds, C. J.**  Total laryngectomy: indications for and results of operation.
J. Laryngol., Lond., 1920—XXXV—257.

**Trotter, W.**  Method of lateral pharyngotomy for exposure of large growths in epilaryngeal region.
J. Laryngol., Lon., 1920—XXXV—289.

## SECTION 12.—TRACHEA AND BRONCHI.

**Bard, L.**  Compression of trachea from aerophagia with idiopathic dilatation of esophagus.
Arch. de mal. de l'appar. digest., Paris, 1920—X—449.

**Burgess, J. L.**  Report of selected cases of foreign bodies in bronchi and esophagus.
Texas State J. M., Fort Worth, 1920—XVI—128.

**Elliott, J. H.**  Dilatation of bronchi.
Med. Rec., N. Y., 1920—XCVIII—253.

**Freudenthal, W.**  Bronchoperiscope.
Laryngoscope St. Louis, 1920—XXX—527.

**Goodloe, A. E.**  Laryngo-tracheo bronchoscopy.
Tenn. M. Ass. J., Nashville, 1920—XIII—141.

**Hofer, G.**  Chronic stenosis of larynx and trachea.
Kien. klin. Wchnschr. Vienna, 1920—XXXIII—515.

**Mitchell, W.**  Case of broncho-esophageal fistula.
Arch. Radiol. & Electroth., Lond., 1920—49.

## SECTION 13.—VOICE AND SPEECH.

**Head, H.**  Aphasia and kindred disorders of speech.
Brain, London, 1920—XLIII—87.

**Richardson, C. W.**  Demonstration of reconstruction of section of defects of hearing and speech.
Laryngoscope, St. Louis, 1920—XXX—487.

**Stern, H.**  Laryngectomy and retraining of the voice.
Wien. klin. Wchnschr., 1920—XXXIII—540.

**Venables, J. F.**  Stammering.
Seala Hayne Neurological Studies, London, 1920—I—331.

## SECTION 14.—ESOPHAGUS.

**Axhausen, G.**  Reconstruction of esophagus.
Beit. z. klin. Chir., Tübing., 1920—CXX—163.

**Bard, L.**  Compression of trachea from aerophagia with idiopathic dilatation of esophagus.
Arch. de mal. de l'appar. digest., Paris, 1920—X—449.

**Burgess, J. L.** Report of selected cases of foreign bodies in bronchi and esophagus.
Texas State J. M., Fort Worth, 1920—XVI—128.

**Forbes, H. H.** Use of radium in esophageal cancer.
N. York M. J., 1920—CXII—568.

**Mitchell, W.** Case of broncho-esophageal fistula.
Arch. Radiol. & Electroth., Lond., 1920—49.

**Oettinger and Caballero.** Mega-esophagus.
Bull. Soc. med. d. hop., Paris, 1920—XLIV—1052.

**Ringsdorff, H.** Esophageal stenosis with multiple spasms.
Monatschr. f. Kinderh., Berlin, 1920—XIII—131.

**Rossi, F.** Foreign body in esophagus.
Policlin., Rome, 1920—XXVII—696.

## SECTION 15.—ENDOSCOPY.

**Burgess, J. L.** Report of selected cases of foreign bodies in bronchi and esophagus.
Texas State J. M., Fort Worth, 1920—XVI—128.

**Freudenthal, W.** Bronchoperiscope.
Laryngoscope St. Louis, 1920—XXX—527.

**Goodloe, A. E.** Laryngo-tracheo bronchoscopy.
Tenn. M. Ass. J., Nashville, 1920—XIII—141.

**Jackson, C.** Peroral endoscopy and laryngeal surgery.
Laryngoscope, St. Louis, 1920—XXX—520.

## SECTION 16.—EXTERNAL EAR AND CANAL.

**Carpenter, E. R.** Surgical problems in otologic work.
Texas State J. M., Fort Worth, 1920—XVI—121.

**Moraes, E.** The ear and the hearing.
Brazil med., Rio de Jan., 1920—XXXIV—460.

**Neville, S.** Tetanus due to ear infection.
China M. J., Shanghai, 1920—XXXIV—381.

**Romanos, Mesonero.** Herpes zoster of ear and neck, with peripheral facial paralysis.
Siglo med., Madrid, 1920—LXVII—401.

**Tanaka, F., and Yoshida, C.** Vital fixation of auricular organs and staining of nerves.
Japan Med. World, Tokyo, 1920—X—.

**Wood, A.** Moth in ear.
Lancet, London, 1920—II—600.

## SECTION 17.—MIDDLE EAR, INCLUDING TYMPANIC MEMBRANE AND EUSTACHIAN TUBE.

**Bacher, J. A.** Surgical treatment of acute otitis media in children, with report of fifty consecutive cases.
Calif. State J. M., San Fran., 1920—XVIII—327.

**Bardes. A.** Aural aftermaths of influenza.
Med. Rec., N. Y., 1920—XCVIII—810.

**Carpenter, E. R.** Surgical problems in otologic work.
Texas State J. M., Fort Worth, 1920—XVI—121.

**Cecilia, J. Santa.** Eye sign of facial paralysis.
Bravil med., Rio de Jan., 1920—XXXIV—444.

**Frey, H., and Orzechowski, K.** Otosclerosis in relation to tetany.
Wien. klin. Wchnschr., 1920—XXXIII—697, 754.

**Guttman, J.** Case of carcinoma of middle ear.
N. York M. J., 1920—CXII—675.

**Lapat, Wm.** Catheterization of eustachian tubes through the mouth.
J. Am. M. Ass., Chicago, 1920—LXXV—1498.

**Leegard, F.** Otogenous pyemia, sinus phlebitis and sinus thrombosis.
Norsk Mag. f. Laegevidensk., Kristiania, 1920—XXCI—745.

**McKenzie, D.** Aqueduct of fallopius and facial paralysis.
J. Laryngol., Lond., 1920—XXXV—244, 271, 296.

**Moraes, E.** The ear and the hearing.
Brazil med., Rio de Jan., 1920—XXXIV—460.

**Neville, S.** Tetanus due to ear infection.
China M. J., Shanghai, 1920—XXXIV—381.

**Sorenson, S. T.** Operations for scarlatinal otitis.
Hosp.-Tid., Khenh., 1920—LXIII—457.

**Tanaka, F., and Yoshida, C.** Vital fixation of auricular organs and staining of nerves.
Japan Med. World, Tokyo, 1920—X—.

## SECTION 18.—MASTOID PROCESS.

**Bardes, A.** Aural aftermaths of influenza.
Med. Rec., N. Y., 1920—XCVIII—810.

**Barnhill, J. F.** Anomalous sigmoid sinus thrombosis; report of cases.
Med. Rec., N. Y., 1920—XCVIII—388.

**Carpenter, E. R.** Surgical problems in otologic work.
Texas State J. M., Fort Worth, 1920—XVI—121.

**Dittman, G. C.** Paralysis of abducens nerve secondary to mastoiditis.
Minnesota Med., St. Paul, 1920—III—439.

**Glogau, O.** Mastoidectomy (perisinus abscess, exposure of dura) followed by attacks of toxic insanity; recovery.
Laryngoscope, St. Louis, 1920—XXX—566.

**Granthamhill, C.** Symptomless influenzal (streptococcal) mastoiditis.
Lancet, London, 1920—II—241.

**Hill, Frederick T.** Lateral sinus thrombosis, with report of seven cases.
Ann. Otol., Rhinol. and Laryngol., St. Louis, 1920—XXIX—829.

**Jones, W. D.** Two atypical cases of acuet mastoiditis.
Texas State J. M., Fort Worth, 1920—XVI—123.

**Jordan, L. G.** Mastoid cases.
Mil. Surgeon, 1920—XLVII—310.

**Leegard, F.** Otogenous pyemia, sinus phlebitis and sinus thrombosis.
Norsk Mag. f. Laegevidensk., Kristiania, 1920—XXCI—745.

**Molinari, G.** Mastoid versus vertebral suppuration.
Riforma med., Naples, 1920—XXXVI—550.

**Robinson, J. A.** Cavernous sinus thrombosis following a secondary mastoidectomy.
Laryngoscope, St. Louis, 1920—XXX—574.

**Rott, Otto M.** Concerning the question of jugular ligation in sinus thrombosis.
Ann. Otol., Rhinol. & Laryngol., St. Louis, 1920—XXIX—820.

**Salinger, S.** Mastoiditis without tympanic involvement.
Laryngoscope, St. Louis, 1920—XXX—573.

**Salinger, Samuel.** Primary periostitis of the mastoid.
Ann. Otol., Rhinol. & Laryngol.. St. Louis, 1920—XXIX—943.

**Stoops, R. P.** Mastoidectomy in presence of erysipelas.
Nebraska State M. J., Norfolk, 1920—V—217.

## SECTION 19.—INTERNAL EAR.

**Aynesworth, H. T.** Vertigo.
Texas State M. J., Fort Worth, 1920—XVI—243.

**Cantaloube, P.** The function of the vestibule.
Revue neurologique, Paris, 1920—XXVII—305.

**Crane, C. G.** Neurootology.
Ann. Otol., Rhinol. and Laryngol., St. Louis, 1920—XXIX—879.

**Edmunds, T. W., and Dudley, G. B., Jr.** Case of mastoiditis, with necrosis of bony lamina covering sigmoid portion of lateral sinus.
Virginia M. Month., Richmond, 1920—XLVII—317.

**Frey, H., and Orzechowski, K.** Otosclerosis in relation to tetany.
Wien. klin. Wchnschr., 1920—XXXIII—697, 754.

**Grahe, K.** The internal ear in léthargic encephalitis.
Münchener med. Wchnschr., Munich, 1920—LXVII—629.

**Heitger, Joseph D.** The present status of neurootology from the borderline standpoint.
J. Am. M. Ass., Chicago, 1920—LXXV—800.

**Kerrison, P. D.** Vestibular vertigo; prognosis in different types of cases. Reports of cases.
Ohio M. J., Columbus, 1920—XVI—726.

**Lyons, Horace Raymond.** Barany tests in supratentorial tumors proved by operation or necropsy.
Ann. Otol., Rhinol. & Laryngol., St. Louis, 1920—XXIX—898.

**Martel, Fred J., and Jones, Isaac H.** The education of the vestibular sense.
Ann. Otol., Rhinol. & Laryngol., St. Louis, 1920—XXIX—859.

**McKenzie, D.** Aqueduct of fallopius and facial paralysis.
J. Laryngol., Lond., 1920—XXXV—244, 271, 296.

**Milesi, G.** Auditory neuritis in meningitis.
Policlin., Roma, 1920—XXVII—924.

**Moraes, E.** The ear and the hearing.
Brazil med., Rio de Jan., 1920—XXXIV—460.

**Pearson, W. W.** Vestibular manifestations in neurologic cases.
Iowa M. J., Des Moines, 1920—X—303.

**Scott, S.** Ear in relation to certain disabilities in flying.
J. Laryngol., Lond., 1920—XXXV—225.

**Tanaka, F., and Yoshida, C.** Vital fixation of auricular organs and staining of nerves.
Japan Med. World, Tokyo, 1920—X—.

**Vail, H. H.** Studies by Barany rotation and caloric tests of tumors of nervus acusticus.
Laryngoscope, St. Louis, 1920—XXX—505.

## SECTION 20.—DEAFNESS AND DEAFMUTISM, AND TESTS FOR HEARING.

**Aymard, J. L.** Problem of the deaf.
South African M. Rec., Cape Town, 1920—XVIII—243.

**Booth, F. W.** Education of deaf.
Nebraska State M. J., Norfolk, 1920—V—261.

**Goldstein, M. A.** Deaf child.
Laryngoscope, St. Louis, 1920—XXX—479.

**Krukenberg, H.** Operative treatment for deafness.
München. med. Wchnschr., 1920—LXVII—835.

**Love, J. K.** Origin of sporadic congenital deafness.
J. Laryngol., Lond., 1920—XXXV—263.

**Moraes, E.** The ear and the hearing.
Brazil med., Rio de Jan., 1920—XXXIV—460.

**Peck, A. W.** How the deafened rebuild their lives.
Laryngoscope, St. Louis, 1920—XXX—490.

**Richardson, C. W.** Demonstration of reconstruction of section of defects of hearing and speech.
Laryngoscope, St. Louis, 1920—XXX—487.

**Samuelson, E. E.** Ears and job.
Laryngoscope, St. Louis, 1920—XXX—501.

**Seligmann, A.** A case of deafness in infantile scurvy.
Monatschr. f. Kinderh., Berlin, 1920—XVIII—221.

**Storey, J. de R.** Psychology of deafened people from a layman's point of view.
Laryngoscope, St. Louis, 1920—XXX—496.

**Wright, J. D.** The deaf.
Laryngoscope, St. Louis, 1920—XXX—597.

**Yearsley, M.** Can acquired deafness lead to congenital deafness?
J. Laryngol., Lond., 1920—XXXV—270.

## SECTION 21.—FOREIGN BODIES IN THE NOSE, THROAT AND EAR.

**Burgess, J. L.** Report of selected cases of foreign bodies in bronchi and esophagus.
Texas State J. M., Fort Worth, 1920—XVI—128.

**Goodloe, A. E.** Laryngo-tracheo bronchoscopy.
Tenn. M. Ass. J., Nashville, 1920—XIII—141.

**Orendorff, Otis.** Foreign body in nasopharynx.
J. Am. M. Ass., Chicago, 1920—LXXV—1343.

Rossi, F. Foreign body in esophagus.
Policlin., Rome, 1920—XXVII—696.

Wood, A. Moth in ear.
Lancet, London, 1920—II—600.

## SECTION 22.—ORAL CAVITY, INCLUDING TONGUE, PALATE AND INFERIOR MAXILLARY.

Arnone, L. Prosthesis for cleft palate in nurslings.
Riv. di clin. pediat., Florence, 1920—XVIII—347.

Ballenger, Edgar G., and Elder, Omar F. Orchitis from mumps: the need of conserving the testes by incision of the tunica albuginea.
J. Am. M. Ass., Chicago, 1920—LXXV—1257.

Bercher, J. Indications and technic for blocking inferior dental nerve.
Paris méd., 1920—X—193.

Blair, V. P. Treatment of advanced carcinoma of mouth.
J. Missouri M. Ass., St. Louis, 1920—XVII—395.

Bonnet-Roy, F. Treatment of ranula.
Paris méd., 1920—X—184.

Bowen, C. F. Fractures of bones of face.
Am. J. Roentgenol., N. York, 1920—VII—350.

Brown, G. V. I. Plastic work in surgery of the jaw.
Wisconsin M. J., Milwaukee, 1920—XX—143.

Cobb, C. M. Tooth brush a cause of repeated infections of mouth.
Boston M. & S. J., 1920—CXXVIII—263.

Cole, P. P. Surgical treatment of malignant disease of lip and jaw.
Lancet, Lond., 1920—II—845.

Comby, J. Scurvy in infants.
Medicine Paris, 1920—I—673.

Courbon, P. Recurring dislocation of jaw from bullet close to angle.
Revue neurologique, Paris, 1920—XXVII—337.

Cushing, H. Experiences with 332 Gasserian operations.
Am. J. M. Sc., Phila., 1920—CLX—157.

Davidsohn, H. Hutchinson's teeth.
Deutsche med. Wchnschr., Berl., 1920—XLVI—295.

Dorrance, Geo. M. Epithelial inlays versus skin or mucous membrane flaps for replacing lost mucous membrane in the mouth.
J. Am. M. Ass., Chicago, 1920—LXXV—1179.

Dunning, Henry S. Surgical treatment of chronic maxillary sinusitis of oral origin.
J. Am. M. Ass., Chicago, 1920—LXXV—1391.

Fargin-Fayolle, P. Stomatology in 1920.
Paris méd., 1920—X—188.

Floyd, C. Study of streptococci obtained from mouth in cases of chorea.
J. Med. Research, Bost., 1920—XLI—467.

Friesell, H. F.  Progress in dental education.
    J. Am. M. Ass., Chicago, 1920—LXXV—1247.

Ganley, J. E.  Vincent's angina-stomatitis.
    Boston M. & S. J., 1920—CLXXXIII—466.

Gompertz, L. M.  Relation of teeth to general medicine.
    Med. Rec., N. Y., 1920—XCVIII—217.

Guthrie, Haidee Weeks.  A dental clinic for children in a settle-
    ment.
    J. Am. M. Ass., Chicago, 1920—LXXV—1245.

Hallez, G. L.  Scurvy in infants.
    Medecine, Paris, 1920—I—123.

Harms. C.  Etiology of actinomycosis of the tongue.
    Munchen. med. Wchnschr., 1920—LXVII—903.

Hatton, Edward H.  Adenoma of mucous glands of mouth, and
    macrocheilia.
    J. Am. M. Ass., Chicago, 1920—LXXV—1176.

Hochschild, H.  Chronic large parotid glands in children.
    Jahrb. f. Kinderh., Berl., 1920—XCII—360.

Jacobson, A. C.  Practical mouth hygiene.
    Boston M. & S. J., 1920—CXXCIII—264.

Jamieson, J. K., and Dobson, J. F.  Lymphatics of tongue: particu-
    lar reference to removal of glands in cancer of tongue.
    Brit. J. Surg., Lond., 1920—VIII—80.

Kranz, P.  Hutchinson's teeth (a reply).
    Deutsche med. Wchnschr., Berl., 1920—XLVI—773.

Lain, Everett S.  A clinical study of epithelioma of the lower lip.
    J. Am. M. Ass., Chicago, 1920—LXXV—1052.

Leulero.  Radiography of lower jaw.
    J. de radiol. et d'electrol., Paris, 1920—IV—36.

Macht, David I.  Benzyl alcohol for toothache.
    J. Am. M. Ass., Chicago, 1920—LXXV—1205.

Miller, A. L.  Gradual reduction of fractures of the maxilla and
    mandible.
    J. Am. M. Ass., Chicago, 1920—LXXV—1255.

Newall, W. A.  Case of infantile scurvy.
    Am. J. Roentgenol., N. Y., 1920—VII—371.

Novitsky, J.  Dead teeth and antral pathology.
    Illinois M. J., Oak Park, 1920—XXXVIII—143.

Peters, W.  Operative treatment of carcinoma of the lip.
    Zentralb. f. Chir., Leipz., 1920—XLVII—564.

Potts, H. A.  Treatment of comminuted fractures of the mandible.
    J. Am. M. Ass., Chicago, 1920—LXXV—1178.

Robertson, H. E.  Local amyloid with special reference to socalled
    amyloid tumors of the tongue.
    Ann. Otol., Rhinol. & Laryngol., St. Louis, 1920—XXIX—773.

Schulze, W.  Etiology of postoperative parotitis.
    Zentralb. f. Gynäk., Leipz., 1920—XLIV—613.

Seligmann, A.  A case of deafness in infantile scurvy.
    Monatschr. f. Kinderh., Berlin, 1920—XVIII—221.

**Strettiner, H.** Note on operation for harelip.
Zentralbl. f. Chir., Leipz., 1920—XLVII—952.

**Thompson, J. E.** Relationship between ranula and branchiogenetic cysts.
Ann. Surg., Phila., 1920—LXXII—164.

**Tousey, S.** Dental infection.
N. York M. J., 1920—CXII—353.

**Welty, Cullen, F.** Closure of fistulous openings through alveolar process into antrum of Highmore.
J. Am. M. Ass., Chicago, 1920—LXXV—867.

**Wesselhoeft, C.** Orchitis in mumps.
Boston M. & S. J., 1920—CLXXXIII—425, 458, 520.

## SECTION 23.—FACE.

**Cole, P. P.** Surgical treatment of malignant disease of lip and jaw.
Lancet, Lond., 1920—II—845.

**Hochschild, H.** Chronic large parotid glands in children.
Jahrb. f. Kinderh., Berl., 1920—XCII—360.

**Lain, Everett S.** A clinical study of epithelioma of the lower lip.
J. Am. M. Ass., Chicago, 1920—LXXV—1052.

**Peters, W.** Operative treatment of carcinoma of the lip.
Zentralb. f. Chir., Leipz., 1920—XLVII—564.

**Zacherl, H.** Malformations of the face.
Arch. f. klin. Chir., Berl., 1920—CXIII—374.

## SECTION 24.—CERVICAL GLANDS AND DEEPER NECK STRUCTURES.

**Geymüller, E.** Actinomycosis of neck and brain.
Deutsche Ztschr. f. Chir., Leipz., 1920—CLI—200.

**Jones, E. G.** Surgery of the neck.
Med. Rec., N. Y., 1920—XCVIII—386.

**Romanos, Mesonero.** Herpes zoster of ear and neck, with peripheral facial paralysis.
Siglo med., Madrid, 1920—LXVII—401.

**Thompson, J. E.** Relationship between ranula and branchiogenetic cysts.
Ann. Surg., Phila., 1920—LXXII—164.

## SECTION 25.—THYROID AND THYMUS.

**Alamraine, A.** Surgical anatomy of nerves of the thyroid.
Rev. de chir., Par., 1920—XXXIX—403.

**Berkeley, W. N.** Preliminary report on new method for clinical diagnosis of toxic thyroid states; serologic technic.
Ohio M. J., Columbus, 1920—XVI—754.

**Bingham, G. H., and Richards, G. E.** Corelation of results of treatment of goiter by surgical and roentgen ray methods.
Canad. M. Ass. J., Toronto 1920—X—988.

**Canelli, A. F.** Anatomy and pathology of the thymus in young children.
Pediatria, Napoli, 1920—XXVIII—573.

**Cottis, G. W.**  Practical points in goiter surgery.
N. York State J. M., 1920—XX—290.

**Coulaud, E.**  Thyroid and pituitary organotherapy.
Bull. méd., Par., 1920—XXXIV—859.

**Crile, G. W.**  Special consideration of toxic adenoma in relation
to exophthalmic goiter.
Ann. Surg., Phila., 1920—LXXII—141.

**Crotti, A.**  Etiology and pathology of exophthalmic goiter: their
hearing on prevention. prognosis and treatment.
Ohio M. J., Columbus, 1920—XVI—738.

**Förster, W.**  Nerve blocking for goiter operation.
Munchen. med. Wchnschr., 1920—LXVII—904.

**Frazier, C. H.**  Management of toxic goiter from surgical point of
view.
Ann. Surg., Phila., 1920—LXXII—155.

**Freeman, L.**  "Tourniquet operation" in toxic and other goiters.
Ann. Surg., Phila., 1920—LXXII—161.

**Fussell, M. H.**  Diagnosis and treatment of hyperthyroidism.
N. York M. J., 1920—CXII—205.

**Gandy, C., and Piedelievre, R.**  Cancer of the thymus.
Bull. soc. méd. d. hop., Paris, 1920—XLIV—867.

**Garibaldi, A.**  The thyroid and production of antibodies.
Cron. med., Lima, 1920—XXXVII—200.

**Goetsch, Emil.**  Diagnosis and treatment of thyroid disease based
on use of epinephrin hypersensitiveness test.
N. York State J. M., 1920—XX—282.

**Goetsch, E.**  Disorders of thyroid: hypersensitiveness test with
special reference to "diffuse adenomatosis" of thyroid.
Endocrinology, Los Angeles, 1920—IV—389.

**Hoppe, H. H.**  Treatment of hyperthyroidism with corpus luteum:
a second report.
Ohio M. J., Columbus, 1920—XVI—749.

**Ishihara, M.**  Effect of experimental extirpation of thyroid body.
Bull. Naval Med. Ass. Japan, Tokyo, 1920—I.

**Jaeger, H.**  Parathyroid implants in postoperative tetany.
Zentralb. f. Chir., Leipz., 1920—XLVII—565.

**Janney, N. W., and Henderson, H. E.**  Diagnosis and treatment of
hypothyroidism.
Arch. Int. Med., Chicago, 1920—XXVI—297.

**Johnston, C. H.**  Diagnosis of hyperthyroidism.
J. Mich. M. Soc., Grand Rapids, 1920—XIX—456.

**Juarros, C.**  Hyperthyroidism and the Bloch syndrome.
Siglo med., Madrid, 1920—LXVI—417.

**Judd, E. S.**  Results of operation for adenoma with hyperthyroidism and exophthalmic goiter.
Ann. Surg., Phila., 1920—LXXII—145.

**Judd, E. S.**  Results of surgical treatment of exophthalmic goiter.
N. York State J. M., 1920—XX—287.

**Kottmann, K.** Colloid chemistry and the thyroid problem.
Schweiz. med. Wchnschr., Basel, 1920—L—644.

**Larson, J. A.** Further evidence on functional correlation of hypophysis and thyroid.
American J. Physiol., Baltimore, 1920—LIII—89.

**Loeb, L.** Compensatory hypertrophy of thyroid. V. Effect of administration of thyroid, thymus gland and tethelin and meat diet on hypertrophy of thyroid in guinea pigs.
J. Med. Research, Bos., 1920—XLII—77.

**Loeb, L.** Studies on compensatory hypertrophy of thyroid gland.
J. Med. Research, Bost., 1920—XLI—481.

**Mayo, C. H.** Adenoma with hyperthyroidism.
Ann. Surg., Phila., 1920—LXXII—134.

**Mieres, J. F.** Exophthalmic goiter in the tuberculous.
Semana med., Buenos Aires, 1920—XXVII—507.

**Marine, D.** Physiology of normal thyroid and physiology of thyroid in exophthalmic goiter.
Ohio M. J., Columbus, 1920—XVI—735.

**Marine, D., and Kimball, O. P.** Goiter survey work in Ohio; incidence of simple goiter in school children of Cleveland, Akron and Warren.
Ohio M. J., Columbus, 1920—XVI—757.

**Moore, R. F.** Exophthalmos and limitation of eye movements of exophthalmic goiter.
Lancet, London, 1920—II—701.

**Morris, M. F., Jr.** Therapy of hyperthyroidism.
Med. Rec., N. Y., 1920—XCVIII—431.

**Pearson, J. M.** Goiter; its medical treatment.
Cana. M. Ass. J., Toronto, 1920—X—983.

**Porter, M. F.** Goiter.
Ann. Surg., Phila., 1920—LXXII—129.

**Porter, M. F.** Hyperactivity of thyroid.
J. Indiana M. Ass., Ft. Wayne, 1920—XIII—295.

**Poppens, Peter H.** Tetany following thyroidectomy.
J. Am. M. Ass., Chicago, 1920—LXXV—1068.

**Rachford, B. K.** Substernal goiter, with pressure symptoms.
Am. J. M. Sc., Phila., 1920—CLX—410.

**Ribbert.** Necropsy of sarcoma of thyroid.
Arch. f. klin. Chir., Berl., 1920—CXIII—248.

**Rogers, J.** Organ therapy in thyroid and allied disorders.
Med. Rec., N. Y., 1920—XCVIII—631.

**Rowe, A. H.** Basal metabolism in thyroid disease aid to diagnosis and treatment; utility of modified Tissot apparatus.
Calif. State J. M., San Fran., 1920—XVIII—332.

**Russell, W. B.** Toxic goiter in Orientals.
National M. J., China, Shanghai, 1920—VI—101.

**Schiassi, B.** Outcome with exophthalmic goiter.
Policlin., Roma, 1920—XXVII—285.

**Sergent, E.** Exophthalmic goiter mistaken for tuberculosis.
Paris méd., 1920—X—80.

**Sloan, E. P.** Tubercular goiter patient.
Illinois M. J., Oak Park, 1920—XXXVIII—144.

**Starr, F. N. G., Graham, R. R., and Robinson, W. L.** Goiter.
Cana. Ass. J., Toronto, 1920—X—977.

**Stiell, W. F.** Subthyroidism.
Practitioner, Lond., 1920—CV—146.

**Terry, W. I.** Toxic goiter.          ·
Ann. Surg., Phila., 1920—LXXII—152.

**Tourneux, J. P.** Acute suppurative thyroiditis.
Progres méd., Par., 1920—XXXV—371.

**Van Meter, B. F.** Goiter.
Kentucky M. J., Louisville, 1920—XVIII—297.

## SECTION 26.—PITUITARY.

**Behse, E.** Pituitary tumor.
Finska läk-sällsk. handl., Helsingfors, 1920—LXII—382.

**Coulaud, E.** Thyroid and pituitary organotherapy.
Bull. méd., Par., 1920—XXXIV—859.

**Engelbach, Wm.** Classification of disorders of hypophysis.
Endocrinology, Los Angeles, 1920—IV—347.

**Larson, J. A.** Further evidence on functional correlation of hypophysis and thyroid.
American J. Physiol., Baltimore, 1920—LIII—89.

**Lissner, H. H.** Hypopituitarism; report of case.
Endocrinology, Los Angeles, 1920—IV—403.

**Mieres, J. F.** Exophthalmic goiter in the tuberculous.
Semana med., Buenos Aires, 1920—XXVII—507.

**Redwood, F. H.** Some disturbances of pituitary gland.
Virginia M. Month., Richmond, 1920—XLVII—301.

**Seaman, E. C.** Presence of iodin in large quantities of sheep pituitary gland.
J. Biol. Chem., Baltimore, 1920—XLIII—1.

## SECTION 27.—ENDOCRANIAL AFFECTIONS AND LUM-
## BAR PUNCTURE.

**Barnhill, J. F.** Anomalous sigmoid sinus thrombosis; report of
cases.
Med. Rec., N. Y., 1920—XCVIII—388.

**Edmunds, T. W., and Dudley, G. B., Jr.** Case of mastoiditis, with
necrosis of bony lamina covering sigmoid portion of lateral
sinus.
Virginia M. Month., Richmond, 1920—XLVII—317.

**Geymüller, E.** Actinomycosis of neck and brain.
Deutsche Ztschr. f. Chir., Leipz., 1920—CLI—200.

**Glogau, O.** Mastoidectomy (perisinus abscess, exposure of dura)
followed by attacks of toxic insanity; recovery.
Laryngoscope, St. Louis, 1920—XXX—566.

Grahe, K. The internal ear in lethargic encephalitis.
Münchener med. Wchnschr., Munich, 1920—LXVII—629.

Hassin, G. B., Levy, D. M., and Tupper, W. E. Facial pontine
diplegia (traumatic).
J. Nerv. & Men. Dis., N. Y., 1920—LII—25.

Head, H. Aphasia and kindred disorders of speech.
Brain, London, 1920—XLIII—87.

Hill, Frederick T. Lateral sinus thrombosis, with report of seven
cases.
Ann. Otol., Rhinol. and Laryngol., St. Louis, 1920—XXIX—829.

Leegard, F. Otogenous pyemia, sinus phlebitis and sinus thrombosis.
Norsk Mag. f. Laegevidensk., Kristiania, 1920—XXCI—745.

Lobell, Abraham. A case of cerebellar abscess diagnosed postmortem.
J. Am. M. Ass., Chicago, 1920—LXXV—600.

Lyons, Horace Raymond. Barany tests in supratentorial tumors
proved by operation or necropsy.
Ann. Otol., Rhinol. & Laryngol., St. Louis, 1920—XXIX—898.

Milesi, G. Auditory neuritis in meningitis.
Policlin., Roma, 1920—XXVII—924.

Rivers, T. M. Indol test on the spinal fluid for rapid diagnosis of
influenzal meningitis.
J. Am. M. Ass., Chicago, 1920—LXXV—1495.

Robinson, J. A. Cavernous sinus thrombosis following a secondary
mastoidectomy.
Laryngoscope, St. Louis, 1920—XXX—574.

Rott, Otto M. Concerning the question of jugular ligation in sinus
thrombosis.
Ann. Otol., Rhinol. & Laryngol., St. Louis, 1920—XXIX—820.

Speidel. Late results of encephalitis after influenza.
Münchener med. Wchnschr., Munich, 1920—LXVII—630.

Vail, H. H. Studies by Barany rotation and caloric tests of tumors
of nervus acusticus.
Laryngoscope, St. Louis, 1920—XXX—505.

## SECTION 28.—CRANIAL NERVES.

Bercher, J. Indications and technic for blocking inferior dental
nerve.
Paris méd., 1920—X—193.

Cecilia, J. Santa. Eye sign of facial paralysis.
Bravil med., Rio de Jan., 1920—XXXIV—444.

Cushing, H. Experiences with 332 Gasserian operations.
Am. J. M. Sc., Phila., 1920—CLX—157.

Dittman, G. C. Paralysis of abducens nerve secondary to mastoiditis.
Minnesota Med., St. Paul, 1920—III—439.

Ellett, E. C. Optic neuritis, associated with disease of the nasal
sinuses; report of two cases.
J. Am. M. Ass., Chicago, 1920—LXXV—805.

**Garland, J., and White, P. D.** Paralysis of left recurrent laryngeal nerve associated with mitral stenosis.
Arch. Int. Med., Chicago, 1920—XXVI—343.

**Hassin, G. B., Levy, D. M., and Tupper, W. E.** Facial pontine diplegia (traumatic).
J. Nerv. & Men. Dis., N. Y., 1920—LII—25.

**Heitger, Joseph D.** The present status of neurootology from the borderline standpoint.
J. Am. M. Ass., Chicago, 1920—LXXV—800.

**Marriott, W. McKim.** Postdiphtheritic paralysis of the respiratory muscles: Report of case treated by prolonged artificial respiration.
J. Am. M. Ass., Chicago, 1920—LXXV—668.

**McKenzie, D.** Aqueduct of fallopius and facial paralysis.
J. Laryngol., Lond., 1920—XXXV—244, 271, 296.

**Rich, A. B.** Innervation of tensor veli palatini and levator veli palatini muscles.
Johns Hopkins Hosp. Bull., Balt., 1920—XXXI—305.

**Romanos, Mesonero.** Herpes zoster of ear and neck, with peripheral facial paralysis.
Siglo med., Madrid, 1920—LXVII—401.

**Vail, H. H.** Studies by Barany rotation and caloric tests of tumors of nervus acusticus.
Laryngoscope, St. Louis, 1920—XXX—505.

## SECTION 29.—PLASTIC SURGERY.

**Brown, G. V. I.** Plastic work in surgery of the jaw.
Wisconsin M. J., Milwaukee, 1920—XX—143.

**Chubb, G.** New method in rhinoplasty.
Lancet, London, 1920—II—354.

**Cohen, L.** Correct rhinoplasty.
Surg., Gynec. & Obst., Chicago, 1920—XXXI—412.

**Dorrance, Geo. M.** Epithelial inlays versus skin or mucous membrane flaps for replacing lost mucous membrane in the mouth.
J. Am. M. Ass., Chicago, 1920—LXXV—1179.

**Oppenheimer, S.** Condemnatory note on use of paraffin in cosmetic rhinoplasty.
Laryngoscope, St. Louis, 1920—XXX—595.

**Oppenheimer, S.** Implantation methods in cosmetic rhinoplasty.
Boston M. & S. J., 1920—CLXXXIII—329.

## SECTION 30.—INSTRUMENTS.

**Imperatori, C. J.** Apparatus for irrigating nasal cavities. useful in home treatment.
Laryngoscope, St. Louis, 1920—XXX—550.

**Shapiro, A. F.** Instrument for simplifying tonsillectomy by snare.
N. York M. J., 1920—CXII—681.

**Unger, M.** New instrument and method for washing and draining nasal sinuses.
Laryngoscope, St. Louis, 1920—XXX—561.

## SECTION 31.—RADIOLOGY.

**Aikins W. H. B.** Radium in toxic goiter.
Am. J. Roentgenol., N. Y., 1920—VII—404.

**Bingham, G. H., and Richards, G. E.** Corelation of results of treatment of goiter by surgical and roentgen ray methods.
Canad. M. Ass. J., Toronto 1920—X—988.

**Bowen, C. F.** Fractures of bones of face.
Am. J. Roentgenol., N. York, 1920—VII—350.

**Leulero.** Radiography of lower jaw.
J. de radiol. et d'electrol., Paris, 1920—IV—36.

**Mitchell, W.** Case of broncho-esophageal fistula.
Arch. Radiol. & Electroth., Lond., 1920—49.

**Sonnenschein, Robert.** Radium in the treatment of malignant tumors of the nose and throat: its use and possible abuse.
J. Am. M. Ass., Chicago, 1920—LXXV—860.

**Von Dworzak, Z.** Radium therapy in diseases of nose, ear and throat.
Colorado Med., Denver, 1920—XVII—238.

## SECTION 34.—EYE.

**Beck, J. C., and Deutsch, E.** Interrelation between eye, ear, nose and throat with presentation of cases.
Am. J. Ophthalmol., Chicago, 1920—III—349.

**Berens, C., and Uren, C. T.** Effect of nose and throat infections on ocular functions of aviators.
Am. J. Ophthalmol., Chicago, 1920—III—170.

**Cecilia, J. Santa.** Eye sign of facial paralysis.
Bravil med., Rio de Jan., 1920—XXXIV—444.

**Crile, G. W.** Special consideration of toxic adenoma in relation to exophthalmic goiter.
Ann. Surg., Phila., 1920—LXXII—141.

**Crotti, A.** Etiology and pathology of exophthalmic goiter: their bearing on prevention, prognosis and treatment.
Ohio M. J., Columbus, 1920—XVI—738.

**Ellett, E. C.** Optic neuritis, associated with disease of the nasal sinuses; report of two cases.
J. Am. M. Ass., Chicago, 1920—LXXV—805.

**Forbes, H. H.** Use of radium in esophageal cancer.
N. York M J., 1920—CXII—568.

**Judd, E. S.** Results of operation for adenoma with hyperthyroidism and exophthalmic goiter.
Ann. Surg., Phila., 1920—LXXII—145.

**Judd, E. S.** Results of surgical treatment of exophthalmic goiter.
N. York State J. M., 1920—XX—287.

**Liebault, G.** Acute frontal sinusitis and ptosis.
Bull. méd., Par., 1920—XXXIV—815.

**Loeb, H. W.** Two cases of blindness relieved by ethmoid exenteration; case of keratoiritis due to tonsil infection.
J. Missouri M. Ass., St. Louis, 1920—XVII—409.

**Meller.**  Relation of retrobulbar neuritis to nasal cavity.
Wien. klin. Wchnschr., 1920—XXXIII—205.

**Marine, D.**  Physiology of normal thyroid and physiology of thyroid in exophthalmic goiter.
Ohio M. J., Columbus, 1920—XVI—735.

**Moore, R. F.**  Exophthalmos and limitation of eye movements of exophthalmic goiter.
Lancet, London, 1920—II—701.

**Nagel, C. S. G.**  Congenital atresia of lacrimal duct.
Am. J. Ophth., Chicago, 1920—III—406.

**Potts, J. B.**  Nasal infection basis of certain ocular lesions.
Am. J. Ophthalmol., Chicago, 1920—III—195.

**Schiassi, B.**  Outcome with exophthalmic goiter.
Policlin., Roma, 1920—XXVII—285.

**White, L. E.**  Diagnosis of accessory sinus disease causing loss of vision.
Laryngoscope, St. Louis, 1920—XXX—551.

**Wiener, Meyer and Sauer, W. E.**  A new operation for the relief of dacryocystitis through the nasal route.
J. Am. M. Ass., Chicago, 1920—LXXV—868.

# ANNALS

OF

# OTOLOGY, RHINOLOGY

AND

# LARYNGOLOGY

INCORPORATING THE INDEX OF OTOLARYNGOLOGY.

| VOL. XXX. | JUNE, 1921. | No. 2. |

## SOME POINTS IN THE ANATOMY OF THE HUMAN TEMPORAL BONE.

BY JOSEPH GOLDSTEIN, M. D.,

DEPARTMENT OF ANATOMY OF THE STANFORD UNIVERSITY
MEDICAL SCHOOL,

STANFORD UNIVERSITY, CALIF.

### I.—THE WEIGHT AND DENSITY OF THE TEMPORAL BONE.

The weight of the bones of the skull in both sexes is greatest from twenty to forty-five, according to Gurriere and Massetti, 1895. Hence the maximum weight of 63.5 grams found in No. 119, among one hundred cleaned, dried temporal bones, probably approaches the maximum weight of the dry disarticulated adult bone quite closely. The lightest adult bone, No. 133 of this series, weighed but 22.5 grams, giving a difference of 41 grams.

Specimen 119 displaced 43 grams of water, its density hence being 1.48, but specimen 133 displaced but 10.5 grams of water, indicating a density of 2.14. Hence the lighter bone apparently had a far greater density. But the weight and density of bones, even when dried by years of exposure in a dry atmosphere, depends upon a great number of factors. One must consider the age and possibly racial characteristics of the individual bone and especially the method and the extent of the cleaning. Hence for this and other reasons the results obtained from these two specimens probably are only roughly indicative of the true density.

The average weight of fifty intact right temporal bones in Table I, regardless of sex and including the ear ossicles and the styloid and zygomatic processes to the point of articulation of the latter, in the dried state is 41.5 grams. Fifty left temporal bones average 41.6 grams. Hence asymmetry in form, even though present to a marked degree as described by Cheatle in 1913, in certain skulls, does not give one side a preponderance in average weight, even if one takes only a relatively small number of temporal bones.

## TABLE I.

| Right Side | | | Left Side | | |
|---|---|---|---|---|---|
| No. of Specimen | Weight | | No. of Specimen | Weight | |
| 1 | 39 | grs. | 7 | 52 | grs. |
| 44 | 47 | " | 15 | 29 | " |
| 10 | 48 | " | 18 | 31 | " |
| 16 | 52 | | 44 | 47 | |
| 19 | 27 | " | 45 | 47 | |
| 22 | 46 | " | 55 | 47 | |
| 24 | 57 | | 60 | 38 | |
| 25 | 51 | | 63 | 34 | |
| 27 | 33 | | 71 | 43 | |
| 32 | 53 | | 75 | 51 | |
| 38 | 34 | | 76 | 43 | |
| 40 | 32 | | 79 | 49 | |
| 49 | 49 | " | 80 | 53 | |
| 51 | 36 | | 85 | 37 | |
| 52 | 30 | | 92 | 43 | |
| 58 | 61 | " | 94 | 31 | " |
| 59 | 48 | | 109 | 35 | |
| 64 | 30 | | 116 | 37 | |
| 65 | 39 | | 119 | 63 | " |
| 66 | 43 | " | 120 | 48 | " |
| 68 | 38 | | 121 | 47 | |

TABLE I.—Continued.

| Right Side | | Left Side | |
| No. of Specimen | Weight | No. of Specimen | Weight |
| --- | --- | --- | --- |
| 69 | 52 " | 130 | 52 " |
| 70 | 62 " | 145 | 50 " |
| 105 | 47 | 146 | 47 ' |
| 106 | 32 | 148 | 42.5 ' |
| 107 | 37 | 153 | 38 ' |
| 108 | 30 | 156 | 25 |
| 114 | 52 | 157 | 36 " |
| 115 | 39 ·· | 163 | 27 " |
| 122 | 35 " | 166 | 31 ' |
| 124 | 27.5 " | 167 | 36.5 ' |
| 125 | 37 ' | 168 | 36.5 ' |
| 131 | 36 | 323 | 43 ' |
| 133 | 22 | 325 | 38 |
| 134 | 31 " | 327 | 38 |
| 142 | 46 | 328 | 34 |
| 147 | 57 " | 333 | 38 |
| 152 | 35.4 " | 341 | 47 |
| 154 | 38 " | 345 | 33 |
| 164 | 37 | 347 | 36 |
| 322 | 39 | 349 | 40 |
| 326 | 32 | 352 | 49 |
| 329 | 50 | 353 | 40 |
| 331 | 52 | 357 | 44 |
| 335 | 40 | 359 | 30 |
| 340 | 50 | 361 | 48 |
| 342 | 48 | 364 | 36 " |
| 343 | 40 | 369 | 40 |
| 344 | 41 | 372 | 55 |
| 348 | 32 | 373 | 59 |

Average wt., 41.5 "        Average wt., 41.6 "

II.—TORSION OF THE PETROUS PORTION.

As is well known, the temporal bone represents three elements—the petrosal, squamous and tympanic elements—which
usually can be separated at birth. The external acoustic

canal is largely unformed. At this time the tympanic ring is circular in outline and the tympanic membrane directly continuous and lies in the same plane as the external surface of the squamosa. Canal formation begins by the rapid growth of the anterior and posterior margins of the tympanic element, which are much thicker than the rest of the tympanic portion of the canal at this time. In adult bones, as we shall see later in the discussion of the osseous external acoustic orifice, we sometimes find a thickening at these very points, although this border usually becomes very thin in the adult condition.

At birth the petrous portion seems to show no torsion. In cross section it assumes the shape of an isosceles triangle— the anterior superior and the posterior superior surfaces forming straight sides. The inferior surface is quite irregular due to its articular surfaces, to the numerous foraminæ and the jugular fossa. The superior angle of the triangle is slightly rounded.

In the adult bone certain changes have occurred in the contour of the petrous portion. The medial extremity which articulates with the basilar portion of the sphenoid is directed anteriorly. This gives the superior border of the petrous bone a slightly bent direction, because it remains in juxtaposition with the sphenoid. But the superior margin, viewed from a median plane, also is rotated, anteriorally or clockwise, looking medially. The change that has taken place during this period of torsion has modified somewhat the structures underlying and contained within this portion of the bone, which forms the superior surface of the external auditory canal and envelops a part of the tympanum. The torsion which modifies the petrous portion modifies the form of the canal, as we shall see also, that of its external orifice.

In calculating the amount of rotation that the medial portion of the petroum element makes, I used the styloid process to fix the bone. It is impossible to determine the angle that the petrous portion makes with the styloid process in the newborn, on account of the absence of the process, but in the adult bones this process, when intact, is usually very definite and constant in direction.

The method used in calculating the angle of torsion is as follows: The bone was fixed by placing the styloid process in a vertical position in a board with vertical holes graded as to size.   The processes which are of variable size were fitted very snugly into suitable holes.   In this manner, one can eliminate error to a great decree and can be relatively sure that all angles are measured from a fairly definite base line.   The surface of the board is at right angles to the process, and the superior margin of the petrous portion is adjusted parallel to the edge of the board.   By using the plane surface of the board as a base line, one can measure the angle of rotation of the petrous portion quite accurately with a protractor.   In order to reduce error to a minimum, the angle of rotation was measured on a line passing through the center of the orifice of the internal auditory canal.   This surface of the bone sometimes is irregular, due to a ridge just over this orifice.   In these cases the arm of the protractor was placed as nearly parallel to the entire surface as possible.   Such a procedure was rarely necessary, however, for usually the arm of the protractor could be rested on the side of the petrous bone, placed parallel to the surface with little difficulty and the angle read.

## TABLE II.

| Specimen No. | Angle of Rota'n | Specimen No. | Angle of Rota'n |
|---|---|---|---|
| 3 | 118° | 122 | 117° |
| 7 | 113° | 126 | 105° |
| 16 | 117° | 127 | 118° |
| 17 | 113° | 131 | 116° |
| 20 | 118° | 134 | 110° |
| 22 | 116° | 139 | 115° |
| 24 | 122° | 145 | 119° |
| 28 | 116° | 149 | 115° |
| 31 | 114° | 154 | 113° |
| 35 | 125° | 159 | 114 |
| 46 | 115° | 163 | 113° |
| 59 | 115° | 166 | 120° |
| 65 | 113° | 170 | 114° |
| 66 | 112° | 322 | 115° |
| 67 | 116° | 343 | 112° |
| 75 | 117° | 345 | 115° |
| 76 | 115° | 346 | 113° |

TABLE II.—Continued.

| Specimen No. | Angle of Rota'n | Specimen No. | Angle of Rota'n |
|---|---|---|---|
| 78 | 122° | 354 | 121° |
| 82 | 115° | 355 | 117° |
| 89 | 112° | 359 | 113° |
| 93 | 121° | 365 | 114° |
| 117 | 118° | 369 | 116° |
| 118 | 120° | 374 | 114° |
| 120 | 113° | 1169 | 112° |
| 121 | 113° | 1350 | 120° |

It was interesting to find that there is a correlation between the angle of rotation of the petrous portion, measured as above, and the direction of the long diameter of the osseous external auditory orifice. When the long axis of the external orifice approaches a vertical plane—that is, when it is almost parallel to the styloid process, the anterior superior surface as measured above makes an agle of approximately 120° with the plane surface of the board. In specimens with the long axis approaching a horizontal position. the anterior superior surface makes an angle of approximately 110° with the plane surface of the board. In by far the commonest form. the long axis lies between the two extremes. the angle being about 115°. An average of the fifty specimens in Table II, calculated by this method, gave an angle of 115.7°. The maximum amount of rotation as measured above was 20°, which is the difference between 105° in specimen No. 126 and 125° in specimen No. 24. As the accompanying photographs show, one can determine the amount of rotation of the petrous portion with considerable accuracy by noticing the direction of the long diameter of the osseus external acoustic orifice. Furthermore, if the styloid processes of any series are placed parallel and opposite. the lines indicating the direction of the long diameter of the external orifice will be parallel.

Specimen 149, Fig. 1. the opposite surface of which is represented in Fig. 2. illustrates the usual condition of rotation. In specimen No. 126. represented in Figs. 3 and 4. the direction of the string or the long diameter of the external acoustic orifice is almost parallel to the styloid process, thus repre-

senting a totally different angle of rotation.  In specimen No.
24, represented in Figs. 5 and 6, on the other hand, the direction of the long diameter of the external acoustic foramen
forms almost a right angle with the styloid process.

There are numerous factors to be considered as to the
cause of this rotation, which is always in the same direction—
the superior margin being directed anteriorly, but it occurs
after birth.  At birth and shortly afterwards, no torsion was
observed in looking over 125 fetal and infantile specimens.
It will be recalled that the basilar portions of the occipital
bone also is more vertical and only slightly grooved at this
period, the deep hollowing found in  adult bones apparently
being coincidental with the torsion of the petrous element.

By the sixth month of fetal life, the skull, though smaller,
is in much the same condition as at birth, except that the
occipital region is relatively larger.  The most striking differences are the insignificance of the facial portion and the
flatness of the base.  In the cranium the frontal region is
relatively small.  According to Dwight, '07' Merkel divided
the growth of the head into two periods, with an intervening
one of rest.  The first period ends with the seventh year and
is followed by inactivity till puberty, when the second period
begins.  Our interest lies in Merkel's first two stages of the
first period, which are said to end at the fifth year.  In the
first stage, reaching to the end of the first year, the growth is
general, but the face gains on the cranium.  At six months
the basilar process rises more sharply, which, with the downward growth of the face, may have an important effect on
the torsion of the temporal bone, since the greatest degree
of rotation occurs at this time.  In the second stage, to the end
of the fifth year, the vault grows more than the base, assuming a more rounded and finished appearance.  The face still
gains relatively, but grows more in breadth than in height.  It
is quite probable from my observation that with the termination of this period the maximum degree of torsion has been
attained.

As stated above, the torsion begins after birth and apparently continues quite rapidly, for as far as I could observe, in
specimens a few years old, the maximum amount of torsion

already had been reached. Hence torsion occurs during infancy at a time the brain grows most rapidly. We have a rapidly growing brain and growing bones which envelop it. We also know that the brain molds the skull to a certain extent and that the skull also modifies the shape of the brain. Since these two conditions appear at the same period in development, the brain factor may have a great deal to do with these modifications of the petrous element at this time. It is possible that the cerebellum and the medulla oblongata exert a pressure by their rapid growth, forcing the basilar portion of the sphenoid and the superior margin of the petrous portion of the temporal bone anteriorly, thus accelerating the growth of the anterior portion of the skull which responds to the marked development of the frontal lobes.

The rapid growth of the cerebrum after birth also may exert a pull upon the dura at its close attachment to the superior margin of the petrous portion of the temporal bone, thus deflecting the medial extremity forward. Not only is the direction of this portion changed during this period, but the superior margin is molded somewhat, for this border is sharper in the adult form than it is in the infantile condition.

### III.—THE ANGLE BETWEEN THE PETROSA AND SQUAMOSA.

The angle that the superior margin of the petrous portion makes with a tangent parallel in the main, with the squamosa also, is greater in the adult condition than it is in the new-born. The squamous portion of the temporal bone has the general direction of the lateral surface of the calvarium—the squamosa itself occupying about one-half of the lateral surface in length. The suture between the parietal and temporal bone immediately over the mastoid process is generally very low, and one can readily measure the angle that the petrous element makes with the squamosal by means of a protractor, upon disarticulated bones. Using the external surface of the squamosa immediately above the posterior root of the process as a base line for one arm of the protractor, the angle which the petrous element makes with this arm can be measured directly.

About the time of birth there apparently is a very slight variation in the angle. It varied from 66 to 70 degrees in a small series of 20 infantile and newly born temporal bones. In the adult condition there is a greater variation, however, for an angle of 52 degrees was found as a minimum and one of 64 degrees as a maximum. The average of the angles between the petrous and squamous portions in 50 specimens in Table III is 57.2 degrees.

TABLE III.

| No. of Specimen | Angle | No. of Specimen | Angle |
|---|---|---|---|
| 1 | 59 | 35 | 56 |
| 2 | 53 | 39 | 53 |
| 3 | 55 | 40 | 60 |
| 4 | 60 | 42 | 58 |
| 6 | 60 | 43 | 58 |
| 7 | 52 | 44 | 60 |
| 9 | 55 | 45 | 60 |
| 14 | 54 | 46 | 64 |
| 15 | 58 | 47 | 60 |
| 16 | 58 | 48 | 56 |
| 17 | 55 | 49 | 60 |
| 18 | 60 | 51 | 58 |
| 20 | 55 | 53 | 58 |
| 21 | 58 | 56 | 60 |
| 22 | 59 | 58 | 60 |
| 23 | 58 | 61 | 55 |
| 24 | 56 | 71 | 60 |
| 25 | 53 | 152 | 55 |
| 26 | 60 | 159 | 55 |
| 27 | 60 | 321 | 62 |
| 28 | 60 | 326 | 61 |
| 29 | 60 | 341 | 56 |
| 30 | 60 | 374 | 57 |
| 31 | 57 | 1114 | 55 |
| 34 | 56 | 1168 | 58 |

IV.—VARIATIONS IN THE MASTOID FORAMEN.

The mastoid foramen, when present, has a greater uniformity in position than one infers from a textbook description. Piersol, 1907, gives a typical description in saying that a small canal, the mastoid foramen, transmitting a vein, runs from the sinus to the outside of the bone, and sometimes reaches as far back as the suture between the temporal and the occipital. Cheatle, 1906, described the vein as leaving the lateral sinus in its descending part and usually running upwards, backwards and outwards with a curved course, to emerge at the posterior edge of the base of the mastoid process. I believe it would be more nearly correct to limit the area of emergence, for after looking over more than 250 adult temporal bones I find that it usually emerges directly over the digastric groove, on a level with the upper margin of the osseus external acoustic orifice. When the lambdoidal suture at its lower extremity forms a convex surface on the mastoid portion of the etmporal bone, the foramen is found slightly medial to the digastric groove. If the lambdoidal suture is straight at this region, which is the more common form, the foramen may even appear in the suture, or within a centimeter of the suture, thus appearing directly above the digastric groove. It would appear from this that the suture between the temporal and the occipital bones had a great deal to do with determining the position of the foramen. One very rarely finds the foramen lateral to the digastric groove.

By tabulating the occurrence of the common forms of canal, we find some interesting data, as judged by 250 specimens in Table 4, chosen at random from our collection. In 68 specimens, or 27 per cent of the bones, there was no indication of a canal from the lateral sinus to the outside of the bone. One can always find emissary foraminæ, variable in number and size, over the mastoid process and at its base, but I do not include any canals that cannot be traced to the lateral sinus. It also is relatively common to find a canal apparently for a vein, entering and leaving on the lateral surface of the base of the process without penetrating deeply into the bone.

In 167 specimens, or 67 per cent of the 250 bones, the canal is single and usually can be traced with very little difficulty from the sinus to the outside of the bone. It is common to find one opening of the canal on the inner table, which divides within the spongiosa and emerges by two openings. This was observed in 11 specimens, or 4 per cent. Four specimens had two separate canals traceable from the sinus to the outside.

In one case the canals were fully two centimeters apart, and both appeared above the digastric groove, being due to two separate veins leaving the lateral sinus.

When the foramen divides within the diplöe to emerge as two canals, one finds them emerging almost parallel. In a few cases, the canal is directed straight out from the lateral sinus, and the distance between the lateral sinus and the external surface of the bone is no greater than the thickness of the bone.

Cheatle, 1906, in discussing the size of the canal described it as being as "big as a pencil" in some cases, and so small that it would not admit a pin in others. Myer, 1913, reported an abnormally large unilateral foramen mastoideum with a diameter of 6 mm. on the inner surface, and a sulcus emissarium on the exterior with an oval mouth with a long diameter of 8 mm. In the 1500 adult temporal bones examined I found none with an abnormally large canal, thus indicating that large canals are very uncommon.

TABLE IV.

| | No. | Per Cent. |
|---|---|---|
| Absence of emissary canal | 68 | 27 |
| Single emissary canal | 167 | 67 |
| Bifurcating emissary canals | 11 | 4.4 |
| Double canals | 4 | 1.6 |
| Total | 250 | 100 |

V.—THE PROCESSES IN THE MASTOID REGION.

The pars mastoidea, which forms the posterior part of the temporal bone, is continued below into a conical projection, the mastoid process, the size and form of which varies somewhat and which is said to be larger in the male than in the female. The mastoid process is relatively small at birth and contains no air cells except at the antrum. It becomes distinct about the first year, coincident with the obliteration of the petrosquamous suture. The suture is frequently found not wholly fused in the adult temporal bone. Toward puberty the process becomes pneumatic. This process, which serves for the attachment of the sternocleidomastoideus, splenius capitis and the longissimus capitis muscles, is sometimes divided by a deep groove, the digastric, for the attachment of the posterior belly of the digastricus. Just medial to this groove is a small shallow furrow which lodges the occipital artery.

So much diversity of opinion exists among authorities as to the correct names of the processes of the mastoid region that one is hardly safe in describing this region without first referring to matters of terminology. Gray, 1905' edition, makes no reference to paramastoid or paroccipital processes in man, but in the edition revised by Lewis, 1913, the paramastoid is described in connection with the occipital bone, as an eminence which sometimes projects downwards from the rough under surface of the jugular process, where the rectus capitis lateralis muscle and the lateral atlantooccipital ligament are attached. It is stated that this eminence may be of sufficient length to reach and articulate with the transverse process of the atlas. The last edition of Gray does not mention the par-occipital process, and neither Piersol, 1907, nor Allen, 1884, describe either process. Morris, 1899, says that a process of bone projects rarely from the under surface of the quadrilateral shaped jugular process "homologous to the par-occipital process present in many animals." Thomson, 1917, also described a rough or smooth elevated surface, or else a projecting process springing from the under surface of the extremity of the jugular process, the extremity of which may articulate with the transverse process of the atlas. When this process is met with, he terms it paramastoid or par-occipital. According to Corner, 1896, Macalister, regarded the jugular process and its extension as the paramastoid or par-occipital. Bryce, 1914, described a distinct ridge occurring normally on the medial lip of the groove for the digastric muscle, which may be developed into a process of considerable dimensions and may even be rendered bullous by containing an air cell. This process he calls paramastoid. The term par-occipital is not mentioned in this text.

Corner, 1896, examined 304 mastoid processes and called attention to the existence of a process of the temporal bone on the inner side of the digastric groove which was present in some form in 93 per cent of the specimens he examined. He also found a similar crest, ridge or process present on the temporal bones of 20 monkeys and in the skulls of 3 lemurs. He proposed in the consideration of the constant presence of this process, that the name "par-occipital" should be confined to the downward expansions of the occipital bones, and the name "paramastoid" should be applied to the process at the inner lip of the digastric groove.

Waldeyer, 1909, in discussing processes of this region, wrote that "Der Processus retromastoideus ist diejenige Bildung, welche mich zu einer erneuten Untersuchung der Regio occipitalis und mastoidea des menschlichen Schädels veranlasst hat und den Kernpunkt dieser Abhandlung darstelt." He added that the retromastoid process is "einen meist stumpfen, bald mehr rundlichen, bald mehr länglichen Fortsatz von durchschnittlich 0.5 bis 2 cm. Höhe, der sich an der Stelle des Zusammenstosses des oberen queren Nebenschenkels der Linea nuchæ inferior mit der Linea semicircularis superior entwickelt."

Other processes also have been described in this region. Waldeyer, 1909, stated that von Haferland described a rounded process which develops on both sides from the angulus mastoideus of the parietal and which projects laterally directly above the parietomastoid suture. Von Haferland termed this projection the processus astericus, but Waldeyer preferred the designation tuberculous supramastoideum posterius.

Since the prefix *para* means beside, beyond, accessory to, apart from, and against, the paramastoid process should by definition be near the mastoid process. When one examines this region in a series of temporal bones, one can find the mastoid process with the digastric groove in all degrees of depth —from a mere slight sulcus in cases in which the process shows no indication of division, to that of a deep groove a centimeter or even more in depth, where the process is well divided. This seems to indicate that this process, though frequently divided by a deep grove, is in reality one and the same process developmentally. Hence it would seem that when the process is bifid due to the presence of a deep digastric groove, the outer portion should preferably be called the lateral and the other the medial portion of the mastoid process. And in cases where there are two grooves, as described later, the terms lateral, intermediate and medial could be used.

In Table 5, 500 adult temporal bones showing indications of a mastoid-occipital suture are classified with reference to the appearance of the medial portion of the mastoid process. The lateral portion of the mastoid process is present in all. Specimen 32 has a definite retromastoid process, and in three others it was indicated. In 37 cases two grooves were observed, one the digastric and the other the occipital, thus splitting the mastoid process into three portions with the presence of an intervening ridge or tubercle.

It is stated that in rare cases the extremity of this process may articulate with the transverse process of the atlas. The corresponding atlas is not present in our collection, but the length of the jugular process is such that this could well have been the case in this specimen, although its character suggests that this was not so.

The triplicate condition or that in which the medial portion of the mastoid process is divided, may be confined entirely to the temporal bone; or as in Figure 7, it may be more extensive, occupying the adjacent lateral portion of the occipital. In this particular case the medial portion of the mastoid process exists as two marked ridges. The jugular process articulated with a superior articular process of the atlas obliterating the jugular notch entirely, the condyloid and jugular processes being continuous.

Fig. 8 shows an abnormally large jugular process, more than .1 cm. in length, extending from the quadrilateral shaped space on the under surface of the occiptal bone. This process has been described by Thomson, 1917, and by others.

Other conditions within the process also may be of unusual interest. Fig. 9 shows a single large mastoid cell, more than 1 cm. in diameter, occupying the medial portion of the mastoid process, while another cell, Fig. 10, same specimen, occupies the entire lateral portion of the process. This latter cell was 1½ cm. in length, 1 cm. wide and 1 cm. in depth.

## TABLE V.

Character of the portion of the mastoid process medial to the digastric groove in 500 specimens:

| | | |
|---|---|---|
| Ill defined or absent | 118 | 23.6% |
| Bullous | 69 | 13.8% |
| Short crest | 79 | 15.8% |
| Long crest | 107 | 21.4% |
| Rough irregular prominence | 21 | 4.2% |
| Tubercle | 65 | 13. % |
| Divided (by occipital groove) | 37 | 7.4% |
| Retromastoid process (1 definite, 3 indicated) | 4 | 0.8% |
| Total | 500 | 100. % |

### THE OSSEOUS EXTERNAL ACOUSTIC MEATUS.

Of all the variable features of the normal temporal bone, the osseus meatus reveals the greatest number. One finds so many grades of variations in the size and contour that the determination of the normal form is quite difficult. Harrison Allen, 1884, in describing the relationship of the tympanic ring to the antrum, stated that "the curve of the U is much roughened and produced downwards." In Morris, 1899, it is stated that the external auditory meatus assumes the form of an elliptical bony tube. Toldt, 1908, depicted as typical an antrum nearly circular in outline. Cheattle, 1906, who wrote extensively on various aspects of the temporal bone, did not describe the form of the antrum. Thomson, 1917; in Robinson's Revision of Cunningham's Anatomy, fifth edition, described the meatus as oval in form with its long axis almost vertical near the orifice. Neither Piersol, 1907, nor Bryce, 1915, mention its form.

The specimens examined by me include all the above forms —from those almost round in appearance to those of an extremely oval type. The round forms are of various sizes, some measuring no more than 0.5 cm. in diameter at the orifice, although the maximum diameter at this point was 1.5 cm., a variation in size of 300 per cent. From the round form the picture changes by degrees to that of a decided oval. All gradations in form can be seen, even if one observes only a relatively small number of bones. The shortest diameter of an oval form was 0.5 cm., and the longest, a little less than 2.0 cm. Between these figures one can find all possible forms and dimensions.

Oval forms were observed extending in a vertical plane. practically parallel to the styloid process. The opposite condition with the long axis in a horizontal plane and almost at angles to the styloid also was observed. Specimen 126, Fig. 4, illustrates the former condition, with the string over the long axis, and specimen 24, Fig. 5, approaches the opposite form. The intermediate form, which is the more common condition. is seen in Fig. 1, specimen 149. No form was observed in which the superior margin of an oval orifice lay posterior to a line drawn vertically through the center of the orifice of the meatus.

The size of an orifice may be greatly modified by exostoses. Cheattle, 1913, said that these always occur on the tympanic portion of the bone. Welcker, 1864, was one of the earliest anatomists to describe this form of exostosis. He found it far more common in skulls from American Indians than in any other race. Although exostosis had been observed by otologists in Europe at that time, their presence was regarded as quite rare. According to Welcker, 1864, who described three exostoses of the tympanic portion of the ring, Seligman had noted their presence in five out of six temporal bones from South American Indians.

An exostosis of the tympanic portion of the antrum may develop to a state of almost total occlusion of the meatus. as is seen in the accompanying photographs. Figs. 11 and 12. of an Indian skull found on Blaylock's Island, Columbia River, near Umatilla, Oregon. In the left meatus, Fig. 11, the extremities of the superior margin of the ring have become so thickened that they almost touch. Fig. 12 of the right meatus, shows a third somewhat smaller exostosis appearing at the inferior border of the ring, midway between two marginal thickenings. It is very doubtful whether a patent canal was present during life, for it probably was completely occluded by the exostoses with the overlying soft parts.

The failure of otologists and anatomists in general to record these exostoses would indicate that they are quite rare. Yet specimen 100, Fig. 13, has an exostosis present on the posterior margin—the anterior being normal. This, too, came from an Indian. But on looking over 75 more Indian skulls I failed to find another specimen with exostoses at these points.

Another structure which tends to diminish the size of the orifice is the postauditory tubercle which develops downwards from the superior margin of the external auditory orifice and may reach a goodly size. Although frequently absent, it may be modified and project outwards and downwards as a shelf or laminum. Specimen 1228, Fig. 14, presents such a case. In specimen 331, Fig. 15, this tubercle has a base of almost one centimeter, and is in the form of an equilateral triangle, the apex of which is directed downwards and slightly outwards.

The tympanic portion of the meatus may be generally thickened, even to one-half a centimeter, thus occupying some of the orifice, as the petrous portion is the denser bone of the two and yields least, hence diminishing the size of the orifice.

SOME POINTS IN THE ANATOMY OF THE HUMAN TEMPORAL BONE.

1. The average weight of 100 clean, dry, temporal bones was found to be 41.5 gms. and approximately the same on both sides.

2. The average angle between the superior margin of the petrous portion and the squamosa is 67.2° in the adult and 78° in the infant.

3. The angle between a horizontal and the posterior superior surface of the petrous portion varied between 105 and 125 degrees and coincided with the long diameter of the osseus external acoustic foramen.

4. A mastoid emissary canal was absent in 27 per cent of 250 specimens; was single in 67 per cent and quite variable in direction and number in 6 per cent. The external foramen usually is located above the digastric groove on a level with the upper margin of the osseus external acoustic orifice. Tubercles and exostosis were observed in the meatus.

5. In view of the present confusion in use of the terms paramastoid and par-occipital, it is suggested that we speak

of lateral and medial portions of the mastoid, and also in cases of triplicate division, of an intermediate portion, designating the other paramastoid processes as jugular and retromastoid.

## REFERENCES.

Allen, Harrison: 1884. Human Anatomy, Philadelphia.

Bryce, T. H.: 1914. Osteogoly, Vol. 4, Part 1. Elementary Human Anatomy, Philadelphia. Quain's edition.

Cheattle, Arthur H.: Surgical Anatomy of the Temporal Bone. Hunterian Lectures, 1906.

Corner, E. M.: 1896. "The Processes of the Occipital and Mastoid Regions in the Skull." Journal of Anatomy and Physiol., London, Vol. 30.

Dwight. Thomas: 1907. Osteology, Human Anatomy. Piersol. G. A. Philadelphia.

Gray, Henry: 1899. Human Anatomy, London.

Gurriere and Masetti: Rivista speriment. di Freniatria e de Med. legale, 1895. Quoted after Piersol, Human Anatomy, Philadelphia, 1907.

Meyer, A. W.: Spolia Anatomica. Journal of Anat. and Physiol., Vol. 48, 1913-14.

Morris, Henry: 1899. Human Anatomy, Philadelphia.

Qualn's Anatomy. 1914.

Thomson, Arthur: 1917. Osteology, Human Anatomy. Cunningham, D. J. New York, Edition 5.

Toldt, Carl: 1908. Anatomisher Atlas, Suchste Auflage.

Waldever: 1909. Der Processus retromastoideus. Abh. der Königl. Preuss. Akad. d. Wiss.

Welcher, H.: 1864. "Un'ber knöchern Verengerung und Verschliessung des äussern Gehörganges." Archiv. für Ohrenheilkunde, Vol 1-2.

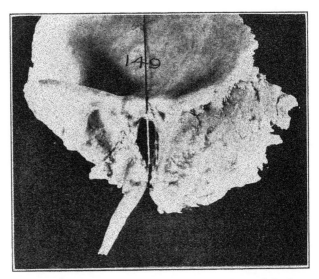

Fig. I.  Specimen 149.  Exemplifying the relation of the long axis
of the external acoustic orifice to the styloid process, the usual
condition.

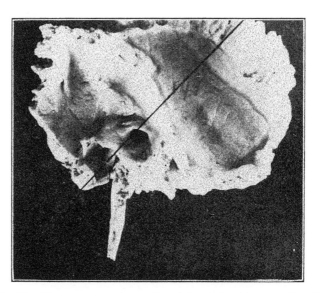

Fig. II. The same specimen, the string indicating the direction of the posterior superior surface of the petrosa, the usual condition.

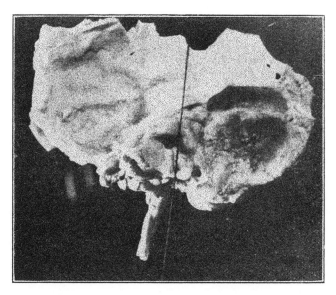

Fig. III. Specimen 126. Showing the direction of the posterior superior surface of petrosa almost parallel to styloid process.

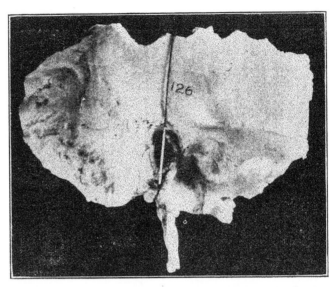

Fig. IV. The same specimen, showing the long axis of external acoustic orifice almost parallel to styloid process.

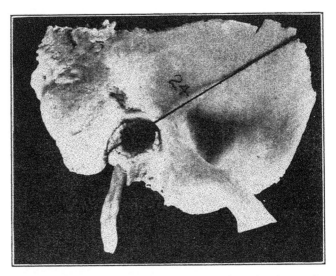

Fiv. V.  Specimen 24.   The long diameter of meatus forms almost
a right angle with styloid process.

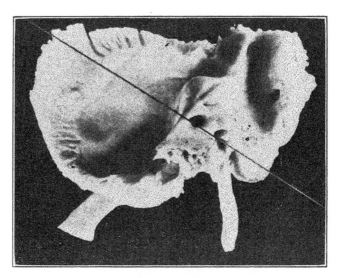

Fig. VI. The line across the posterior superior surface of petrosa forms almost a right angle with styloid process.

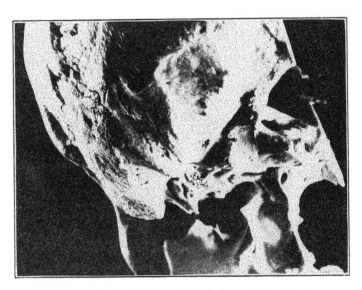

Fig. VII.   Triplicate division of the left mastoid process.

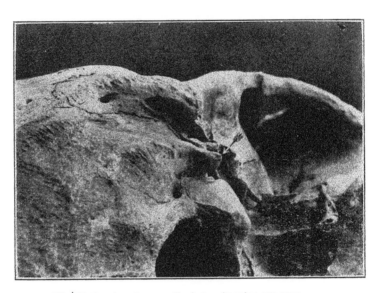

Fig. VIII.   An abnormally large jugular process.

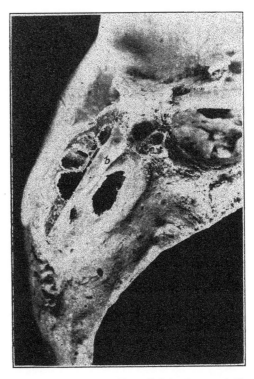

Fig. IX.   A single mastoid cell medial to the mastoid process.

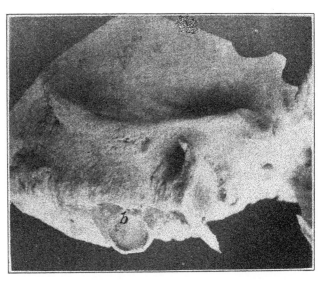

Fig. X.  A single large air cell lateral to the mastoid process.

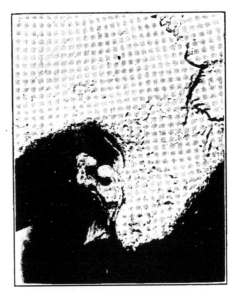

Fig. XI. Marked exostoses of the tympanic element in a left external auditory orifice.

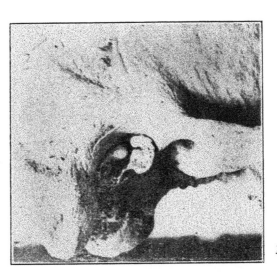

Fig. XII.  Right meatus with three points of exostoses.

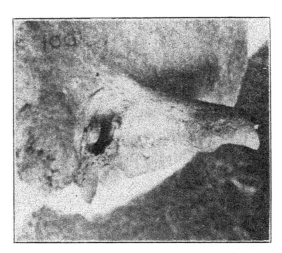

Fig. XIII.   Exostosis of the posterior portion of tympanum.

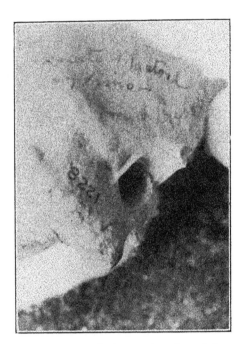

Fig. XIV.  A laminum projecting outwards and downwards from the superior margin of the external auditory orifice.

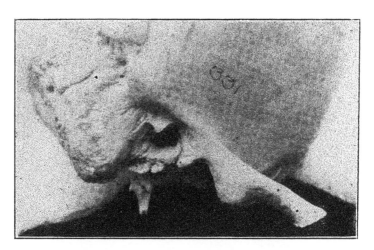

Fig. XV.  A large post-auditory tubercle.

# XVII

# THE ROENTGENOGRAPHIC STUDY OF THE ACCESSORY SINUSES WITH SPECIAL REFERENCE TO THE NEW TECHNIC FOR THE EXAMINATION OF THE SPHENOID SINUSES.*

By George E. Pfahler, M. D.,

Philadelphia.

The accessory sinuses are demonstrable by the Roentgen rays because they contain air and are surrounded by bony walls. They are, therefore, more transparent than the surrounding tissues. By means of the Roentgen rays one can demonstrate their size, outline, position and the condition of the walls and the septa. The sinuses on the two sides of the head can be projected in such manner that they can be used for direct comparison as to their transparency or density. In this connection it must be borne in mind that if the sinus on one side is smaller than that of the opposite side, it is normally less transparent and must, therefore, not be interpreted as being diseased.

Disease of the accessory sinuses may consist of exudate within the cavities, of tumor formation within the cavities, or of any of the bone diseases involving the bony walls. Exudate within the accessory sinuses causes a decrease in transparency. One cannot determine the nature of the exudate by the Roentgen rays, and we must expect mucus, pus or blood to cast similar shadows. If this exudate involves only the sinuses on one side, there will be shown a striking contrast when compared with the opposite side. If both sides are involved, as for example in the case of the maxillary sinuses, one would compare the transparency or opacity with the sphenoids and the frontals above. If all of the sinuses are diseased and filled with exudate, one must consider the opacity of the sinus areas as compared with the detail of structure in the remainder of the skull. In this connection, care must

---

*Read before the Section on Otology and Laryngology of the College of Physicians at its regular meeting March 16, 1921.

be taken that a poor roentgenogram is not interpreted as a general opacity of all of the sinuses.

Absence of one or more of the sinuses will also show a lack of transparency, and this frequently involves both sides, especially in the frontal region. This must not be confused with the diagnosis of total opacity due to exudate, and can be definitely differentiated by a lateral view compared with the frontal views. In practically all instances, even in the posteroanterior view or frontal view of the frontal sinuses, the outline of the sinuses can be demonstrated, even though both sides are totally filled up with exudate.

The great advantage to the rhinologist of a complete examination of the accessory sinuses consists in the accurate information which he can obtain as to the exact size of the sinuses, the location of the septa, and the localization of the exudate. Sometimes this exudate is confined to a definite pocket. Localized pockets of pus within the ethmoids are especially difficult to determine by any other means.

Tumors of the accessory sinuses may be either primary or secondary. If secondary the disease is usually an extension of an epithelioma from surrounding structures. If primary, it is usually some form of sarcoma. In practically all instances there is, in addition to the exudate within the sinus, a destruction or expansion of the walls of the sinus. If of slow growth there may be simply expansion or even increased bone formation such as occurs in the osteomas. When these tumors are malignant there is practically always an actual destruction of the surrounding walls. Most frequently these tumors involve the maxillary sinuses and a pressure inward of the inner wall, a destruction of the outer wall, and very commonly a destruction of the alveolar process may be recognized. Frequently there is invasion backwards into the ethmoid cells.

Disease of the bony walls of the accessory sinuses will present the characteristics peculiar to the nature of the disease, but most frequently it consists of an osteomyelitis either pyogenic or syphilitic. In both these instances there is associated exudate within the sinuses and destruction or sclerosis depending upon the acuteness of the infection and the differentiation of these two conditions must be made by other clinical means.

## TECHNIC.

It is my recommendation and custom to make a complete examination of all the accessory sinuses rather than to attempt to confine the study to one particular group. A more extended study, however, can be made when special information is required concerning one particular group. As a routine I make three posteroanterior views. I prefer to have the patients lying down because they are more liable to keep perfectly still, and absolute stillness is essential. Complete fixation of the head is also essential, for any slight movement disturbs detail. I make three posteroanterior views. First, for the best demonstration of the frontal sinuses, I pass the central ray at an angle of 35 degrees from the plane passing through the glabella and external auditory meatus and directed towards the frontal sinuses. This view demonstrates the lateral and vertical limits of the frontal sinuses best, but also gives some information with regard to the outline of the sphenoids and the upper ethmoid cells. The second view is taken with the central ray passing in a line connecting the external auditory meatus and the external canthus and of course centered over the median line. This demonstrates to the best advantage the vertical and lateral outline of the sphenoids. The third posteroanterior view is taken with the central ray passing immediately below the level of the mastoid processes in the median line and directed toward the maxillary sinuses. This projects the base of the skull above the maxillary sinuses and gives a clearer view, obstructed only by the overlying shadows of the vertebra and the tissues of the neck. It is very important in making the posteroanterior views that the head be perfectly level. That is, the vertical plane passing through the external auditory meati must be parallel to the film. This can be accomplished by means of the head leveler previously described by me.[1]

I then make a lateral view of one or both sides, and these lateral views can be made stereoscopically. Sometimes a stereoscopic view is of advantage, but in general I have gained little from the stereoscopic study of these sinuses. This lateral view will demonstrate the depth of the frontal sinuses and the thickness of their walls together with any modification

in their normal transparency. The condition of the bony walls
can be ascertained, especially the frontal sinuses, and also of
all of the other sinuses. This lateral view also shows the vertical and anteroposterior dimensions of the sphenoid sinuses,
but it does not permit a differentiation of one from the other.
At times, when the two are not of uniform size and one is
opaque, this latter can be recognized because of the projection
of a clear space surrounding it made by the clear and larger
sphenoid sinus. In this lateral view one is able to study the
outline of the maxillary sinus in its vertical and anteroposterior
dimensions, but since one is superimposed upon the other, little
differentiating value is obtained. This lateral view also gives
considerable information as to disease in the ethmoids, but
because they are superimposed upon one another the disease
on one side or the other cannot be differentiated. In addition
to these views, the sphenoids may be studied by oblique views
by which the shadow of the sphenoids are projected alternately
into the orbital space, first on one side and then on the other,
as previously described by me.[2] One can also study with advantage the maxillary sinuses obliquely, this study being especially desirable when there is suspicion of infection from the
teeth or when there is disease of the walls of the sinuses. This
has also been previously described by me.[3]

### NEW TECHNIC FOR THE VERTICAL EXAMINATION OF THE SPHENOIDS AND MASTOIDS.

Much difficulty and dissatisfaction has been encountered in
the demonstration of the sphenoids and ethmoids by vertical
view; that is, in the demonstration of the horizontal plane of
these sinuses, so as to project them side by side in horizontal
section. Heretofore it has been necessary to project the outlines of these sinuses through the vertex of the skull or downward within the submaxillary space and below the tissue of
the neck. In either instance the position of the sinuses is so
far away from the photographic film that there is much distortion and great want of definite detail. With the object of
bringing the films nearer to the sphenoid and ethmoid cells
to be photographed I have devised a method of placing a special film into the mouth, pushing it backward firmly against
the pharynx. This gives a definite level for the projection of

the outlines of these sinuses and eliminates mo.t of the irregular extraneous shadows of overlying bones.  One has then
above this film only the base of the skull and in this small area
one practically obtains only the outlines of the sphenoid sinuses
and the ethmoid cells surrounded by a border of teeth in the
upper jaw.  A preliminary report on this method of study was
made by me before the American Roentgen Ray Society in
discussion.[4]

Many difficulties have been involved in this procedure.  In
the first place it is necessary to cut the films to the exact size
and shape that will fit the average mouth and pharynx.  I
obtained this first by finding a size that would best fit my own
mouth and which I could hold in position comfortably when
pushed entirely against the posterior wall of the pharynx.
This size is 2 by 3 inches.  It is square at one end and curved
at the end which is pushed against the pharynx  I then found
great annoyance from the secondary radiation of the tissues
about the mouth, which caused a great deal of fog.  This was
partially overcome, even as early as 1915, by the use of metal
placed underneath the film, yet there was still much disturbance from the secondary radiations of the tissues of the head
because it was necessary to use, as in all vertical examinations,
a comparatively hard ray.  More recently I have overcome
this by using double screens, which I have cut to exactly fit
this special film.  The double screens are attached by means
of a hinge, the lower one being attached to a layer of brass.
Special black paper envelopes are made to fit these holders
and they are rendered waterproof by covering them with rubber.  This double screen technic permits the use of much
softer radiation, which gives rise to less scattered rays.  Fig. 1.

This examination is made with the patient in the sitting posture (Fig. 2).  The chin is rested upon the headrest.  The film
is then pushed back into the mouth against the pharynx and
held in place by the teeth.  The distance from the target to the
top of the head is 18 inches, using a 3 inch cylinder, and a
vacuum corresponding to a 4 inch parallel spark gap, and an
exposure of approximately 8 seconds, with 30 milliamperes
of current.

By this technic we can now demonstrate clearly the outline
and size of these sphenoid sinuses projected side by side, and

this gives the operating surgeon a definite idea as to the position of the septum, for in many instances the septum is distinctly to the right or the left of the median line. By this process one can also demonstrate a horizontal projection, or in horizontal section, the ethmoid cells. At times large ethmoid cells in the region of the sphenoids are involved by exudate which, by all other means, leads one to suspect disease of the sphenoids. With the definite demonstration of the location of exudate by this means, or even the demonstration that these various cells are normal, I am sure that a great advance can be made in the study and treatment of the diseases of the posterior accessory sinuses. On account of illness since developing this technic, I have not made this study as extensive as I propose to do, but I have already been greatly surprised at the great variations in the outlines of the sphenoid sinuses as well as the great variation in the size and outline of some of these posterior ethmoid cells. It is rare that the two sphenoid sinuses are of equal size, and it is very common to find the septum on one or the other side of the median line. This technic, combined with the posteroanterior and the lateral views, permits one to make a very exact and definite demonstration of the sphenoid sinuses in every plane and in every direction, and surely such exact information must be of distinct value to the clinician.

REFERENCES.

1. Head Leveler for the Study of the Pituitary Fossa and the Accessory Sinuses. American Journal of Roentgenology, April. 1917, Vol. IV No. 4.

2. The Roentgen Rays as an Aid to the Diagnosis of Diseases of Sphenoid Sinus. Annals of Otology, Rhinology and Laryngology, December, 1912.

(3) Die isolierte Aufnahme einer Oberkieferhälfte und die isolierte Aufnahme des Processus styloideus. Fortschritte auf dem Gebiete der Róntgenstrahlen, Band XVII, p. 369-371, Jour. Am. Med. Ass., February 8, 1908.

(4) The Annual Meeting of the American Roentgen Ray Society. Chicago, Ill., September 27-30, 1916. The American Journal of Roentgenology, Vol. IV, p. 411.

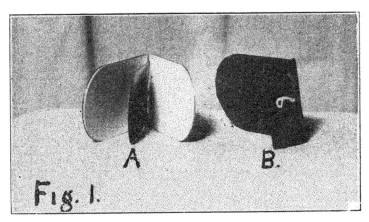

Fig. 1. (a) Shows double screen with film standing between. (b) Black envelope for holding the screen. This must then be covered with rubber or other material to keep the film dry.

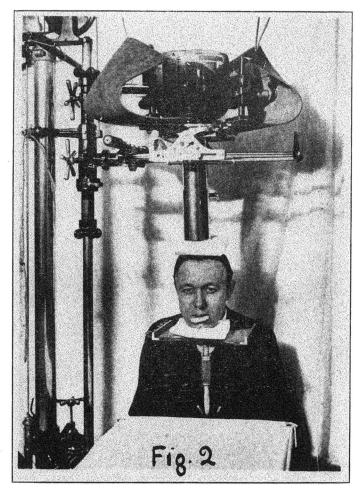

Fig. 2. Film and double screen in position in the patient's mouth, showing the position for making the Roentgenogram.

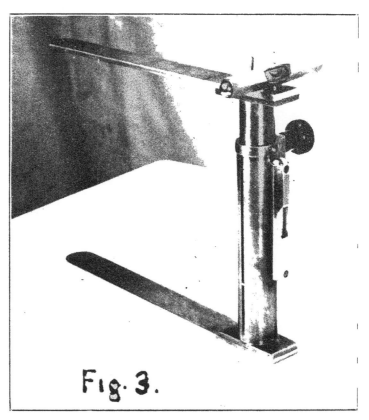

Fig. 3.

Fig. 3. Leveler for getting the position of the head in sinus work, the ends of these arms to be inserted against the small concha of the ears.

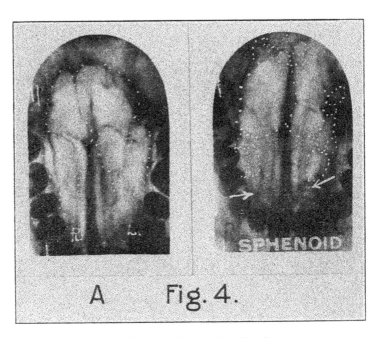

Fig. 4.  (a)  Normal sphenoid and ethmoid cells.
(b)  Normal sphenoid and posterior ethmoid cells. with exudate
in the anterior ethmoid cells.

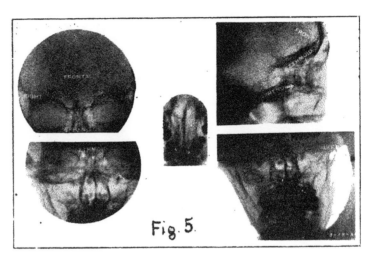

Fig. 5. Showing a complete set of sinus films and demonstrating exudate in the anterior ethmoid cells.

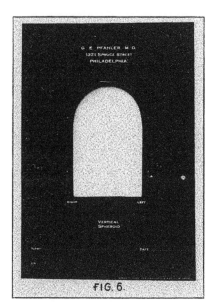

Fig. 6.   Cardboard mount specially designed to hold the vertical sphenoid film.

## XVIII.

## SOME EXPERIMENTS TO SHOW THE FLOW OF FLUID FROM THE REGION OF THE TEGMEN TYMPANI, EXTRADURAL TO AND MEDIAL TO THE PASSAGE OF THE SIXTH CRANIAL NERVE THROUGH THE DURA MATER TO THE LATERAL WALL OF THE CAVERNOUS SINUS.

By H. J. Prentiss, M. D.,

Iowa City, Iowa.

The reason for this study followed an inquiry from Doctor Cobb of Marshalltown, Iowa. He stated that he had an involvement of the external rectus following a mastoid operation and went into some detail regarding the case. The actual work of this experiment was carried on by Doctor I. N. Crow, who has had large experience in this department, both as an instructor and as a graduate student.

. I present photographs of a head showing the flow of a colored fluid from the region of the tegmen tympani to the dorsum epiphii. Photograph I is a picture of the floor of the brain box with the dura intact. Owing to the light reflections, the shadow of the india ink in the middle cerebral fossa is not as plainly shown as over the dorsum epiphii, remembering that the glistening dura was between the fluid and the camera. Nevertheless the shadow is quite plainly seen in the right cerebral fossa and very plainly in the region of the dorsum epiphii. Photograph II is a picture of the same head showing the lines of incision through the dura. Photograph III is a photograph of the same head with the dura lifted away, exposing the india ink directly. The injections were made before the calvarium had been removed. Therefore the brain was in contact with the dura as in life. A complete evisceration of the mastoid cells was made exposing the tegmen: a small opening was then made in this roof, but not injuring the dura. A graduated syringe was inserted in this opening, and seven cc. of india ink injected. The calvarium and brain were then removed with the results as shown by the photographs. We notice in a general way that the fluid circulated medially, reached the cavernous sinus and flooded the dorsum epiphii. Lateral to the foramen spinosum and the course of the middle meningeal artery, the fluid lifted up the dura periosteal membrane broadly. It was limited posteriorly by the course of the large superficial petrosal nerve, from the hiatus Fallopii and along the groove leading to the middle lacerated foramen. The fluid passed medially over and under the Gasserian ganglion, but outside the periganglionic connective tissue sheath. The fluid continued its course medially until it reached the cavernous sinus and was then directed backward through the isthmus between the apex of the petrosa and the posterior clinoid process, thus reaching the dorsum epiphii, where it diffused between the dura and the periosteum. Here it was continuous with the injection from the other side. At the isthmus the sixth nerve grooves the lateral edge of the dorsum epiphii, and is iot not conceivable that direct pressure on this nerve in this notch may cause impairment of its function?

We experimented upon twelve specimens and succeeded in four in getting the above results.

February 28, 1921.

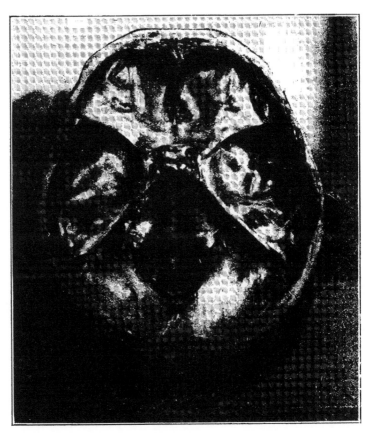

Fig. 1.

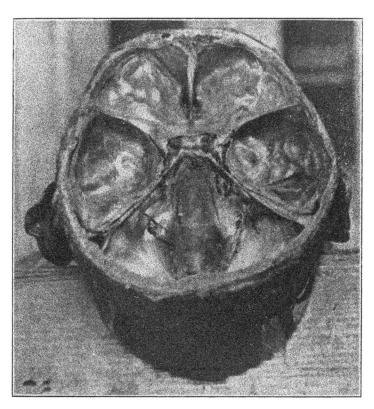

Fig. 2.

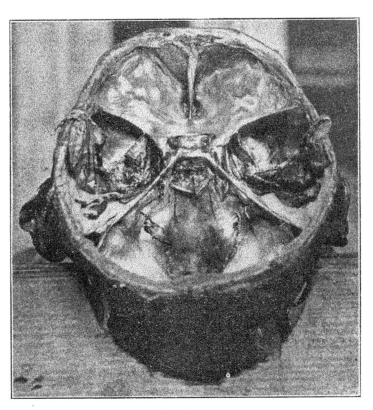

Fig. 3.

# FOSSA OF ROSENMUELLER.

By H. J. Prentiss, M. D.,

Iowa City, Iowa.

The head specialists are so boldly exploring the remote regions of their specialty that it occurs to the writer some observations on the anatomy of the fossa of Rosenmueller may be helpful. The texts are curiously obscure, and though some have excellent illustrations of this region, yet the descriptive discussion is far from satisfactory.

The fossa of Rosenmueller is a lateral extension of the nasopharynx, dorsal to the Eustachian tube and the levator palati. It would seem to be a part of the first visceral pouch, the other part being the Eustachian tube, carried into the expanded middle ear. The nasopharynx is described as hourglass in shape, being expanded above at the base of the skull, contracted at the attachment to the dorsal edge of the internal pterygoid plate, and then expanding into the oral pharynx by its attachment to the inner surface of the mandible at the posterior limit of the mylohyoid ridge. Fig. I shows a posterior view of one-half of the pharynx suspended from the skull. The skull is markedly flexed or depressed. The left side illustrates the bony structure, the dotted line presenting the pharyngeal attachments. We know that the musculature of the pharynx is applied over a very powerful submucosa called the pharyngeal aponeurosis. Of course, where the pharynx ceases ventrally, this aponeurosis ends, the mucosa only being continued into the nasal, oral and laryngeal cavities.

What are the attachments of this aponeurosis? Beginning in the median line, on the basilar process of the occipital bone, is the middle pharyngeal spine to which is attached the pharyngeal raphe. From this point the pharyngeal aponeurosis swings laterally and somewhat posteriorly over the rough quadrilateral surface on the under surface of the petrous portion of the temporal bone, to attach to the lateral pharyngeal spine. This name is given to the inner and anterior limit of the tympanic plate or annulus of the temporal bone, which is quite massive at this place and overhangs the pharyngeal crest which runs from this point to the apex of the petrous bone. Figs I, II, III. The pharyngeal crest divides the under surface of the petrosa into two unequal parts. The anterior and smaller surface or tubal surface helps support the Eustachian tube. The posterior surface presents the eleven points of interest so well known or unknown. This pharyngeal crest runs from the lateral pharyngeal spine to the apex of the bone and continues into the inner plate of the pterygoid process, medial to the scaphoid fossa. Fig. II. Along this crest the delicate mucosa of the pharynx attaches, separating the fossa of Rosenmueller from the tube and beneath from the levator palati. These two structures are entering the pharynx above the sinus of Morgagni, and where, therefore, the pharyngeal aponeurosis ceases as such. Figs. II, IV, V.

Leaving this crest the mucosa passes directly to the inner pterygoid plate, down this plate to its hamular process, and from there swings laterally to the inner surface of the mandible, along the pterygomandibular raphe. At the mandible it attaches by a small attachment at the posterior limit of the mylohyoid ridge. Fig. 1. The superior constrictor muscle does not follow the pharyngeal mucosa to the lateral pharyngeal spine, but swings forward beneath the fossa of Rosenmueller to attach to the lower half of the internal pterygoid plate, as a rule. Fig. I.

Viewing the pharynx from behind, one observes how the nasopharynx swings around the internal pterygoid muscle in reaching its attachments. Fig. I.

Due to this definite lateral attachment of the fossa of Rosenmueller, the foramen ovale for the passage of the inferior division of the fifth cranial nerve is anterior, being separated only by the eustachian tube. The carotid foramen for the internal carotid artery is directly behind this lateral attachment with nothing intervening. Fig. 1, II.

Summary.—The fossa of Rosenmueller is a contracted cone (contracted ventrodorsally). Its apex reaches to the lateral pharyngeal spine. Its base opens into the general cavity of the nasopharynx. Its anterior wall is a delicate mucosa covering the eustachian tube and levator palati. Its posterior wall is the mucosa covering the dense pharyngeal aponeurosis. At its apex, in front is the inferior maxillary division of the fifth

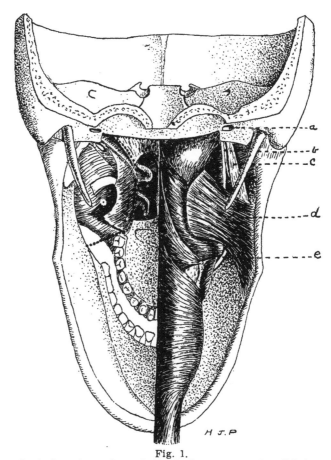

Fig. 1.
Posterior view of one-half of pharynx.  a—Carotid foramen.
b—Third division of fifth cranial nerve.  c—Spheno-mandibular ligament.  d—Internal pterygoid muscle.  e—Lingual nerve wrapping
around attachment of pharynx mandible.

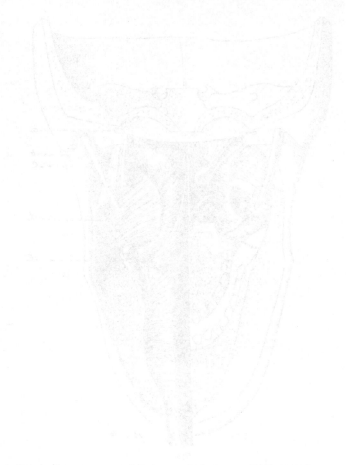

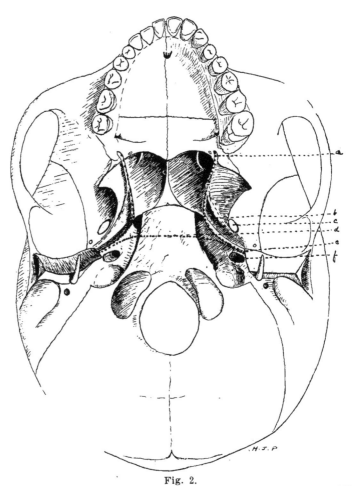

Fig. 2.

To show naso-pharyngeal attachments. a—Hamular process.
b—Scaphoid fossa. c—For. ovali. d—Medial pharyngeal spine.
e—Lateral pharyn. spine. f—Carotid foramen.

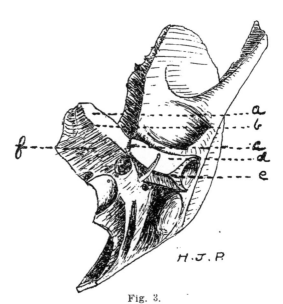

Fig. 3.

Under surface of temporal bone to show lateral pharyngeal
spine and pharyngeal crest. a—Tubal surface. b—Pharyngeal
crest. c—Lateral pharnygeal spine. d—Annulus or tympanic plate.
e—Vaginal process. f—Rough quadrilateral posterior surface.

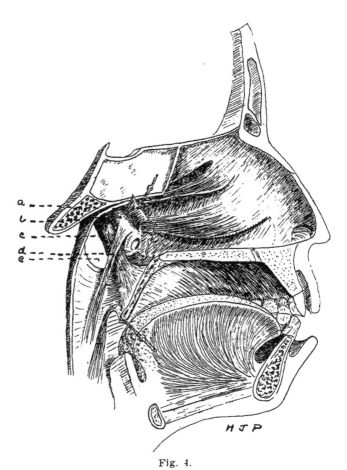

Fig. 4.

Fig. 4. To show the eustachian tube and lev. palati in anterior wall of fossa of Rosenmueller. Mucosa removed. a—Reflected mucosa. b—Eust. tube. c—Lev. palati. d—Salpingo-pharyngeus muscle. e—Sinus of morgani.

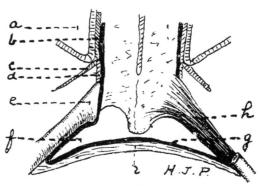

Fig. 5.

Fig. 5. View from above, diagramatically showing fossa of
Rosenmueller. Right side—Eustachian tube removed to show lev.
palati beneath. a—Antrum. b—Vert. plate of palate bone. c—Ex.
pterygoid plate. d—Internal pterygoid plate. e—Eustachian tube.
f—Fossa of Rosenmueller. g—Mucosa. h—Lev. palati. i—Pharyngeal aponeurisis.

# XX.

# SOME OBSERVATIONS ON THE MASTOID PROCESS AND ITS CELLS.

By H. J. Prentiss, M. D.,

Iowa City, Iowa.

The various texts call attention to the presence of small cells in the apex of the mastoid process of the temporal bone and small cells at the base. The department of anatomy in the University of Iowa finds a goodly number show large cells toward the apex and small cells in the region of the triangle of election or Macewen's triangle. (Fig. 1).

A study of this quite common variation from the text has led to a study of the reason for this variation in the two types of cells. As the result of these findings we believe that the point should be emphasized that the mastoid process is a petro-squamo-mastoid process and not a petro-mastoid process.

Referring to Figures 2, 3, 4, 5 and 6A and B, we observe sketches of temporal bones or parts of these bones at term. Fig. 2 is a lateral view of the entire bone. Note that the squamosa extends well down, posterior to the external auditory canal. Fig. 3 shows the squamosa removed, leaving the petrosa. Note that the dependent portion of the squamosa closes in the lateral side of the mastoid antrum, forming therefore its lateral wall in the complete bone. The roof, floor and medial wall is formed by the petrosa. Fig. 6A.

Fig. 4 shows the lateral view of the squamosa and annulus. Fig. 5 shows a medial view of the same two bones. Note how this view indicates that the squamosa has two tables which separate in the region of the antrum and attic, leaving the single outer table as the lateral wall of the antrum and attic. This inner table at the place of separation articulates with the tegmen tympani and the outer table, at a lower level, with the petrosa, in the region of the antrum and with the drum membrane in the region of the epitympanic recess. (Figs. 6A and B). Fig. 6A is a schematic vertical section through the antrum at term, and Fig. 6B, through the drum membrane.

With the great lateral growth of the brain, after birth, the squamosa develops a horizontal portion, there being only a vertical portion at term. This horizontal portion develops into the eminentia articularis, glenoid fossa, roof of the external auricular canal, besides the mass of cells leading from the lateral wall of the antrum. (Figures 7D and C). Fig. 8 is one of a series. A vertical section was made through the external auricular canal, not injuring, therefore, the posterior wall of this canal and also exposing the antrum. The lateral wall of the antrum was painted with a wax, making it impervious to fluids. Pouring a colored fluid into the antrum, the apical cells were invaded, but not the lateral cells. Removing this wax, thus opening into these lateral cells, and then painting the remaining walls with a melted wax, on pouring into the antrum a differently colored fluid, the lateral cells were invaded, but not the apical cells. After these injections were made, the cortex was ground away with the resulting picture of the two sets of cells. Fig. 8.

In a certain number of specimens this sharp differentiation was not obtained, the two fluids mingling. That a few specimens showed this sharp differentiation indicates that there is a tendency for a persistence of this separation in the adult bone. The clinical men note that apical cells may be involved, and not basal cells, and vice versa.

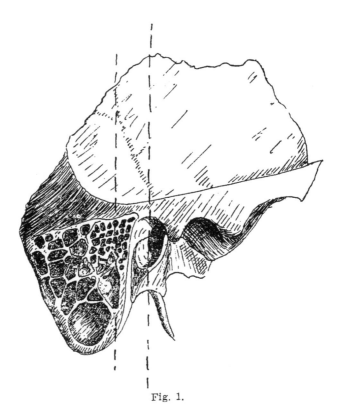

Fig. 1.

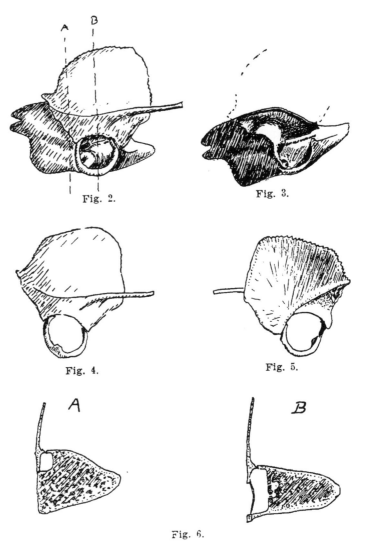

Fig. 2.

Fig. 3.

Fig. 4.

Fig. 5.

Fig. 6.

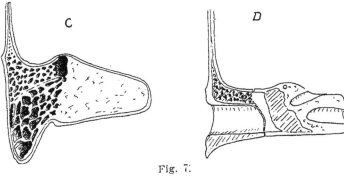

*C*       *D*

Fig. 7.

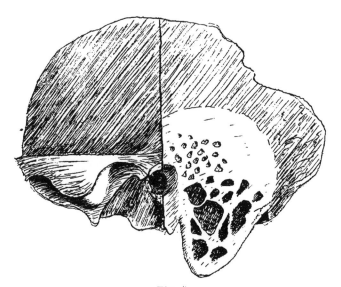

Fig. 8.

## XXI.

## FURTHER REPORT ON THE USE OF RADIUM, THE X-RAY AND OTHER NONSURGICAL MEASURES, COMBINED WITH OPERATIONS ABOUT THE HEAD AND NECK.*

By Joseph C. Beck, M. D.,

Chicago.

In presenting for your consideration the material with which I have busied myself for the past twenty years or more, in other words, since X-rays, radium and other similar modes of treatment have been in vogue, I am hoping to elicit a discussion so that I may learn more.

While I am sure that I shall not be able to bring out anything new or original, I do know that I am presenting a fair amount of material, most of which is malignant disease. and unfortunately accompanied by an enormous mortality. I am further cognizant of the fact that my report is accurate although pessimistic as to the ultimate results. If reporters on malignant disease will carry out this plan they will go a long way towards progress and assist that grand society, organized principally for control of cancer.

It is only by following up our cases and repeatedly making reports upon them that any sort of statistics can be prepared.

In order to save the reader looking up my previous papers, I wish to state that in 1904 I reported on the "Use of X-ray and Radium in Cancer About the Nose, Throat and Ear" (1) with negative results. In 1907 I reported on "X-ray, Radium and Fulguration in Malignant Disease of the Nose, Throat and Ear" (2). In this report I found no result—that is, cures from these remedial agents. In 1912 I reported on the "Use of Autolytic Solution in Combination of Operations and X-ray in Cancer of the Head and Neck" (3), with encourag-

*Read before the College of Physicians and Surgeons. Philadelphia. Also Middle Section of the American Laryngological, Rhinological and Otological Association, Cincinnati, February, 1920.

ing results in a limited number of cases.  Subsequent application of this treatment (autolytic solutions of cancer) in a large group of carcinoma cases proved it to be of no specific value.

In 1914, I reported on "Carcinoma of the Larynx With Special Reference to Radium Therapy" (4), in which one case was described in detail.  Extensive study was reported upon the microscopic changes of the carcinoma by the use of radium; no startling results were reported in this paper, nor any cure of extensive carcinoma.

In the same year (1914) I reviewed the entire literature for the last twenty years, of "Nonoperable Methods of Treatment of Inoperable Malignant Disease" (5), and showed in the conclusions that authentically no cures had been reported from any of these procedures, but that X-rays, radium and allied agents and chemical substances, like the colloidal, copper, silver, etc., also eosin compounds, promised results.

In 1917, I presented "Experience With Suspension Laryngoscopy in Over Two Hundred Cases, With Report" (6), in which I cited a most encouraging case of carcinoma of the larynx that apparently was cured by surgical procedure, carried out through the intralaryngeal raute, by suspension laryngoscopy, and the employment of deep X-ray therapy, both before and after operation.  As will be shown later, I was too hopeful in this case.

In the same year I presented two papers entitled "Further Report on the Treatment of Malignant Disease of the Larynx" (7) and "Management and Statistics of Malignant Disease of the Upper Respiratory Tract" (8).  These papers were profusely illustrated, especially with case reports, many of which are again presented in this paper, because at that time many had just been operated upon, whereas I report on their subsequent course now.

The region to which I confine my treatment is the head and neck, which comprises ophthalmologic, otolaryngologic, stomatologic, oral and general surgery, as well as the dermatologic field.  The pathologic conditions that I have treated are:

1. Carcinoma, epithelioma and adenocarcinoma.
2. Sarcoma.
3. Endothelioma.

4. Papilloma.
5. Angioma.
6. Lymphangioma.
7. Fibromyxoma.
8. Neuroma.
9. Chloroma.
10. Fibroma.
11. Adenoma.
12. Lymphoma.
13. Lypoma.
14. Cystoma.
15. Epulis.
16. Osteoma.
17. Verruca.
18. Rhinophima.
19. Leucoplakia.
20. Paraphinoma.
21. Syphiloma.
22. Keloid.
23. Tuberculoma.
24. Exostosis and osteitis.
25. Hematoma.
26. Abscess.

The forms of treatment employed were:
1. Surgical.
2. X-ray (surface and deep).
3. Radium (surface and deep).
4. Surgical diathermia.
5. Cautery (sprays and galvano- and electrolysis and ionization).
6. Lysins and chemotherapy.

To bring out details in the management of these various pathologic conditions, I have decided to pass in review some of the cases which I have treated and observed, selecting one case of each type, stating the history in the briefest possible manner, omitting the reports of negative findings or laboratory tests, as for instance, Wassermann, etc. (some of the conditions cannot be presented in illustrations because nothing showed externally). In the conclusion of your discussion, I will be pleased to answer any question which may have been omitted in the presentation.

Case 1 (Fig. 1).—Male, age 53 years. Clinical diagnosis: Epithelioma of right lower lid. Applied 50 mg. of radium

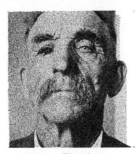

Fig. 1.

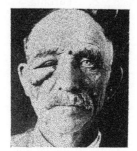

Fig. 2.

element screened by 1/10 mm. of aluminum, this for eight hours.

The following morning I excised the growth wide of the involvement and immediately performed a plastic (pedicle method) operation for reconstruction of the lid. (Fig. 2.) Two weeks later I rearranged the flap to make a better cos-

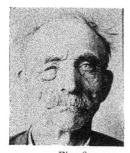

Fig. 3.

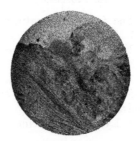

Fig. 4.

metic effect. (Fig. 3.) The microscopic examination of the mass removed showed a distinct epithelioma and areas can be made out of changes due to the radium application.

Case 2 (Fig. 4).—Male, age 48 years. Clinical diagnosis: Epithelioma of the inner canthus and lower lid, side of nose and face on left side. This I removed surgically wide of its point of involvement. After the wound was healed and observed for a short time a recurrence was found about the nasal margins. Fifty mg. of radium pure was applied, screened by 1.4 mm. of aluminum for six hours, once a week

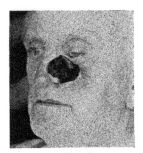

Fig. 5.

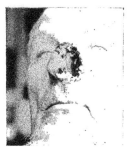

Fig. 6.

for five weeks. (Fig. 5.)    Three months later, no recurrence.

Case 3 (Fig. 6).—Man, aged 67. Diagnosis, clinically and microscopically: Epithelioma of dorsum, left side of nose as far as the upper lip. Spontaneous ulceration. Fifty mg. radium pure, screened by 1/10 mm. of aluminum applied for

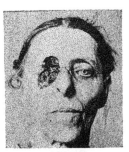

Fig. 7.

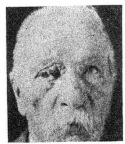

Fig. 8.

four hours, at different portions of the involved surfaces. Each surface received from three to eight applications of the same amount of radium. After one and one-half years he was finally declared well. It is now over one year, and there has been no recurrence.

Case 4.—Female, age 46 years. Epithelioma of the lids,

secondary involvement of eye and orbital tissue of right side. Attending ophthalmologist was compelled to exenter- ate the orbit and remove both lids. The growth recurred. I applied 150 mg. of radium pure, screened by 1/10 mm. of

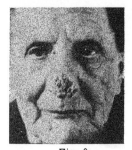

Fig. 9.

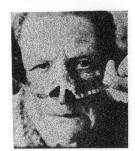

Fig. 10.

aluminum all over the cavity and margins for ten hours. Two months later all evidences of epitheliomatous structure was gone from the orbital cavity, but on two points at the inner canthus there was still evidence of suspected growth. (Fig. 7.) Fifty mg. of radium pure, screened by 1/10 mm. of alumi- num, was applied for six hours. (Patient returned to her

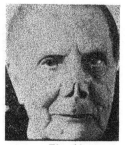

Fig. 11.

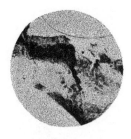

Rig. 12.

home and I have not seen her since.) Subsequent use of par- tial mask in Cases 2, 3 and 4, to replace the defects, is prefera- ble to plastic operations for these old people.

Case 5 (Fig. 8).—Male, age 61. Microscopic and clinical diagnosis: Epithelioma of right inner canthus. Two erythema doses of X-ray treatment given within a period of nine weeks.

Not alone did the growth fail to diminish, but actually grew. The patient passed out of my hands.

Case 6 (Fig. 9).—Female, age 66 years. Epithelioma of the tip of the nose. Treated by X-rays for two months (type

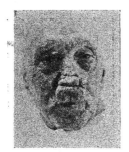

Fig. 13.

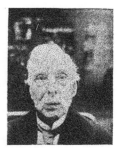

Fig. 14.

of treatment not known). Stated that the growth was rapidly increasing. The growth protruded for half an inch. Patient refused to submit to anything else than the radical removal -of the growth. I removed the growth wide of its margins by means of the Percy cautery. (Fig. 10.) After about two months the nose appeared healed. (Fig. 11.) Patient refused

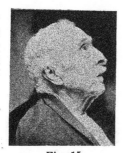

Fig. 15.

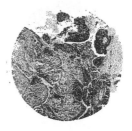

Fig. 16.

any kind of plastic cosmetic operation. Fig. 12 shows the growth to be a true epithelioma, very much inflamed and possibly changed by reason of X-ray treatment.

Case 7 (Fig. 13).—Male, age 71. Rhinophima, with secondary epitheliomatous degeneration. The growth is seen to hang down over the man's lip and he was compelled to hold it up by a sort of sling in order to be able to breathe, speak and eat. A thorough decortication with adaptation of the surrounding healthy skin in order to cover the raw surface, produced an excellent cosmetic and physiologic result. (Figs. 14

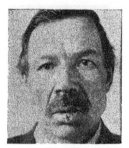

Fig. 17.

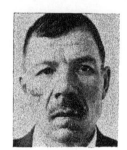

Fig. 18.

and 15.) The microscopic examination (Fig. 16) showed the typical histologic picture of hypertrophy of the epithelium, blood vessels, glands and connective tissue, but also in spots suspicious areas of an epthelioma. Consequently I had him X-rayed for three erythema doses within six months. He lived five and one-half years longer, dying from cardiovascu-

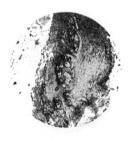

Fig. 19.

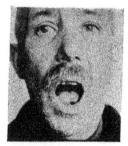

Fig. 20.

lar disease, with no recurrence or evidence of carcinoma in any other part of the body.

Case 8 (Fig. 17).—Male, age 46 years. Epithelioma of the lip. This was excised and the parts immediately approximated. (Fig. 18.) X-rays were subsequently employed for three erythema doses over the submental and submaxillary regions (glands tributary to this region), as well as the operated area. There has been no recurrence now for over two and one-half years. Fig. 19 gives the microscopic proof of the epithelioma. It has been the rule and still is, in some of

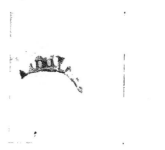

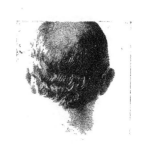

Fig. 21.                              Fig. 22.

the clinics, to remove the lymph glands and block from the submental region and make a greater sacrifice of the lower lip than in this case. This makes the operation much more formidable, causing considerable deformity of the mouth, and from observation of the cases treated like the one illustrated here it would appear that it was unnecessary. Time alone will

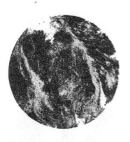

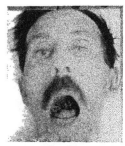

Fig. 23.                              Fig. 24.

tell. The question also arises whether one may not treat the epithelioma of the lip simply with the X-rays or radium without surgery. Conflicting reports make me choose the procedure as outlined in this case. I have treated twenty-six cases of facial epithelioma similar to these illustrated, by means of surgery, X-ray, fulguration, carbon dioxid and radium, and I must say that nothing will compare to the use of radium. Some of the early cases were operated upon several times and finally developed into true cancers with fatal results.

Case 9.—Male, age 45 years. Carcinoma of the anterolat-

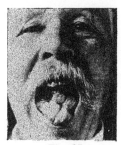
Fig. 25.

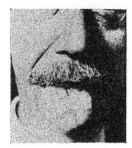
Fig. 26.

eral part of the tongue and that portion of the floor of the mouth (no photograph obtainable). (Operated away from home.) By means of a Percy cautery the growth was removed wide of its involvement. Lips and mouth were protected by speculum containing running cold water. Six weeks later the wound was healed and the tip of the tongue was fixed to the

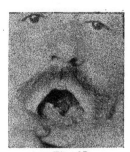
Fig. 27.

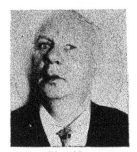
Fig: 28.

floor of the mouth. (Fig. 20.) During the healing process a sequestrum came off due, no doubt, to the extreme heat of the cautery. This was a portion of the alveolar process of the lower jaw. (Fig. 21.) Patient's neck region was X-rayed for a period of two weeks, when he disappeared from observation. About two months later he returned with a recurrence in the neck (Fig. 22), but none at the site of original growth. Fig. 23 showed a typical alveolar carcinoma. The subsequent course of the case was rapidly developing metastatic condition, which caused the patient's death.

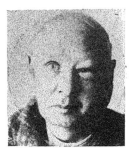

Fig. 29.

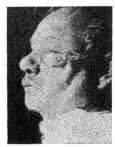

Fig. 30.

Case 10 (Fig. 24).—Male, age 53 years. Carcinoma of the base of the tongue and soft palate, tonsil and pharynx, also glands of neck. Preliminary X-ray treatment (one erythema dose to the neck) to attempt to block off further invasion of the lymphatics. Radical operation. Lived for about six

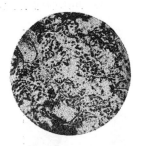

Fig. 31.

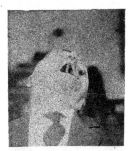

Fig. 32.

weeks, in a miserable condition: feeding possible only with a stomach tube.

Case 11 (Fig. 25).—Male, age 61 years. Microscopic diagnosis: Carcinoma of the half of the tongue. There were no glands of the neck present. Advised operation, removal of tongue. Patient refused operation. Under deep X-ray treatment the neoplasm grew to such proportions as to make breath-

ing impossible through the mouth or nose. A tracheotomy was
performed. One hour after this the patient disappeared and
was never traced with the aid of relatives and police.

Case 12.—Male, age 55 years. Suspected epithelioma of

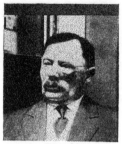

Fig. 33.

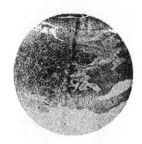

Fig. 34.

dorsum and lateral portion of tongue. No glandular involvement of the neck. . Consulted the clinic at Johns Hopkins.
and being a prominent physician from the South, he was
given special attention by Dr. Barker, etc. A piece of the
tissue was removed by them and diagnosticated papilloma
or nonmalignant growth. He received very intensive treat-

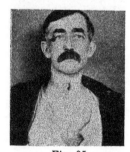

Fig. 35.

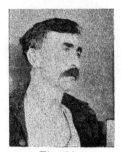

Fig. 36.

ment by radium (exact dose, etc., not stated in their report).
Patient presented himself to me with two very agonizing symptoms, namely, hyperesthesia and excessive salivation. It was
impossible for him to eat anything but the blandest food, and
even this caused pain. There was a history of lues, although
the Wassermann was always negative. The tongue looked

white and felt hard on the surface. There was an enlargement on the left side near the base (Fig. 26), with a distinct
line of demarcation. I diagnosticated the condition as a radium burn and treated it as such. The line of treatment was

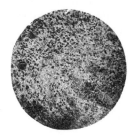

Fig. 37.

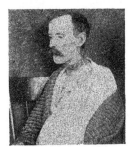

Fig. 38.

absolute rest to the tongue by insisting on feeding him with
an esophageal tube and coating the tongue with various substances that could be made to stick, such as starchy pastes containing tragacanth. This was, however, without any lasting
benefit. Atropin proved to be of most value. Recently he
consulted the Mayos and more radium treatment was advised.

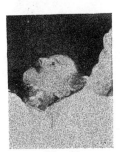

Fig. 39.

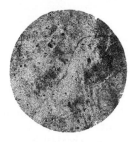

Fig. 40.

They believed that he had a malignant disease engrafted upon
a luetic tongue. There were no enlarged glands present in the
neck.

Case 13.—Male, age 58 years. Sarcoma of tonsil. Came to
me with a severe radium burn of the right side of the base of
the tongue and pillar and cheek. (Fig. 27.) The radium had

been applied by means of needles into a tumor of the tonsil microscopically diagnosed sarcoma. The growth had entirely disappeared when he presented himself to me and showed only a dirty slough within the tonsillar fossa. He gave a history of having been operated upon for peritonsillar abscess with pus discharge. The physician who made the diagnosis of sarcoma and had the radium applied had not seen any pus. The radium burn healed very readily following the application of bismuth subiodid powder.

Statistical: I have treated seventeen cases of carcinoma of the tongue, either surgically or combined with X-rays, radium, diathermia, cautery, etc. All the cases have succumbed to the disease or some immediate complication, bronchopneu-

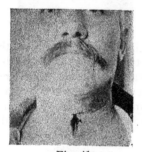

Fig. 41.

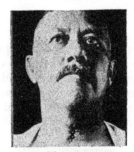

Fig. 42.

monia and sepsis occurring in more than one case.

Case 14.—Male, age 60 years. Epulis in the left first upper molar. Transillumination and radiograms showed the greater portion of the antrum involved. (Fig. 28.) Sublabial operation, wide resection of the growth, removal of the greater portion of the superior maxilla. One hundred mg. of radium element, screened by ¼ mm. of silver filter, was placed into the cavity created by the operation and allowed to remain for twelve hours. The wound healed slowly, and in about two weeks a recurrence was observed. He was X-rayed intensively, but the growth progressed so rapidly in spite of this (Fig. 29) that a more radical procedure was decided upon, namely, total resection of the upper jaw (Fig. 30). Subsequent to this operation the patient received 50 mg. of radium screened as above, at periods of three days apart, for from three to

six hours. The recurrence was kept in abeyance and great
hopes were entertained for his cure, but, as usual, after two
months glands began to develop in the anterior and posterior
triangle and nothing could stop the final fatal termination.
Fig. 31 shows the microscopic section.

Case 15.—Male, age 52 years. Carcinoma of the upper jaw
simliar to the one just described. A radical total resection
of the upper jaw was performed; Figs. 32 and 33 show the
end result, Fig. 34 the microscopic section. This case never
received any X-ray or radium treatment, either before or after
operation, and is shown as one of the cases to prove my contention in the introduction, that perhaps what we consider
good treatment in the use of the X-ray and radium in car-

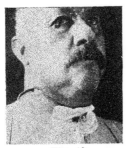
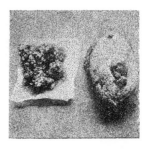

Fig. 43.                              Fig. 44.

cinoma may be just the opposite. The patient is living, fourteen years after operation.

Statistical: I have had 19 cases of carcinoma of the upper
jaw, all operated; most of them belonged to the inoperable
type. In the majority, X-rays, radium, Percy's cautery or
some other nonsurgical measure was employed in conjunction with operations. Only two cases lived and can be spoken
of as cured. Most of the patients died from carcinoma
metastasis.

Case 16 (Fig. 35).—Carcinoma of the larynx. Male, age
46 years. When I saw him first, he had a well developed
neoplasm, but entirely within the larynx and confined to one
side. Laryngotomy was performed and the growth removed,
the wound being immediately closed except for the retention
of a tracheal canula. Six weeks later he returned with a

marked recurrence. Laryngeal fissure was then performed, all the growth removed and the fissures opened for subsequent X-ray and radium treatment. This was instituted almost immediately after operation, but in spite of this fact recurrence was noticed, especially about the left posterior part of the larynx. During this intensive X-ray and radium treatment (16 mg., all that was obtainable at the time) pieces of the growth were removed at an average of once a week for microscopic examination as to control of the effect ·of the treatment. These sections clearly demonstrated slow but positive destruction of cancer cells. At the end of one year the laryngeal cavity appeared free from carcinoma, both macro- and microscopically (Fig. 36). Patient returned to his home

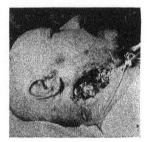 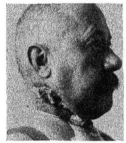

Fig. 45.                    Fig. 46.

town, his physician reporting that there was no recurrence in situ, but he developed marked neurotic and neuritic symptoms, including pains radiating down the arm, chest and legs, so ·severe that morphin had to be administered. The neurotic symptoms were very peculiar and ordinarily would be considered as hysterical. They were so unusual and constant that I may be pardoned for mentioning them again in detail. "Always before a thunderstorm appeared he became very restless and panicky and insisted on locking himself in a dark room, until the storm passed. He would frequently do this twenty-four hours before the storm came on." These neuritic painful conditions usually followed such a nervous spell and the pain would center itself in the big toes. He died three years from the time I first diagnosed his case as carcinoma, or over two years after X-ray and radium were employed.

A postmortem examination was made, and no evidence of any metastasis could be found. I received the entire larynx and made a thorough macroscopic and microscopic examination, but could not demonstrate any carcinomatous tissue. (Fig. 37.)

Case 17.—Male, age 53 years. Came with a rapidly growing swelling on side of neck (Fig. 38). Examination within the throat and mouth revealed no primary growth. He was given deep X-ray treatment intensively, but the growth continued to increase until a tracheotomy was necessary. The tumor finally ulcerated (Fig. 39) and a microscopic section (Fig. 40) showed a typical carcinoma. The subsequent course was an early metastases into both lungs in spite of very active

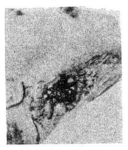

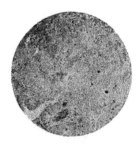

Fig. 47.                              Fig. 48.

X-ray treatment, from which death ensued.

Case 18.—Male, age 47 years. Well advanced carcinoma of the larynx. A laryngofissure was performed and the growth thoroughly removed by the Percy cautery, allowing the fissure to remain open for after-treatment. (Fig. 41.) Within two weeks the fissure healed (Fig. 42). The interior of the larynx shows no evidence of any growth (Fig. 42). He left for his home in Wyoming. One month later he returned with an enormous recurrence, both in the neck as well as within the larynx, requiring tracheotomy. The neck tumor had broken down so as to appear like an abscess and this was opened and drained. Shortly after I removed a part of the mass from the neck, including the skin, which was involved in the process (Fig. 44). There remained, however, quite a bit of growth in situ (Fig. 45). This was now treated by

means of the surgical diathermia, as described by Nagel-
schmidt. At first it appeared as though this line of treatment would be effective, because the growth was shrinking
and appeared healthy (Fig. 46). However, suddenly there
occurred a marked change, and in spite of the treatment the
growth spread very rapidly (Fig. 47)' and caused great difficulty in breathing and swallowing. Suddenly one day he had
a severe arterial bleeding that exsanguinated him and he died
within an hour. Fig. 48 shows a microscopic section of a
carcinoma.

Case 19.—Male. Was referred to me with a diagnosis of
laryngeal carcinoma confined to the right cord. A microscopic
section accompanied the patient. The physician as well as the

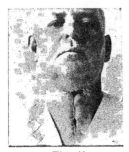
Fig. 49.

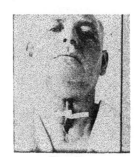
Fig. 50.

patient pleaded for intralaryngeal operation and nonsurgical
measures should be given a trial. Consequently I performed
a suspension laryngoscopy and removed what I thought to
be the entire growth by that method. Subsequent to this
operation the patient was given intense deep X-ray treatment
over the thyroid region. The laryngeal condition appeared
to heal very rapidly and his voice became quite clear. After
the second erythema dose he developed marked symptoms of
myxedema, which no doubt were due to the action of the X-
rays on his thyroid gland. Therefore this line of treatment
was discontinued, and he was put on large doses of thyroid
extract, which corrected the myxedematous state. He then
returned to his home in Vancouver, where he was observed
by his physician (otolaryngologist). After nearly one year
he was again sent back to me with a suspected recurrence

within his larynx. As he still insisted that he did not wish any operation upon the larynx externally, and was willing to take his chance on the former line of treatment, I removed all that I thought was diseased and had his larynx region X-rayed but not as intensively as the first time, as I feared to cause the myxedematous symptoms. This time, however, he did not improve; on the contrary, the growth took on a rapid development. At this time the patient agreed to an operation, and I found that laryngectomy alone could be of any value. This was performed under local anesthesia with very little difficulty. The usual technic differed in that I placed a dermal lined fistula (Fig. 49) subhyoidally to accommodate a tube which communicated with his trachea, making

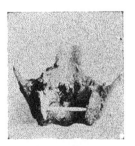

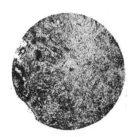

Fig. 51.                    Fig. 52.

a sort of an artificial larynx (Fig. 50). Whenever he bent his head forward so as partially to kink this tube he could produce sounds that were quite audible and understood as speech. Fig. 51 shows the larynx, in which the growth extends anteriorly, but is confined within the larynx. Fig. 52 shows the microscopic section of a carcinoma. The patient again returning to the coast to be observed by his otolaryngologist, who reported about eight months later that the patient developed abdominal symptoms that proved to be due to cancer, from, which he soon died. The larynx did not show any recurrence.

Case 20.—Male. Well developed neoplasm confined to the larynx. Microscopic examination (Fig. 56) proved it to be a carcinoma. A laryngeal fissure was performed and the growth removed wide of its development (Fig. 53). As soon as practicable an intubation tube carrying one hundred mg. of radium element, screened by a filter of 1.10 mm. of aluminum was inserted by way of the mouth and held in place by two threads (Fig. 54). These are tied over a piece of gauze, as suggested by Iglauer. The radium was removed after six hours, but the intubation tube was allowed to remain. These radium applications were repeated twice more within the next two weeks. The intubation tube was now left out and the fissure permitted to close (Fig. 55). Weekly inspection showed no recurrence for over two months, but at the end of that time a small growth appeared on one side which, however, was not at all influenced by either radium, X-rays or operation, and the usual termination of a metastasis and cachexia followed.

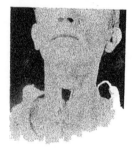

Fig. 53.

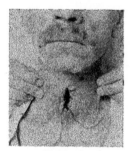

Fig. 54.

Case 21.—Male. Advanced carcinoma of the larynx, base of tongue and esophagus, upper part. Under local anesthesia I performed a tracheotomy. By means of pharyngotomy I removed a tumor mass, including the larynx, in the obliteration of the upper end of the trachea (purse string closure), base of tongue and the esophagus contiguous to the posterior portion of the larynx. A permanent esophageal intubation by way of the nostril was instituted, through which the patient was fed (Fig. 57). I wish to state that that was the most comfortable way of alimentation in such an extreme case under my observation. The remaining portion of the wound was closed by primary intention. The secretions that accumulated within the esophageal cavity were removed by the aid of suction. There were no X-ray, radium or other electrical measures employed. The patient made a splendid recovery

from the operation.   Three weeks after the operation I removed the esophageal tube and allowed the patient to swallow
liquids.   On the third day, following this natural mode of
feeding, the patient experienced while swallowing a glass of
milk a sudden sharp pain in the middle of·his back and into
the neck.   Within a few hours he developed classical symptoms of a septic mediastinum and died.   Most probably the
permanent esophageal tube caused a decubitus, followed by
rupture during efforts of deglutition.   It must be remembered
that the base of his tongue had been removed, therefore swallowing was not normal.   Fig. 58 shows the microscopic section
of the carcinoma.

Case 22.—Male, age 60 years, had posttyphoidal laryngeal

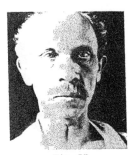
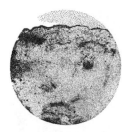

Fig. 55.                                  Fig. 56.

abscess when a young man requiring tracheotomy and incision
of abscess.   Twenty-six years later, after all the symptoms
of the abscess had entirely disappeared, he developed a most
rapidly growing tumor, both within·the larynx and on both
sides of the neck.   It was somewhat indurated,·and I thought
that I had a case of Reclus' disease or woody phlegmon.   A
hurried tracheotomy had to be performed (Fig. 59), and at
the same time I obtained a piece of tissue for microscopic
examination, which proved to be a very active carcinoma (Fig.
60).   I began the use of autolytic solution, obtained from
fetal tissue, as recommended by Fichera and published by me
(ANNALS OF OTOLOGY, RHINOLOGY AND LARYNGOLOGY, March,
1912).   The result was most gratifying, and for some time it
appeared as if the growth was going to melt away, but liver
· metastasis appeared, with the usual ending.

Case 23.—Man, age 53, a public speaker for many years, with a hoarse voice for the past ten years, noticed in the last two months that this hoarseness was increasing.

Examination showed a unilateral swelling along the entire cord. Removal of a small portion and microscopic examination revealed a typical epithelioma (Fig. 62). An operation was performed under local anesthesia in the form of a laryngeal fissure, removal of the entire cord and considerable normal neighboring tissue. An immediate closure without tracheotomy or intubation was undertaken. There developed considerable edema within the larynx, causing embarrassment in respiration; however, this lasted only a day, when he began to breathe with comfort. Fourteen years later he still was

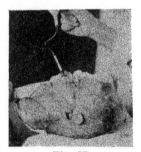

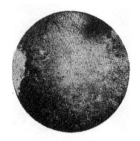

Fig. 57.                              Fig. 58.

free from recurrence. He is an insurance man and requires a good voice, which he still has. He has some little difficulty when he swallows, characterized by a sort of pull on his thyroid cartilage, which is due to marked cicatricial bands developed in the healing (Fig. 61).

Case 24.—Man, for about six months has considerable difficulty in speaking and for the past month some slight embarrassment in breathing when walking fast.

Examination shows a unilateral growth of one cord which appears to dip under into the subglottic region. Under suspension laryngoscopy a small piece of tissue from the tumor was removed; microscopic examination showed it to be a typical quite rapidly growing carcinoma (Fig. 64). The physician referring the patient requested that if an operation was to be performed a preliminary application of a lethal dose of .

radium, say 200 mg. of the element, be placed over the region
of the larynx and allowed to remain for about ten hours.   The
term lethal had reference to the local destruction of the activity
of the cancer cells so that in operating implantation carcinoma
would be avoided.   This is the advice of Wood and P——,
New York, based upon experiments, and the physician mentioned above had more than five years' experience in cases
where radium was employed.

Operation under local anesthesia.   A thyrotomy was performed, and the growth was removed with considerable
healthy neighboring tissue.   A preliminary tracheotomy having been made, it was deemed advisable to allow the tube to
remain for a day or two, especially so since two radium

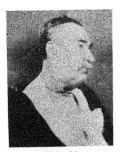

Fig. 59.

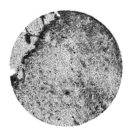

Fig. 60.

needles, each 12½ m., were introduced into the wound caused
by the excision of the growth.   The patient exhibited unusual
symptoms on the operating table, having several attacks of
projectile vomiting, also being extremely nervous, although
never complaining of pain.   On being returned to his bed he
showed symptoms of shock, from which he never rallied.   He
had very unusual toxic symptoms, which I could not quite
understand, consequently called in an expert internist (physiologic chemistry), who was of the opinion, as was I, that the
patient was suffering from a toxemia due to the massive dose
of radium employed just before the operation.   In less than
thirty-six hours' time from the time of the operation the patient was dead in spite of all efforts.   An immediate postmortem examination revealed locally an absolutely reactionless

area about the thyroid region (Fig. 63). No other post-mortem examination was performed.

Statistical: I have treated fifty-nine cases of cancer of the larynx, surgically alone or in combination with X-ray, radium,

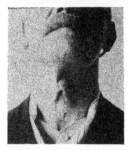
Fig. 61.

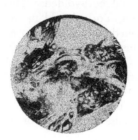
Fig. 52.

fulguration or surgical diathermia, Percy's cautery, galvano-cauteries, autolytic and colloidal solution. Also a limited number of cases in which only radium or X-rays were employed. Operative measures were intralaryngeal, both by indirect and by means of suspension laryngoscopy, laryngo-fissure, hemilaryngectomy, laryngectomy and extensive resec-

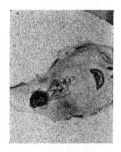
Fig. 63.

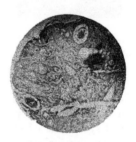
Fig. 64.

tion of glands and tumors of the neck secondary to the laryngeal growth.

Nine cases are alive, the longest since the operation, fourteen years. One case twelve years, one seven and one-half years, one six years and one five years and two months. The remaining four cases are between four years, and, the most recent one, three months ago. These last four cases will not be considered cured until at least five years have passed without recurrence, either locally or metastatic. Strange to say, the oldest case which I have alive since operation was oper-

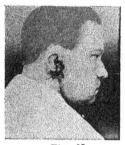

Fig. 65.

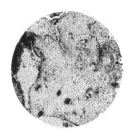

Fig. 66.

ated upon by the indirect laryngoscopic method. I see the man once or twice a year in order to keep him under control, and each time I review his microscopic section. The next oldest case, now twelve years, had a laryngofissure with immediate closure. The next two were laryngectomies, and the fifth a hemilaryngectomy and partial resection of esophagus,

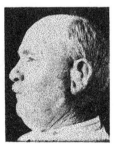

Fig. 67.

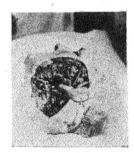

Fig. 68.

but no glands. The four cases not yet considered cured because of the short duration were treated by laryngofissure or radium alone.

Case 25.—Epithelioma of auricle. Man, age 53 years. Two years before he was referred to me he noted a small swelling within his ear, which he had removed by a surgeon, who had

it examined microscopically and pronounced cancer. He recommended thorough surgical removal, to which the patient
objected and consulted a "paste cancer cure specialist" in
Iowa. He was treated just once. The ear became sore, then

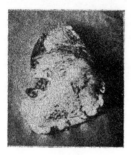

Fig. 69.

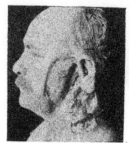

Fig. 70.

healed and deformity resulted. (Fig. 65.) He was free from
pain or recurrence for over two years. Now (1914) he no-
tices a swelling in his neck and some pain in his arm. I found
a recurrence within the external auditory canal and a mass on
the side of the neck. I removed a piece from the canal
which showed a true epithelioma (Fig. 66). I had him X-

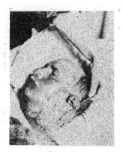

Fig. 71.

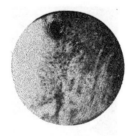

Fig. 72.

rayed for a period of six weeks without any special benefit,
except perhaps the control of the pains. He finally consented to a more radical operation, which was performed by
the excision of the growth within the canal and radical removal of the mass in the neck. He was subsequently rayed,
but recurrence appeared almost immediately. The pains be-

came excruciating, even after the use of opiates. He went back to his home town, where he lived about six weeks longer and his physician reported his death from a gradual exhaustion with symptoms of esophageal involvement.

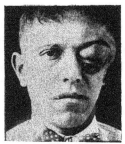

Fig. 73.

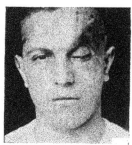

Fig. 74.

Case 26.—Man, age 51 years. A year ago had a small growth curetted from his external ear, followed by X-ray and radium treatment. There was a rapid recurrence and a marked swelling developed in his neck, as far as the clavicle. With this history, he was referred to me (Fig. 67) by Dr. Emil Beck, to whom he was recommended owing to the fact that he

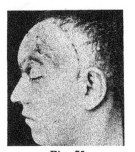

Fig. 75.

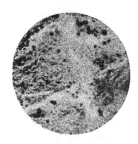

Fig. 76.

described a method of treatment of epithelioma and carcinoma for which this case was suitable. This method consists of the removal of all or as much of the growth as possible, including the overlying skin, fat and muscle, and subsequent X-ray and radium treatment. As many secondary removals of the growth as necessary are undertaken, so that the rays act

directly on the cancer without any screening or absorption of
the beta rays by skin, muscle, fat or destroyed tumor. The
work of Dr. Emil Beck is described in detail, including experimental work by G. W. Arner of the Ryerson Laboratory, University of Chicago, in surgery, gynecology and obstetrics. In October, 1919, I performed this extensive resection
of skin, muscles and as much of the tumor as was safe, and
left the area exposed for subsequent X-ray and radium treatment. Part of the pinna was sewed in for possible subsequent reconstruction. (Fig. 68.) The excised tumor mass
is shown in Fig. 69, and Fig. 72 shows the microscopic section. It is a true carcinoma. He received seven erythema
doses of X-rays within a period of nine weeks, also 40 mg.

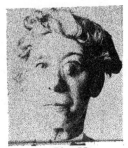

Fig. 77.

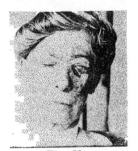

Fig. 78.

of radium, screened by only 1/10 mm. of aluminum and often
the needles were unscrewed within the tumor. This combined
treatment appeared to be of some benefit about the margins
of the exposed area (Fig. 71), but the growth deeper down
continued to develop so that more of the mass was removed,
including the lower half of the auricle (Fig. 72). Shortly
after this the patient developed difficulty in swallowing and
hoarseness, also great pains in his arms and hand. Three
months later, after a miserable existence on large doses of
morphin, with but little relief from pain, he succumbed from
exhaustion.

Statistics: I have had seven cases of epithelioma of the
external auditory canal and auricle, of which three are living,
one now eight years since operation, one three and one-half,
and one seven months since he was discharged as cured. The

first one was operated upon and subsequently treated with X-rays. The second one was treated by carbon dioxid (snow) and radium, employing six seances of the snow and four applications of radium 10 mg., screened by ¼ mm. of brass, for one hour at each application. The third was treated by radium alone, 50 mg., screened by 1/10 mm. of aluminum, for six sittings, each half an hour.

Case 27.—Man, age 27 years. Sarcoma of orbit. Received a slight trauma about one year before, which left a swelling above the left eye. About two months ago this swelling started to grow, and the last two weeks it grew so rapidly as to close his eye and cause considerable headache and pain. (Fig. 73.) A small section was removed and the microscopic exam-

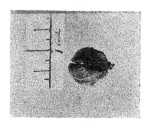

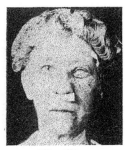

Fig. 79.                    Fig. 80.

ination proved it to be a large spindle celled sarcoma. (Fig. 76.) He was immediately operated upon, and Figs. 74 and 75 show the condition just after operation. It was necessary to resect part of the orbit and temporofrontal bone, but the dura was not involved. It was not more than two weeks when he developed a recurrence. He was immediately put upon intensive X-ray treatment. In spite of everything that was done, Cooley's toxins, salvarsan, etc., he went from bad to worse and very soon developed an intracranial growth from which he died.

Case 28.—Woman, age 30. Melanosarcoma about the orbit. Referred to me with a growth on the inner canthus of eye close to the tear sac, also complaining of nasal obstruction, for more than three months. The growth has been rapidly developing for the past month (Fig. 77). It appeared very

dark in color, as though it was a very vascular neoplasm
fixed to the bone. The eyeball was absolutely free from any
involvement. Under local anesthesia the neoplasm was easily
removed, including the periosteum, and left open for subsequent radium treatment (Fig. 78). Fig. 79 shows the size
of the growth, and Fig. 82 its microscopic appearance—a
small spindle and round celled sarcoma, numerous blood
lakes and many masses of pigment. Immediately after operation 50 mg. of radium pure, screened by 1/10 mm. of aluminum and rubber tissue, was placed into the wound for six
hours. Two weeks later two radium needles, each 12½ mg.,
were thrust into a mass which filled the greater portion of the
left side of the nose and pushed the cartilaginous septum over

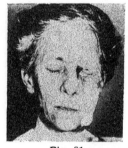

Fig. 81.

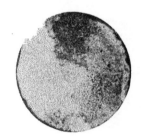

Fig. 82.

to the other side, and these needles were allowed to remain
for four hours. Fig. 80 shows them in place. The area of
the excised tumor practically healed and an ectropion of the
lower lid developed. I now noted a small swelling in the
upper inner corner of the orbit which felt elastic. Into this I
thrust two radium needles of the same dosage as before, but
only left them in place three hours. There now developed
two radium scorches on the cheek from the first application
which was kept from irritation by a gutta percha dressing
(Fig. 81). At the end of six weeks the patient markedly
improved in every way. She could breathe through the nose,
the wound healed, the small mass in the upper inner corner of
the orbit disappeared, and the radium scorch cleared up. She
returned to her home for observation by her physician. One
month later she returned with a swelling in her neck, and on

examination I found what appeared to be a gland, also some increase in the size of her alveolar process of the left superior maxilla. I removed the suspected gland and found it to be a very fleshy appearing mass, but I was able to remove it in toto without very much difficulty. The microscopic examination proved it to be a pigmented sarcomatous degeneration of the gland. I immediately placed her on deep X-ray treatment; March 21, 1920, two weeks after treatment, shows the swelling of her jaw and neck to be diminished rather than increased.

Case 29.—Male, age 37. Nasal sarcoma. Referred to me eleven years ago as an inoperable case, on account of rapidity of growth and profound anemia resulting from continuous

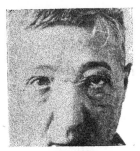

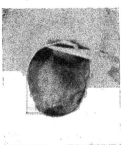

Fig. 83.                    Fig. 84.

hemorrhages. The growth was protruding through the external nostril, apparently pushing the eyeball laterally, while the bridge of the nose was spread out and the hard and soft palate were depressed into the mouth. X-ray examination showed the both antra filled. Under local anesthesia I severed the nose, by a sublabial incision, from its attachment to the apertura pyriformis and the nasal septum, thus exposing both antra and both nasal cavities, which were filled up by the tumor mass. Bleeding was quite profuse. Retracting the face upwards, so to speak, made it possible to work fast. By means of an electric burr, the anterior wall of the antra was removed, and then a greater portion of the tumor mass was removed from the nasal cavity and the antrum on both sides. It was impossible to completely clear the nose on account of the loss of blood. The bleeding was stopped by packing and

the face brought down again and sutured by two stitches below the upper lip. This operation stopped the constant hemorrhages and patient rapidly gained so that six weeks later a
second operation was performed under local anesthesia. This

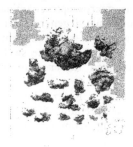

Fig. 85.

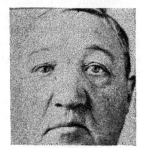

Fig. 86.

time the nose was turned down by making a transverse incision
across the root of the nose and severing the nasal bones and
nasal process of the superior maxillæ. More tumor mass
was removed, but again the operation could not be completed
on account of hemorrhage. Figs. 83 and 84 still show the
spread nose and depressed palate. Two months later I finally

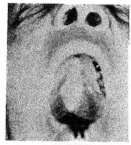

Fig. 87.

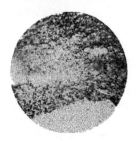

Fig. 88.

removed the remaining parts of the tumor (Fig. 85) by way
of the natural nasal passage, which resulted in very free nasal
breathing. The remaining tags of the growth were now treated by the aid of two radium needles each 12½ mg., once a
week for six weeks, when the patient was considered cured.
It is now eleven years since treatment was begun, and over

a year since any recurrence has been observed. Figs. 86 and 87 show the appearance much improved. Fig. 88 proves the growth to have been a small spindle cell sarcoma.

Case 30.—Male, age 33. Sarcoma of palate and postnasal

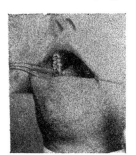

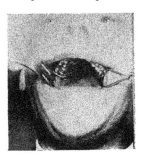

Fig. 89.                    Fig. 90.

space. For about three months this patient noticed a small growth on the inner surface of the alveolar process of the superior maxilla at the first molar tooth. (Figs. 89 and 90.) A piece of tissue was removed for microscopic examination and it proved to be a small round celled sarcoma. (Fig. 92.) Fifty mg. of radium, screened by 1/6 mm. of silver and cov-

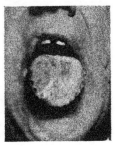

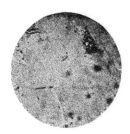

Fig. 91.                    Fig. 92.

ered by rubber tissue, were properly applied by the radium expert and permitted to remain for six hours. I have never seen anything disappear as rapidly and the surface looked absolutely normal. Keeping the patient in Chicago for a few days in order to observe the condition, I noticed on the third day a very bright red colored spot to the side of his tongue and cheek. The patient complained of a burning sensation which soon increased to pain, so that it pained him to eat anything. It was necessary to cocainize the tongue and cheek each time before eating. Fig. 91 shows an area of burn

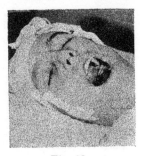

Fig. 93.

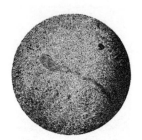

Fig. 94.

from the radium, and the radium expert (Dr. Wolpert) declared that the rubber covering of the radium capsule must have been defective and that we had a radium burn from secondary rays. He returned to his home city, where his physician reported to me that he had a great difficulty in eating. It was necessary to use cocain sprays and morphin.

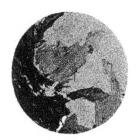

Fig. 95.

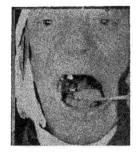

Fig. 96.

This pain or fear of taking food caused great emaciation. The surface of the previously existing neoplasm was fairly normal. One morning the doctor called in a hurry to the patient's home, and when he arrived found the patient had died. The family declared that he gave a sudden moan out of his sleep, breathed very laboriously and was blue in the face. No postmortem was permitted and cause of death is unexplained.

Case 31.—Young man, age 19. (Fig. 93.) When a small boy had tonsil and adenoid operation performed. The adenoids were said to have returned and he was operated on a

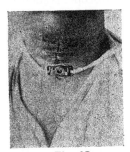
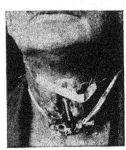

Fig. 97.                              Fig. 98.

second time. The same complaint of nasal obstruction was noted very soon after the second operation. Patient consulted another specialist, who thought he had a tumor back of his nose. Microscopic examination of a piece removed showed fibrosarcoma. When he was referred to me he had a mass very firm to the touch in the vault of the pharynx.

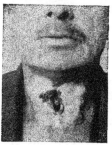
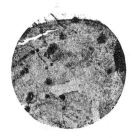

Fig. 99.                              Fig. 100.

A piece removed for microscopic examination verified the previous examination. (Fig. 94.) A slight positive Wassermann reaction was reported. Antiluetic treatment had no effect, and in order not to lose much time it was considered best to reexamine by the aid of the microscope. (Fig. 95.) Two needles, each 12½ mg., were thrust into the mass with the soft palate retracted and a capsule containing 10 mg., screened by ¼ m. of brass and covered by rubber, was placed for three hours into the posterior portion of the left nasal cavity which was obstructed by the tumor. An exudate appeared the next day, and I made a microscopic section that showed it to be a very pronounced fibromatous meshwork with many leucocytes. One month later, patient returned to me and I found that more than one-half of the growth had disappeared and left a deep, sloughy surface. No treatment was applied; when he returned one month later the surface was clean. The remainder of the growth was now treated by thrusting two needles of 12½ mg. each into it directly through the soft palate and allowed to remain for four hours. Fol-

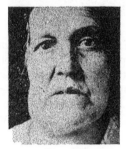 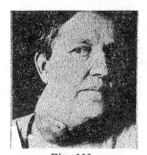

Fig. 101.                    Fig. 102.

lowing their removal there resulted a very brisk bleeding which required a postnasal tampon. This bleeding did not stop entirely after twelve hours of tamponade and another tampon was necessary. Patient again left the city for his home town, and his physician reported by letter that the boy was losing a little blood right along. The last inspection showed the growth to have practically disappeared, allowing nasal breathing and clearing the nasal tone to his speech. The surface, however, still bleeds when touched.

Case 32.—Man, age 62, came to see me with symptoms of a radium burn of his tongue, cheek and soft palate (Fig. 95). The history showed that he had a peritonsillar abscess, evacuation of which had been several times attempted. It finally ruptured spontaneously. Dr. Sonnenschein, who saw him after the rupture, suspected malignancy and removed a piece of tissue which the laboratory reported as sarcoma. He had the radium expert put in two needles, each 12½ mg., for six hours. Following this, the patient experienced great pain in swallowing, for which difficulty he consulted me. I found a whitish membrane on the inner surface of the cheek, anterior pillar of the tonsil and posterior lateral surface of the tongue on the right side (Fig. 96). Inserting an esophageal tube and allowing it to remain all day, he was fed through it, thus giving his strength which he lost from not taking any nourishment for several days owing to pain. The surfaces of the burn were covered with emulsion of scarlet red, which appeared to assist in the healing very much. In two weeks he was cured. There is no evidence of any neoplasm, and the

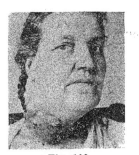

Fig. 103.

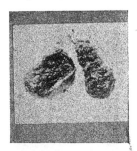

Fig. 104.

tonsillar area appears as though he had had a Pynchon cautery dissection of the tonsil.

Case 33.—Man, age 49, for the past six weeks had difficulty in breathing and speaking, but in the past week had two severe choking spells. Examination showed a firm tumor, apparently pedunculated, and attached to one side of the larynx, covering both vocal cords. Placing the patient in a recumbent position, head over the edge of the table, immediately relieved his obstructive breathing. Consequently I suspended him, and under local anesthetic (spray) removed the growth. A most distressing accident occurred which came near to causing the patient's sudden death during this suspension operation. While grasping the growth the Killian forceps cut through the pedicle, and in that moment the patient inspired and sucked the growth into the trachea. Fortunately, having his lungs sufficiently filled with air, he made a violent effort to clear the trachea and the tumor hit me in the face. It certainly was a great relief to both the patient and myself.

The surface from which the growth was removed healed very rapidly; and the patient returned to his home city in less than a week very much encouraged. I was sure there would be a recurrence, because the microscopic examination of the growth proved it to be a large celled sarcoma. Less than a month later the patient returned with his larynx filled up so that he required an immediate tracheotomy. I decided to do a laryngotomy at the same time and remove as much of the growth as possible and anticipated subsequent radium treatment by way of the mouth (Fig. 97). This operation

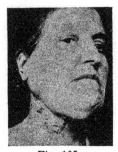
Fig. 105.

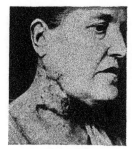
Fig. 106.

proved to be of little value, consequently I reopened the larynx and treated the process through the external route both by radium and X-ray. Fig. 98 shows 100 mg. of radium properly screened, 1/6 mm. of silver and rubber. This was continued for six hours, every other day. Alternating with this treatment the patient received X-ray treatment. After two weeks he developed a marked erythema, so that all treatment was stopped. There was now no evidence of any growth, and the area that had been rayed showed marked effect like a burn (Fig. 99). The noticeable thing was the marked symptoms of absorption of that toxemia that I suspect is due to the destruction of radium and X-rays. He went back to his home and his physician reported that he lived only for about one month, dying apparently of absorption of poison and weakness.

Case 34.—Sarcoma of the neck.   Female, age 51, noticed a small lump below her right jaw which was growing very rapidly (Fig. 101).   I had her placed under the deep X-ray treatment, which had the opposite effect—it made the tumor grow (Figs. 102 and 103).   I decided to try and stop this growth by operation, and by means of local anesthesia removed two large masses of characteristic sarcomatous tissue (Fig. 104) which proved to be microscopically a large spindle cell sarcoma (Fig. 108).   The result from the operation was gratifying (Fig. 105).   This result, however, did not remain very long; in fact, in less than two weeks there was a rapid reformation of the growth (Fig. 106), and in another month the patient was so weakened that she could not sit up, and the

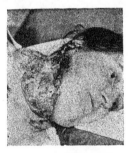

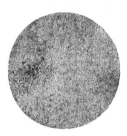

Fig. 107.                              Fig. 108.

growth was enormous (Fig. 107).   Other means, as Coley's toxins, were also employed, without the slightest benefit, the patient dying of exhaustion.

Case 35.—Sarcoma of the parotid.   Female, age 23, a month previously noted difficulty in opening the mouth, with a tight feeling on the left side of her face.   Suddenly the swelling appeared, which increased her pain (Fig. 109).   A tentative diagnosis of retention in the parotid gland was made, but this had to be changed, as the swelling extended to the back of the neck.   She was directed to use deep X-ray for six erythema doses, which was followed by disappearance of the swelling with all the symptoms.   This, however, lasted only for about a month when the tumor returned with greater rapidity.   It was now decided to operate, and so an incision was made retroauricularly (Fig. 110) and a fair amount of the tumor removed, but not radically, on account of the large vessels and facial nerve. (Fig. 111.) She was again put on X-ray treatment, but the growth continued to develop until after four months the patient succumbed to a general toxemia

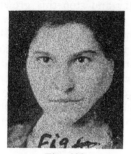

Fig. 109.

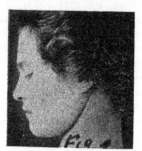

Fig. 110.

without any temperature. The microscopic diagnosis was that of a mixed cell sarcoma (Fig. 112).

Case 36.—Chloroma of the face. `Boy, age 4. Mother noted a number of swellings about the face which made the skin overlying them look pale blue or green (Fig. 114). Routine blood examination gave me a picture that was most surpris-

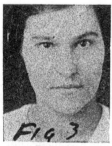

Fig. 111.

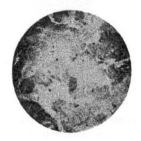

Fig. 112.

ing and led to the diagnosis. It was the following:
1. Leucocyte count, 210,000.
    (a) Neutrophilic myelocytes, 38 per cent;
    (b) Polymorphonuclear leucocytes, 40 per cent;
    (c) Lymphocytes, 16 per cent;
    (d) Eosinophiles, 20 per cent;

(e) Large mononuclears, 10 per cent;

(f) Eosinophilic myelocytes, 3 per cent.

2. Red count, 2,900,000.

3. Color index, .8.

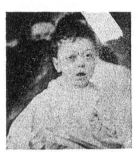

Fig. 113.

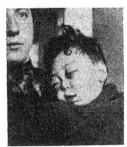

Fig. 114.

He was immediately put on deep X-ray treatment and Fowler's solution, but the disease progressed uninterruptedly, and in less than three weeks he had the appearance shown in Fig. 113. It was very difficult to rouse him and there resulted a great emaciation and anemic appearance of the rest of the body. Terminal state was associated with subcutaneous

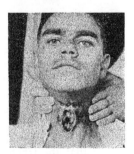

. Fig. 115.

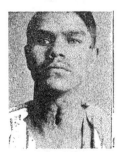

Fig. 116.

bleeding about the abdominal wall and the extremities. One large hematoma occurred in the quadreceps exterior on the right side. The child succumbed seven weeks from the time the mother noted the swellings about the face.

This is the only case of chloroma I ever saw. It is unfortunate that a microscopic section could not have been ob-

tained.  The literature on this point shows the tumor to be
a fibroblastic structure resembling a sarcoma, but instead of
blood lakes there are actual blood vessels.

Case 37.—Papilloma of the larynx.  Male, age 23, when
seven years of age developed hoarseness, which persisted.
The laryngologist of his home town diagnosed it papilloma
and in conjunction with a general surgeon performed a thyrotomy and removed a mass of papillomatous material.  He
kept the larynx open for a long time, also a tracheotomy tube
in place.  When the larynx finally closed, he removed the
tracheotomy tube and permitted its opening to close.  It became, however, necessary to reinsert the tracheotomy tube in
a day or two, the larynx having again filled up with papil-

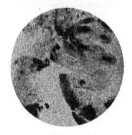

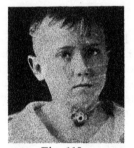

Fig. 117.                              Fig. 118.

loma.  For the next three years there was nothing done for
the boy.  At that time another laryngofissure was performed,
the growths removed and the larynx again left open for some
time for after treatment.  When finally the larynx closed the
tracheotomy tube was not removed.  When he was presented
to me, sixteen years from the time of his first operation, I
found his larynx filled completely with a mass, and when the
tracheotomy tube was removed it was found that the trachea
had collapsed and patient could get no air.  This was no doubt
due to the low grade infection of the cartilage rings and subsequent absorption.  It was decided, after a suspension laryngoscopy and removal of some of the tissue for microscopic
confirmation, again to open the larynx, remove all the papilloma and then give him a massive dose of radium.  Under
local anesthesia the laryngofissure was performed, and it was

discovered that most of the thyroid cartilage was replaced by
scar tissue. The growth was also much firmer than ordinary
papilloma. Into the cavity created by the removal of all of
the growth 100 mg. of radium element, screened by 1/10 mm.
of silver, was placed and allowed to remain for eight hours.
There resulted almost immediately a most profound toxemia,
with marked symptoms of mental depression which never had
been observed in the patient before. He refused food and
talked of suicide. The wound itself was of fairly healthy
appearance, although a great deal of discharge was present.
(Fig. 115.) As soon as this diminished and the wound permitted, I inserted an up and down Jackson's laryngostomy
tube which he wore for three weeks, when the trachea ap-

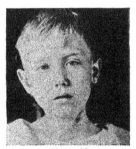

Fig. 119.

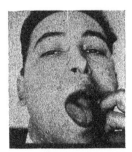

Fig. 120.

peared firm enough not to collapse. (Fig. 116.) The fissure
will be kept open for some time to be sure there is no recurrence. He will finally have a plastic closure of the laryngostomy. Fig. 117 shows a typical papilloma with considerable
round cell infiltration.

Note.—Six months later. His physician writes that the
patient has regained his normal state of general health, and
locally there appears no recurrence.

Case 38.—Boy age 7, when two years old had the first
symptoms of laryngeal obstruction and hoarseness, which soon
developed into severe choking spells, so that his laryngologist
had to do a tracheotomy. This tracheotomy tube could never
be removed or left out but for a minute, and at his presentation to me it had not been removed for over two years.

Examination. About the tracheal canula there was seen

a typical papilloma of considerable size. (Fig. 118.) I performed suspension laryngoscopy under vapor anesthesia and found the entire larynx filled with papillomatous masses. I removed as much as I deemed advisable and immediately inserted a hard rubber intubation tube which carried 25 mg. of radium screened by 1/10 mm. of silver. This intubation tube was held in position at the tracheal wound by means of a ligature as first suggested by Iglauer. The radium was permitted to remain for twelve hours, when he was reintubated without the radium. The following day 25 mg. of radium element screened by 1/10 mm. of silver was applied over the papillary excrescences about the tracheal opening and allowed to remain six hours. In less than a week the trachea was closed and

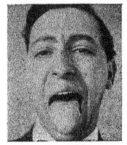

Fig. 121.

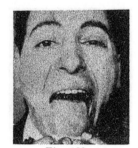

Fig. 122.

the intubation tube removed. (Fig. 119.) It appeared to be a striking result; however, the patient had some difficulty in breathing in the next day or two, especially when sleeping, so that I decided to reinsert a small tracheotomy tube and allowed him to return to his home city. The larynx remained free from papilloma and reports from his laryngologist are that he recovered completely, now over three years ago.

I have the records of thirty-nine cases of papilloma, principally of the larynx, of which sixteen cases received either X-ray or radium treatment in conjunction with operative interference. I am convinced that the best way is to treat the cases early, by intubation, the tube carrying the radium as described. When once the papilloma is of greater size and has lasted a longer time or perhaps has been previously operated upon, I think that operative interference, preferably by suspension laryngoscopy, followed by radiation of radium, is best. The X-ray treatment of papilloma of the larynx has been anything but satisfactory to me, especially when the larynx is not opened. I have made several attempts with fulguration or surgical diathermia in cases but without satisfaction. I have the records of three cases of papilloma of the adult diagnosed by microscope, which were treated as such, but the subsequent course proved them to be malignant. Of course it is possible that a papilloma may become a malignant growth.

Case 39.—Lupus of the tongue. Male, age 25. For the past six or eight months noticed a hardening of his tongue, with nodular formations, especially towards the left side. Exam-

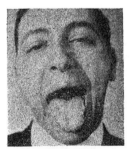
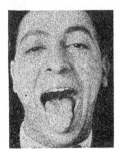

Fig. 123.                    Fig. 124.

ination showed swelling and several hard nodules can be made out in different parts of the tongue. (Fig. 120.) After one course of X-ray treatments there was noticed a marked change in that the whole tongue softened. (Fig. 121.) After a rest of two weeks from treatment, I noted a very soft spot near the dorsum (Fig. 122), which finally broke down, discharging a yellowish material but containing nothing but contamination organisms. Following the healing of this abscess he was again subjected to a course of X-ray treatments. (The radiologist stated he was using a medium tube for fifteen minutes at each seance.) The tongue had a much healthier appearance, following this treatment. (Fig. 123.) Treatment was then discontinued because I noted a sort of a shrinking of the whole tongue. (Fig. 124.) Six months later he presented himself and the tongue looked smooth and more like normal. (Fig.

125.) The microscopic examination of a particle of tissue removed at the time of the ruptured abscess showed a granulation with no typical giant cells present. (Fig. 126.)

I have treated three cases of this nature, although one of

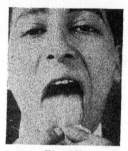
Fig. 125.

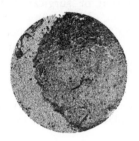
Fig. 126.

the cases no doubt was true primary tuberculosis of the tongue. In that case I had excellent results from the use of radium. It required two years to determine that the condition was cured. The end result was a tongue much deformed and restricted in motion. The third case is practically the same as Case 39, only that radium instead of the X-ray was employed.

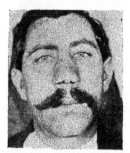
Fig. 127.

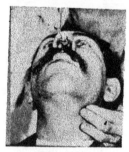
Fig. 128.

I employed from 10 to 20 mg. screened by 1/10 mm. of silver, leaving it in place one to two hours. These applications were made every three days. The case is still under treatment but progressing favorably.

Case 40.—Tuberculosis of external nose. Male, age 33. For two years noted a swelling about the tip of his nose, which finally opened up and discharged. Examination showed a granulating mass in the columella of the septum and extending to the floor, where it was severed by the ulcerative process. (Figs. 127 and 128.) A piece of tissue was removed for

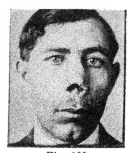

Fig. 129.

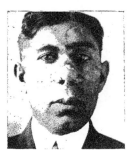

Fig. 130.

microscopic examination and found to be indicative of true tuberculosis.

He was put on X-ray treatment (daily), medium tube, ten minutes. It did very little good—in fact, the process continued to ulceration. I finally applied 30 mg. of radium element screened by 1/10 mm. of aluminum, and allowed it to remain

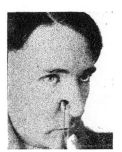

Fig. 131.

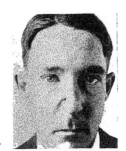

Fig. 132.

for six hours. Following this treatment there was a rapid improvement, so that in three weeks the nose was healed in scar formation as seen in Fig. 129. To correct the defect Dr. Carl Beck during my absence in France performed an Indian plastic operation which partially restored the cosmetic part of his nose. (Fig. 130.) I am now performing secondary operations to help him to breathe through his nose as well as further to improve its appearance.

Case 41.—Male, age 29 years, presented himself to me with a swelling on the side of his nose and face, which finally broke

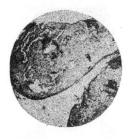

Fig. 133.

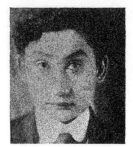

Fig. 134.

down at the alar region. (Fig. 131.) The interior of the right side of his nose was entirely blocked, and had the appearance of a luetic condition. A Wassermann was found strongly three plus, but the tissue removed was distinctly tuberculous and had a striking similarity to that removed from the nose of Case 40. (Fig. 133.) He was given several intravenous

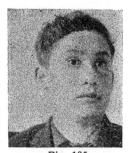

Fig. 135.

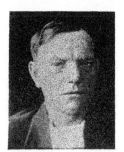

Fig. 136.

injections of salvarsan and a thorough mercury and iodid medication, but with only partial benefit. Not until he received intensive X-ray treatment did the process finally heal. (Fig. 132.)

There are five true tuberculosis cases of nose which have come under my observation, all living, the longest fifteen years.

This case is recorded in Ballenger's textbook. It is interesting to note in connection with this case that the ultimate cure or nonrecurrence followed direct sunlight treatment brought in concentrated rays into the nasal cavity by the aid of a series

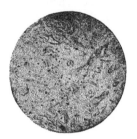

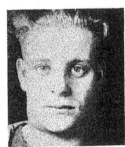

Fig. 137.                            Fig. 138.

of magnifying loops catching sunlight and bringing it into concentrated form on the lesion.

The other two cases were subsequently operated on with actual cautery with the result of marked cicatricial contractions.

Case 42.—Blastomycosis of face. Rhinoscleroma of nose.

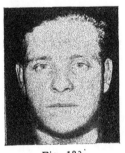

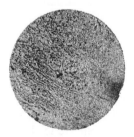

Fig. 139.                            Fig. 140.

Tuberculosis of glands of the neck. Boy, age 14, for several months had an eruption about his face, especially the margins of his eyelids; all efforts of treatment by various physicians. including dermatologists and ophthalmologists, failed and the process was getting worse. Examination showed small ulcerations covered by dirty scabs. (Fib. 134.) When these crusts were removed and slight scraping made from the ulcer, smeared and cultured (special media prepared) it was found to be practically pure blastomyces.

He was immediately put on X-ray treatment. He received six ten minute applications of the light tube when the face was healed and remained so. (Fig. 135.)

Case 43.—Male, age 46, suffered with nasal obstruction for nearly a year, during which period he has had several intranasal operations. He suffers considerable pain and headache. His general health has been very much affected by this condition and he appears anemic. Examination shows the external nose very much broader, especially at the root of the nose. (Fig. 136.) The entire nasal cavity on both sides is firmly

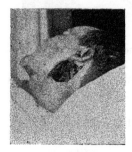

Fig. 141.

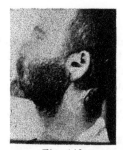

Fig. 142.

packed with the neoplastic structure. Looking into the throat, the postnasal space was found filled out with a mass which is verified by palpation. A piece of tissue was removed for microscopic examination, which bled very freely. The examination of this specimen justified, the diagnosis of large spindle celled sarcoma, with a very peculiar type of cells throughout the section. (Fig. 137.) It was decided to do a radical operation, and consequently I severed the external nose sublabially from the margins of the apertura pyriformis, and thus was enabled to remove all the growth from both sides of the nose very rapidly. Bleeding was considerable and hard to control. As a result of the operation there recurred a marked discharge. Examination showed the presence of a capsulated organism, the bacillus of Frish, and those peculiar cells seen in the section not previously recognized, the socalled Mikulicz cells. The patient was immediately put on X-ray treatment and no recurrence followed. He went back to his home city, and I was subsequently notified that he succumbed probably to his secondary general condition rather than from the rhinoscleroma.

This was the first case of rhinoscleroma confined to the nose I have ever seen. I have treated four other cases of rhinoscleroma, all confined to the larynx, and aside from the dilation, intubation, tracheotomy and laryngostomy, they were also treated by X-ray and radium. I have observed that these treatments had a very decidedly beneficial effect on the local condition. Yet in all the cases it was necessary to use mechanicosurgical treatments as described above.

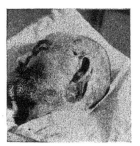 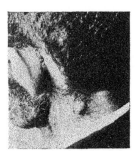

Fig. 140.                                   Fig. 144.

Case 44.—Young man, age 23, has had a unilateral swelling on the side of his neck for several months, recently becoming larger and giving him some pain. Examination showed a number of glands enlarged and matted together, extending from the lower jaw to the clavicle and almost the entire half of the neck. (Fig. 5.) The interior examination was negative, both tonsils and adenoids having been thoroughly removed. Removal of one gland revealed a true tuberculous change in it. (Fig. 140.) He was treated with deep X-rays, receiving three erythema doses within a period of four months. All but one of the glands disappeared. This one broke down and I had to open and drain it. Following this treatment the patient was and is cured. Fig. 139.)

I have treated many such cases just this way, except that in most of them the work within the nose, mouth and throat was of great importance to remove the original focus to prevent secondary infection of the tuberculous glands with pyogenic organisms. Very satisfactory results followed this line of treatment, and the radical resection of glands of the neck is practically unheard of in the large clinics in this country.

Case 45.—Neuroma of postauricular region. Man, age 52, for six months previous to his consulting a physician, noted a gradually increasing swelling below and behind his left ear. The surgeon who first saw him diagnosed the case as probable malignant growth of the parotid gland and operated for this. Two months following that operation the patient presented himself to me, with a recurrence of a semielastic growth at the angle of the lower jaw, which was associated with excruciat-

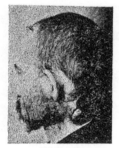

Fig. 145.

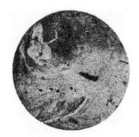

Fig. 146.

ing pains, locally as well as deep in the head and radiating to the vertex. I excised the growth down to the deep fascia. (Fig. 141.) The cavity thus created was left open for subsequent X-ray treatment, believing it to be malignant. A peculiar fact brought out by the operation was that the growth apparently had a capsule and the muscles were not infiltrated. Microscopic examination proved it be a true neuroma. (Fig. 146.) The wound healed very rapidly by the aid of a plastic, and the patient was apparently well (Fig. 142), but this only lasted three weeks, when another recurrence was noted with all the symptoms only more severe. (Fig. 143.) Several separate nodules now appeared in the old operated field. (Fig. 144.) He was now put on intensive X-ray treatment, with the result that the growth increased, but the pain was affected somewhat, especially right after each treatment. (Fig. 145.)

I finally decided to do a Gasserian ganglion operation, having failed with injections of alcohol into the foramen uvale. The operation consisted in the resection of the posterior root of the ganglion. Two years later the tumors were much larger, but there was no pain present.

I have had a number of these and allied forms of neoplasms, some of which were treated in conjunction with X-rays, and I have never observed any marked beneficial changes from X-ray treatment alone. The control of the pain was about the best that could be said for it.

Case 46.—Paraffinoma of external nose. Female, age 23, being displeased with the shape of her nose, which from a photograph appears not to have been deformed (Fig. 147),

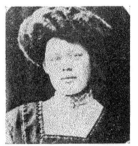
Fig. 147.

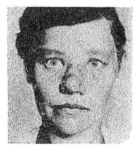
Fig. 148.

consulted an advertising quack (beauty parlor), who injected the bridge of her nose with paraffin. Two or three months later her nose began to pain her and showed a tendency to a bluish red discoloration. Shortly after that she noted that the mass injected was growing. She went back to him and he made an incision into it without any benefit. With this condition she presented herself to me, and I found that the mass was not confined to the place injected, but extended to the tip and side of her nose, with a small mass near the center of the forehead. Large blood vessels traversed the overlying skin. (Fig. 148.) Wishing to determine the histologic nature of the growth, I excised a small mass from the center (Fig. 149), which I allowed to remain open. I made a very interesting observation while dressing the wound, namely, an oozing out of paraffin proven microscopically. The swelling in

the center became much smaller and less red, whereas the
sides were growing and extending into the orbital cavities and
side of the face. (Fig. 150.) She had a great deal of pain in
the infiltrated parts, as well as radiating pain. The later conditions were not at all influenced by X-ray, radium or any
other applications, consequently I determined to operate—
that is, radically to resect all the paraffinoma possible. Under
general anesthesia, because it was impossible, either by local
infiltration or ethyl chlorid spray, to anesthetize the parts, I
dissected the apparently healthy overlying skin to either side,
as well as over the forehead (Fig. 151), and with considerable difficulty dissected out a number of fibrous masses. (Fig.
15.) These microscopically examined showed atypical paraf-

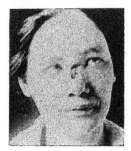

Fig. 149.

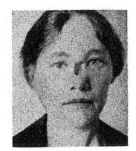

Fig. 150.

finoma in the proliferation stage—that is, many new blood
vessels forming throughout the tumor, rapidly obliterated by
active growth of connective tissue about these vessels. This
connective tissue acted differently from the usual inflammation. (Fig. 153.) Readapting the dissected flaps of skin, they
were held together by two or three horse hair stitches. They
healed very promptly, as shown in Fig. 154. There remained
a central defect which healed by cicatrization. The subsequent course is very interesting in that a slow ·regrowth may
be observed which, however, is not associated with pain. I
am employing 10 mg. of radium element, screened by ¹⁄₄ mm.
of aluminum for one hour every day, over different areas involved, and can see some effect from the treatment. The final
result will be most interesting.

I have had one other case that approached anything like the

one described. It is illustrated in my chapter in Loeb's Operative Surgery of the Nose, Throat and Ear. That case terminated in suicide. I have seen a number of ugly paraffin masses injected for cosmetic purposes, but not that grew like the two reported.

Case 47.—1. Leucoplakia of the tongue. 2. Lymphoma of the tongue. Female, age 41, had observed a white spot on the side of her tongue for about a year, which came shortly after she had some teeth drawn on that side. (Fig. 155.) Recently this white spot increased, consequently she consulted a physician, who diagnosed the condition. Fearing the possibility of a carcinoma developing, he referred her to me for radium treatment. I found that the healed alveolar process

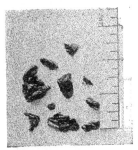
Fig. 151.

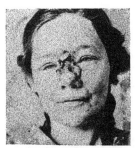
Fig. 152.

of the lower jaw had a very sharp edge, and when the mouth was closed the affected portion of her tongue came directly over this sharp edge. (Fig. 156.) Therefore I concluded that this was a case of decubital necrosis. I correspondingly advised her dentist to make a hard rubber plate (Fig. 157), which would prevent the tongue from coming in contact with this sharp edge of the jaw. At the same time I applied 10 mg. radium element, screened by 1/10 mm. of silver for one hour, every three days. This was held against the tongue by the dental plate. After two weeks there was nothing seen on the tongue.

Case 48.—Man, age 33, presented himself on account of a swelling of his tongue, which had been present for about two months. There was a great deal of itching in his tongue, causing him to consult a physician a week previous, who in-

serted a red hot electric needle into the tip. Examination revealed a triangular area of ischemic tissue at the tip, with a
central dark spot; within twenty-four hours there was a line
of demarcation of a slough. (Fig. 158.) At this time he com-

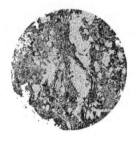

Fig. 153.

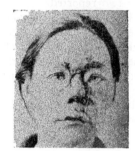

Fig. 154.

plained more of inability to swallow, and the whole of the
tongue felt boardlike and his tonsils like two tumors, almost
shutting off the breathing. There was no evidence of pus or
even inflammation. The patient was very pale, and the blood
examination showed a picture of a secondary anemia. There
was a leucocytosis present. The process of necrosis of the

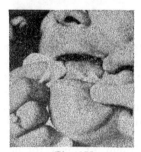

Fig. 155.

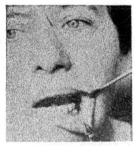

Fig. 156.

tongue rapidly progressed and completely sloughed off at the
tip. (Fig. 159.) I have had his tongue X-rayed, and to my
astonishment there was a marked effect on the healing of the
tongue ulcer, as well as a reduction in size of the tongue as a
whole. (Fig. 160.) The swelling of the tonsils was also
markedly reduced. He was given a general X-ray treatment,

arsenic internally and blood transfusion. For a day or two it looked as if he would recover. However, there was a sudden change for the worse, marked cerebral symptoms of anemia developed and he died. A section taken of the tongue

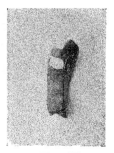

Fig. 157.

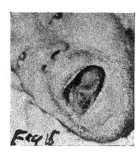

Fig. 158.

immediately after death showed microscopically a marked lymphocytic infiltration throughout the substance of the tongue. (Fig. 161.)

This is the only case of this type that I have seen, but I have had eleven cases of Hodgkin's disease, in which the tonsils were markedly enlarged, with symptoms to some extent

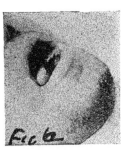

Fig. 159.

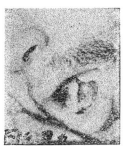

Fig. 160.

referable to the tongue. All these cases received X-ray treatment and also the other customary general treatment. The tonsils, like the glands in the neck, were beneficially influenced, but all the cases finally died.

My records show that I have seen and treated eighteen cases of marked leucoplakia of the tongue alone, and seven additional cases of tongue and cheeks. Nothing has ever affected them better than radium applications. Antiluetic treatment was absolutely of no value. X-ray was of some value, but I do not recall a single case that was permanently cured. I

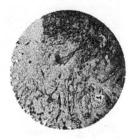

Fig. 161.

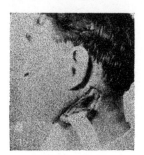

Fig. 162.

have seen four cases develop into an epithelioma, and one case very rapidly destroyed a patient's life by metastasis of a jaw cancer. Discontinuance of smoking had some effect on the denseness of the patches.

Case 49.—1. Chronic deep neck abscess, or woody phlegmon. Suspected malignant disease. 2. Perichondritis of the

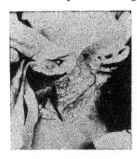

Fig. 163.

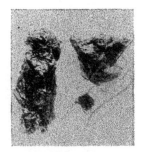

Fig. 164.

larynx. 3. Scleroderma involving larynx. Male, age 53, was referred with a swelling of the left side of the neck, located below the lower jaw and extending backwards to the occiput. It was hard, not painful, and had a somewhat inflamed skin surface which was adherent to the underlying mass. He gave a history that he had a mastoid operation three years before this swelling appeared. There was no evidence of any focus of invasion in the nose, mouth or throat. Removing a piece of the mass for microscopic examination, the wound was left open for X-ray treatment. (Fig. 162.) The mass was then

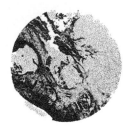

Fig. 165.

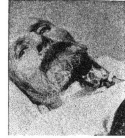

Fig. 166.

X-rayed by deep penetrations for one erythema dose, but no appreciable difference was noted following this. The microscope revealed the growth to be inflammatory. Patient being a physician, was anxious to return to his western home, and urged me to remove the mass by radical surgical procedure. To this I acquiesced, and under a general anesthesia removed

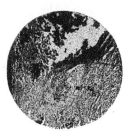

Fig. 167.

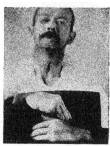

Fig. 168.

all I was able of the mass (Fig. 164), being compelled to liberate the vital structures of the neck, as the carotid artery, internal jugular vein and pneumogastric nerve. In the dissection there were areas that appeared suspicious, consequently I permitted the wound to remain open for subsequent X-ray treatment. I prepared a flap of the overlying skin, which I hoped to use in covering the wound, after being certain that there remained no cancerous tissue. (Fig. 163.) Examination of the resected mass at various points showed nowhere any microscopic evidences of malignant disease, only

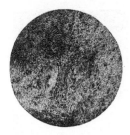

Fig. 169.

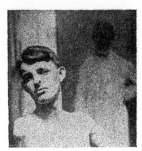

Fig. 170.

chronic inflammation with areas of necrosis. (Fig. 165.) The day following the operation, the wound discharged unusually much, and the discharge escaping over the healthy skin of the chest and shoulder caused a marked pustular formation. Examination of the pus showed a pure culture of a diplococcus. On the third day after operation there appeared a most dis-

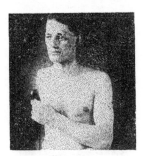

Fig. 171.

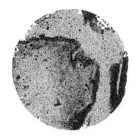

Fig. 172.

agreeable complication, namely, a softening of the internal carotid artery, threatening rupture. I immediately ligated low down near the sternoclavicular articulation. However, I did not shut off all the blood at once, not wishing to produce cerebral anemia. The same day the softened arterial wall ruptured with a very free bleeding, but the nurse stopped it by

hard pressure until I was able completely to ligate the artery.
Following immediately this ligation he developed a hemiplegia
on the right side.  He lived for two more days, dying, I believe, from weakness due to the shock and hemorrhage.

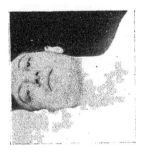

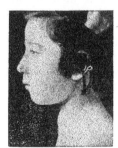

Fig. 173.                              Fig. 174.

I believe this patient had originally a Bezold's mastoiditis
with a sinking abscess of the neck.  This remained chronic.
the organism being inactive during all that time, but becoming very active under the influence of the X-ray and operative intervention.  The extreme lytic action of these bacteria

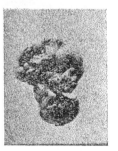

Fig. 175.                              Fig. 176.

I believe was responsible for the softening of the arterial wall
and other complications.  The lesson to be learned from this
case is that the socalled woody phlegmon or chronic cellulitis should never be subject to radical operation.  I have observed several cases of this woody phlegmon and have treated
them with X-rays.  Two of these became malignant, the

patient succumbing to the disease, however, more slowly than in the usual secondary neck carcinoma.

Case 50.—Male, age 62 years, was referred to me as a case of cancer of the larynx for radium treatment. He had considerable difficulty in breathing and his voice was much affected. Clinically it had the appearance of a carcinoma of the larynx.

Desiring to remove a piece of tissue from the larynx for microscopic examination as well as to introduce an intubation tube loaded with radium, I attempted to do a suspension laryngoscopy, but this was impossible on account of his struggles for air. Consequently a tracheotomy was performed. The examination of the microscopic examination was negative as

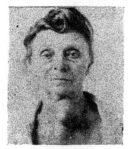
Fig. 177.

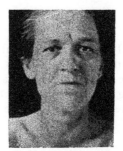
Fig. 178.

to cancer, and all it showed was an inflammation. (Fig. 167.) Patient received, on general principles, a crossfire application of radium element 25 mg. on the intubation tube and 100 mg. on the outside of the thyroid cartilage on the left side where the suspected malignant growth was located. The screening at the intubation tube was 1/10 mm. of aluminum, whereas outside there was a screen of silver ¼ mm. The radium was left in position for six hours. The immediate result on the breathing was good, but I considered it due to the mechanical effect of the intubation tube. Patient went back to his home town and his otolaryngologist reported to me that there appeared to be a steady progress for the worse. Three weeks later he returned and there appeared to be a marked increase both within the larynx and externally. Another piece of tissue was removed from the larynx and examination was again reported negative as to cancer. It was inflammatory; nevertheless, I advised a thyrotomy. On dissecting down on the swelling, my associate, Dr. Pollock, noted a sort of a fluctuation of the mass. Incision permitted the escape of a large quantity of thick pus, which contained very few microorganisms. This abscess was drained and the thyrotomy postponed. (Fig. 166.) The result now was striking in that the intralaryngeal growth entirely disappeared, and the patient began to gain in strength and voice. However, there recurred a most distressing and wholly unexpected complication. About two weeks after operation the patient had a chill, followed by high temperature (105°), evidences of swelling about the abscess cavity and a very septic appearance. From that time on for about

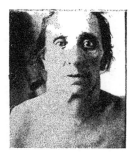

Fig. 179.

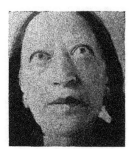

Fig. 180.

six weeks he had repeated chills and rises of temperature with a gradual loss of vitality, so that he finally succumbed to that complication. The wound itself did not demand any surgical interference and there was no doubt that the infection got into the system through the internal jugular vein. Ligation would have been the proper thing, but the patient was not a good risk for any operation.

I have seen not less than twenty-five cases of similar character that had all the clinical appearance of carcinoma, but later showed abscess; most of these cases are syphilitic perichondritis in the old. At present I have two cases of this form that are tuberculous in nature. The microscopic examination, however, reveals simply an inflammatory process not characteristic of either lues or tuberculosis, nor is there any other characteristic, physical or blood finding.

Case 57.—Male, age 43, for more than two years noted a scar formation in his skin all over the body, especially about the face, hands and feet. These scars contracted and produced a crippled condition of his hands and fingers, toes and eyelids. (Fig. 168.) He also noted that his voice and breathing became difficult. Examination of the larynx showed contraction and thinning of the mucous membrane. It became necessary to open the larynx to relieve these symptoms. A piece of tissue from within the larynx showed under the microscope it was purely connective tissue of chronic variety. (Fig. 169.) The thyrotomy was kept open for a long period (several weeks), during which time the patient received X-ray and radium treatment. The result was very satisfactory and he recovered

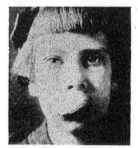

Fig. 181.

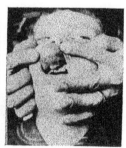

Fig. 182.

a fair voice and good breathing. The body as a whole received X-ray treatment with benefit. It must be added that large doses of thyroid extract was given during his stay at the hospital and after he left.

Case 52.—Keloid about the face. Man, age 26, while crossing an elevated railroad, tripped and fell on the third rail, which was highly charged with electricity. The accident caused a severe burn about the face and arm, necessitating the amputation of the arm. The resultant deformities from the loss of the alæ nasi, part of the upper lip and lid are shown in Fig. 170. The scars were distinctly keloid in character, and their removal was always followed by recurrent keloid. Fig. 172 shows a typical section of such scar formation, with the unusual hypertrophy of the epithelium covering the scars. I finally had applied X-ray and radium over these keloid areas, using always a screen of aluminum and leaving it in situ for two hours. Subsequent to this sort of treatment, I noted a softening of the scars, but the best thing noted was the non or slight reformation of the keloid after plastic operations of correcting the ala, lip and lid. (Fig. 171.)

I have treated a fair number of keloids about the face and have found nothing approaching the value of radium applications. From the X-ray I have not seen very much benefit, and surgically there is usually a failure, no matter how carefully one approximates the skin incisions. The internal administration of thyosinamin is perhaps of some value. I make use of it in every case.

Case 53.—Thyroid gland. A. Hyperthyroidism and exoph-

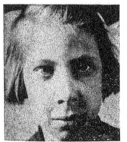

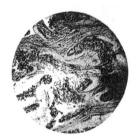

Fig. 183.                    Fig. 184.

thalmus. B. Lipoma. C. Malignant disease. Man, age 27, for more than a year has been suffering with nervousness, headaches and weakness and for the past month can scarcely walk. Also noted a swelling about his neck and a bulging of his eyeballs.

Examination shows a typical extreme thyrotoxic state with all the signs of a markedly progressed case. (Fig. 173.) He was immediately placed on appropriate X-ray treatment, with the result that within six weeks I could remove his tonsils, devitalized teeth and ligate the superior thyroid arteries. He recovered completely without any further thyroid operation.

Case 54.—Woman, age 48, has had for more than a year all the classical symptoms of hyperthyroidism, but no glands enlarged. The most marked symptom was the exophthalmos. (Fig. 180.) After seven erythema X-ray doses, it was noted that we could attempt to remove the various points of chronic infection. Consequently her tonsils and teeth were removed, and practically all her thyrotoxic symptoms disappeared, but the exophthalmos remained the longest—in fact, they never went back to normal. It was, however, noticed that whenever she received a diathermic treatment to the neck (over the region of the sympathetic ganglion) there was a temporary recession of the eyeball, as proven by the exophthalmometer.

I have treated many cases of thyroid gland disease not thyrotoxic, adenomatous and colloidal degeneration, and have observed but very transient benefit. However, the toxic symptoms were always favorably influenced.

Case 55.—Female, age 8. Mother noticed that the daughter

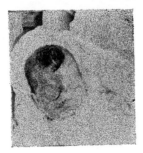

Fig. 185.

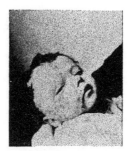

Fig. 186.

developed a swelling in the center of her neck, which for the past two months was growing. It caused no other symptoms. Examination revealed a soft nonpulsating tumor that extended from the thyroid cartilage below the sternal notch and quite a ways laterally. (Fig. 174.) Believing it to be a thyroid gland enlargement, she had received adequate X-ray treatment for three erythema doses without the least particle of effect. Consequently I operated and found a lobulated tumor indicative of lipoma. (Fig. 175.) The microscopic examination showed it be a lipoma. (Fig. 176.)

Case 56.—Female, age 59, had a neck swelling for several years, but recently it began to grow quite rapidly. She consulted a physician, who attempted to remove the growth, but the patient stated the doctor said he had to desist on account of uncontrollable hemorrhage. When she presented herself to me there was a hard nodular swelling extending the whole anterior part of her neck, causing considerable difficulty of swallowing. An old scar bisected the swelling. (Fig. 177.) Suspecting a malignant growth, either sarcoma or carcinoma, I had her given treatments, but after five erythema doses there was not only no benefit, but she became worse, especially in her breathing, so that I had to perform a tracheotomy. This was accomplished with considerable difficulty, because I had to plough through a very bloody tumor. I performed practically the whole operation with the Percy electric cautery, thus minimizing the bleeding. The patient lived fairly comfortably, so far as breathing was concerned, for about one month, but she lost rapidly in weight because she could not

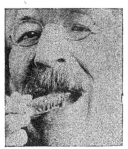
Fig. 187.

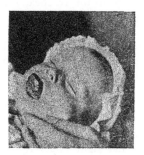
Fig. 188.

swallow. She refused a gastrostomy. The microscope demonstrated a highly vascular epithelial growth.

Case 57.—Female, age 61, had a large neck for many years, but noticed that during the past six months it grew more rapidly and became hard and nodular. She also had difficulty in breathing. (Fig. 6.) Suspecting malignant change, I had her treated by intensive X-ray for three erythema doses, but with no appreciable result. Desiring to relieve the pressure upon the trachea by lifting the gland away, I placed the patient on the table for a local operation. I had barely injected two drachms of apothesin and made the incision when the patient developed marked nervous symptoms, a very rapid heart beat, general tremors and vomiting, which I could not control. There developed a marked acetone breath, and in spite of all my efforts she died in less than twenty-four hours from symptoms of exhaustion.

Case 58.—Female, age 63, always had a swelling of her neck, but quite recently it began to grow very rapidly, so that when she presented herself for examination she could scarcely breathe or swallow. She had been for several weeks under the treatment of a competent physician, who said she received ray treatments without any benefit.

There was a very hard nodular mass practically surrounding the neck. (Fig. 179.) Attempts to intubate her with a stiff rubber catheter were futile, and since there was no time to lose I attempted to cut down to her trachea. In the attempt of going through a mass of soft, excessively bleeding tissue to the trachea, I found myself embarrassed by inability to stop the bleeding except by pressure, and when doing this I shut off her breathing entirely. In a frantic effort to reach the trachea I finally did open it, but the patient was exsanguinated and died on the table. I made an immediate postmortem and found that the growth had extended into the mediastinum.

Case 59.—Female, age 9. (a) Lymphangioma of lip. (b) Hemangioma of face and tongue. (c) Varices of the tongue. Ever since she was a little baby the parents noticed a swelling of her right upper lip, which had periods of enlargement and recession. Figs. 181 and 182 show the patient when she presented herself to me. It had a fairly firm doughy feeling and was not painful. Puncture revealed nothing. Suspecting a lymph vessel growth, I had her placed under X-ray treatment, which had absolutely no effect. I then put on 50 mg. of radium element, screened by ⅓ mm. of silver, for four, five and six hours, respectively, within two months. After a month of waiting I noted but very little change for the better, consequently I excised an encapsulated growth, following which I had a very good cosmetic effect. (Fig. 183.) The microscope verified my clinical diagnosis of lymphangioma. (Fig. 184.) There were many changes of an inflammatory character, which probably were due to the X-ray and radium treatment.

Case 60.—Child, age 1½. A few days after the baby was born the mother noted a small red spot about the right upper eyelid and this grew so rapidly that within a month the entire eyelid was involved. Various treatments were tried by the family physician, but nothing appeared to stem the progress. When I saw it, the appearance was as in Fig. 185. I decided to try out various modes of treatment, selecting the different portions involved and confining the particular treatment to that part. I applied the carbon dioxid snow over the area of the forehead. The eyelid I treated with 10 mg. of radium element, screened by ¼ mm. of aluminum. The cheek I injected with boiling hot water, the upper lip with X-ray, and the outer part of the cheek, ear and neck with minute ligations subcutaneously placed. The result, after very uphill and persevering treatment for nearly one year, was the complete disappearance of the growth, leaving a healthy but much scarified face. (Fig. 186.) The eyelids which received the radium treatment gave the best cosmetic and physiologic result. She had more than twenty applications of radium, always an hour duration, and there remained a perfectly transparent cornea. It is my intention when I am sure there will be no recurrence to do a facial plastic operation on her.

Case 61.—Male, age 64, complains of thickening of his tongue, especially on the sides. This condition has been in existence for the past two years, gradually getting worse. Examination shows a marked dilatation of the veins from the tip to the base, extending towards the floor, on either side. (Fig. 187.)

The base of the tongue veins were equally dilated. I could find neither a local nor general condition explaining this condition. Application of 25 mg. of radium, screened by 1/10 mm. of aluminum, and well covered by rubber tissue, placed between the tongue and floor of the mouth for six one-hour periods caused a marked diminution in the size of the veins.

The base of the tongue showed no particular change.

Case 62.—Baby, age 2 years, was born with a blue tongue, which gradually grew until there was not room enough within the mouth, and it protruded. (Fig. 158.) There were no great difficulties in breathing, but some trouble in feeding. Following one application of X-ray for 15 minutes by a medium tube, the tongue grew so rapidly that it became necessary to retract the cheek to allow air to pass for breathing.

The nasal breathing appeared to be shut off by pressure against the soft palate. The child weakened so rapidly and nothing could be done to stem the tide. It died in less than a week from the time the X-ray treatment was given.

I have treated eighteen cases of angiomata about the head and neck with very satisfactory results by various methods as indicated in the case. There is no question that the radium is the best means of treating it, especially if one has the larger plaques to apply over greater areas.

CONCLUSIONS.

1. Comparing cases treated before radium and the X-ray were in vogue, I find my records show a higher percentage of cures of malignant disease when these were not employed. This is contrary to the general belief.

2. There appears to be a toxemia develop in cases of malignant disease wherein large doses of radium and X-ray are employed which differs from the ordinary toxemia found in cancer or toxemia from X-ray and radium in nonmalignant disease. I am trying to determine if in the chemistry of the blood there could be isolated a substance and possibly prevented or neutralized. I have asked Dr. Gradwohl to assist me in determining this fact, and he has already shown me that one substance appears to be increased in the blood following treatment of malignant disease by means of massive dosage of radium and X-ray.

3. The earliest possible diagnosis of malignant disease with as thorough early operation without X-ray or radium treatment, either before or after operation, would be, in my judgment at the present, to the best interest of the patient.

4. I fully realize the greatness of X-ray and radium as to the possibilities of curing malignant disease, but thus far in my experience of nearly sixteen years, it has not demonstrated this value.

5. Realizing the great possibilities, I shall continue to experiment with them as well as any other substance or mode of treatment that promises at all any possibility of a cure of cancer.

6. As stated in the beginning of the paper, following up the cases and re-reporting on them is of the utmost importance.

7. In nonmalignant conditions there should be every effort made to determine the value of X-ray and radium, because there is everything to be gained and nothing lost but time. There are exceptions, as, for instance, thyroid gland enlargements without toxic states have been often treated by X-ray, procrastinating until these symptoms appeared.

8. The proper technic of applying X-ray and radium is essential; furthermore, the technic employed should be reported.

NOTE.—Since the presentation of this paper, more than a year ago, a number of cases here reported have undergone marked changes, and many new cases have been observed, upon whom the radium treatment associated with operation was employed. It would be well if I were able to amplify this article by reporting these cases, but there is neither time nor space at the present for such a publication; it will, therefore, be reserved for a future occasion. I have learned one or two very important facts which do not appear in the paper in regard to the mode of application of the radium needles. I refer to the danger of causing marked destruction in the close proximity to the radium needle applied within the center of the growth, and if at the same time there is a stimulating action of the radiation from the center to the periphery of the growth. Therefore in the employment of radium needles or, for that matter, any other applicators, it is best to treat from the periphery to the center. Another observation that is important is that while one may demonstrate microscopically true cancer cells in cancer areas treated by radium, I have noted in a number of instances that no regrowth occurred from these for a period of nearly a year. Are we to assume that such cancer cells are innocuous? Time only will tell.

I have treated a number of cases of malignant diseases of the upper respiratory tract with radium only, and without operation, and in several instances most remarkable results were noted. How permanent these will be again only time will tell.

## BIBLIOGRAPHY.

1. Reprinted from·Annals of Otology, Rhinology and Laryngology, June, 1916.

2. X-ray, Radium and Fulguration in Malignant Diseases of the Nose, Throat and Ear, 1907.

3. Annals of Otology, Rhinology and Laryngology, March, 1912.

4. Annals of Otology, Rhinology and Laryngology, March, 1914.

5. Annals of Otology, Rhinology and Laryngology, March, 1912.

6. Annals of Otology, Rhinology and Laryngology, June 1, 1916.

7. Read before Illinois State Medical Society, May, 1917.

8. Read before Middle Section American Laryngological, Rhinological and Otological Society, February 26, 1917.

## XXII.

## THE TONSIL QUESTION—RELATION TO DUCT-LESS GLANDS—FUTILITY OF OPERATIVE INTERFERENCE IN THE EXUDATIVE DIATHESIS TYPE OF CHILDREN.

By Grant Selfridge, M. D.,

San Francisco.

The modern tonsil operation had its birth twenty centuries ago, and to Celsus one must give the credit of performing the enucleation with his finger.

History does not tell us why the complete enucleation operation went into the discard, but it lay there in a state of "innoccuous desuetude" until it was resurrected by the late Dr. John Farlow of Boston, thirty-odd years ago. Apparently progressive Boston did not follow in Farlow's footsteps, and it remained for Chicago to relocate the operation, and it fell to Dr. Chas. M. Robertson to describe a new method of removing tonsils at the New Orleans meeting of the American Medical Association in 1903.

It was my privilege to meet Dr. Robertson and see his method of procedure, prior to the New Orleans meeting. On my return home I undertook to work out an operative technic, and to start a propaganda, based on observations made in the eastern states, that no tonsil was a good tonsil, and therefore should be removed forthwith.

Since that time we have watched the game progress, participating in it, to be sure, and have seen it claimed, in many articles on "Tonsils," that all diseases, between "fallen arches" and alopecia areata, including deformities of the nasal septum, high arched palates, as well as deformities of the teeth and jaws, are attributed to the tonsils, whether diseased or not

Even the layety, with and without medical advice, frequently have insisted on the entire removal of the tonsils for almost every conceivable infirmity, and frequently for self made diagnoses.

It is not surprising that mistakes in diagnosis have been made by the laity, when we note that rheumatisms have proved on more careful medical study to have been classified as syphilis, neuritis, flatfoot, pellagra, arteriosclerosis, etc.

Shambaugh of Chicago, in his public utterances and published articles, does not decry the reckless removal of tonsils, and yet he states in one article that one must not omit the precaution of emphasizing the fact to the patient about to have his tonsils removed that the operation may have no influence on his disorder. His private utterances, however, suggest that a large percentage of tonsils should only be removed under exceptional circumstances.

During the past ten or twelve years I frequently have had children brought to my office after operation on the tonsils, by the mother, to be told, "My child is no better," and after hearing this many times and reading the unexpressed thought —"we wish you would repay the expenses we have been put to," I began to inquire of myself, if there was not somewhere an explanation of this surgical failure. My inquiry has taken me to many places and made many interviews with some of the internationally famous laryngologists, and my final conclusion is that the evidence points to an interrelation of the tonsil with the ductless gland system, and that the failure to recognize such relationship helps to explain, to my mind at least, the cause of failures such as have been encountered by myself.

I do not wish to decry the value of the removal of tonsils in properly selected cases, but I do wish to say that my belief is that there is a well founded physiologic interrelation between the tonsils and adenoids, and the ductless glands, and think that the signs of dysfunction of the latter, as evidenced in the child and frequently in the parent, should have proper attention and proper medication first before the child is rushed to the operating room.

We believe, too, that the apparent gland dysfunction in many cases is sufficiently predominant and offers a satisfactory explanation for the many reinfections, colds, etc., seen in large numbers of children, grouped under the socalled exudative diathesis by Czerny, Lyman and others.

It is largely to this type of children, who have a history of beginning life with an eczema, drippy, watery noses, asthma, who have difficulty in digesting milk, fats, carbohydrates, eggs; who may have big heads and big bellies, fat pads, are slow in their mental development, and who may have signs of spasmophilia, or on the other hand, may be precocious, sway-backed, flat footed, have winged scapulæ, thin, velvety or dry skin, deformities of the ears, high arched palate, sex organ deficiencies, and perhaps other signs of status lymphaticus, that our attention, therefore, is particularly directed.

We must include in the above the sign of slight hypothy-roidism set forth in McGarrison's recent work, "The Thyroid" —i. e., "infantile constipation, unusual coldness of limbs; fail-ure of fontanelles to close with normal period, slowness in learning to balance the head or sit up; delayed eruption of the teeth, and their malformation, early caries of the milk teeth, lack of vivacity, intelligence and slowness to learn to smile, somnolence, lordosis, scoliosis, slowness to walk, small and weak muscles, mouth breathing and snoring, adenoids and lymphatic enlargement, slowness to talk, rickets, tetany, neu-resis, poor luster and growth of hair."

McGarrison in his book, quoting from Leonard Williams (Encyclopedia of Medicine, Surgery, London, 1912, page 265), summarizes his views as follows: "Adenoids and enlarged tonsils occur in children who have an inadequate supply of thyroid secretion. The hypertrophic condition in each case is apparently the result of an endeavor on the part of the organism to supply an internal secretion as nearly allied as possible to the one which is lacking. If the hypertrophy is not very pronounced, and if it has not been very long in exist-ence, great enough and protracted enough, that is, to produce complications, such as disease in the tonsils themselves or in the ears, then the exhibition of thyroid extract will cause their regression."

Otts (Alienist and Neurologist, 1913, page 116, 120) reports some interesting experiments with the powdered dried tonsil of the calf, and the evidence from the experiments "suggest that they (the tonsils) yield to the blood a hormone which influences the contractility of involuntary muscles (uterus) and the blood pressure, and possesses also a powerful diuretic action." (McGarrison.)

The frequent rather marked hypertrophy of other lymphoid structure in Waldeyer's ring, i. e., lingual tonsil and lymphoid masses behind the posterior faucial pillars—following the removal of the tonsils (complete enucleation) and the frequent filling in of the tonsillar spaces with lymphoid masses free from crypts—as mentioned by Bordley of Baltimore, as well as the persistent and oftentimes protracted vasomotor and vasotrophic changes seen in the pharynx and nose following operation, particularly in the exudative or anaphylactic type— above described—suggest strongly nature's effort to give to the economy a needed substance which surgery has removed. And the fact that the exhibition of minute doses of thyroid overcomes many of these symptoms lends support to this view.

The writings of Burt Shurley, S. P. Beebe and many other writers deal with the relationship of acute infection of the nose, nasopharynx, and particularly the tonsils, to hyperthyroidism with or without exophthalmus, though Shurley calls attention to certain pathology in the nose itself, present in hyper- and hypo-thyroidism.

While it is a well known fact that a case of simple goiter may be changed over night into an active hyperthyroid, through a sudden acute infection or a sudden shock, the fact of the patients having been probably a hypothyroid of years' standing, with parents perhaps of thyroid deficiency. is, I believe, frequently lost sight of, if considered at all, in this tonsilductless gland relationship.

That the recognition of the slight thyroid deficiency in early life and the treatment thereof might alter or prevent the advent of hyperthyroidism with exophthalmus, is evident.

Jules Glover (Paris) has called particular attention to the type of child presenting vasomotor disturbances of the nose. with watery discharge, and associated with recurrent swelling of the tonsils, unaccompanied by any signs of bacterial invasion and no increase in the bacteria normally found in the nose or on the tonsils. He also calls attention to a vasomotor condition of the nose following the removal of the adenoids. in subjects with subnormal pulse and temperature and signs of arrested development or general dystrophy. He finds the giving of thyroid in combination with phosphoric acid and with occasionally the addition of an extract made from the tonsil, result in marked improvement of the vasomotor condition, as well as improvement in general conditions and reduction in the size of the faucial tonsils.

Harvey Cushing ("Pituitary Body," page 247) says: "In view of the unquestionably close relation of many states of dyspituitarism, particularly those of primary glandular insufficiency, to lymph hyperplasia (status thymolymphaticus), it is quite probable that there may be a tendency toward adenoid formation in the pharynx, irrespective of the presence of a pharyngeal rest."

Citelli, who has produced more readable articles on the relation of adenoids to the pharyngeal hypophysis and central hypophysis in dyspituitarism, than any living laryngologist, seems to have proved by his anatomic studies of the region of the pharyngeal pituitary and central pituitary an anatomic connection between the two—a craniopharyngeal canal—occurring not infrequently in subjects showing a large adenoid development. His histologic studies have convinced him of a hypersecretion of the pituitary in several of the cases studied.

As a result of these studies and clinical observation, he has called attention to a psychic syndrome occurring in childhood and adolescence "which may be complete or partial, as follows:

1. More or less marked deficiency of memory.
2. Somnolence or sometimes insomnia.
3. Intellectual defects.
4. Difficulty in fixing the attention.

He has found that some of these cases improve after removal of the adenoid but finds the addition of pituitary extract feeding gives better results.

Among case reports, he mentions a man of thirty years of age, complaining of "heaviness in the head, loss of memory, sleepiness." Examination showed adenoids, hypertrophy of lower turbinates, nasal stenosis. Improvement in thirty days on pituitary feeding without operation.

Another case, boy of fifteen, with adenoids, loss of memory, sleepiness, intellectual torpor, aprosexia, weakness in legs. Removal of adenoids, but after 40 days little improvement of psychic symptoms. Then pituitary extract; soon great improvement.

Caliceti writing on "Hypophysary Feminism in Adenoid Subjects" seems to confirm the views of Citelli.

Whether the presence of adenoids in these cases causes the hypophysary symptoms or results from infections of the posterior nares or adenoids primarily, does not seem a settled question. It would seem to me from a careful study of Cushing's cases and my own, that there are evidences that the state of status thymolymphaticus was either acquired very early in life or was due to hereditary conditions, and thus the large size of the adenoids is simply an index of the dystrophy present.

Spolverini, writing about a series of nineteen cases of asthma seen in children, whose ages varied from six to ten years, says: "These children all showed more or less hypertrophy of the superficial or deep lymphatic glands, accompanied by tonsillar or pharyngeal hypertrophy, occasionally splenic or other tumefaction, pallor, facial eczema, low arterial pressure," etc. In other words, a status lymphaticus.

Haven Emerson, commenting on quite a large number of autopsies done on status lymphaticus adults, mentions the enlargement of lymphoid structures, the faucial, pharyngeal and lingual tonsils, and states definitely that these cases are especially prone to be overwhelmed by acute infections.

Ewing, "Military Aspect of Status Lymphaticus," says: "In infants, and before puberty, lymphatic hyperplasias, large thymus and signs of rickets are prominent, as well as hyperplasias of the lymphatic tissue in the tonsillar ring, intestine (Peyer's patches) and spleen."

Schlutz and Larson in "Anaphylaxis and Its Relation to Some Diathesis Common to Infancy and Childhood," have, as a result of their experimental work with guinea pigs, come to the final conclusion that "in at least one type of cases studied (inflammatory exudative diathesis, Czerny), definite anaphylaxis to foreign proteids exists, and probably the majority of the phenomena occurring in the condition are truly anaphylactic."

During my studies of the past three or four years I have tried to discover the underlying factors which help to explain the anaphylaxis occurring in hay fever and asthma, and it seems to me that such phenomena are more prone to occur in individuals of the status lymphaticus type.

This type of individual (exudative diathesis) should be properly classified among the "vagatonics," and he fits in well with the understood description of status lymphaticus. In addition to other physical signs, he does not stand the stress of life, he is not a good soldier, withstands infections poorly (as shown in the recent pandemics of influenza), and is easily overwhelmed by shock, whether from shell fire, food, animal hair or pollen proteins. His blood picture in a very large percentage of cases shows a neutrophile eosinophile increase.

Therefore, this type is entitled, in our opinion, to a careful hunt for the causes related to the anaphylaxis before surgery is resorted to. It goes without saying, however, that any focal infection, whether of the ear, nose, throat, teeth, gall bladder or appendix, should be removed, wherever found.

During the past year or so, I have seen some twenty-five children, from three to fifteen years of age, in addition to a fair number of adults, who have come with histories of hay fever, asthma and cold catching, nonbacterial in type. Most of these cases had their tonsils and adenoids removed prior to seeing me, and in none of these children had there been any improvement in their hay fever, asthma or "colds."

Few of these children were found sensitive to foods. Twenty-five per cent of the asthmatics have been found sensitive to animal hair protein, principally horse dander. Several to the orris root of face powder, a few to pollens, and some gave no reaction whatever.

The following cases may be of interest:

1. Child of four years, born at eight months, had a great deal of disturbances in early life from foods, was on a very carefully selected diet when I saw her.

Examination showed a serous catarrh of both ears, of two or three weeks' duration; a large adenoid and moderately sized tonsils. Opening both ear drums several times and treating the nose and throat did no good. The adenoids and tonsils were removed—the latter only on the insistence of the pediatrist. Improvement for a few days and then the ears were as bad as ever. A more careful study showed the child anaphylactic to orange juice, which was in her dietary. On removing this the ears cleared up in twenty-four hours and the child has had no recurrence in one year.

2. An adult, about thirty-five years old, seen four years ago during my active service at the Southern Pacific Railway Hospital for recurrent attacks of colds, watery in type, and serous catarrh of both ears. I had Dr. George Willcutt open both ear drums repeatedly. He straightened a deflected septum and removed the tonsils without effect. · The patient was then investigated for dietary disturbance and was finally found sensitive to potatoes. These were removed from his dietary and his ears cleared up. Two years later a similar attack following eating potatoes cleared up on removing the cause. This man had a thin, delicate skin, feminine in type, hair distribution also feminine in type, and shaved infrequently. He could be classified as a status lymphaticus type. His case is mentioned, as well as the preceding, to illustrate the need of careful study before operating. I am not the only one guilty of having followed an opposite course. I might say in extenuation, I was very early in the protein sensitization testing.

3. A boy of fourteen was put in the hospital for removal of his tonsils, principally because he had colds and because he was backward in school, and the operation had been advised by the family physician. I did not see him until he was under the anesthetic. Some cheesy material was found in his tonsils, otherwise nothing of moment about either the adenoids or tonsils. The boy looked like a little old man, his face was oldish, he had very dry skin, was thin, sex organs the size of a five-year-old. He was somewhat backward in school, but very fond of outdoor sports. He only had erupted four of his second teeth, and X-ray examination showed the congenital absence of six of the second teeth germs, and all the rest of the second teeth were unerupted and are scattered around in various directions in his jaws. What teeth he had are baby teeth except as noted.

He was not seen for several months following the operation, when the greatest changes were noted. The senile look had disappeared, the skin had become normal in texture and color, sex organs normal for age, except for feminine hair distribution. No change in teeth and no change in desire for study; twenty pounds gain in weight. Whole pituitary has .been given with some apparent improvement, and some thyroid, but neither have been taken with any regularity, perhaps due to parental indifference or lack of belief in the necessity of treatment. Both parents show signs of ductless gland deficiencies.

The results in this case are rather striking and unusual, especially the stimulation of growth of sex organs. The latter is hard to explain on any other basis than either the removal of an infection in the adenoid or relief of pressure on the pharyngeal pituitary from the adenoid. The improvement in metabolism is probably based on the removal of an infection in the tonsil which had a further influence on a hereditary hypothyroid subject.

5. Boy, aged thirteen, rather tall for his age; unusual sex organ development. Blood picture, polys. 54 per cent; lymph. 33 per cent; large monon. 2 per cent; eosinoph. 11 per cent. He gives a history of asthma, first beginning at the age of nine months. apparently following pneumonia and pleurisy at this time. The asthma has only occurred at long intervals and curiously only when there was a cat in the house.

For three years prior to September, 1919, when Admiral Rodman's fleet arrived, there had been no asthma. The gift of a cat from one of the officers brought on violent asthma.

On one occasion, three years ago, he had a severe attack of hives, following playing with a cat. No asthmatic history in family. The history shows that teething, talking, walking and school progress were normal. No apparent nervousness and the boy is quite even tempered. He has lordosis, flat feet, prominent scapulæ, long thorax, drop ears, high arch. palate, deflected septum and irregularities in teeth, slightly dry skin, unusual sex organ development. Tonsils and adenoids have not been removed. Eating rolled oats gives him hives. so his mother says, and eggs disagree. Skin tests for these are negative. He was tested with all foods, bacteria, some pollens and animal hair, and proved to be sensitive to cat hair, crab, veal and ray grass. He was given immunizing doses of cat hair protein, the cat was sent away, and as the boy was apparently thin for his age and height, was put on small doses of thyroid extract.

The net result for eight month is: No asthma, infrequent colds, gain in weight of fifteen pounds. Tonsils and adenoids appear reduced in size and without surgery.

6. Boy, aged fourteen, 5 feet 3½ inches in height, weight 106 pounds. Blood picture: hemoglobin, 90 per cent; polys. 42 per cent; lymph. 45 per cent, large monon. 3 per cent, eosin. 10 per cent. His mother's emphatic announcement to me was "all my boy's troubles have followed the removal of the tonsils!" The history briefly is: Was bald until one year old. Had frequent colds. Tonsils partly removed at the age of seven; after that bronchitis began to develop, and severe sneezing colds occurring with great frequency during the year. In January, 1919, he had influenza. Following this asthma developed. In April, 1919, the tonsils and adenoids were re-operated, and the lower turbinates partly resected to relieve the sneezing and asthma, without benefit.

His mother says he was slow in every way except in his school. His personality was somewhat of a supercilious make up, rather irritating in type.

Examination showed a deflection of the septum with hypersensitive tubercle of the septum, nothing else in the nose and throat. He had flat feet. lordosis, prominent scapulæ, sex organs very much undeveloped for his age. He was put on anterior lobe pituitary extract, grs. 4, daily. A few days of this gave him some headache, insomnia and nausea. The dose was reduced to gr. ½ daily, and in a short time increased to gr. 4. Locally two drops of 95 per cent alcohol were injected into the tubercle of the septum (both sides), which seemed to relieve the sneezing for a few weeks, but returned in about six weeks.

The pituitary extract has been continued to date (seven months), and the result is that the asthma seems to have stopped, the sneezing gone and the cold catching tendency vastly improved. He has had but two severe attacks of asthma during this period, one of which appears associated with eating a lot of indigestible food, the other with an attack of bronchitis. Sex organs have begun to develop in a very satisfactory way, disposition has improved. He is in the hands of a gymnasium teacher, to be taught proper breathing and exercises to strengthen his abdominal and back muscles, and there is every hope of making a fairly normal young man.

## CONCLUSIONS.

Physicochemistry has to do with the origin and evolution of life, and if the chemical actions, reactions and interactions in the human body are controlled by the various ductless glands, then any alteration of the chemical interactions of the body may bring about disturbances of the body growth and disturbance of metabolism.

Inasmuch as the thyroid appears to be the great regulator of metabolism and particularly of carbohydrates, and as disturbances of metabolism as well as disturbances of the autonomic nervous system are outstanding in the anaphylactic type of individual, we believe such evidence of pathologic physiology should influence the medical man of today to a more careful study of the patient before ordering surgery directed to the nose and throat, that may result in harm and do the patient no good.

## BIBLIOGRAPHY.

Byant, W. S.: "The Clinical Possibilities of the Pharyngeal Pituitary," Medical Rec., Sept., 1916.

Beck, C. J.: "Evolution of the Tonsil and Adenoid Operation." Surg. Gyne. and Obs., 1914.

Cushing, Harvey: "Pituitary Body and Its Disorders."

**Citelli: "Sui rapporti fisio-pathologico tra sistema ipoficario e varie lesione di lunga durata sia del faringe nasale che dei seni sphenoidali su una special sindrome psichica ela sua cura 'hivist'," Ital. di neuropat, 1911, IV, 481; 529.

**Citelli: "On the physio-pathological relations between the hypophysic system and various chronic diseases of the naso-pharynx and sphenoid cavity." Leitschr. f laryngal. Rhinol. Wurzl, 1912. V. p. 513,—5.

**Citelli and Caliceti: "Three Adenoid Patients with Hypophysary Feminism." Policlin. Rome, 1918. XXV. Sez. Pra 245, 250.

**Citelli: "Sull" effecacia terapeutica deli 'estratto d'lpofisilenla sindrome psichia de ma descritta' Boll, d.mal. d areech d. Gola e dnaso Firenga 1914, 169, 176.

**Caliceti: "Hypophysary Feminism in Adenoidal Subject." Pediatria, Naples, March, 1919. XX/ V. II 16.

Emerson, Haven: "Status Lymphaticus in Adults." Arch. Int. Med., January, 1914.

Ewing: "Military Aspect of Status Lymphaticus." J. A. M. A., November 9, 1918.

**Glover, Jules: "Tonsillar Function, Nasal and Pharyngeal Vaso-Motor Disturbances." Opotheraphy. Aun de med. et. chir. infant, February, 1909.

Lyman, Geo.: "Dietetics of Eczema." Arch. Ped. 1915.

McGarrison: "Thyroid Gland." Wm. Wood & Son, 1917.

Osborn, H. F.: "Origin and Evolution of Life." Scribner & Sons, 1918.

Ott, Isaac: "Action of Tonsil." Alienist and Neurologist, May, 1913.

Shurley, Bert.: "Manifestation of Thyroid Disease in the Upper Respiration Tract." Laryngoscope, March, 1911.

Schultz & Larsen: "Anaphylaxis and Its Relation to Some Diseases Common to Infancy and Childhood." Arch. Ped., December, 1918.

Shambaugh, Geo.: "Discussion of Clinical Problems Relating to the Faucial Tonsils." Surgical Clinics of Chicago, December, 1918.

**Spolverini: "Sulla etiologia e pathogenesi della nervosi asthmatica infantile la Pediatric." Napali, 1918. XXV: 569.

---

**These articles were translated for me by Mr. W. A. Brennan of the John Crerar Library, Chicago.

# XXIII.

## THE NORMAL AND PATHOLOGIC PNEUMATIZA-
## TION OF THE TEMPORAL BONE—
## A REVIEW.*

By Norval H. Pierce, M. D.,

Chicago.

It may seem to you rather extraordinary that a whole evening should be devoted to a consideration of a single man's work on one subject. I feel, however, that the matter is of such vast importance, and is so intimately connected with the practical, everyday work of otologists, that the time will not be misspent.

The work which we are to review was published in 1918 and consists of two volumes—one a volume of text containing 296 pages; the other, a volume of illustrations and 111 microphotographs of serial specimens of mastoids on which the conclusions of Wittmaack are based. I have had fifty of them reproduced for stereopticon demonstrations. The work was commenced about twelve years ago when Wittmaack began to accumulate his anatomic material for the study of cholesteatoma.

In order to bring before your mind the far reaching revolutionary character of these conclusions, it will be necessary for me to recall to you that up to the time of the appearance of Wittmaack's work anatomists divided the pneumatic portion of the temporal bone into three normal types: (1) The pneumatic mastoid, (2) the mixed form, in which the pneumatic structure was more or less equally divided with the spongy structure of the bone, and (3) the compact mastoid, in which few or no pneumatic cells were present. This was considered normal, just as the color of the various types of irises is considered normal. Variation in the pneumatic structure was not in any way regarded as the result of disease.

---

*Read before the Chicago Laryngological and Otological Society, January 3, 1921·

It is true that Wittmaack drew upon the work of various investigators in support of his thesis. He accepts the mode of pneumatization as described by Wildermath and others of the Strasser school, in their studies of the pneumatization of the bones of birds; in the pathologic processes he draws upon the work of such men as Bezold, Siebenmann, Toubert, Moure. Canapele, Lombard, Kanasugi, Preysing, Görke, Reitschel and others.

He divides the normal pneumatization of the temporal bone into three stages. Under undisturbed conditions the mastoid process at the end of the first or beginning of the second year consists of spongiosa. From then until about the fifth year it is a mixed spongiosa pneumatic structure, and from then on we have a complete pneumatizing proceeding. In the first period we have the formation of the cavum, recessus and antrum. At birth these cavities are filled with a myxomatous tissue which is covered with cuboid epithelium. At first there is a mere slit existing between this gelatinous tissue and the tympanic membrane. Gradually the embryonal tissue is absorbed or disappears, and the epithelium following it lines the air containing cavities: first, the cavum, then the recessus and at last the antrum. Normally when this pneumatization is undisturbed the submucous tissue consists of a very thin layer over the bone, and the epithelium changes from the cuboid type, normal in the embryo, to the endotheliated epithelium of one or two cells in depth.

At the end of the first or beginning of the second year the second stage begins and consists in the entrance of myxomatous tissue in the marrow cavities of the underlying spongiosa. The cells of these cavities are absorbed and at a given time the epithelium from the antrum dips down, and as it dips down the myxomatous tissue is resorbed until it becomes the submucous layer with the epithelium covering it. Thus an air space is made. This process goes on continuously by the invasion of marrow spaces by the myxomatous tissue until consecutively the air cells are completed at the end of the fourth or beginning of the fifth year.

The third stage extends through life and is denominated by Wittmaack as the stage of interstitial pneumatization. This consists of the formation of small pneumatic spaces communi-

cating with the larger spaces which are formed in early childhood in the nodal points of the network which forms the cells
of the preexisting pneumatic spaces.

His conclusions are: (1) The development of pneumatic
systems in the temporal bone—that is, the tubal cells, the
tympanic cells and the mastoid cells follows a more fixed mode
of developmental process with far greater regularity than has
heretofore been believed. (2) The normal structure of the
pneumatic process is characterized by a far reaching pneumatization and not by a sclerosing process. The individual
peculiarities in the formation of the pneumatic system in later
life—that is, after the fifth year, is not manifested by the
peculiarity of the mastoid as a whole, but only as an interference in the peripheral structure of the pneumatic system. It
will be seen, therefore, that he recognizes but one type of
normal mastoid and that is one in which complete pneumatiza-
tions occur. The presence of spongiosa is a sign of arrested
development.

What is the cause of this arrested development? And here
perhaps we have the corner stone of Wittmaack's deductions.
In seeking for the cause of this disturbance of pneumatization
he reasons that the cause must primarily be searched for in
the middle ear mucosa, the osseous structures evidently playing a secondary part in the process of pneumatization. Even
in the normal process it is quite evident that the bone is sub-
ordinate to the changes which are wrought in it by the submucous myxomatous tissue. It has been known for a long
time and written about by many authors that the middle ear
of the newborn and sucklings is subject to a peculiar inflammatory process which has been denominated the otitis media
of the newborn, otitis media concomitans, etc. It is latent in
its character and course and is discovered most frequently at
the postmortem table. According to Solowzow, over ninety
per cent of all newborn children and infants are subject to
this inflammatory process in the middle ear. Preysing, Görke,
Rietschel and more lately Göffert have extensively investigated this form of otitis media. The frequency with which
it is found in children or infants rendered it difficult for Wittmaack to secure a large number of undoubtedly normal temporal bones in the first year of life. Much more easily could

temporal bones with this inflammatory process of the mucous membrane be secured. He concludes that the process is not physiologic but is undoubtedly a pathologic condition, and this view is supported by the presence of pus in the cavities of the middle ear and the known anatomic changes in the mucosa. These anatomic changes have been especially studied by Görke and Rietschel, and they agree that there are two definite types, a plastic and an exudative form, and Wittmaack suggests as a result of his investigations that these may be divided into a latent insidious type and a more acute form with a relatively rapid course. To these forms Wittmaack adds the hyperplastic changes in the plastic otitis media and an atrophis form with an exudate. It is evident that in the majority of cases we have a mixed type of these pathologic changes. The pure type of the first group is, however, clinically without symptoms and is, therefore, unsuspected during life. How this can affect the pneumatization will appear later.

The cause of this latent, symptomless, insidious form of inflammation was ascribed first by Aschoff to the aspiration of amniotic liquor, vernix or meconium into the tube and then into the cavum. The entrance of this irritant may occur in fetal life (aspiration of amniotic liquor), or during the time of birth (aspiration of amniotic liquor, vernix and meconium). The pollution of the cavum with amniotic liquor is, according to Aschoff, the cause of the presence of leukocytes in the cavum of the newborn. According to this view, otitis media neonatorum is not an infectious process, but rather a reaction to a foreign body. It does, however, according to Hartmann and other authors, render the structures more disposed to bacterial invasion. This is in agreement with the frequency with which bacteria are found in the exudate of the middle ear of newborn children. However, the foreign body reaction with sterile exudate may effect changes in the mucosa which will interfere with or check pneumatization. In fact, Preysing in a great number of all ears which he examined in the newborn found an exudate which was sterile. Among the infected cases the pneumococcus was by far the most frequently found. The changes wrought by the inflammatory process in the mucosa are characterized by a more or less intensive infiltration of the superficial layers of the mucosa and the epithelium with round cells, dilatation of the blood cells and production of an exudate containing more or less pus corpuscles. The epithelial strata is changed to an extent that the ciliated epithelium (forming the tube) is found in places far removed, in the recessus and even in the antrum, areas in which the ciliated epithelium is never found in normal conditions. On this point Wittmaack differs from Preysing and Görke. His conclusion, based on a study of a large amount of material, is that the extension of ciliated epithelium over the mucosa of the middle ear must be regarded as a pathologic process. He has proven by experiments on the lower animals—rabbits, cats, etc.—by his production of a purulent inflammation in the ear that he can produce a spreading of ciliated epithelium.

The normal epithelium of late fetal or early infantile life in the cavum is cuboidal-in character, which changes under normal conditions to the epithelioid type. The persistence of the cuboidal epithelium and the presence of ciliated epithelium Wittmaack regards as a mark of pathologic changes. The persistence of the cuboidal and ciliated epithelium coincides with other evidences of pathologic conditions in specimens showing interference with pneumatization, to a degree that suggests that his views are correct. Moreover, these abnormal epithelial types are not present in normal pneumatization.

Allowing for a relatively broad individual latitude in normal regression of the submucous tissues, there comes a time in the third to the fourth month where a normal type may be differentiated from an abnormal type. There can be no doubt that in the presence of the inflammatory process under consideration the superficial layers of the mucosa and the deep subepithelial myxomatous tissue shows no tendency to regression but, on the contrary, displays a tendency to thicken. Wittmaack differs from Preysing in this regard and criticises one of his illustrations which Preysing displays as a normal mucosa as being evidently an abnormal condition dependent upon an inflammatory process. Wittmaack believes that a normally developed mucosa cannot be differentiated into various layers, and when this is possible it is due to disease.

We have, then, the persistence, more or less complete, of the embryonal subepithelial myxomatous tissue, but undoubtedly a proliferation of the same. We have then an exquisitely hyperplastic mucosa rich in blood vessels. The superficial layer under the epithelium shows marked infiltration with round cells. Also there is a typical formation of lymph follicles. This thickening of the subepithelial tissue is especially to be found in the niches of the cavum and recessus. Another change which is characteristic of this condition is the formation of granulation nodules.

The point is made by Wittmaack that this inflammatory process causes the total or partial arrest of the recession or disappearance of the myxomatous embryonal tissue. This does not occur in a regular manner over the entire surface, but in a very irregular manner depending largely upon the inflammatory intensity at a given point. It can be readily understood how bridges of membrane may thus be formed by an incomplete resorption or abnormal strands of tissue, especially in the recessus epitympanicus and about the foot of the stapes—anywhere where there are sharp corners and depressions.

Granting that the inflammatory process causes persistence of the thick subepithelial portion of the mucosa represented largely by a hyperplastic type derived from the former myxomatous tissue, and remembering the manner in which the epithelium follows the myxomatous tissue into the marrow spaces of the bone, it can be readily understood how the process of pneumatization is arrested. It seems that the subepithelial tissue is deprived of its power of invading the marrow spaces, and where this does occur in a limited manner the epithelium has no power of penetrating, but remains as a level layer on the thickened submucous tissue.

He concludes, first, divergences from the normal structure of the mastoid depend without exception upon typical processes in consequence of changes in the character of the mucosa in the first and second years of life.

Second, the changes in the character of the mucosa may be grouped under the hyperplastic and fibrous types.

Third, the hyperplastic type develops from a latent insidious plastic inflammatory process in the mucosa.

Fourth, the fibrous type depends on an acute exudative inflammatory process.

Fifth, whether disturbance of the pneumatization is partial or complete depends upon the intensity of the changes in the mucosa.

Sixth, every type of disturbance of pneumatization gives a typical structure picture of the mastoid—

    I. Complete arrest of pneumatization.
        a. By hyperplastic.
        b. By fibrous mucosa.
    II. Partial arrest of pneumatization.
        a. In the hyperplastic inflammation (severe, intermediate and light grade).
        b. By fibrous mucosa (prolonged pneumatization).

Seventh, the concurrence of hyperplastic with fibrous changes in the mucosa occur with relative frequency and lead to mixed forms of structure types, sometimes with one and sometimes with the other component predominating.

What relationship does pathologic pneumatization bear to changes in the tympanic membrane? As the tympanic membrane is the one visible portion of the otic structures, it is interesting and important to know whether the changes in this membrane bear any relationship to pathologic pneumatization. Wittmaack is unable to say at the present time just what relationship slight and moderate anomalies in the tympanic membrane bear to the pneumatization process. This is readily understood when we remember that changes occur rapidly in the tympanic membrane after death. He believes, however, that he is safe in saying that the manubrium in the otoscopic examination lies in a course that is nearer to the posterior external auditory canal than in normal cases and the circumference of the tympanic membrane appears more oval and is smaller than normal in cases of disturbance of pneumatization. In other words, the infantile type of the tympanic membrane persists. Changes in the tympanic membranes themselves may or may not have a relationship to the character of the mucosa within the cavum. He points out, however, that slight diffuse and regular cloudiness of the tympanic membrane with a diminution in the luster is an indication of disturbance of pneumatization, together with the other changes in the mucosa which accompanies these disturbances. This cloudiness is due to increase in the cuticle layer of the tympanic membrane and the decreased luster is due to a greater desquamation of the superficial layers. The cuticle layer of an entirely normal adult consists of a single layer of perfectly flat epithelium and this gives a bright luster. In hyperplastic changes of the mucosa we often find the deep cuticle layers composed of cuboid cells. The subepithelial layers show a thicker and richer vascularity. The superficial layers of epithelium are raised in lamella, which give them a rougher surface. This gives the cloudiness and lack of luster of the tympanic membrane on otoscopy. This is a normal condition in the first period of development and reaches frequently into the second period. In this way it is explained why in sucklings and small children we seldom find a tympanic membrane with the luster of the adult tympanic membrane. We very frequently find by otoscopy atrophy of the tympanic membrane in connection with the fibrous changes in the mucous membrane with complete or marked arrest of pneumatization. This is due to the arrest of the membrana substantia propria.

Abnormalities in the tympanic membrane are associated with arrested pneumatization indicated by spotting of the tympanic membrane by areas of thickening associated with areas of atrophy, the areas of thickening appearing as whitened islands, while the areas of atrophy give a darker tone to their translucence and the color of the membrane within the tympanic cavity.

Calcareous deposits in the tympanic membrane are not associated with changes in pneumatization. Peripheral cloudiness of the tympanic membrane is frequently associated with changes in the mucosa accompanying pathologic pneumatization.

What is the relation of pathologic pneumatization to the accessory mucous membrane bands and folds? It is known that in the recessus epitympanicus is found a number of ligaments and duplicatures of the mucosa. Wittmaack attempts to answer the question. What is the absolutely normal anatomic content of the epitympanic space? If we confine ourselves to the temporal bone with a completely undisturbed development we can say that in the recessus we find, besides the two folds, the ligamentum malei externum sive laterale, the ligamentum malei superior and the ligamentum malei anticum. Occasionally one or the other of these ligaments is lacking. Especially is the ligamentum malei superior inconstant. It is absent with relative frequency in high tegmens and well developed pneumatic cells.

When the bones are examined at a time when the myxomatous tissue is not yet completely absorbed, the anlage of these ligaments can be discerned within the tissue in the form of fibrillary strands and presents a resistance to the ingrowing epithelium similar to that displayed by the ossicles.

The development of the inconstant socalled accessory folds frequently occurs from the incomplete absorption of the subepithelial tissue. In this way small bridges of tissue or sheets of tissue originate, reaching from one wall to the other of the epitympanic space. Zuckerkandl has previously described the development of accessory folds in a similar manner.

The arrest of pneumatization in the mastoid has a tendency to draw the sigmoid sinus forward, a very practical fact to remember in our operations on such cases. Especially noteworthy is the protocol in one of his cases (No. 38), in which complete arrest of pneumatization is pictured, and where the displacement forward of the sigmoid sinus is most marked.

In summing up the relationship which arrested pneumatization bears to other parts of the temporal bone, we find:

1. There undoubtedly exists a certain relationship between pathologic pneumatization and certain anomalies of the tympanic membrane, lusterlessness, cloudiness, atrophies, scars, etc.

2. Changes in the tympanic membrane cannot be regarded as always constant accompaniments of pathologic pneumatization.

3. In entirely normal pneumatized temporal bones we find only the constant ligaments in the epitympanic space. The development of accessory folds is a sign of pathologic pneumatization.

4. The displacement forward of the sigmoid sinus is found in pathologic pneumatization. The higher grades of displacement only with the worst form of disturbance of pneumatization.

5. The persistence and unusual breadth of the fissures is an accompaniment of pathologic pneumatization.

It is apparent that the work of Wittmaack explains many hitherto unexplained problems. It explains, for instance, the socalled chronic catarrhal otitis media which arises from apparently no cause and which has been explained on the hypothesis of an acute diathesis ' or a catarrhal inflammation. It explains the chronic tubotympanal inflammation, or at least places these conditions in an entirely new light.

The more important conclusions as regard the relation of arrested pneumatization to inflammatory disease of the ear may be summed up as follows:

I. Practically all severe forms of suppurative middle ear involvement develop in temporal bones with pathologic pneumatization insofar as this depends on continuous extension from the tube.

II. Chronic middle ear suppuration exists on the basis of complete arrested pneumatization, or the severest forms of disturbance of pneumatization, with markedly hyperplastic mucosa and develops in the child:

A. Chronic suppuration of the mucosa on the ground of the acute exacerbations of the suckling.

B. The chronic cholesteatoma suppuration, either (a) after acute necrosing otitis through ingrowth of the epithelium in consequence of large peripheral defects of the tympanic membrane, or (b) as an insidious process with intake of the pars tensa after sequestration of the antrum recessus from the cavotubal cavity in consequence of adhesions from Shrapnell's membrane, or an atrophy above, or adhesions above or below the posterior folds; (c) middle ear suppuration with epithelization or combination recessus cavum and cavum cholesteatoma suppuration and a combination of the process which leads to cholesteatoma formation.

III. The form which the chronic suppuration and its course pursues is preordained by the anatomic changes within the several cavities of the middle ear before the appearance of the clinical symptoms. Also, the secondary and end processes, such as the extent of perforation, epidermization, polyp formation, scarring, etc., depend upon a preformed anatomic substratum.

IV. The acute middle ear suppurations develop with predilection in medium and lighter grades of disturbance of mucosa and corresponding character of the mucous membrane.

V The greater the hyperplasia, the thicker the epithelium, and the less the pneumatization, the greater is the tendency toward the occurrence of acute inflammatory processes and eventually a protracted course, and the less, on the contrary, is the tendency to frank mastoiditis and vice versa.

VI. The character of the secretion in an acute otitis media stands in direct relationship to the character of the mucosa. Thick, highly hyperplastic mucosa with ciliated epithelium is especially apt to produce a mucous or mucopurulent secretion. Slight hyperplasia with flat epithelium gives thick, purulent, tenacious secretion. Fibrous changes predispose to a thin fluid, serous or seropurulent secretion.

VII. Normally pneumatized temporal bones are most frequently infected in acute middle ear disease with resulting frank mastoiditis.

VIII. Middle ear inflammations of tubercular and luetic character exist on the anatomic substrata of the mucous membrane and its accompanying disturbance of pneumatization. Their course depends also on the changes in character of the mucosa as it occurs in the course of pneumatization.

The relation which pathologic pneumatization bears to endocranial complications is most interesting and important. In the pictures which I shall cause to be thrown on the screen you will find how frequently abnormal vascular communications persist between the abnormal mucosa, the meninges, the bulb of the jugular and the sigmoid sinus.

It would be impossible to give a complete account of the monumental work performed by Wittmaack. We must be content with this short and incomplete sketch.

Before closing I must, however, accentuate the very kernel of Wittmaack's deductions, namely, that nearly all inflammatory diseases of the middle ear, in their genesis, nature and course are dependent in certain anatomicodevelopmental changes in structure of the mucosa and osseous structures of the ear. Most of these alterations in structure are caused by a latent, insidious, inflammatory process which occurs in early life. In other words, if in late life an individual develops middle ear inflammation (catarrhal) with adhesions, fixation of the stapes, etc., or the special suppurative type of inflammation is predestined when the occasional cause arrives by the changes which have occurred in the first years of that individual's infancy. On this fundamental principle he has erected a plausible, logical structure which must be proved or disproved by future investigations. True, there are discrepancies, and here and there we discover findings and conclusions which are susceptible of quite different interpretations, but on the other hand he throws light on many dark corners of otology and explains in a logical manner many points of pathogenesis which have heretofore been merely surrounded with meaningless words.

# XXIV.

## SARCOMA OF THE MASTOID.

By Harry Friedenwald, M.D., and Joseph I. Kemler, M.D.,

Baltimore.

Malignant tumors of the middle ear and mastoid are very rare. This is especially true of sarcomata. Haug[1] found only fifteen cases of malignant growth of the middle ear and neighboring structures in all the literature written during the period of twenty years from 1870 to 1890, while Neuhart[2] could find only eight cases published in the United States up to 1918. Bezold[3] observed one case of sarcoma in a series of 5,227 cases of ear diseases. In the records of the London Hospital,[4] averaging 200,000 general patients per annum for a period of ten years, not a single one occurred. There was no case found in the ear clinic of Vienna[5] among 10,157 patients.

Some of the latest textbooks on diseases of the ear, such as Kerrison,[6] Barnhill,[7] and Politzer,[8] make no mention of sarcoma, while Dench,[9] Urbantschitsch[10] and Ballenger[11] refer to it briefly under the differential diagnosis of such conditions as retroauricular abscesses.

While carcinoma occurs more frequently after the age of forty, and sarcoma in the young, yet several cases of carcinoma have been reported in very young persons by Alexander,[12] Knapp[13] and Nager.[14] On the other hand, Milligan[15] reported a case of angiosarcoma in a patient sixty-three years of age.

In 1898 Brose[16] reported a case of sarcoma in a child three and a half years of age. Patient had slight pains in the ear for six months without otorrhea. Then a growth appeared in the canal with very offensive discharge. It was looked upon as an ordinary polypus and removed, but it recurred very quickly. This procedure was repeated several times until the mastoid became greatly enlarged. There was neither fever nor other ill health. An operation for simple mastoid was undertaken; neither pus nor cheesy matter was found, but instead a soft reddish gray fleshy mass which upon compression yielded a pale grayish white juice. This mass was easily removed with a sharp curette. Bleeding was not severe. The tumor filled the mastoid cavity, antrum and ear canal and was completely cleaned out. It recurred very quickly, and signs of new growth were observed at the end of one week. The facial nerve soon became paralyzed. Dysphagia and aphonia developed. Patient died nine months after the first symptoms appeared. Microscopically the growth proved to be round and spindle cell sarcoma.

Christinneck[17] reported two similar cases in 1894 and 1896. Another case reported by Haug[18] in 1894 was that of a girl eighteen years of age with a chronic otorrhea of fifteen years' standing. The canal was filled with granulations which were removed with profuse bleeding. These granulations recurred in great masses, involved the surrounding tissues and, in six months' time, extended to the lower maxilla. The mass became ulcerated and discharged pus. Masses of tumor also made their appearance in the mouth and nose. The hearing became very bad. The facial nerve was not attacked. No sound could be heard upon catheterization of the eustachian tube on the affected side. The submaxillary glands were enlarged. An operation was performed nine months later, namely, a thorough exenteration of the tumor masses. There was no excessive bleeding. Recurrence, however, was rapid. Meningitis developed and the patient died two months after operation. On pathologic examination the growth was found to be a small round cell sarcoma.

Kipp[19] in 1902 reported a case of a boy five years of age with a chronic otitis media and polypi of several months' duration. He was treated for three weeks, when the mastoid became involved and an operation was necessary. On opening the mastoid a large cavity above and in front of the tip was found, filled with granulations of large size and greenish color. The cavity extended far in towards the pharynx. The bone was found exceedingly soft. A radical mastoid was performed. From every part of the wound there was an unusually rapid and very abundant growth, which was again removed three months later. This procedure was repeated several times, when the patient began to complain of severe pain in the head. Paralysis of the facial nerve followed, optic neuritis also became evident and the growth assumed a very large size. The patient died six months after operation. The tumor, removed after death, weighed six pounds, eight ounces and measured 25 inches in circumference. Microscopically it proved to be a small round cell sarcoma.

In 1903 Dench[20] reported a case of endothelial sarcoma occurring in a child of eighteen months, with paralysis of the sixth nerve. X-ray therapy was applied, with temporary disappearance of the tumor. The patient, however, died ten weeks later from recurrence. This case was not operated upon.

One case of carcinoma has been reported by Treitel[21] and Danziger,[22] which followed closely upon an attack of influenza. A history of trauma from four weeks to nine months before onset of symptoms was noted in two cases reported by Milligan.[23] All the reported cases resulted in death within one year from the time the growth appeared except a case published by Tobey,[24] which was seen four years after operation with no signs of recurrence.

Chronic otitis media is not necessarily present, but on the contrary, sarcoma has usually been found in previously healthy ears. As a rule the beginning is unattended by any marked symptoms, but as soon as the canal is perforated there is a fetid discharge with the formation of polypi and granulations filling out the entire canal and extending into the mastoid, causing softening and destruction of the bone cells. These soon break down and fluctuation results. This has been mistaken for retroauricular abscess. The origin of the tumor can rarely be ascertained, as it grows very rapidly and infiltrates the neighboring tissues. According to Schwartze,[25] it may arise from the mucous membrane of the middle ear or from the antrum and then involve the entire mastoid, the parotid gland and eventually extends down the neck.

The superficial tissue ulcerates, while deeper down it involves the facial nerve, penetrating into the temporal fossa and resulting in death from six to eight months after onset. The granulations when removed cause more or less bleeding and there is rapid recurrence. Histologically round and spindle cell sarcoma is the type commonly found.

The case we wish to report occurred in a man 42 years of age, well built, a singer by profession, who sought medical aid November 5, 1918, on account of a slight reduction in hearing in the left ear. The family, history was negative. He is married and has four children. There was no history of tuberculosis or cancer in the family.

Past history: Patient had had a facial paralysis on the right side three years before, of which he still presents some evidence. He remembers no other serious illness during his entire life. Patient had been examined by one of us six months previously and found to be in perfect health except for a slight laryngitis, which cleared up very quickly under treatment. During the epidemic of Spanish influenza of 1918 he suffered a rather severe attack with no ear complications at the time, but upon recovery claims to have noticed a defect in hearing in the left ear .which still persists. He has neither pain nor discharge from the ear. Neither has he lost weight. At this time, three months after his illness, he has recuperated perfectly.

Upon examination the right ear is found normal. The left ear: The auricle is of the same size as the right. Half way in the canal a perfectly round fibromalike mass is seen filling out a little over two-thirds of its lumen and is attached to the posterior wall by a rather broad pedicle. Through a small speculum the tympanic membrane can be seen to be intact.

Hearing test: With "A" tuning fork, Weber to the left, Rinné positive both sides, Schwabach lengthened five seconds on the left side; $C^2$, $C^4$ tuning forks and Galton whistle heard perfectly on both sides; whisper heard at eighteen inches on left; watch heard only three inches on the left and eighteen inches on the right.

Looking upon the growth as a simple fibroma, it was removed with cold snare. Bleeding was so profuse that a suspicion of malignancy arose, and much to our surprise the microscopic section showed "spindle cell sarcoma." The growth recurred quickly and filled up the entire canal. The patient began to complain of slight pains in the ear and mastoid region, although there was very little swelling and tenderness. There was a fetid discharge of bloody and purulent matter.

The operation was delayed for two months on account of the indecision of the patient.

On January 2, 1919, two X-ray plates taken gave the following information: "There is an absence of bone destruction in the auditory canal, the upper mastoid cells present but hazy, the lower cells are absent, and in their stead there is a large area of lessened density." Diagnosis given by roentgenologist was as follows: "There has been destruction of mastoid cells from some cause, either mastoiditis or malignant tumor."

The operation was performed January 7, 1919, three months after onset. An incision was made as in simple mastoid operation; the periosteum was found normal; the cortex was very thin. The cells of the mastoid process and antrum were destroyed and replaced by masses of tumor and an exudate of a pale yellowish color filling out its lower half. The growth did not extend into the aditus, and therefore the middle ear was not explored. The dura over the posterior fossa was found exposed. The lateral sinus wall was so eroded that while cleaning off tumor masses from its surface there was profuse bleeding. Otherwise there was little bleeding during the operation. The posterior wall of the auditory canal was partly removed. The entire cavity was packed with gauze and dressed as usual.

The dressings were changed on the fourth day. There was no bleeding, but a fetid discharge was found. Patient was subsequently dressed daily and the odor disappeared quickly. Recovery was slow, the wound closing in three and one-half months. The auricle became much enlarged soon after the operation, swelling subsiding slowly and by the time the wound was healed the auricle had returned to normal size. The canal was still very much narrowed and a minimal discharge was present. This also disappeared three months later.

The patient was last seen in April, 1921, more than two years after operation. He has had no recurrence and is apparently in good health. Hearing is the same as when he was first examined. He has been carefully examined by competent internists and neurologists, and metastasis have not been discovered. There has been no facial paralysis on the side of the tumor.

This case is of especial interest for the following reasons:

First, it is the only case on record where the origin is definitely known to be somewhere in the mastoid cells. Second, it follows closely upon an attack of influenza. Third, this case has survived a period of more than two years and shows neither

### BIBLIOGRAPHY.

1. Archives fuer Ohrenheilkunde, XXX, p. 126.
2. Laryngoscope, Vol. XXVII, p. 543.
3. Cited by Brose, Archives of Otology, Vol. XXVII, No. 4.
4. Cited by Neuhart, Laryngoscope, Vol. XXVII, p. 543.
5. Cited by Brose, Archives of Otology, Vol. XXVII, No. 4.
6. Diseases of the Ear, Philip D. Kerrison, 1913.
7. Principles and Practice of Modern Otology, John F. Barnhill, 1911.
8. Diseases of the Ear, by Edward Bradford Dench, 1919.
10. Lehrbuch der Ohrenheilkunde, Victor Urbantschitsch, 1910.
11. Diseases of the Nose, Throat and Ear, Ballenger, 1911.
12. Diseases of the Ear in Infancy and Childhood, Gustave Alexander, 1914, p. 363.
13. Cited by Behrens, Transactions Amer. Laryngol., Rhinol. and Otol. Soc., 1905, p. 452.
14. Ueber die bildung von Labyrinth sequester bei Mittelohr carcinom, Verh. d. Deuchen Otol. Geselschaft, 1908, p. 130.
15. Archives of Otology, 1896, Vol. XXV, p. 263.
16. Archives of Otology, Vol. XXVII, No. 4.
17. Christinneck, Archives f. Ohrenheilkunde, Vol. XVIII, p. 291, and Archives f. Ohrenheilkunde, Vol. XX, p. 34.
18. Archives fuer Ohrenheilkunde, XXX, p. 126.
19. Kipp, Transactions of Amer. Otol. Soc., Vol. VIII, p. 63.
20. Zeitschrift f. Ohrenheilkunde, Vol. XLV, p. 172.
21. Ueber das Karzinom des Ohres, Zeitschrift f. Ohrenheilkunde, 1898. Vol. 33, p. 152.
22. Beitrage zur Kentniss des Felsenbeinkarzinom Archives f. Ohrenheilkunde, 1896, Vol. 41, p. 35.
23. Journal of Otol., Rhinol. and Laryngol., 1911, p. 258.
24. Boston Medical and Surgical Journal, 1911, Vol. CLXV, p. 726.
25. Handbuch der Ohrenheilkunde, Vol. II, p. 609.

# XXV

# THE MINOR ROLE OF THE CONDUCTION APPARATUS IN SLOWLY PROGRESSIVE DEAFNESS.*

By Francis P. Emerson, M. D.,

SURGEON MASSACHUSETTS CHARITABLE EYE AND EAR INFIRM-
ARY, OTOLOGIST MASSACHUSETTS GENERAL HOSPITAL,

Boston, Mass.

' The function and relative importance of the conduction apparatus, given a normal end organ and normal hearing, is well understood. The physics of sound production, transmission and perception in health obey definite laws that are accepted by all aurists in principle, if not in detail. The object of this paper is to ask your consideration to the relation of the conduction apparatus to certain pathologic conditions that have resulted in or are causing deafness.

Our present conception of the etiology of nonsuppurative deafness has been influenced by the gradual differentiation of the function of the perception and conduction apparatus. Among the many questions that could not logically be explained by attributing to the conduction apparatus the cause for the progressive loss of hearing through interference with the sound waves, was the difficulty in accounting for the upper part of the scale always being lost first. This was usually accompanied by tinnitus—that is, labyrinthine irritation. Again, in progressive deafness there was a tendency for the hearing test to become equal, until by the time the low limits had been raised to about 512C² the Rinné and low limits would not vary even a few seconds for the two sides. It was not conceivable that the pathology of the eustachian tube and middle ear could result in equal loss of function in so many cases. Third, when suppuration had resulted in the destruction of the membrana propria, with necrosis and sloughing of the malleus and incus, it was observed that in many cases the hearing was

---

*Read before the American Laryngological, Rhinological and Otological Society at Boston, June 3, 1920.

exceptionally good, especially if the process was of the fulminating type. At times even sound perception might be painfully acute, although the conduction apparatus was disorganized. This leaves only the stapes. Is this indispensable to normal hearing? If we have an immovable stapes with a normal end organ, even this condition, if it were possible, would not preclude fairly good hearing for the spoken voice. When the stapes become fixed in the oval window, as the result of fibrous bands formed during the course of a chronic nonsuppurative otitis media, the perception apparatus has been functionally impaired long before the stapes loses its mobility. When fixation of the stapes is accompanied by profound deafness there is also an associated perception deafness that is more important than the condition of the oval window. It is then outside the concduction apparatus that we must look for the real cause in progressive loss of hearing. In the experience of the writer, there is no such thing as a pure conduction deafness. In every case of deafness, in whatever category you may classify it, there is diminished tone perception from the beginning. It is this impairment of tone perception that is the important problem in any attempt to arrest or restore lost hearing. Lastly, it is common knowledge that nerve deafness frequently follows acute and chronic systemic poisons and that certain drugs in full dosage have a disastrous effect on the organ of Corti. These findings make it necessary to reconstruct our otologic concept to conform to the newer pathology, or, as so often happens, confirm our clinical findings but explain the etiology in accordance with our recent views. It is true that certain types of infection show inflammatory reaction that in one case is confined to the mucous membrane, in another to the fibrous tissue and in still others to the osseous elements as end results. These manifestations of involvement of the middle ear are of secondary importance, however, as compared to the question of damage, temporary or permanent, to the end organ. Let us take the nomenclature of the last international congress and try and interpret it along these lines. In the child obstructed with adenoids, or in the adult with tubotympanic catarrh, the deafness is not due so much to the closure of the eustachian tube and the interference with the conduction apparatus as such, but rather that the closure of the tube is followed by absorption of air in the middle ear, indrawing of the membrana tympani, impaction of the stapes in the oval windows and labyrinthine disturbance. This is accompanied by tinnitus and a loss of tone perception in the upper part of the scale which is functional for a time, but is ultimately followed by nerve degeneration. To be sure, in a child with adenoids, the low tone limit may be raised temporarily. This becomes normal, however, as the eustachian tube opens, but the loss in the upper tone limit continues if the loss of hearing is progressive. When, therefore, in a case of chronic catarrhal otitis media the low limits are again raised, the upper limits have been markedly cut down. This would indicate that the progress of chronic deafness was not because of increasing obstruction in the middle ear, but because of further impairment of tone perception.

In those cases of (O. M. C. C.) chronic tubotympanic catarrh we find not only that the upper tone limits were lost first, but that where the course has extended over a number of years there may be also areas of tone deafness with the lower limits unchanged. These findings are accompanied by a ground glass appearance of the membrana tympani, loss of the light reflex and indrawing. Where the changes in the membrana tympani were characteristic there was no question as to diagnosis. There was a type of case, however, that did not show changes in the membrana tympani and where we were accustomed to find a clean nasopharynx. These cases were classified as catarrhal adhesive otitis media, or, if the deafness was pronounced, with changes in the bone conduction, they were called by some beginning otosclerosis. It was not uncommon to find typical changes on one side and a clear membrana tympani on the opposite side, and yet the hearing, after a number of years, might be almost identical. This type of case, whether atypical chronic catarrhal otitis media or not, begins with loss of the upper tone limits and tinnitus. There may or may not be areas of tone deafness. As the disease progresses the hearing gradually tends to become the same on both sides, the tinnitus becomes more high pitched, and there may or may not be vertigo. The progress of the disease is not, in the judgment of the writer, influenced very much by the changes in the conduction apparatus. The primary step is a closure of the tube, causing intralabyrinthine changes in the perception apparatus, and a raising temporarily of the low limit. The process in the eustachian tube may then run its course and yet the deafness goes on, influenced by the acute exacerbations of a toxic focus, i. e., after the deafness is once established it is progressive, not because of increasing mechanical obstruction from adhesions, tissue thickening or bony deposits in the conduction apparatus, but because of loss of tone perception from damage to the end organ, from the reaction to a definite chronic infection. That the upper conversational limit is first impaired has been confirmed by the audiometer of Dr. Dean.

Silent areas occur so often in nonsuppurative otitis media that the hearing test may be misleading. If we happen to test our bone conduction with a fork corresponding to the silent area it would, of course, not be heard or be transmitted to the other side. Even an approximately correct conclusion in regard to hearing cannot be reached without using all the forks from 96a to $2048C^4$, nor without several tests by the same observer in a given case. As before stated, the upper part of the scale is lost first, and, as we would expect, both air and bone conduction are lowered for certain forks unless there is a concurrent middle ear, for sound waves, produced by the striking of a given fork, are registered in the same part of the perception apparatus, whether passing through a media of air or bone. It follows, then, that with no obstruction in the middle ear any lowering of bone conduction must be accompanied by a lowering of air conduction for the same fork. On the other hand, any obstruction in the middle ear would raise the bone conduction and lower the air conduction for forks below $512C^2$. The higher the fork required to register a lowering of bone conduction the better the prognosis (Miss C. G.) The hearing test alone with all the forks is the only guide in estimating the remaining function in any given case of deafness. This is only a help, for no hearing test and no aural examination now known can tell us whether nerve degeneration has actually commenced. The evidence increases that while we may have pure nerve deafness we never have pure conduction deafness; the fact that some nerve impairment exists in every case of deafness was not recognized, as in the usual tests we rarely resorted to all the forks. The loss of the upper register, whose lower limit is roughly indicated by the whispered voice, is then prima facie evidence that the deafness is due to damage to the end organ.

Inspection of the membrana tympani gives us no information as to the function of hearing, neither does it enable us to form any conception as to whether we can hold out any hope for the future. The immobility of the membrana tympani, malleus or incus, areas of atrophy, or even the absence of the membrana propria, do not justify a gloomy prognosis nor give much information that is helpful to the patient. These are end results, and unless we have some definite pathology that explains the different steps that have led up to this condition and can determine whether the cause is still active, we are not in a position to do the patient any good.

Etiology.—From the experience of the writer, the primary infection, so far as the deafness is concerned, is usually in the lymphoid tissue. In children, primarily, in tonsil and adenoid infection. In adults, without regard to age limit, usually in the tonsils, especially the supratonsillar fossa, with secondary involvement of the surrounding lymphoid tissue, especially in the pharynx. These foci date back to the infectious diseases and are subject to repeated exacerbations. Even when there is obvious sinusitis or bony necrosis in the mandible, in the majority of cases there had been a preceding chronic infection in Waldeyer's ring, which apparently started in the tonsil. The lymphatic connection between the supratonsillar fossa and the middle ear is direct, and there is usually a history of sore throats as a child but none of late years.

Prognosis.—The writer is willing to admit that he does not know from the first examination whether an advanced case will improve or not. It all depends on the amount of damage to the perception apparatus. The membrana tympani, malleus and incus may be gone and the promontory bare, and yet if this was the result of a sudden explosion of a virulent infection the nerve function would be but little impaired. On the other hand, the membrana tympani may appear almost normal, with a progressive secondary nerve atrophy so far advanced that the case is beyond help. It is rarely the case that one ear (usually the one last infected) does not improve. We have much to learn in the treatment of those cases where nerve degeneration has actually commenced. After the cause has been removed, whether we can, in these advanced cases, reclaim any lost function by auditory reeducation, electricity, the use of strychnin, etc., is still an open question. The removal of toxic foci thoroughly must always be an individual equation. The war experience has taught us that much can be done by perseverance in restoring lost function. In the judgment of the writer no department of otology offers so much encouragement or so large a field of usefulness as the treatment of slowly progressive deafness.

Treatment.—Treatment of the eustachian tubes, either by bougies or inflation through a septic field, is never justifiable as a routine and never does any good in chronic cases. It can readily be understood that anything causing a secondary pharyngitis would have a bad effect on the hearing. As a matter of fact, the writer has never seen marked improvement in hearing in chronic deafness from any treatment that did not include freeing the supratonsillar fossa of infected tissue, whether this be in patients of ten or sixty-five years of age. Do not try to increase the mobility of the ossicles or pay any attention to the conduction apparatus except to free it of infection. Remember that toxic products are being constantly thrown into the circulation and that the perception apparatus suffers first from toxemia and then from nerve degeneration. In a certain number of cases the writer believes that after all sources of reinfection have been removed that much can be done by reeducation of the perception centers. That is, the central end organ does not seem to interpret the sound waves on account of functional disuse. On the other hand, it looks as though the highly specialized nerves, like the nerve of hearing, when degeneration has commenced, was uninfluenced by treatment. Experience has shown that very many cases given up as hopeless on account of nerve degeneration, were only functionally crippled. These cases will improve and stay improved with no other treatment than removal of the cause of the deafness. Moreover, these cases are not unusual, for it is the exception if one ear or the other does not gain if the low tone limit is still unchanged.

B.—O. M. C. C.  S. S.: Eight years; school; Dec. 27, 1919. P. H.: T. and A. operation at Massachusetts General Hospital three months ago.  Measles two months ago and since then she has been deaf with ringing in both ears.  Examination: Ears—A. D., membrana tympani indrawn; dull; no thickening.  A. S., membrana tympani indrawn; light reflex present but not clear.  Pharynx: Epipharynx blocked by a large adenoid.  Sinuses: Transillumination clear except over ethmoids.  Diagnosis: Infective O. M. C. C.

| R | | L |
|---|---|---|
| 2/25 | W. V. | 2/25 |
| 14/6 | R 256C | 16/6 |
| — | W | — |
| 64 | L. L. | 64 |

Treatment: Adenoid removed under gas.  Feb. 24, 1920. Has ha da cold for two weeks.

| R | | L |
|---|---|---|
| 25/25 | W. V. | 25/25 |
| 20/9 | R 256C | 15/7 |
| | W>+ | |
| 40/13 | 512C$^2$ | 45/18 |
| 62/22 | 1024C$^3$ | 40/20 |
| 22/7 | 2048C$^4$ | 18/10 |
| 32 | L. L. | 32 |

(Hearing tests made by A. M. A.)

Result.—This case improved in hearing distance twenty-three feet without Politzerization or any direct treatment of the ears.  The noises still continue.

Terminal stage in a case of slowly progressive loss of hearing extending over twenty years:

Mrs. R.—Fifty-two years; married.  P. H.: Always well. No history of acute infections.  Under constant treatment directed especially to the tubes by a competent aurist.  No history of vertigo or tinnitus.  A. U.: Ground glass appearance. L. R. gone.  No areas of atrophy or thickening.  No stapes fixation.  Examination: Transillumination negative; no pus in nares; M. M. normal; septum straight; breathing free; no infection.  Pharynx: Lateral pharyngitis marked, but whole pharynx shows a low grade pharyngitis.  Tonsils: Cryptic tonsillar disease and mucopus in both.  Pharyngeal secretions changed and patient gets up every morning to clear her throat and sometimes during the night.

P. S.—The chronic focal infection in the tonsil, low-grade pharyngitis and infection of the lymphoid tissue in the mouth of the tube followed by deafness would seem obvious.

| R<br>Shout<br>7/15 | W. V.<br>R 512C²<br>W>+<br>Galton | L<br>Shout<br>5/15 |
|---|---|---|
| — | L. L. | — |
| 256 | 1024C³ faint in A. D. | 256 |
| | 2048C⁴ not heard in A. D. | |
| | 2048C⁴ faint in A. S. | |

Fulminating case with great damage to middle ears. Marked improvement in hearing (without inflation), because the perception apparatus was not injured sufficiently to be followed by nerve degeneration.

Miss C. G., 28 years; B. Sweden; single; salesgirl. Ref., Dr. N. P. H.: Measles four years; aural discharge from both ears until 15 years old; then T. & A. operation and ears were dry until six months ago. Has colds every winter with swellings under jaws and soreness back of ears. No general illness since the measles but does not feel strong.

Examination: A. S.—O. M. S. Ch.; A. D.—Eff. O. M. S. Ears examined by Dr. C. T. P.

Considerable tonsil tissue in supratonsillar fossæ containing mucopus. Transillumination negative. Band passing from left eustachian tube to posterior pharyngeal wall. Low grade pharyngitis.

| R<br>Shout<br>27/45 | W. V.<br>R 512C²<br>W | L<br>1 1/2/25<br>28/46 |
|---|---|---|
| 256 | L. L. | 256 |
| N | U. L. | N |

A. S.: Directly ahead promontory is covered with granulations of watery pink color. The membrana tympani is entirely absent in the posterior half. Posteriorly can be seen niche of round window. Anteriorly and above remains of malleus. Shrapnel's membrane is covered with grayish membrane. Slight discharge. Diag.: O. M. S. Ch.

A. D.: Dry. Horseshoe shaped perforation involving entire portion of membrana tympani up to anterior and posterior ligament. Malleus intact with lower end tied down to promontory by band of adhesions. Underneath posterior superior border of perforation can be seen incudostapedial joint. Along posterior border of perforation can be seen niche of round window. Promontory is covered by mucous membrane. Tinnitus like steam. Diag.: Eff. O. M. S. Teatment: Tonsillectomy at Massachusetts Charitable Eye and Ear Infirmary, October 31, 1919.

Miss C. G.—

| | Jan. 8, 1920 | | | Jan. 19, 1920 | |
|---|---|---|---|---|---|
| R | | L | R | | L |
| 8/25 | W. V. | 3/25 | 8/25 | W. V. | 4/25 |
| 7/17 | R 256C | 16/23 | 12/21 | R 256C | 11/21 |
| 20/32 | 512C$^2$ | 18/30 | 34/45 | 512C$^2$ | 20/40 |
| 20/33 | 1024C$^3$ | 21/31 | 32/20 | 1024C$^3$ | 45/33 |
| 14/10 | 2048C$^4$ | 12/7 | 16/9 | 2048C$^4$ | 19/9 |
| 128 | L. L. | 128 | 96 | L. L. | 96 |

| | Feb. 17, 1920 | | | Feb. 24, 1920 | |
|---|---|---|---|---|---|
| R | | L | R | | L |
| 25/25 | W. V. | 8/25 | 25/25 | W. V. | 20/25 |
| 10/19 | R 256C | 13/19 | 9/15 | R 256C | 9/15 |
| 43/33 | 512C$^2$ | 35/29 | 22/17 | 512C$^2$ | 15/33 |
| 42/30 | 1024C$^3$ | 32/27 | | $+<$W | |
| 10/16 | 2048C$^4$ | 7/10 | | | |
| 96 | L. L. | 64 | 256 | L. L. | 64 |
| | $+<$W | | | | |

Result: In this case the conduction apparatus, if compared to a chain, has two or three links missing in its most vital part. The left ear still has a scanty discharge. The patient has had active ear involvement from childhood until twenty-eight years old, and yet the right ear gained twenty-five feet in four months and the left nineteen feet. No inflation at any time. After removal of the tonsils the accompanying infection in the pharynx and tube was treated as long as improvement continued. (Hearing tests made by A. M. A.)

B. O. M. C. C. (INFECTIVE).

Sept. 27, 1919. Miss R. A., 23 years; in college; home, California. P. H.: For six to eight years catarrhal colds. Last year throat infections; T. and A., two years ago; rheumatism in arms and shoulders at fourteen years; measles at seven years. Four years ago A. D. commenced to be dead; A. S., one year later. No tinnitus or vertigo. Thinks hearing is not so good as one year ago.

Examination: A. D.—Membrana tympani dull and indrawn; L. R. broken. A. S.—Membrana tympani indrawn; L. R. faint. No areas of atrophy or thickening. Palate pale.

| R | W. V. | L |
|---|---|---|
| 3/25 | | 2/25 |
| 18/32 | 512C² | 22/37 |
| 32 | L. L. | 32 |

Treatment.—Infection cleared up. No inflation or any direct treatment of the ears.

Result.—From the first test one would hardly have expected the hearing to return to almost normal. The whispered voice improved from 3 feet to 25 feet.

| R | W. V. | L |
|---|---|---|
| 25/25 | | ·25/25 |
| 12/21 | R 256C | 10/18 |
| 27/16 | 512C² | 28/15 |
| 25/35 | 1024C³ | 26/39 |
| 14/7 | 2048C⁴ | 11/17 |
| | W>+ | |
| 64 ? | L. L. | 32 |

The tonsils were removed two years ago, but apparently she had no after-treatment for the epipharyngitis and tubes.

Miss A. M. C. Nov. 26, 1919. Single; 38 years. P. H.: Puffing tinnitus in right ear for seven years. Much worse for last two or three years. Slight vertigo. No history of aural discharge. Deafness has gradually developed. Has had an impacted molar removed: Tonsils and adenoid operation, also had tonsillar crypts burned with cautery recently. Duration of deafness uncertain.

Examination: A. D.—O. M. C. C.; M. T., dull, indrawn; L. R., broken. A. S.—O. M. C. C.; M. T., dull, indrawn; L. R. broken. X-ray of sinuses shows slight increase in density over the right antrum. The left ethmoid cells are hazy. Teeth negative.

Throat: Low grade pharyngitis. Tonsil remains, especially in upper part of fossa. Mucopus present.

Operation Dec. 30, 1919. Fenway Hospital. Tonsillectomy. Right antrum found negative.

| | Feb. 2, 1920 | | | March 2, 1920 | |
|---|---|---|---|---|---|
| R | | L | R | | L |
| 1 1/2/25 | W. V. | 4/25 | 1/25 | W. V. | 25/25 |
| 0/7 | R 256C | 0/7 | 7/8 | R 256C | 8/7 |
| — | W | | | W>+ | |
| 13/33 | 512C$^2$ | 13/26 | 14/22 | 512C$^2$ | 17/31 |
| 13/37 | 1024C$^3$ | 25/35 | 26/15 | 1024C$^3$ | 31/39 |
| 18/9 | 2048C$^4$ | 14/10 | 5/8 | 2048C$^4$ | 7/7 |
| 512 | L. L. | 128 | 256 | L. L. | 96 |

(Hearing tests made by A. M. A.)

Result.—In the right ear the lower limit was reduced from 512 to 256. The left ear gained 21 feet for the whispered voice and the low limit was reduced from 128 to 96.

N. H. B., 42 years; mill superintendent, Maine. Jan. 22, 1920. P. H.: Weight, 210 pounds. Nose broken when a child and deflected to the right. Deformity includes the bony framework. Deviation of septum to right occludes that side completely. Any nasal irritation is now followed by lacrimation, anterior nasal discharge and redness of the nose, accompanied by sneezing. Sleeps with his head raised and cannot stand much cold air. Has been growing deaf for seven years. Cannot hear his watch in the right ear by air conduction. Does not consider that his right ear is of any use in conversation. Two sisters are deaf. No general illness.

Examination: A. D.—Membrana tympani dull and indrawn; L. R. broken and faint. A. S.—Membrana tympani indrawn; L. R. faint; no areas of thickening or atrophy. A. U.—Stapes movable.

| R | | L |
|---|---|---|
| Shout | W. V. | Shout |
| N | U. L. | N |
| 0/10 | R 256C | 7/12 |
| | W>+ | |
| 2/18 | 512C$^2$ | 4/16 |
| 27/15 | 1024C$^3$ | 22/14 |
| 15/5 | 2048C$^4$ | 9/5 |
| 512 | L. L. | 256 |

Treatment.—Jan. 31, 1920. Operation at Brooks Hospital: (1) Submucous resection of septum. (2) Refracture of nasal bones and correction of external deformity. (3) Tonsillectomy.

Result.—In twenty-five days the hearing for the whispered voice in the right ear (which he considered of no use to him for conversation) has gained 25 feet and the low limit had changed from 512 to 256. The left ear had improved 3 feet. No inflation used. (Hearing tests made by A. M. A.)

February 24, 1920.

| R | W. V. | L |
|---|---|---|
| 25/25 | | 3/25 |
| 5/10 | R 256C | 5/8 |
| | +<W | |
| 12/16 | 512C$^2$ | 5/11 |
| 26/18 | 1024C$^3$ | 22/30 |
| 15/7 | 2048C$^4$ | 11/3 |
| 256 | L. L. | 256 |

### CONCLUSIONS.

1. There is always a nerve element in every case of so-called conduction deafness of the progressive type.

2. The prognosis in regard to restoration of hearing is dependent upon the perception and not upon the conduction apparatus.

3. Toxic deafness and that due to beginning nerve degeneration cannot be differentiated by any aural examination.

4. Silent areas or islands of deafness are quite common in O. M. C. C.

5. The etiological factor is usually active in the lymphoid tissue as a chronic infection with acute exacerbations.

6. In some cases of long standing deafness it would seem necessary to reeducate the central perception centers by exercises, after all sources of infection have been eliminated.

# XXVI.

## ACUTE HEMORRHAGIC OTITIS MEDIA.*

### By H. C. Ballenger, M. D.,

#### Chicago.

In February and the latter part of January and early part of March, 1920, it was my privilege to pass through an epidemic of, for lack of a better name I might call an acute hemorrhagic otitis media. A better name might be an "acute streptococcic otitis media." This epidemic seemed to be confined to a few villages of the North Shore. Whether the proximity of the Great Lakes Naval Training Station or the camp at Fort Sheridan had anything to do with it or not I do not know. The epidemic apparently came from the North and appeared to reach its apex in Glencoe and Winnetka. It seemed to recede as it approached Chicago. At least I found very few other otologists who experienced this epidemic.

Altogether in a period of about three weeks, with a few cases preceding and following this period, I saw about fifty-six cases (a total of 72 ears) of various degrees of severity of this socalled hemorrhagic otitis media.

The onset was fairly sudden, with pain and temperature usually from 100 to 103 degrees. The ear drum became red and bulging quite early. The shortest time from a normal to a red bulging drum, which I witnessed, was two hours. In all these cases, with the exception of perhaps half a dozen, I was able to do an early paracentesis before rupture occurred. In 75 per cent of these cases, following the paracentesis, there was a sudden rise of temperature, usually in children, to 103°. In many cases the temperature rose to 104° and in a few to 105°. One of these cases I wish to report in some detail later. In very few of these cases did the paracentesis relieve the head pain.

I mention head pain because that more nearly described the discomfort than an earache. They would complain of a

*Read before the Chicago Laryngological and Otological Society February 7, 1921.

throbbing or aching head. They would not tolerate the twist-ing or undue motion of the head. The tenderness on press-ure over the mastoid and vicinity was very marked in the more typical cases. Traction on the pinna also caused pain. As a rule this pain subsided in from three to seven days. A few cases had it for two or three weeks.

The most striking feature following the paracentesis was the profuse bleeding, which usually persisted for two to seven days, gradually changing to a pink serous discharge. In one case the bloody serum persisted for two weeks. As a rule this discharge appeared to be without trace of pus which could be discerned with the naked eye. However, a typical pus dis-charge would eventually occur. In most of these cases the bloody serum could be seen pumping through the incision synchronous with the heart beat. The canal could be cleaned out and would fill almost immediately. In the more marked cases pads of cotton would have to be kept over the ear to take up this excessive discharge, and in some cases it was necessary to change this pad every half hour.

The examination of the canal and ear drum did not reveal a typical sinking down of the posterior superior canal wall in any case of this series. Only one patient showed a swelling behind the ear and that for one night only. This case was interesting and I wish to report it in some detail.

E. C., girl, age 7 years, first complained of pain in her left ear January 26, 1920. I saw the child about two hours after the onset and found a red bulging ear drum on which I did a paracentesis without anesthesia. The ear bled very pro-fusely. The following morning the mother called and said that the child still had a high temperature and had pain in the other ear. Saw child again and the first ear.was still bleed-ing quite profusely. Examination of the opposite ear showed a red bulging ear drum similar to the first. Paracentesis was done on this ear without anesthesia. It also bled very pro-fusely as had the first. The child complained of her head hurting very much. Both ears seemed to be tender over the mastoid region on pressure. The following morning I saw the child and both ears were still bleeding, although a some-what lighter color than the previous day. The mother stated quite a hemorrhage had occurred during the night from the left ear. So much so that one or two towels were soaked. The head pain still persisted and her temperature was still high, 103.5°. An attempt was made by the nurse to irrigate the ears with a warm saturated solution of boric acid, but so much discomfort was created and it seemed so futile, as five minutes after having it done the ears were discharging bloody serum as profusely as before, that I directed the nurse to do nothing but keep the cotton changed as soon as saturated.

The high temperature persisted and on the fourth day consultation was had with a pediatrician (Dr. Helmholtz) and with Dr. G. W. Boot. It was decided that no meningitis existed and that there was no involvement of the lateral sinus, but that there was a mastoid involvement on both sides.

The urinalysis taken the day before revealed albumin and pus. The leukocyte count was 13,000. A blood culture was taken by Dr. Helmholtz and he reported a streptococcus with a suggestion of a capsule.

On the fifth day, about 10 p. m., the mother reported a swelling behind the left ear, and as she was unable to get me she called Drs. Blatchford and Boot. They decided to operate immediately and took her to the hospital that night. Upon her arrival at the hospital she showed some improvement and the operation was postponed until the following morning. At that time I saw her and the swelling had disappeared and the temperature was down to normal. The child was feeling much better. It was then decided not to operate at the present time, due primarily to the presence of pus in the urine and the absence of any of the usual indications for the operation. For two weeks following this flareup there was a temperature varying from 99 to 100 degrees, and with a continuation of the bloody pus. The urine continued to show pus and albumin, and the blood count showed a leukocytosis varying from twelve to seventeen thousand. There was an occasional flareup of temperature to 102°, but an absence of all signs of edema of the canal wall. No further swelling occurred behind the mastoid. The mother would not consent to an operation at this time, and on March 7, about six weeks following the onset, consultation was had with Dr. Gordon Wilson, and it was decided at this time that the simple mastoid operation was indicated due to the persistent otorrhea. Ten days later, with

Dr. Wilson assisting, I did the simple mastoid operation on the left ear. Recovery was rapid and uneventful. The operated ear was dry in two weeks' time. The right ear continued to discharge for three weeks following, when it dried up. Both ears have remained dry until the present date and the hearing in both ears is normal. The urine cleared up following the advent of the dry ears.

Another interesting case was Mrs. P., age 35, who called me about 2:30 in the morning, January 29, 1920, complaining of a very bad earache. She was just recovering from influenza, and on examination I found a typical red bulging drum with tenderness over that side of the face. I did a paracentesis on the affected ear which bled profusely. The opposite ear appeared normal. The following morning I was called and the patient complained of severe pain in the opposite ear. This ear drum was red and bulging, on which I did a paracentesis. It also bled profusely. The bloody discharge still persisted from the first ear. Her temperature following the paracentesis rose to about 104°. The pain was not lessened by the paracentesis, and on the following five nights it was necessary to give her opiates to control her, despite the fact that in my opinion opiates are contraindicated in this condition. The bloody discharge persisted for about a week, when it gradually changed to the purulent form. During this time she was running a temperature of 99 to 103 degrees and suffered extreme pain. However, there was no local signs of a breaking down, though extreme tenderness was present. Three weeks after the onset one ear healed up and the other was reduced to a minimum of discharge. She had a sudden recurrence of pain and a second paracentesis was done to enlarge the then present small opening. The ear at this time did not bleed and in ten days the second ear was dry. There has been no recurrence to date and her haring is normal.

I wish to describe briefly a third case, Baby M., age 5, on whom a double paracentesis was done, followed by excessive bleeding from both ears, which persisted as a bloody serum for several days following the opening. Pain and tenderness persisted in both ears; temperature of 100 to 102 degrees was present for two weeks following. However, no local sign of a breaking down of the mastoid process was present. The most striking feature in this case was the advent on the third day of black urine. Microscopic examination revealed pus and blood cells. Albumin was also present. The hemorrhagic urine was diagnosed by Dr. Aldrich and Dr. Wall in consultation as coming from an acute hemorrhagic nephritis. The child appeared toxic and the advisability of an operation was considered. However, an operation was postponed, due primarily to the presence of the hemorrhagic nephritis. The urine gradually cleared up, and in eight weeks both ears were dry with normal hearing. Her tonsils and adenoids were subsequently removed.

In view of the above typical cases and in the ultimate outcome of the remaining cases, the question would arise as to the advisability of an early operation when the general and local symptoms are so marked. It is my opinion that surgical interference during the early stages is a mistake, due primarily, as I believe, to a nonclotting in the small vessels, with the resultant danger of the infection being transmitted to the meninges, the sinus, or directly into the blood stream. In fact, in many cases I believe that doing a paracentesis is sufficient to create an avenue of entrance into the blood stream, as the profound symptoms could be explained satisfactorily in no other way. However, this is largely a surmise on my part, and I hope in the discussion this point will be mentioned. The two cases that came to operation were both operated upon some weeks following the onset, after all symptoms had subsided, with the exception of the persistent otorrhea. Both cases made a very rapid recovery and were left with dry ears and normal hearing.

All of the cases in this group have dry ears at the present time and so far as I know they all have normal hearing.

A few cases of this type which were operated early of which I have indirect knowledge had many an alarming complication, two cases developing multiple abscesses.

### CONCLUSIONS.

I believe an early and free paracentesis is indicated, despite the subsequent rise in temperature and the hemorrhage, as all of my cases recovered with dry ears and normal hearing.

A minimum amount of interference during the bloody serous stage, whether swabbing or subsequent enlargement of
the ear drum should be done.

The time of election for operation should be after the ear
has quieted down and it is done for a persistent otorrhea.

25 E. WASHINGTON ST.

# XXVII.

## BACTERIAL FLORA AND WEIGHTS OF A SERIES OF EXCISED TONSILS.

By E. J. Lent, M. D., and M. W. Lyon, Jr., M. D.,

South Bend, Ind.

During the eleven months from August, 1919, to June, 1920, about half of all the tonsils removed at the clinic were weighed in pairs and a culture on blood agar was made from one of the crypts of one tonsil of a pair. In all 218 pairs of tonsils were weighed; 214 were cultured. The individuals from whom the tonsils were removed represent patients of the private practice in the city of South Bend and vicinity. The organs were removed for the usual causes, such as recurrent attacks of tonsillitis, sore throat, removal of foci of infections, hypertrophy, etc. The series includes persons of all ages, from early childhood to early old age, both sexes, and individuals of the various social conditions found in a prosperous industrial center.

In the last three years several important papers on the occurrence of hemolytic streptococci in the crypts of excised tonsils have been published. Nichols and Bryan[1] in 1918 reported hemolytic streptococci as found in 75 per cent of tonsils cultured; Blanton, Burhans and Hunter,[2] in 1919 reported 80 per cent; Pilot and Davis,[3] 1919, 97 per cent; Tongs,[4] 1919, 83 per cent; Maclay,[5] 1918; Cummings,[6] Spruit and Atem, 1919, 82 per cent, reported the presence of hemolytic streptococci among other bacteria found in the crypts of a large number of tonsils, the percentage not being stated. The results of the present study show little not found by other workers and serve to confirm their observations. The average percentage (61 per cent) of hemolytic streptococci in this series is somewhat less than that represented by other authors, though in some months it was as great as that reported by Nichols and Bryan.[1]

The technic of making the culture was as follows: Each pair of tonsils was brought to the laboratory in a clean tin box. The two tonsils were then weighed together. One tonsil of a pair was then selected and a sterile wire loop was pushed into the bottom of a conspicuous crypt, rotated once or twice inside of the crypt and then smeared on the surface of a blood agar plate. If the tonsil was covered with mucus it was washed off with sterile water or salt solution. If the surface of the tonsil was merely moist and the crypt mouth well disclosed the wire loop was pushed into the crypt without preliminary washing. The blood agar plates were ordinarily made by adding 1 cc. of whole human blood to 10 cc. of melted agar in tubes and pouring into sterile culture dishes. In some cases a weaker proportion of blood was used. Each plate was divided by wax pencil lines into eight sectors and a loop of material from a crypt spread over one of the sectors. Plates were incubated aerobically for 24 hours and the resultant growth observed. Subcultures were ordinarily not made, and the character of the organisms present was determined by their appearance on the blood agar plate and by staining them by Gram's method. This method seems to be satisfactory for the demonstration of hemolytic streptococci. For the satisfactory demonstration of pneumococci and streptococcus viridans the method is not entirely satisfactory for complete identification. Here the colonies which yielded Gram positive cocci arranged in pairs and short chains, and which caused no change in the blood agar were identified as pneumococci, while those appearing in pairs and short chains and producing a greenish discoloration about the colonies were identified by streptococcus viridans. The results of these cultures of 214 pairs of tonsils are found in table 1.

The most commonly found organism was streptococcus hemolyticus, occurring a total of 129 times, or 61 per cent. The next most common organism was nonhemolytic staphylococci, occurring 122 times, or 57 per cent. These were followed in order of frequency by Gram positive diplococci or short chained streptococci provisionally regarded as pneumococci, 55 times, or 26 per cent, and by streptococcus viridans, 28 times, or 14 per cent. Other organisms occurred in small numbers and corresponding low percentages. Organisms apparently identical with influenza bacilli occurred only three times, or about 1½ per cent. Fusiform bacilli and spiral organisms were found twice. In these two instances these organisms were so numerous on the surface of the agar that they must have grown there and not have been left when the smear was made. As the plates were incubated aerobically and other organisms were present at the same time, the resultant growth must have been one of symbiosis.

In table 2 is shown the incidence of hemolytic streptococci in this series of tonsils from month to month. The total number of tonsils examined during any one month appears in most cases to be entirely too small to make reliable figures, there never having been 50 cultures in any one month. The percentage of streptococcus hemolyticus present ranged from 26 in November to 75 in February. The next largest number occurred in August and May when 72 per cent of the tonsils cultured showed the presence of hemolytic streptococci. The percentage of hemolytic streptococci in January and February, the months when there were many cases of epidemic influenza in this vicinity, are 63 and 75 respectively, but being based on very small numbers of tonsils removed during these months these figures do not have much significance. During the actual period of the epidemic no tonsils were removed.

Seventy-five percent in February is essentially no different from 72 per cent in August and in May. The three times in which influenza-like bacilli were found occurred once in September, twice in April. Most other work done on the culturing of tonsils appears to have been limited to an examination during a comparatively short period of time, but Maclay[5] noted considerable variation at different periods of the year. It would appear, superficially at least, that hemolytic streptococci in tonsils shows some variation from month to month, when one considers the low figures in November with the higher figures obtained in other months. With such small numbers of cultures to deal with one must be cautious, however, in drawing conclusions.

The weights of the tonsils in pairs ranged from two to nineteen grams. The average weight of 218 pairs was 7.08

grams. The usual weight of the tonsils lay between five and seven
grams, which includes 32 per cent of all the tonsils weighed;
75 per cent ranged from four to nine grams. The various
weights and their frequency are shown in table 3. As many
of the tonsils were removed because of an hypertrophied condition, the average weight of all the tonsils is somewhat higher
than the usual weight, the average being brought up by a comparatively small number of heavy tonsils appearing at the end
of the table. That the usual weights represent fairly well the
weight of normal tonsils is shown by the uniformity of the
curve of the frequency of the weights. If the figures in the
table are plotted out in a graph a maximum is found at 16.4
per cent, with a fairly uniform slope on either side until the
excessively heavy tonsils are reached. The bluntness of the
apex is an indication that there is considerable latitude in the
weight of the normal pair of tonsils. The current belief that
the largest tonsils are found in children was substantiated
in collecting these figures, but the heaviest pair in this series
came from an adult. The very light ones also came from
adults.

### CONCLUSIONS.

During a period of eleven months 214 pairs of tonsils were
cultured. The most common organism found was streptococcus hemolyticus, 61 per cent. The next most common organisms were nonhemolytic staphylococci, 57 per cent; pneumococci, 26 per cent, and streptococcus viridans, 14 per cent.

The percentage of hemolytic streptococcus appears to vary
from month to month.

During the same period 218 tonsils were weighed in pairs.
The average weight was found to be 7.08 grams. The usual
weight ranged between five and seven grams.

Since writing the foregoing, a paper dealing with the pathologic histology of tonsils containing hemolytic streptococci
by Kellert[7] has come to our attention. He found streptococcus hemolyticus of frequent occurrence in tonsillar crypts. In
our series a considerable number of tonsils at the beginning
of the investigation were sectioned and examined microscopically. Like Kellert, we were unable to detect any characteristic pathologic change in those tonsils which yielded large
numbers of hemolytic streptococci. The sectioning was aban-

doned after having examined about 25 or 30 tonsils. Our findings swere essentially the same as those of Kellert, although polymorphonuclear leucocytes were not so abundant and cartilage was not found. In the crypt of one tonsil was found a bit of vegetable material with a cell arrangement suggesting leaf structure.

NUMBER AND PER CENT* OF ORGANISⅠS CULTURED AEROBICALLY
FROM TONSIL CRYPTS.

| Organisms | Relative Abundance | | | | | | | |
|---|---|---|---|---|---|---|---|---|
| | Predominating | | Common | | Few | | Total | |
| | No. | Pct. | No. | Pct. | No. | Pct. | No. | Pct. |
| Streptococcus hemolyticus ....87 | | 42 | 24 | 11 | 18 | 9 | 129 | 61 |
| Streptococcus viridans............12 | | 6 | 14 | 7 | 2 | 1 | 28 | 14 |
| Pneumococci ........................13 | | 6 | 24 | 11 | 18 | 8 | 55 | 26 |
| Staphylococci nonhemolytic..14 | | 66 | 44 | 21 | 64 | 30 | 122 | 57 |
| Staphylococci hemolytic.......... 3 | | 1.5 | 8 | 4 | 6 | 3 | 17 | 8 |
| Gram positive, tetracoccus forms........................ 0 | | 0 | 0 | 0 | 2 | 1 | 2 | 1 |
| Gram negative diplococci...... 4 | | 2 | 9 | 4 | 5 | 2 | 18 | 8 |
| Bacilli of Friedlander group.. 2 | | 1 | 2 | 1 | 1 | 0.5 | 5 | 2 |
| Influenza-like bacilli ................ 1 | | 0.5 | 2 | 1 | 0 | 0 | 3 | 1.5 |
| Other Gram negative bacilli.. 2 | | 1 | 5 | 2 | 3 | 1.5 | 10 | 5 |
| Diphtheroid bacilli .................. 0 | | 0 | 3 | 1.5 | 2 | 1 | 5 | 2 |
| Bacillus subtilis ...................... 0 | | 0 | 0 | 0 | 1 | 0.5 | 1 | 0.5 |
| Other Gram positive bacilli.. 1 | | 0.5 | 0 | 0 | 0 | 0 | 1 | 0.5 |
| Organism of Vincent's angina 0 | | 0 | 1 | 0.5 | 1 | 0.5 | 2 | 1 |

MONTHLY INCIDENCE OF HEMOLYTIC STREPTOCOCCI CULTURED
FROM TONSIL CRYPTS.

| Month | Percent | Number Cultured |
|---|---|---|
| January ................................ | 63 | 8 |
| February ................................ | 75 | 8 |
| March ................................ | 48 | 27 |
| April ................................ | 54 | 22 |
| May ................................ | 72 | 11 |
| June ................................ | 70 | 10 |
| July ................................ | 0 | 0 |
| August ................................ | 72 | 43 |
| September ................................ | 60 | 30 |
| October ................................ | 62 | 24 |
| November ................................ | 26 | 21 |
| December ................................ | 40 | 10 |

*Fractions of a per cent have been as a rule disregarded

### WEIGHTS OF 218 PAIRS OF TONSILS.

| Weights | Number | Percent |
|---|---|---|
| 2—2.9 grams | 2 | 0.95% |
| 3—3.9 | 16 | 7.35 |
| 4—4.9 | 25 | 11.40 |
| 5—5.9 | 36 | 16.40 |
| 6—6.9 | 35 | 16 |
| 7—7.9 | 24 | 11 |
| 8—8.9 | 24 | 11 |
| 9—9.9 | 23 | 10.05 |
| 10—10.9 | 14 | 6.40 |
| 11—11.9 | 8 | 3.65 |
| 12—12.9 | 0 | 0 |
| 13—13.9 | 3 | 1.75 |
| 14—14.9 | 1 | 0.45 |
| 15—15.9 | 2 | 0.95 |
| 16—16.9 | 3 | 1.75 |
| 17—17.9 | 1 | 0.45 |
| 18—18.9 | 0 | 0 |
| 19 | 1 | 0.45 |

### BIBLIOGRAPHY.

1. Nichols, H. J., and Bryan, J. H.: Journ. Amer. Med. Ass., Vol. 71, p. 1813, November 30, 1918.

2. Blanton, W. B., Burhans, C. W., and Hunter, O. W. Journ. Amer. Med. Ass., Vol. 72, p. 1520, May 24, 1919.

3. Pilot, I., and Davis, D. S.: Journ. Infect. Dis., Vol. 24, p. 386. April, 1919.

4. Tongs, M. S.: Journ. Amer. Med. Ass., Vol. 73, p. 1050, October 4, 1919.

5. Maclay, O. H.: Laryngoscope, Vol. 28, p. 598, August, 1918.

6. Cummings, J. G., Spruit, C. B., and Atem: J. Am. M. Ass., Chicago, 1919—LXII—704.

7. Kellert, Ellis: J. Med. Research, 1920—XLI—387.

# XXVIII.

## EPIDEMIC MASTOIDITIS.

By JAMES E. REEDER, M. D.,

SIOUX CITY, IOWA.

Any man who professes to practice otology and was not in the service during the fall and winter of 1917 and 1918, in my mind missed a great opportunity to witness one of the events in the annals of otology.

I happened to be in charge of the operative service at Camp Cody when the epidemic of streptococcus, pneumonia and mastoiditis hit us like a bolt out of a clear sky at the time we least expected such an unheard of and unprecedented catastrophe. Most certainly it was unprecedented, as it has been shown by other writers that precedent was set both as when to interfere surgically in acute mastoiditis as well as the postoperative care.

Just why such an epidemic should occur, there are a number of etiologic factors to be considered, but as yet of all the theories which have been advanced, none are satisfactory in explaining the true cause. True, it seems environment played a very important role, as the men were taken from all walks of life and thrust into an intensive training which they had to endure, and were not allowed to rest for some slight indisposition, but had to be quite sick to be admitted to the base hospital, no doubt all of this resulted in a lower physical resistance for some time until they became acclimated or had become hardened physically to stand the military routine. It was during this readjustment period these men were good subjects for any acute infection which might arise, notably acute streptococcic sore throat.

The streptococcus in its different types was the most important infection we had to contend with. This particular organism was not only an important etiologic factor in all primary infections, but played an important role as secondary infections following the acute exanthemas, such as measles and scarlet fever. It seems this organism may be dormant, as it were, only waiting for an opportunity to become active upon any lowered resistance of its host.

I am convinced of this, as a number of the ward attendants had repeated cultures from the nose and throat, and they all showed a predominant streptococcus growth as well as a slight leucocyte count. These cultures and blood counts were taken weekly, and as long as the blood count showed a good resistance they were kept on ward work, but if a slight indisposition was apparent with low resistance these men were placed on other duty for a few days. In this way we were always able to keep our help in the mastoid ward up to very good efficiency.

It is not surprising, when one considers the foregoing, that we virtually had an epidemic of mastoiditis or at least sporadic, as we frequently had a number of cases from one company and not any from another, but from different battalions.

It was during December, 1917, and January, February, March and April, 1918, that we had such a large series of cases of (operative) streptococcus mastoiditis. From my observations I am convinced the mastoid is more frequently involved through the blood stream than was thought probable in the past.

Symptomatology.—Cases where the otitis media symptoms seemed to predominate and, say, slight pain over the antrum and a high temperature with a timely paracentesis, although the great percentage of these cases had gone on to rupture before they were admitted to the hospital—as a rule, this class will undergo resolution without surgical interference of the mastoid.

There is another class of cases in which the otitis media and mastoiditis appears simultaneously. A paracentesis is done at once, but the case is one of those fulminating types, and it is necessary to do a mastoidectomy in four or five days to relieve the pain. While the patient is very septic and may show a leucopenia, you then wonder how it is possible so much destruction could be done in such a short time.

Another class of cases were those complicating systemic diseases, such as measles. These cases would become involved

. and the patient not aware of it until necrosis had taken place. These no doubt were infected through the blood stream.

Blood counts, if these were above 12,000, we watched the mastoid very closely. Headache is a symptom that to my mind is more important than is given credit, relative to complications of acute mastoiditis. A constant headache always means to me a dural irritation or a beginning meningitis.

Where precedent was set in this epidemic of streptococcus mastoiditis was the assurance of knowing just when to interfere surgically. This was determined by the following points, which I wish to emphasize: First, as a case was admitted, a culture was taken of the discharge, or at the time of the paracentesis a culture was taken. If this proved to be either pneumococcus or streptococcus, and at the end of the third or fourth day pain and tenderness still persisted over the mastoid along with a leucocytosis, also an occasional leucopenia asserted itself, we immediately opened the mastoid. A leucocytosis meant to us only an increased resistance, for some of the worst cases had a normal count or a leucopenia. Second, if the X-ray showed a large pneumatic mastoid along with history of sudden onset and continuous severe pain, this always meant early operative procedure. There is just one factor that stands out in acute mastoiditis which has always been more or less of guesswork, and that is bone necrosis. It is this factor alone that determines when we shall operate. If this could always be determined I believe our mortality following acute suppurative mastoiditis would be lessened. I believe we are nearer to this goal than ever before.

We have those classical cases. In these we have no difficulty, but the classical symptoms do not always appear. It is then we should rely on the X-ray, for it has been shown that when bone necrosis has taken place, in the absence of the classical symptoms operative interference should be instituted at once.

The Operation.—The operation for the removal of the mastoid cells is very much standardized, and I feel it is not necessary to discuss it here. Except I wish to make this statement that in the presence of a streptococcus infection it is best not to use the blood clot, as we tried it in twenty cases, and all but three broke down. Of course this delayed the resolution, and I feel you are endangering the patient possibly to severe complications.

After-care.—We discovered it was best to use dry dressings along with rest and good food. We were disappointed with dichloramin-T. It is possible we did not use the proper technic. In the end we decided it was best to use dry dressings and let them alone.

Complications.—The two uppermost questions in our mind in any acute mastoiditis is the diagnosis of bone necrosis and complications. Our complications consisted of sinus thrombosis, brain abscess, meningitis, arthritis, endocarditis and a general streptococcemia.

Sinus thrombosis is too well known to be taken up in detail, but there is one thing we proved, and that is that a sudden chill followed by a rise in temperature does not always mean sinus thrombosis, but we had so many complications arise that it was the opinion of all that the blood stream no doubt was infected prior to the development of the mastoid or through the lymphatics from the mastoid region and not through the lateral sinus.

Erysipelas was a frequent complication but never proved fatal. It prolonged the period of convalescence.

The one complication which was most dreaded was meningitis. The necropsies show this to be a more frequent complication of pneumonia than was at first suspected. In one case of mastoiditis complicated by meningitis it was shown at postmortem that temporosphenoidal and cerebellar abscesses were found. The heart showed multiple abscesses throughout, and cultures from the pleural cavity were positive for streptococcus.

### CONCLUSIONS.

1. Why such an epidemic of mastoiditis should occur in our army camps, it is difficult to say that any one thing was the etiologic factor, but a number of factors are to be considered. The one important thing which stands out most were the complications associated with the acute contagious diseases, such as measles.

2. The mastoid may become involved through the blood stream or the nasopharynx route.

2. Bone necrosis is the most important thing to keep in mind. This can be determined by constant use of the X-ray along with clinical manifestations.

4. Those mastoids following the acute contagious diseases as complications, in all probability, get their start through the blood stream and give us the most trouble.

# XXIX

# ETHMOID OPERATIONS (DURING THE LATENT STAGE) FOLLOWED BY DEATH. REPORT OF CASES.

By L. Ostrom, A. B., M. D., Major M. R. C., U. S. A.

Rock Island, Ill.

The literature of ethmoid operations presents such a wide difference of opinion that a brief resumé will prove quite interesting. Some surgeons have been very fortunate, while others have had more than their proportion of trouble. Williams[1] in his textbook says: "The mortality is low; I have been fortunate in never having a death." Lenox Browne[27] says: "This measure (curettement of ethmoid cells) is rarely attended by any risk." Packard[2], at our A. M. A. meeting, 1907, remarked that, "Septic infections following turbinal operations are by no means as common as one would believe. When we consider the large blood vessels and lymphatic channels which lie immediately beneath the nasal mucosa and the proximity of the tissues to the brain and its meninges, we would hardly think that the cases of meningitis, cerebral abscess, or thrombosis of the sinuses are as rare as they would seem to be after a diligent search of the literature on the subject." In my limited way I have tried to cover the literature on this subject and come to full accord with Packard, because I find very few references to the subject and remarkably few cases reported. There are, however, numerous hints and warnings that there is danger, and that others have had trouble, so where there is smoke one is sure to find fire.

The tenor of opinion of the dangers attending the operation, at the same time considering it comparatively safe, is well stated by Lack:[21] "I do not wish to exaggerate the advantages of this operation (curettment), but rather to emphasize its dangers and the necessity for caution in performing it. The following, so far as I am aware, is a full account of the ill results that have been reported.

At least three deaths have occurred. Of one I have obtained no details. One was due to polypus forceps having been pushed through the cribriform plate, and therefore was not directly due to this operation at all. The third was due to fracture of the cribriform plate from scraping with the ring knife. 'I have performed the operation myself during the past eight years upon more than 150 patients without any fatal results. Serious ill results, although undoubtedly serious, seem to me small compared with the severity of the disease for which the operation is performed. The fatal results, so far as is at present known, were due to avoidable causes, and prolonged experience proves that the operation, when properly and carefully performed, is both safe and efficient."

Ballenger[25] follows the same tone: "Meningitis following ethmoid operations is rare. The chief point to be mentioned concerning them is that the operation should not be performed if a latent chronic meningitis is already present, as it may cause an acute exacerbation and extension which may prove fatal. The chief subjective symptom of latent meningitis is a severe headache. When this is present the operation should be postponed until it has been proved that it is not due to meningitis."

Loeb[12] admirably advises careful judgment in selection of cases and method of technic. "Operations on the ethmoid cells have been followed by serious results, such as sinus thrombosis, meningitis and death. The possibilities of these untoward results can be lessened by refraining from postoperative packing, postponing operation, when possible, in the presence of an acute infectious process in the nose, and by avoiding any injury in the vicinity of the cribriform plate."

Perhaps Moure[15] expresses the true state of affairs, especially in regard to the reporting of cases. "We should not forget that the number of cases of death from meningitis or subsequent sepsis following surgical interference in the ethmoids is quite considerable (not to mention other unfortunate cases never published), to not make the surgeon careful who ventures to enter this zone, most dangerous, perhaps, from a surgical point of view, for an inexperienced hand or unskillful surgeon."

In their reports some writers suggest that complications, unless induced by faulty technic, seldom prove fatal[9] and that meningitis is seldom a result of sinus suppuration but of an operation to relieve the chronic condition.[29]

That often too much is done is emphasized by Prof. Kuemmel[10] of Heidelburg, after reviewing a fatality following removal of the ethmoid labyrinth, "unless there is some vital indication, too little is better than too much interference in chronic frontal or ethmoid sinusitis." Seymour Oppenheimer[11] agrees with this statement: "If free drainage is present and there are no signs of ill effects on the general health but an occasional headache, and if the patient can be kept under observation, the risks of radical operation more than counterbalance the advantages."

On the other hand, that master rhinologist Hajek[14] takes the opposite view, that too little may be done. In his reports of two deaths he says: "The complications had their origin not in the operated area, but in some overlooked ethmoid cell, some other neglected accessory cavity, especially in some area of pus which had not drained away and which had given rise to an area of infection."

Injury to the cribriform plate or adjoining cranial bones is perhaps the most frequently mentioned cause, yet very few cases are found reported. Thompson[13] says: "The chief danger is from injury to the cribriform plate, as any damage in this area, occurring in the septic conditions which generally call for operation, is generally followed by fatal meningitis."

Douglass[20] in his book writes: "If the brain plate has been wounded or septic material has been conveyed to the dura mater, the patient may slowly develop a pachymeningitis. Sometimes this disease will develop after an operation without the infection or exciting cause having come from the nose. It happens that cases of ethmoiditis often develop a low grade of pachymeningitis and are suffering from it at the same time when they present themselves for operation for the ethmoiditis. Sometimes the operating surgeon in opening the cells of such patients excites an irritation of the dura and a spread of the meningitis, although the instrument has not been outside the proper field of operation."

A number of fatal reports are found where no injury of the cranial bones has taken place. Virulent streptococcus infection with fatal meningitis without injury to the cribriform plate after ethmoid operation is reported by Hajek.[14] A case of purulent meningitis with death is reported by Knutson.[17] Autopsy confirmed the diagnosis and showed that dura nearest the affected bone had not been injured.

Phillips[23] says: "It is contended by some observers that intracranial complications may be induced by the shock and irritation of the operation alone. In a limited proportion of cases of purulent ethmoiditis there is a preexisting latent meningitis or a circumscribed brain abscess, either of which may be excited to renewed activity by the manipulations incident to the operation, especially when carelessly or unskillfully performed." Fatal termination after simple removal of polypi is reported by Voltolini,[3] 2 cases; Broeckaert,[4] 1 case; Rethi,[5] 1 case; H. Knapp,[7] after removal of polypi and orbital tumor; Quinlan,[8] after cautery of middle turbinate. Welty[19] reports two cases following socalled intranasal operations (not his cases but came to his knowledge). Onodi[28] reports 11 cases of cerebral abscess occurring as complication to ethmoid operation. Sluder[24] mentions having 8 cases of meningitis but does not state operative measures.

Fatalities following other intranasal operations, submucous resection, etc., in the presence of latent empyema occur and have been reported.[16] Perhaps a good many more occur than we have any idea of.

•Compared to the radical operations the literature makes one think that these conservative operations are more frequently fatal than are all other intranasal operations put together. When we realize that the radical frontal, ethmoid, antrum or sphenoid operations are seldom performed by the general surgeon or embryo specialist, and that almost every graduate of medicine at some time removes polypi or some parts of the turbinates, and the dangers of sepsis are practically the same, one is apt to conclude that the ratio of ill results should be reversed. Gerber[18] alone gives us the report of 46 cases following the radical Killian operation, more than I can find all together after other reported intranasal operations.

It has been my misfortune to have had three fatal terminations following simple curettement of the ethmoid cells. In each of these.cases I am sure that no injury was done to the cribriform plate or adjoining cranial bones, nor was any septic matter conveyed directly to the dura mater. The operations were carefully executed with the idea only of obtaining free drainage, not of removing every vestige of diseased tissue, laying myself open to criticism of perhaps doing too little rather than too much. The patients were all apparently in good condition for the operation. No packing was used, careful asepsis and antisepsis carried out, and I know of nothing that could have been done to avoid the complications if I could have the opportunity to do them all over again.

Case 1.—Mr. B. M., age 37, Mazon, Ill., Dec. 26, 1906. Severely jolted and stunned in a railroad accident four to six weeks before I saw him. Back has been painful since that time. Has had difficulty in breathing through the left nostril for several years, especially in damp weather. Discharge of pus when he has a cold. Very little headache. Looks sick, very pale, but says he feels O K, except for pain in the back. No temperature. Heart and urine normal. Complains of vague stomach trouble which he thinks comes from his nasal condition. Transillumination shows all sinuses clear. No pus seen in nose, but a small amount of thin serous secretion, such as is seen after sneezing spells, covered the entire mucosa. A large polyp arising by a small pedicle from the middle meatus almost filled the nose. This was removed with a snare, and arrangement was made to do a simple ethmoid operation the next day. •

Dec. 27. Removed cystic and polypoid middle turbinate. curetted ethmoid cells, which were soft and easily broken down, leaving a clean field. Vomited during the operation. The operated area was afterwards swabbed with tr. iodin. No packing was used. Practically no bleeding followed the operation, but a profuse serous discharge, lasting almost two hours, made it appear as if there was an escape of cerebrospinal fluid. This stopped spontaneously and did not recur.

Dec. 28. Feels fine, no bleeding or serous discharge. Said he felt well enough to go to work.

Dec. 30. Found delirious in his boarding house and sent to

the hospital, Dr. Bradford having been called to see him. Temperature, 103. No headache, but severe pain and tenderness in back between the shoulders. Eyes, urine and reflexes normal or slightly exaggerated. Skin very yellow. Nose looks fine. A diagnosis of meningitis had been made.

Dec. 31. Temperature higher, 104 to 105. Eyes normal, no headache, but pressure on the cervical or dorsal vertebræ produced extreme pain. Reflexes of legs abolished. Control of rectum and bladder lost. Has good control of arms.

Jan. 1. Comatose. Died, Jan. 2. Spinal leptomeningitis. Body sent to his home at Mazon, Ill.

Jan. 6. Dr. Bradford informed me that a postmortem would be held to determine the cause of death and advised me to attend. We both went, and I, especially, met a very cool reception because the entire history seemed to point to the operation as the direct cause of death. On the removal of the skull cap, the brain, meninges, and the area about the ethmoids were found perfectly normal, without any evidence of infection or injury. Opening into the ethmoids showed a perfectly executed operation. I insisted that the spinal canal be opened, and when the laminæ and spinous processes were lifted off and the periosteum of the spinal canal incised, the pressure of the contained pus was so great that is squirted quite a ways up in the air. This was extended up to the second cervical and down to the second dorsal vertebra. (There was no pus below the second dorsal.) No culture was made nor was any microscopic examination made of this pus, because the postmortem was conducted for other purposes than merely scientific, matters over which I had no control. Opening the dura showed the cord slightly compressed, dura thick, but no pus was found on or around the cord. The pus was confined exclusively to the epidural space. (Gray's Anatomy[26] gives a minute description of this space: "The spinal dura mater forms a loose sheath around the medulla spinalis and represents only the inner or meningeal layer of the cerebral dura mater; the outer or endosteal layer ceases at the foramen magnum, its place being taken by the periosteum lining the vertebral canal. The spinal dura mater is separated from the wall of the vertebral canal by a space, the epidural space, which contains a quantity of loose areolar tissue and a plexus of veins. The situation of these veins between the dura mater and the periosteum of the vertebræ corresponds therefore to that of the cranial sinuses between the meningeal and endosteal layers of the cerebral dura mater. The spinal dura mater is attached to the circumference of the foramen magnum and to the second and third cervical vertebræ. It is also connected by fibrous slips to the posterior longitudinal ligaments of the vertebræ, especially near the lower end of the vertebral canal. The subdural cavity ends at the lower border of the second sacral vertebræ.") The fact that no pus was found below the second dorsal would have prevented us from obtaining any useful information if we had made a spinal puncture, a procedure which was not done.

The cause of death was a pachymeningitis of the spinal epidural space, caused perhaps by the trauma of the railroad accident, and an acute exacerbation induced by bacterial metastasis through the blood vessels following the operation. Needless to state that the hard feeling toward me changed very much after the postmortem was completed.

Case 2.—P. J., age 24 years, private secretary, has felt bad generally for a long time; nose stopped up, frequently sore throat, and pains in the arms and legs. Chronic ethmoiditis. Antra and frontal sinuses fairly clear on transillumination. May 11, 1914. Tonsillectomy; local anesthesia. Normal reaction and prompt recovery. Felt much better after the operation. May 29. Removed both middle turbinates and curetted ethmoid cells. Turbinates and ethmoids quite dense and firm. There was no pus present, but considerable thick, stringy mucous. Practically no bleeding followed the operation and the operated field seemed to be very satisfactory.

Dr. J. R. Brown, Tacoma, Wash., late president Washington State Medical Society, witnessed the operation. After completing the operation the entire operated field was thoroughly swabbed with tr. iodin, which caused Dr. Brown to remark that he had never seen more care given asepsis and antisepsis in any nasal operation. Patient felt fine for four days and was getting ready to return to Chicago.

June 5. Dr. Bennet, who referred him to me, met him wandering on the street, out of his head, with temperature 103 to 104, and sent him to the Moline City Hospital. When I saw him the next day I recognized a general streptococcus sepsis. Dr. Mock, physician to Sears-Roebuck, was sent down to help us. Autogenous vaccines (hemolytic streptococci from the patient's blood) were made and administered, but in spite of all our efforts he died June 11. Numerous large abscesses had by that time been formed in various parts of the body. Not until some time after his death was I informed that he had had a positive Wassermann. This I consider a general streptococcus septicemia following the operation in spite of all preventives, and not a meningitis. No postmortem was obtained.

Case 3.—Mrs. S. Mc. C., age 62, has had a discharge from nose for twenty years. Not much headache except 'when she has a cold. Health has been good most of the time. Transillumination showed antri and frontal sinuses fairly clear. Chronic ethmoiditis. In as good health at time of operation as she had been for years. Wassermann negative. Was anxious to get rid of the profuse discharge, and to improve nasal breathing. May 15, 1918. Operation. Removed both middle turbinates and curetted ethmoids, all of which were very soft and mushy and easily removed without using any force. The entire field was swabbed with tr. iodin. No packing was used. Was in very good condition following the operation and remained in St. Anthony's Hospital, Rock Island, Ill., for three days, but she felt so well on the third day that she left the hospital without my permission and went to her home, fifteen miles from the city. All next day she felt fine, but by evening went into a stupor and was comatose by midnight. Dr. Moore of Reynolds, Ill., was called, and he talked to me over the telephone about her condition, but I could give him no assistance. Her temperature rapidly rose to 103 and 104.5. At no time was there any headache, convulsions, or other physical signs except high temperature and coma. She died the following morning (five days after the operation) from acute pachymeningitis, in my mind excited by the operation, though there had at no time previously been any symptoms of latent meningeal disease.

## REFERENCES.

1. Watson-Williams, P.: (Rhinology, 1910, p. 224.
2. Packard, Francis R.: (A. M. A., 1907, Meeting.
3. Voltolini: Die Krankheiten der Nase, 1888.
4. Broeckaert, J.: Ann. de Mal d l'Oreille du Larynx, etc.
5. Rethi, L.: Sojous Annual, 1896, IV.
6. Jurgens: Wien Med. Wochenschr., 1899, XLIX, pp. 66-68.
7. Knapp, H.: Arch. of Otology, 1884, XXXIII, p. 51.
8. Quinlan, F. J.: N. Y. Med. Record, 1890, XXXIII, p. 292.
9. Lewis, H. C. B.: St. Paul Med. Jour., 1915, Vol. 17.
10. Kuemmel, Prof., of Heildelberg.
11. Oppenheimer, Simon.
12. Loeb: Op. Surg. of the Nose and Throat, Vol. 2, p. 57, 1917.
13. Thomson: Dis. of the Nose and Throat, 1912, p. 221.
14. Hajek (Arch. f. Laryngol. Bd., XVIII, Heft. 2.
15. Moure, E. J.: Revue Hebd. de Laryngol. XVIII, 5 Mars, 1898, No. 10, p. 273.
16. Hubbard, Thomas: Laryngoscope, Vol. XIII, 1903, p. 682.
17. Knutson: Otol., Laryngol., Meddelanden, Stockholm, Vol. 2, No. 3.
18. Gerber: Die Komplicationen der Stirnhohlenentzundungen, S. Karger, Berlin, 1909.
19. Welty, Dr. C. F.: A. M. A., 1909, Meeting.
20. Douglass: Nose and Throat Surgery, 1906, p. 103.
21. Lack, H. Lambert: Diseases of the Nose, 1906, p. 332.
22. Wright, J.: Laryngoscope, 1903, Vol. XXIII, No. 2, p. 103.
23. Phillips, W.: Diseases of the Ear, Nose and Throat, 1915, p. 619.
24. Sluder: Headaches and Eye Disorders of Nasal Origin, 1918, p. 240.
25. Ballenger: Diseases of Nose, Throat and Ear, 1914, p. 247.
26. Gray's Anatomy, 1918, p. 841.
27. Browne, Lenox: Throat and Nose, 1899.
28. Onodi: Laryngoscope, 1903, Vol. XXIII, No. 2, p. 103.
29. Kyle, J. J.

# XXX

# ABSCESS OF THE FRONTAL LOBE SECONDARY TO SINUSITIS.

By G. W. Boot, M. D.,

Chicago.

F. P., age 41, Bohemian. Admitted to Cook County Hospital complaining of pus discharging from a sinus on the right side of the forehead, of fever and headache.

History: Patient is said to have had some sort of operation for nasal obstruction. The trouble in the forehead followed. (The physician who operated on him stated that this was not true; that he had not done any operation inside the man's nose but had only opened the subperiosteal abscess over the right side of the patient's forehead.) Patient was sick a week before entering the hospital.

Physical examination: Patient is a well developed man of 41. He has an opening on the forehead midway between the right eyebrow and the hair of the scalp above, from which pus is discharging freely. The surrounding area is deeply infiltrated. The scalp is edematous half way to the occiput and past the median line towards the left side. The right upper eyelid is edematous so that the eye can be only partly opened. The pupils are equal.

There is a large amount of pus in each naris, but particularly in the right. The nasal cavities contain crusts. Apparently all four turbinates have been removed either by operation or by disease.

Marked pyorrhea is present and the pharyngeal vessels are injected. The tonsils are small and submerged. There is no cervical glandular enlargement. Both maxillary sinuses light up well on transillumination. The frontal sinuses do not light up well.

Smears from the pus from the nose show a few chains of streptococci of from five to seven members.

Examination of thorax and abdomen is negative. The X-ray report states that there are no frontal sinuses.

Diagnosis: Suppurative right frontal sinusitis.

Twenty-four hours after the above examination was made patient became irrational and held his left forearm strongly flexed at the elbow and with the left upper extremity spastic. The head was turned strongly towards the right with conjugate deviation of the eyes to the right.

The abdominal, epigastric and cremasteric reflexes were absent. The pupillary reflex was present on both sides. Babinski was present on the right side but not on the left. The patellar and triceps reflexes were much exaggerated on the right side. Achilles jerk was present on the right side but not on the left. Ankle clonus and plantar reflexes were absent.

Patient does not remember that he was in the X-ray room yesterday. He points to the doctor, mistaking him for someone else. It is with difficulty that he can be made to fix his attention or do the simplest thing, as, for instance, look upwards, or to one side or protrude his tongue. On irritating patient by pulling his hair there is a coarse tremor set up in the left hand.

Lumbar puncture produces a clear fluid under increased pressure and containing 73 cells per cu. mm. Nonné + + +.

Blood count gave 14,200 whites. Blood pressure S. 130, D. 70. Edema of the right eyelid is greater than yesterday. Pupils are widely dilated but react to light. There is no rigidity and no hemianopsia. Ophthalmoscopic examination was not satisfactory on account of inability to keep the eyes still.

Operation: After the usual preparation the skin over the lower part of the forehead was infiltrated with ½ per cent novocain and an incision made transversely from the midline through the right eyebrow to its outer extremity. The soft parts were retracted upwards and pus was seen oozing through the bone about two inches above the orbital margin. With a gouge the bone was removed over the usual location of the right frontal sinus, and finally a sinus about 2 cm. in diameter and ½ cm. in depth was exposed and found full of pus. After the sinus was well cleaned out its posterior wall was removed and a large amount of pus found between the bone and the dura. This came from every direction for a distance of 5 cm. After enlarging the opening in the frontal bone and evacuating this pus the dura was found red and granulating. It was incised and pus found in the pia in every direction for at least 5 cm. An abscess cavity about 2 cm. in diameter was found in the inner part of the right frontal lobe, lying near the falx cerebri. It was evacuated and a rubber drain inserted. The skin incision was then extended across to the outer extremity of the left eyebrow and search made for the left frontal sinus by means of a gouge. The bone was excavated to a depth of about 2 cm., with no sign of a frontal sinus, so it was concluded that there was no left frontal sinus. The wound was closed with skin clips after inserting drains. The patient seemed a little improved after the operation, but soon relapsed and died in about 48 hours.

The peculiarities in the case were the suppurative rhinitis, the absence of turbinates, the abnormally thick skull, the absence of a left frontal sinus and the extensive involvement of the meninges and brain that must have been present at the time of the first examination without corresponding symptoms. At that time he walked into the examination room just as any other patient would walk and showed no sign of the serious intracranial trouble he was having. Twenty-four hours later he had spasm of the left upper extremity, with turning of the head to the right and conjugate deviation of the eyes to the right, and was comatose. Had he been able to speak English we might possibly have been able to note mental disturbance, but it is not likely.

The frontal lobe is notoriously a silent area. I have seen a sequestrum of the frontal bone 5 by 7 cm. separate as a result of a combination of syphilis and suppurative sinusitis, the dura bathed in foul smelling pus for weeks, with no symptoms referable to the brain.

On the other hand, I have seen suppurative frontal sinusitis on the right side cause a man to write his name upside down and backwards and to set up a sort of double personality so that the patient went to another town without realizing where he was and later "came to" and remembered that he lived in Chicago, and all these disturbances cease in a week after external operation on the sinus with drainage.

Definite symptoms of abscess of the frontal lobe are wanting. There may be the ordinary symptoms of brain abscess, such as headache, choked disc and increased tension of the cerebro-spinal fluid, but, on the other hand, these may not be at all definite. The spinal fluid may be clear or contain but few cells, and changes in the fundus may be absent. Headache, while always present, is a symptom common to so many conditions that it has not much significance in abscess of the frontal lobe. For the present the diagnosis would seem to be best made by exploratory operation in any case of suppuration of the frontal sinus where headache is not promptly relieved by drainage and where lumbar puncture shows changes of an inflammatory type. If we wait until symptoms of involvement of the motor area present themselves the case is apt to have progressed too far for operative interference to be of much avail. In this type of case, when external operation on a frontal sinus is decided upon, exploration of the brain for abscess is justifiable. At least there is no harm apt to result from exposure of the dura. In any case of frontal sinus suppuration, where a subperiosteal abscess has resulted from the pus extending through the bone to its outer surface, remember that the inner wall of the sinus is thinner than the outer wall and fully as apt to be perforated by the pus. Hence in such a case explore inside the skull.

25 E. WASHINGTON ST.

## XXXI.

## REPORT OF CASE OF ORBITAL ABSCESS FROM ETHMOID SUPPURATION.

By Clifton M. Miller, M. D.,

Richmond, Va.

Orbital abscess has been usually considered an ophthalmologic condition, but from the etiology in the majority of nontraumatic cases it appears more properly to belong in the domain of rhinology. The great majority of cases of nontraumatic cellulitis of the orbit, whether they go on to resolution or suppuration, have their origin in infection of one of the nasal accessory sinuses.

The mode of infection from the sinuses varies. It may be through a dehiscence in or by perforation of the bony wall of the sinus. In these cases the abscess, as it were, ruptures into the orbit and the purulent cavity in the sinus and orbit is continuous through the opening. Skillern in his work on the accessory sinuses of the nose, says: "The continual apposition of the purulent secretion results in maceration of the epithelium, which gradually pervades the entire mucosa until it becomes, in certain areas, loose on the underlying bone. The purulent material, thus coming in direct contact with the bone, slowly infiltrates through the canaliculæ and Haversian canals (possibly with the aid of blood and lymph vessels) and eventually reaches the periosteum of the opposite side. From here on but little resistance is opposed to the spread of the infection. The infection may travel along the sheaths of the vessels and nerves." It has seemed to me that a thrombophlebitis of the ethmoid veins has been the cause of the majority of cases which have come under my observation.

Several cases of orbital abscess have been operated upon by me in the past ten years, and in all of them a careful examination of the wall of the sinuses has been made. In none of them could denudation or dehiscence be found, but in all the offending sinus was demonstrated by finding pus.

The ethmoid labyrinth seems to be the cause of orbital cellulitis more frequently than any other sinus. This is particularly true in children.

The offending sinus may be suspected by the direction of the exophthalmos,· but the diagnosis must not be based upon this, a careful examination of the nose being indicated.

Case.—A. J. W. M., age eight years. First seen December 6, 1920. Parents living, in good health. Brothers and sisters healthy.

Boy well nourished, but rather small in stature. Quite bright and active physically.

Has had some of diseases of childhood. Physical examination negative except condition for which he was presented.

Status praesens: Father says that he has had a "bad cold" with profuse nasal discharge, more from right nostril, for the past week. This morning he awoke complaining of the right eye. Condition today has not been good. No appetite and does not want to play.

Examination reveals right nostril filled with profuse mucopurulent discharge. Nostril quickly fills up after being cleared out. Discharge seen coming from below middle turbinate. Gentle suction brings large amount. Slight swelling over upper inner angle of right orbit. Extreme tenderness on pressure over most prominent part of swelling. Motility of eye unimpaired.

With use of rest, hot fomentations over eye, gentle suction and spray containing adrenalin there was no change in the local appearance for three days, and the general condition of the boy seemed better. On the fourth day there was a change for the worse. Swelling more pronounced and painful, some exophthalmos, with cornea directed downward and outward. Marked loss of motility of eye, though there was still some voluntary movement outward and downward. X-ray examination at this time revealed cloudiness in right ethmoid and inner portion of right orbit. Operation was advised but not acceded to for about five days, at which time there was marked increase in the swelling and edema of conjunctiva. Exophthalmos very marked. No motility of eye, cornea turned downward and outward. Discharge from nose almost entirely absent. At no time was there any evidence of a continuity between the ethmoid and orbital abscesses. Pressure over orbital swelling caused no discharge into nose, nor did forcible inflation of nose produce bulging of the orbital swelling.

Under ether anesthesia incision was made into the abscess cavity through the upper lid and about 8 cc. of pus evacuated. Careful search of the inner walls of the orbit was made for denuded bone or an opening into the ethmoid cells but neither could be found. Wick drain inserted and wet dressing applied. Recovery prompt and uneventful with perfect vision and motility of eye. Ethmoid seems entirely free from disease at present.

This case seems to me to have resulted from a thrombophlebitis of one of the ethmoid veins.

STUART CIRCLE HOSPITAL.

# XXXII

# AN ARGUMENT IN-FAVOR OF PRELIGATION OF THE JUGULAR IN SINUS THRO A BOSIS.

By T. H. ODENEAL, M. D

John ———, age 40, laborer, referred to me by a general physician, with swelling and tenderness over the zygomatic area of the right mastoid. Discharging ear for six weeks, during which time he had continued to work. Temperature slightly elevated, felt well with exception of slight pain in swollen area and headaches. No bulging of canal wall or undue sensitiveness on pressure of the mastoid proper (in my opinion, the character of the swelling often indicates sinus thrombosis, swelling high up without being extension from lower down being very suggestive).

On operation the sinus was found thrombosed, with the anterior will necrosed and partly absent.

It is customary for me to ligate the jugular in thrombotic cases before removing the clot, but as the membranous wall of the sinus was partly absent in this case I removed some of the clot before deciding to ligate the jugular and then, having made my decision to ligate, packed the mastoid wound lightly and prepared for the ligation. The incision made, I began separating down to the vein, when the anesthetist informed me the patient had ceased to breathe. About three minutes before, the nurse had taken the pulse and found it normal. Artificial respiration and stimulants failed to revive the patient.

Death no doubt was due to an infarct originating from the sinus thrombus and lodging in a cerebral vessel, causing paralysis of the respiratory center. Had I ligated the jugular in this case before disturbing the clot I have no doubt the patient would be alive today.

I was very much interested in the discussion of the New York Otological Society of March 25, 1919, relative to the merits of ligation of the jugular in sinus thrombosis, and the variety of opinions on the subject stimulated me to report this case, as we have here an actual and not a hypothetical cause for preligation of the jugular in sinus thrombosis.

Whereas formerly the majority of ear surgeons believed in jugular ligation, I believe today they are in the minority, but this case has strengthened me in my former adherence to ligation in all thrombus cases.

In cases of seemingly localized phlebitis, where the sinus is covered with granulations and there is good pulsation, I never open the sinus, and have always had good success with such cases (ligation, of course, is also not done). This case is presented merely as a record, and I hope it will be of assistance as such.

# ABSTRACTS FROM CURRENT LITERATURE.

## I.—EAR.

### Acute Meningitis of Otitic Origin as Observed in the Desgenette Military Hospital During the War.

Lannois and Sargnon.

Rev. de laryngol., d'otol., July 15, 1920.

From November, 1914, to December 31, 1918, 24,600 ear patients were seen. Of these, 5,500 were admitted to the hospital; 630 operations were practiced upon the ear, of which 34 were for otitic meningitis. The number of deaths in the 5,500 cases were 74. Of this number, 26 were due to otitic meningitis. Nothing peculiar was seen in the pathologic anatomy of the cases. Of the eight cases which recovered, in two no microbes could be discovered. The others belong to a variety of serous meningitis with polynuclear action more or less marked. In the fatal cases, on the other hand, the organisms were easy of determination. Ten times pure streptococcus associated with staphylococcus; one case with pneumococcus; meningitis due to streptococcus were decidedly the most grave.

From the standpoint of evolution, three forms can be distinguished: the fulminating, the acute and the subacute. The prognosis varies according to the form. The fulminating type are beyond help; of the acute form, 18 out of 27 had brain abscesses, six recovered; the subacute type furnished two recoveries.

The authors lay great weight upon operating at the earliest possible time. Repeatedly they have operated immediately, day or night, as soon as the lumbar puncture established the diagnosis. Beyond the thorough cleaning out of the mastoid, they practiced only repeated lumbar punctures, at first daily and later every second day until the severe symptoms moderated. In addition to this, they recommend the systematic employment twice daily of hot baths for thirty minutes at a time.                     Harris.

### Paroxysmal Bilateral Suppurative Otitis Media.

Levesque.

Rev. de laryngol., d'otol., April 30, 1920.

The author dwells on the important role which the sympathetic fibers of the trigeminal play in the anatomy and physiology of the nose, throat and ear. Lesions in the eye and in the ear caused by section of the trigeminal in the neighborhood of the Gasserian ganglion have been studied both in the laboratory and in certain cases of brain tumor. They are described under the name of neuroparalytic keratitis and neuroparalytic otitis. The latter is more capable of demonstration than the former. Such a case following tumor of the ganglion has been seen by Levesque. Closely allied to this so-called false otitis is a form of otitis which, in his opinion, is due to an irritation of the sympathetic fibers of the trigeminal. Such a case he has recently seen. It was a young woman who from November, 1911, to the end of 1914 had more than forty attacks of acute suppurative middle ear disease on the right side and more than twenty on the left. The attacks lasted from four to five days and were followed by complete cicatrization of the drum. The onset of the attack is announced by sharp pain in the ear for six or eight hours, accompanied by somnolence hyperacousis and abundant salivation. The face is congested, the conjunctiva injected on the side involved, much lacrimation, profuse discharge from the nose with cough. Paracentesis has been repeatedly performed. Twenty-four hours after the beginning of the attack the drum membrane no longer bulged, gradually resumed its normal color, no perforation persisted, and there was no evidence of scarring. Simultaneously, all the mucopurulent discharge from the nose gradually ceased.

In the author's opinion, this is a case of sympathetic fiber irritation, the cause resting either in the accessory sinuses of the nose or in the teeth. In this particular case, removal of the nasal polyp had no effect upon the attacks. He adds that in another case he has noted the disappearance of the polyp by simple removal of a diseased tooth, and, in many cases, shrinking in the size of the polyp following attention to the teeth.                    Harris.

### What Is to Be Understood by Aberrant Mastoid Cells.

#### Mouret.

#### Rev. de laryngol., d'otol., etc., May 31, 1920.

In the year 1901 Prof. Moure gave the term of aberrant cells as the result of a case at that time under his observation, where a mastoid operation had been performed which was followed a month later by meningitis and death. The autopsy showed a purulent cavity lying on a horizontal plane which passed through the upper pole of the external orifice of the auditory canal and 1 cm. posterior on a vertical plane passing through the summit of the mastoid. A wall of compact bone 0.5 cm., eburnated and healthy, separated this cavity from the antrum.

Based on this finding of Moure, Mouret has made a careful study of the whole subject. In his opinion, Moure's case is one of ostitis. A priori, the separation caused by the thick bone of compact tissue "can only be apparent," although the communication between such a cell and the antrum cannot be direct. In order to determine accurately such a separation, it is necessary in the course of an operation to go to the internal cortex. It is Mouret's custom in his mastoidectomies to make a deep groove in the bone posterior to the antrum and parallel to the line a temporalis. In this way he repeatedly has found deep seated cells which were absolutely isolated from the mastoid. The explanation of the existence of the wall of bone lies in a fusing of the petrosal to the squamous portion of the temporal.

The author describes the embryology of the mastoid and concludes that in its development the bands connecting the petrosa and the squama gradually disappear, although the tendency of both laminae is to grow together. Mouret has carried out extensive experiments with the injection of methylene blue and has demonstrated his contention that these deep seated mastoid cells are really not isolated but connected with the antrum. He makes the following conclusions:

a. That a wandering cell is a pneumatic cell of which the connection with the other pneumatic cavities of the temporal bone does not appear at first inspection and requires in consequence to be sought for. There does not exist in fact an isolated pneumatic cell separated from the entire cavity which communicates with the outer air. A pneumatic cell has need of air in order to live normally.

b. When one encounters an infected mastoid area separated from the large pneumatic cavity, there is a disposition to speak of it as an aberrant cellulitis. Ostitis, however, secondary to a middle ear inflammation, is not rare. Very frequently it constitutes the only mastoid lesion which makes one think of the presence of a wandering mastoid.

c. The presence of cells removed from the antrum is one of the causes which favor strongly a large and deep mastoidectomy as compared with a simple antrotomy.                              Harris.

### Local Anesthesia for Simple Mastoid Operations.

#### Koebbe, E. E.

#### J. Am. M. Ass., Chicago, 1921—LXXVI—1334.

For all of the cases, 1 per cent procain with from 1 to 2 drams of 1:1,000 epinephrin solution to the ounce has been used. The procain and epinephrin are boiled separately. An ordinary 2 cc. Luer syringe with a No. 23 gauge 1-inch needle has been used. The subcutaneous tissues are first infiltrated, beginning at a point directly posterior to the external auditory meatus in the line of incision and following the line of incision to its most upper and anterior point, and then downward anterior to the pinna as far as the level of the tragus. The next infiltration begins at the same point as the first, and extends downward to about 1 inch below the mastoid tip. At this point a slightly deeper injection is made; this effectively blocks the great auricular nerve. Directly below the mastoid tip a deeper injection is now made; this blocks the posterior auricular nerve. The branches of the small occipital nerve are now blocked about 1½ inches posterior to and on a level with the external auditory meatus. The needle is now inserted from behind the ear into the posterior wall of the external auditory canal, nearly to the attachment of the tympanic membrane. This step is very important, as the patient will experience pain when the periosteum around the canal is elevated, and the pinna is pushed forward, if this injection is not made. Finally, the needle is thrust under the periosteum in four or five places so that the anesthetic completely infiltrates all the periosteum that is to be elevated. All this is done before the skin incision is made, and it is not necessary to use any more anesthetic after the operation has been begun.

It requires from 6 to 8 cc. of solution to complete the anesthesia. As soon as the last injection has been made, skin clamps are used to hold the mastoid sheet and towels in position. It is not necessary to wait after the injection has been finished before the incision is made.

A general anesthetic is more or less difficult to administer to a patient undergoing a mastoid operation, on account of the position of the patient, small amount of space and danger of contaminating the field of operation. If the patient's tongue has a tendency to fall backward, or if there is an excess of mucus, the difficulties are still further increased. Then, too, the operator and his assistants usually inhale a considerable portion of the anesthetic. A large proportion of mastoid operations follow an attack of measles, which may also have been complicated with pneumonia and in which a general anesthetic would be given more or less reluctantly. In this series, thirty-five were mastoid cases that followed otitis media complicating measles, and five of the patients had or were recovering from bronchopneumonia at the time of operation. By employing local anesthesia we were able to operate earlier in a large percentage of the cases than would have been possible if it had been necessary to give a general anesthetic. In one case of frank lobar pneumonia, operation was performed on the third day of the pneumonia. The patient recovered uneventfully from the pneumonia and the mastoid wound was healed on the twelfth day.

This method is applicable to all patients except children too young to be reasoned with. In this series the ages range from 15 to 32. However, there is no reason why patients much younger than 15 should not be operated on by local anesthesia, provided they have not been terrorized. Emil Mayer.

## II.—NOSE.

### Trephining of the Frontal Sinus.

#### Mouret.

#### Rev. de laryngol., d'otol., August 15, 1920.

In the last twenty-five years the author has performed all the various operations upon the frontal sinus. The Luc operation has given good results where the sinus is small. It does not allow, however, sufficient room for curetting the entire ethmoid or when the frontal sinus is very large. The Kuhnt gives good results, but the after-appearance is bad. The Killian gives good esthetic results, but as a result of the resection of the orbital roof and especially most of the internal wall, it allows the soft tissues of the orbit to prolapse into the nose and so often sets up a secondary narrowing of the nasofrontal duct.

The radical operation upon the frontal sinus should have these objects in view:

1. Opening the sinus.
2. Removal of all granulation tissue.
3. Curetting the neighboring cells which are diseased.
4. Obtaining the establishment of a permanent opening into the nose.

As the result of his long experience, the author has abandoned all the classical procedures. Of them all, he regards the Killian as the best, but to this he finds the following objections: The prolapse of the soft parts, primary or secondary infection of the periorbital tissues, and stricture of the nasofrontal canal. So far as the first objection is concerned, he states that he has observed in all cases operated on by this method a certain drooping of the soft parts which tends to injure the esthetic result. He lays particular attention upon the primary or secondary infection of the periorbital tissues, and where this does not occur has noted edema of the upper eyelid following the operation, also a denuding and stripping of the orbital floor of the sinus. Even more serious are the inflammatory swellings of the soft tissues of the upper internal angle of the orbit, coming on several weeks, even several months after the operation. Occasionally, a small abscess will form here. His most serious objection, however, is the narrowing of the nasofrontal canal. In small sinuses, the cavity can be obliterated by the method of Killian but not where it is large. It is common to witness the gradual narrowing of a nasofrontal canal, which immediately following the operation was wide open.

As a result of these objections, Mouret favors the Ogston-Luc or the Taptas operation. The former, however, is intended only for small sinuses and possesses the objection that it does not enlarge the nasofrontal canal nor permit of a complete curetting of the ethmoid. The Taptas operation is favorable to sinuses of a larger size and permits of curetting the lateral masses of the ethmoid, as a result of the resection of the ascending process of the superior maxilla. He makes in the anterior wall of the sinus several openings which are separated from one another, permitting the introduction of the curette. This, Mouret believes, is more desirable than the method of Killian. When it is a case of a large sinus with marked development in the roof of the orbit, Mouret favors in addition to the double frontonasal and supraorbital openings a third opening in the external half of the orbital floor of the sinus. He takes great pains, however, not to disturb the inner part of this floor, and especially the orbital portion of the nasal fossa of the frontal which forms the external wall of communication of the sinus with the nose. Operating in this way, one avoids secondary narrowings of this part, upon which depends communication with the nose after operation.    Harris.

### III.—PHARYNX AND MOUTH.

#### Examination of the Throat in Botulism—A Question of Differential Diagnosis.

Vernieuwe.

Rev. de laryngol., d'otol., June 15, 1920.

The author reports the case of a young woman who presented herself to him complaining of a nasal voice, where a paralysis of the soft palate was found. At the same time symptoms of the lack of accommodation showed themselves. A diagnosis of postdiphtheritic paralysis of the soft palate was made. Later, her brother developed the same symptoms. A paralysis of the soft palate was also diagnosed, as well as failure of accommodation. In addition, he complained of a sensation of extreme dryness in the throat during swallowing. There was an elevated temperature, the face was cyanosed, feeble pulse and a paresis of the lower extremities. Inquiry showed that both patients had eaten raw ham as well as six others. All showed lack of accommodation; in four there was paralysis of the soft palate. They all made an uneventful recovery. The paralysis of the soft palate lasted fifteen days; lack of accommodation persisted for a considerably longer time.

The author discusses the resemblance of botulism to postdiphtheritic paralysis and makes the following differential diagnosis:

1. Accommodation and the pupillary sphincter are in botulism generally affected at the same time, if not to the same degree. In postdiphtheritic paralysis,, on the contrary, the pupillary action remains intact.

2. External muscles of the eye are very rarely involved in postdiphtheritic paralysis. In botulism, on the other hand, it is not rare to see, apart from an internal ophthalmoplegia interna, a paralysis of the external muscles.

3. Paralysis of the eye appears often on the first day; more often, on the second or third day after the taking of the poisoning food. Postdiphtheritic paralysis appears much later; on the average, four weeks after the attack of diphtheria.

4. The duration of the paralysis from botulism exceeds in duration that of postdiphtheritic paralysis: "Four to eight weeks in case of diphtheria, five to eight months in paralysis of botulism."

In conclusion, the author refers to the similarity of the symptoms of botulism to those in atropin poisoning: Agittaion, dryness of the throat, notable diminution of the saliva, hallucination of the vision, dilatation of the pupil, but there never exists a paralysis of the external muscles of the eye in atropin poisoning. This symptom is peculiar to botulism.                    Harris.

**The Tonsil and Adenoid Situation in New York City. Report by the Public Health Committee of the New York Academy of Medicine.**

Med. Rec., N. York, 1921—XCIX—845.

The present annual demand for tonsil and adenoid operations can be estimated as of over 55,000. The existing facilities when fully utilized can probably be made sufficient to meet this demand, but the number of operations performed in 1920 was 8,000 below the estimated demand.

There is need for a regulatory system to secure a more uniform distribution of patients among the hospitals and to reduce the excessively long waiting lists in some hospitals.

The standards of operative procedure, as well as the care of children, before and after tonsillectomy, differ considerably in the several hospitals. There is a need of stimulating the institutions to an appreciation of the importance of a thorough physical examination of the patients before operation and of provision for adequate care after operation, as well as for more effective methods of instruction as to care to be taken after the patients leave the hospital.

A longer period of pre- and post-operative care would reduce the number of cases which can be accommodated in hospitals, and an extension of facilities in certain directions or during certain periods of the year might, therefore, be required.          Emil Mayer.

### Induced Atrophy of Hypertrophied Tonsils by Roentgen Ray.

Murphy, James B.; Witherbee, W. D.; Craig, S. L.; Hussey, R. G., and Sturm, Ernest.

J. Am. M. Ass., Chicago, 1921—LXXVI—228.

The factors governing the dose of Roentgen ray given in the region of each tonsil were as follows: The spark gap measured between points was 8 inches; 5 milliamperes; 10 inches distance from the target to the highest point of skin exposed. The time of exposure varied from three to seven minutes, according to the age of the patient. The ray was filtered through 3 mm. of aluminum. The approximate value of this dose was 1 to 1¾ skin units. The patient to be treated was placed on a table in such a position that the ray entered under the angle of the jaw and penetrated through the soft tissues to the region of the tonsil. The area exposed on each side was about 3 square inches, the surrounding parts being protected by heavy sheet lead. For young children a special board was used with retaining straps, and the head secured by means of a gauze bandage.

In all but four cases the treatment was followed by marked improvement. In the majority of cases, two weeks after the exposure to the roentgen ray a distinct shrinkage of the tonsil was noted, this process continuing from one to two months. During this period of atrophy the crypts opened and drained, and, in all but a few cases the exudate disappeared from the throat, and the surface of the tonsils became smooth, pale and of a healthy appearance. With the exception of four cases, no exudate could be squeezed from the deep tonsillar tissue at the end of the period of observation. Later examination of the throat showed the edges of the crypts to be inverted, and in a number of cases white bands resembling scar tissue were noted on the surface.

The results reported here suggest the possibility of utilizing the well known fact that lymphoid tissue is easily destroyed by the roentgen ray for clearing the throat of an excess of this tissue. In the series reported above, only one patient received more than one treatment.

To judge by studies on animals, it should be possible to induce almost any degree of atrophy by repeating the roentgen ray treatments at suitable intervals. It is possible that the hypertrophied condition may return after a lapse of time; but with the mildness of the roentgen ray treatments recommended, there is no reason why it should not be repeated as often as desired, with the proper interval between exposures. The acual amount of roentgen ray used is smaller than that commonly used in the treatment of ringworm of the scalp, from which no bad results have been recorded.

The disappearance of the hemolytic organisms of the throat is attributed, not to the direct action of the Roentgen ray on these organisms, but rather to the proper drainage of the crypts as the tonsil tissue atrophies.

How practicable this treatment will prove can be determined only by the study of a large series of cases followed over a considerable interval of time. Emil Mayer.

### The Value of Vaccine Therapy Versus Tonsillectomy in Systemic Disease of Tonsillar Origin.

Hays, Harold; Palmer, Arthur, and Winslow, Thomas S.

Med. Rec., N. York, 1921—XCIX—304.

1. Systemic disease is often of tonsillar origin, even when the tonsils are small and show little evidence of disease.

2. Cultures from the tonsils should be taken in all cases of systemic disease.

3. Cultures taken from the tonsils, preferably from the supratonsillar fossa, showing any form of streptococcus, should be considered prima facie evidence of tonsillar disease sufficient for their removal, if associated with systemic disease.

4. Tonsillectomy is a better procedure than the administration of vaccines unless operation is contraindicated.

5. A poorly performed operation is no criterion of the value of tonsillectomy. A small piece of tonsil remaining may still keep up the systemic infection.

6. The value of the vaccine as a curative agent is yet to be proved.                                    Emil Mayer.

### Studies of the Nasopharyngeal Secretions From Influenza Patients.

Olitsky, Peter K., and Gates, Frederick L. .

J. Am. M. Ass., Chicago, 1921—LXXVI—641.

From the filtered nasopharyngeal washings, from early cases of uncomplicated epidemic influenza and from the lung tissues of experimental animals, we have cultivated minute bodies of characteristic morphology which are strictly anerobic, are filtrable, and withstand glycerolation for a period of months. The effects on the blood and in the lungs of rabbits and guinea pigs injected with these bodies are similar to those produced by the filtered and unfiltered nasopharyngeal secretions from early cases of epidemic influenza.                                    Emil Mayer.

## IV.—LARYNX, TRACHEA AND ESOPHAGUS.

### Laryngeal Diphtheria. Review of Five Hundred and Fifteen Cases in Which Intubation Was Performed.

Hoyne, Archibald L.

J. Am. M. Ass., Chicago, 1921—LXXVI—1305.

There is probably no more difficult operation in surgery than an intubation properly performed. And whereas almost any one possessing a little surgical skill can make an incision in the neck and insert a tracheotomy tube, very few will succeed in their endeavors to intubate the larynx unless some experience has been acquired in this character of work.

Some of the remarkable results reported for intubated patients in private practice must be totally beyond the comprehension of any one possessing an extensive hospital experience in this type of disease.

Laryngeal diphtheria is the one type of disease in which the general practitioner is most inclined to give massive doses of antitoxin, and yet in cases in which the membrane is confined to the larynx such treatment is seldom required. These patients do not suffer extensively from a toxemia. The ordinary complications of diphtheria, such as the various forms of paralysis and nephritis, are not often encountered when the membrane is limited to the larynx. When death ensues, it is almost invariably due either to asphyxiation, as a result of mechanical obstruction by the membrane or to a complicating bronchopneumonia. From 15,000 to 20,000 units is usually a sufficiently large dose of antitoxin for cases in which the larynx alone is involved. If there are other sites of infection also, as the tonsils or nasopharynx, a considerably larger amount of antitoxin may be demanded.

The following factors may be summarized as having been contributory to the excellent results secured in this series of hospital cases:

1. Permanence of resident physicians.

2. Specially trained nurses, one of whom always has the patients under constant observation.

3. Emergency bell system.

4. An interval of four or five days before the tube is removed after intubation. This has reduced the number of reintubations necessary.

5. Thorough sterilization of instruments, thus lessening to some degree, at least, complicating bronchopneumonias.

6. Thorough cleansing of hands before and after each operation, a simple precaution, which, nevertheless, is often neglected in dealing with intubated patients.

7. The transfer of patients from the tube room as soon as this can be done with safety, thus lessening the chance of crossed infections.                                    Emil Mayer.

## V.—MISCELLANEOUS.

### The Socalled Impassable Cicatricial Stenosis in the Esophagus in Infants.

#### Brindel.

Rev. de laryngol., d'otol., August 15, 1920.

During the present year Brindel has seen five cases of esophageal stenosis in infants. As a result of the study of these cases he is inclined to disagree with Guiseau in his view that the affection is a progressive one. He strongly favors the hypothesis of spasm. In favor of this is the facility with which one can dilate such a stenosis when he has succeeded in passing it for the first time. At the same sitting it is often possible to introduce ten or fifteen numbers of the bougie. If it were a case of purely fibrous stricture, in his opinion, it would not be possible to obtain so rapid a result.

In conclusion, particular emphasis is laid upon the value of the esophagoscope in causing the disappearance, in the great majority of cases, of impassable strictures.                          Harris.

### Roentgenographic Studies of Bronchiectasis and Lung Abscess After Direct Injection of Bismuth Mixture.

Lynah, Henry L., and Stewart, William H.

Ann. Surg., N. York, 1921—LXXVIII—3.

(1) Bismuth mixtures can be injected into the bronchi and lungs of a living patient without danger. (2) The injection of an opaque substance into the lung of the living patient will open an enormous field of usefulness in the study of cough, the expulsion of substances from the lung, and lung drainage. It will also aid in localizing bronchial strictures in the same manner as in the esophagus. Furthermore, it will be of the greatest aid to the thoracic surgeon by mapping out the abscess cavity in the respective lobe of the lung. (3) A definite lung abscess cavity is seldom seen bronchoscopically. Pus is usually seen coming from a branch bronchus, although the abscess may be well around the corner, and not in that portion of the lung from which the pus is oozing. An injection of bismuth mixture or some other opaque mixture will "clear up" this error. (4) Bismuth when it enters the abscess cavity is recognized by its metallic luster, whereas, when it is in the lobular lung structure it is discerned as a dull, opaque area. Pus diffuses and soaks the lobular structure in a manner similar to bismuth; this often makes the involved area appear many times larger than it really is. (5) The bismuth mixture injected in these patients was 8 cc. of bismuth subcarbonate in pure olive oil (1-2). The mixture is rendered sterile by boiling before injection. (6) The injection should be made slowly and not with a "squirt," or else the roentgenographic observations may be spoiled by bismuth soaking the lung structure surrounding the diseased area. (7) It seems from these preliminary studies that cough and action of cilia are not the only means of expelling secretions. (8) While bismuth mixtures were originally injected for the purpose of lung mapping in cases of lung abscess cavities, they seem to have been of therapeutic benefit to the five patients upon whom they were tried. So far the procedure has done no harm. (9) While the fluoroscopic examination is important, stereoroentgenographic examination is the best means of localizing the cavitations. (10) Experience has shown that the Roentgen examination should be made almost immediately after the removal of the bronchoscope, otherwise the patient, in a fit of coughing, will remove much of the bismuth from the involved lung.                    Emil Mayer.

### A Refinement in the Radical Operation for Trigeminal Neuralgia.

Frazier, Charles H.

J. Am. M. Ass., Chicago, 1921—LXXVI—107.

In every respect the results of the radical operation for trigeminal neuralgia are most satisfactory. With the exception of one death from apoplexy of a patient in the convalescent stage, there have been none in my clinic in the last 157 operations (0.6 per cent).

These are the major considerations. Of minor consideration is the "cosmetics." In times past the motor root has been sacrificed with the sensory root, and there followed inevitably atrophy of the temporal, masseter and pterygoid muscles. So far as it affected movements of the jaw it was a matter of inconvenience; but the atrophy of the temporal muscle left a depression above the zygoma that was quite noticeable and prevented what otherwise might have been regarded as a perfect cosmetic result, since the incision was well concealed within the hair line. To meet this objection some surgeons went so far as to resect the zygoma.

In the past the motor root was often sacrificed because the surgeon was afraid he might be leaving a fasciculus of the sensory root with all its unfortunate possibilities. But with the use of the electrode the motor root when exposed can positively be identified as motor by observing the temporal muscle contact.

When the sensory root is adequately exposed, in the course of the operation, it is elevated from its bed with a blunt instrument. Usually the motor root may be seen in contact with the skull, traversing the space behind the root and disappearing behind the ganglion. If recognized or suspected, the electrode is applied; and should it prove to be the motor root, the fibers of the temporal muscle, exposed to view in the wound, will contract. Sometimes at this preliminary inspection the motor root will not be seen because, cleaving to the sensory root, it has been lifted up by the instrument with the sensory root. Under these circumstances I make segmental sections of the sensory root, beginning with the outer fasciculi, and search for the motor root after each section. Usually when half of the sensory root has been divided, one can recognize the motor root as it passes behind the ganglion. But to confirm the observation, the electrode is used. If these directions are followed, the motor root may be conserved in the majority of instances. It has escaped me occasionally, but with continued effort and experience, I believe it will be possible to save the root in every instance. With this refinement in technic the radical operation might be said to be beyond criticism. Symmetry of the face is conserved, as there is no atrophy of the temporal muscle; there is no deviation of the jaw, since the pterygoid muscles are intact; and mastication is in no way interfered with.

Emil Mayer.

### The Mechanism of the Carrier State, With Special Reference to Carriers of Friedlander's Bacillus.

Bloomfield, Arthur L.

Bull. Johns Hopkins Hosp., 1921—XXXII—359.

Bloomfield found it possible to show, in the case of Friedlander bacillus carriers, that the breeding place of the bacteria is in a definite focus—the tonsil. From this point the organisms are discharged into the open pharyngeal cavity, and at times may be introduced into the nose. There is no evidence, however, to indicate that any adaptation takes place between the bacilli and the mucous surfaces. They react as the normal mucous membranes do, both surfaces, leading to actual growth and multiplication on these upon the introduction of the carrier's own strain, or the introduction of a second strain of Friedlander's bacillus.

Of the eighty-five unselected individuals studied in this investigation, 5.8 per cent were found to be carriers of Friedlander's bacillus. The carrier state persisted throughout the observation. There was no tendency for contacts to acquire the carrier state Differential cultures showed the breeding place of the Friedlander bacilli to be in the tonsil. The carrier's own strain or a foreign strain of Friedlander bacillus implanted upon the free surfaces of the mucous membranes disappeared at the same rate of speed as in a noncarrier. It was impossible, artificially, to produce a carrier state by repeated inoculation with B. Friedlander. The general conclusion from these observations is that the carrier state depends on a focus of diseased tissue which affords a breeding place for the bacteria. They do not become adapted to growth on the free surfaces of the mucous membranes. Emil Mayer.

### Pituitary Extract in Conjunction•With Local Anesthesia.

Otrich, G. C.

J. Am. M. Ass., Chicago, 1921—LXXVL—591.

The writer uses a 2 per cent procain solution in combination with pituitary extract, 1 cc. of the obstetric strength, to 5 cc. of the procain solution. "When a larger amount is to be used, I use the surgical strength.

"My preference for pituitary extract to epinephrin is that the action is slower in taking effect and lasts much longer, which is proved by taking the blood pressure curve after the injection. The longer period of vasoconstruction gives a better chance for the organization of the clot. The slow passing effect and the slow returning to normal of the small vessels give the clot a better chance for futher fibrination, thus holding more securely. In epinephrin the action is very rapid and the effect passes with the same rapidity. Therefore, sufficient time is not given for clot formation and fibrination. Furthermore, in the sudden relaxation of the walls of the small vessels and arterioles, the clot will be washed away and the secondary hemorrhage will take place, and it will be harder to control than the original." Emil Mayer.

# SOCIETY PROCEEDINGS.

## CHICAGO LARYNGOLOGICAL AND OTOLOGICAL SOCIETY.

*Meeting of January 3, 1921.*

### THE PRESIDENT, DR. ALFRED LEWY, IN THE CHAIR.

#### Teratoid Tumor of the Floor of the Mouth.

Dr. Otto J. Stein presented the specimen of a teratoid tumor on the floor of the mouth, which he had removed from a patient presented two months previously. Dr. Stein had been asked whether the condition was common or rare as seen by throat specialists. At the time this patient was presented he had seen only two cases but had since seen a third case, the specimen from which he also exhibited.

Dr. Norval H. Pierce presented a paper entitled,

#### "The Normal and Pathological Pneumatization of the Temporal Bone—A Review"* (With Lantern Slides).

### DISCUSSION.

Dr. J. Holinger expressed himself as much interested in Wittmaack's book, which he had only recently received, and tendered his personal thanks to Dr. Pierce for having brought the work to the attention of the Society in this instructive manner. He believed that Wittmaack found well prepared ground in the work of Preysing on the otitis of the newborn. Nevertheless he felt that the work of Wittmaack showed great originality and a very great fascination in its diction. Still he hoped that Dr. Pierce would not expect that all was accepted without criticism.

In the chapter on cholesteatoma, he found that Wittmaack explained that cholesteatoma may form in ears where no suppuration or inflammation had ever occurred. In looking over his own publications Dr. Holinger found that in 1901 he had stated in an article on "Varieties of Cholesteatoma" (read before the Chicago Pathological Society) "Suppuration of the middle ear need not have preceded and yet we have epidermis in the middle ear and cholesteatoma." Ten years ago in a paper on "The Pathology and Prognosis of Internal Ear Complications Resulting from Inflammatory Middle Ear Diseases," he had stated, "It may also occur without even a trace of inflammation or suppuration or granulation being present."

As to the progress of cholesteatoma towards the interior of the skull cavity, the embryonal communications discovered by Wittmaack certainly do not form the only route. The absorption of

---

*See page 509.

bone and consequent disappearance of the walls, as Dr. Holinger had observed, often result in a spreading of the cholesteatoma through perfectly normal bone. The absorption of healthy bone is a process which is general in the cholesteatoma cavities. Dr. Holinger has at least two microscopical specimens of walls of cholesteatoma in which there is no trace of underlying embryonal tissue and where the epidermis is practically on the bone with no more than one layer of subepithelial tissue between it and the bone. Absorption of bone in Howship's lacunae goes on directly under the epidermis, and the epidermis on one place forms a bridge over a Howship's lacuna.

Other points in the course of development of cholesteatoma will be difficult to explain on the basis of faulty pneumatization. Take for example the following cases: A man was 36 years old when first seen. Dr. Holinger observed him for more than ten years. Owing to the fact that the patient could not come regularly for treatment of a very stubborn occlusion of the eustachian tube, the drum-head became more and more retracted. At first it was easy to bring the membrane back to normal, later on hard, then impossible. The retraction was so bad that a regular cholesteatoma formed. It was necessary to perform a radical operation within five years and large masses of cholesteatomous material were found in the antrum. If the man had remnants of embryonal tissue in the antrum and middle ear all the time, why did he have to wait until he was 36 years old before retraction of the membrane began, which finally led to the development of the cholesteatoma after the age of 40?

Furthermore, on December 1st Dr. Holinger read a paper before the Chicago Medical Society on "Perforations of the Drum Membrane," and showed a boy suffering from occlusion of the eustachian tube and retraction of the membrane. The posterior portion of the membrane was deeply drawn up into the antrum but it came back each time after inflation. In that case he could show the cause for the occlusions of the eustachian tube, a scar, perpendicular to the axis of the opening of the eustachian tube, could be seen through the pharyngoscope. This scar distinctly stenosed the eustachian tube. There the process was caused by a visible agent, which produced the occlusion of the tube. So far as he could see, there was no reason to suspect abnormal conditions of the lining membranes of the middle ear or adhesions which form an occlusion of the drum cavity from the upper cavity an antrum. An X-ray picture of the mastoid of this patient showed good pneumatization. So this could not be the cause of the disease. The explanation of this case is clear: In removing the adenoids, the surgeon had injured the orifice of the eustachian tube and the beginning cholesteatoma is the consequence of the stenosis of the tube. The persistent embryonal tissue and incomplete pneumatization is certainly not the cause of every cholesteatoma.

Dr. Joseph C. Beck said that he was at a disadvantage because he had not seen the book of Wittmaack, but he wished to join Dr. Holinger in expressing his appreciation of Dr. Pierce's excellent presentation of a most difficult subject. He was inclined to think that it almost hurt Prof. Siebenmann and a criticism of Wittmaack's work by the professor shortly after its publication was brought out in the leading German journal devoted to otolaryngology, which Dr. Beck had read with great interest. He was sure everyone appreciated the pioneer work of Prof. Siebenmann in otosclerosis and yet were interested in the heated discussions between Siebenmann and Manasse and the former's opposition to Manasse's opinions on otosclerosis, and Manasse has many adherents at present. He had seen Wittmaack in Europe, as a student, and had then the impression that he did not know much more than the others, but his work that had been shown by Dr. Pierce as well as other studies formerly brought out, promised for Wittmaack big things, especially so from the pathologic point of view in such diseases which had not been relieved by previous treatments, as for instance, adhesive processes of the middle ear. The sad part in Wittmaack's work as presented by Dr. Pierce was the inability to prevent this infant spongifying process in the ear. This last work of Wittmaack's was a stimulation for Dr. Beck to go over his microscopic specimens of infant and children mastoid chips again and take, what he thought, from a histologic point of view, to be exudate in the mastoid cells and see if it was not this embryonal tissue which he had probably not stained as carefully as Wittmaack. He intended to study such specimens again and hoped to have the privilege of bringing them before the Society again and emphasizing the points brought out by Dr. Pierce.

Dr. Beck thought he could speak of between 500 and 2000 X-ray pictures of the mastoid taken stereoscopically in regard to pneumatization. These were made in all possible conditions in children, and he was sure that if pneumatization had been inhibited as mentioned by Dr. Pierce, the percentage was too high, because most of the radiograms examined up to five years have been found to have large pneumatized mastoids, usually present on both sides. Many of the children had conditions due to otitis media and adenoids, which should have arrested the pneumatization as stated by Dr. Pierce. If the arrest was due to such tissue changes, why would it not stop pneumatization sooner. In his opinion, the percentage stated to exist was too high.

Another point was the pneumatization of the adult mastoid. The speaker had studied the large pneumatization mastoids and found them having the dumb-bell contraction in and about the antrum mastoidei which was usually diplöic in character. If pneumatization occurred as it was shown by Dr. Pierce from the antrum outwards, how did the pneumatization take place peripherally as can be shown in the X-ray or account for the repneumatization of the pathological mastoid, that is, a mastoid acutely infected and subsequently undergoing resolution? Dr. Beck had a series of X-ray pictures of a physician who had an otitis media with mastoid symptoms and the pictures were taken ad seriatim, showing obliteration of the mastoid as the disease progressed. The patient recovered completely without operation, his drum membrane subsequently showed nothing of the previously existing nipple perforation and the mastoid cells were completely repneumaticized. Whether or not there were any microscopic remains of the pathological process Dr. Beck did not know.

The speaker felt that Dr. Pierce should have the thanks of the Society for bringing the work before them and was convinced that the translation of Wittmaack's work would be of value because it was something in the hope of a new era for otology.

Dr. Alfred Lewy thought that in so widespread an affair as was described by Dr. Wittmaack, especially as it was commonly bilateral, one would think of a failure of development, due to some systemic rather than local process; for instance, failure of some internal secretion. We all know that bony changes can be brought about by pituitary disease. If this disease is found in so high a percentage of sucklings as is claimed by Wittmaack, one would naturally expect a much higher percentage of deafness in children. Of course, our observation of disturbance of hearing in children from causes in fetal life is very inadequate, so Wittmaack's statement, if correct, will explain many cases of deafness in which no inflammatory action has been noticed.

Dr. Lewy asked if any specialized epithelial cell on the order of an osteoblast had been described as causing the erosion or pneumatic spaces. He had found no mention of it in the book.

Dr. Norval H. Pierce (closing the discussion) stated that Wittmaack was especially careful to say that the process he described had nothing to do with otosclerosis. In all his studies he found nothing that bordered on otosclerosis. Otosclerosis occurs in bones that are completely pneumatized, without any changes in the recessus. He thought there seemed to be a great discrepancy between the cases of deafness that occur in adult life and the incidence of otitis media of infants or sucklings. When it was considered that good observers believe that 90 per cent. of infants during the first two years of life have this form of otitis media, it would seem that there would be more cases of deafness and cholesteatomatous formation. However, Zuckerkandl, in his study of 268 cases of adult mastoids, found only 26 per cent. of cases that were perfectly pneumatized, so there was a certain agreement there. A study of the vital statistics might be of some interest and assistance, in determining how many children with this disease were really growing to adult life. Wittmaack admits this discrepancy and did not attempt to explain it, but left it to future developments.

Dr. Pierce thought it seemed a bit fatalistic to say that this condition, occurring in infancy, stamped the individual's auditory fate for life, but if it was true there was no help for it. The matter is not, however, as pessimistic as it would seem. It meant that certain problems must be attacked that had not been attacked so far. If the amniotic fluid found its way into the ear, did that constitute a foreign body? Dr. Pierce thought that it did. It was not normally found in the eustachian tube; that is a closed tube and fluid cannot get into it in fetal life except when the fetus makes extraordinary efforts in swallowing. If it was a normal content of the cavum then that hypothesis would fall down.

Another very practical point in prophylaxis was the proper mode of accouchement. At present the obstetrician holds the head back to save the perineum. They delay labor by anesthetizing the highly developed mother and that might to a certain extent be the cause of the incidence of the condition. All these things must be thought of and prevented or disproved. In the opinion of Dr. Pierce, the book of Wittmaack is a colossal work and he felt that it was largely founded on facts. The occlusion of the tube must be proven or disproven. Dr. Lewy had taken all the joy out of life by saying the thing might be due to the pituitary body, but that also would have to be proven. Wittmaack had not spoken especially of osteoblasts in dealing with the subject.

# CHICAGO LARYNGOLOGICAL AND OTOLOGICAL SOCIETY.

*Meeting of February 7, 1921.*

THE PRESIDENT, DR. ALFRED LEWY, IN THE CHAIR.

### "Fibroma of the Soft Palate"

Dr. George M. McBean presented a patient with a swelling in the right side of the soft palate. There was no complication of any kind, no pain and no history was obtainable. The patient was in the army a couple of years ago and at that time was told he had a large right tonsil. Dr. McBean had put a needle into the growth recently but obtained no fluid. He believed it to be a fibroma of the soft palate.

### DISCUSSION.

Dr. George E. Shambaugh stated that the situation did not look unlike a type of large tonsil which one occasionally encounters, in which the enlargement is for the most part upward between the folds of the soft palate. The enlargement was more exaggerated in this case than he had ever seen from a tonsil. He recalled a case where this type of enlargement of the tonsil existed on both sides in a patient who suffered a great deal from frequent attacks of acute tonsillitis. Tonsils were removed under local anesthesia which was not an easy undertaking. The operation was followed by more or less paralysis of the soft palate resembling the situation observed after diphtheria. The annoyance from fluid getting up into the nose when the patient attempted to swallow persisted a number of weeks. The end results were entirely satisfactory.

Dr. Joseph C. Beck was reminded of two cases, one of which proved to be a calculus (amigdolyth). The case presented much the same appearance as Dr. McBean's but upon opening the supratonsillar fossa he found a mass larger than a small hazlenut, which was made up of a concretion like a stone.

The second case had been seen about two weeks previously and had a growth coming over from the posterior lateral wall. The case was referred to as a sarcoma. Upon exposing the tumor for microscopic examination they found a definite capsule. A piece of the capsule was excised and found to be quite dense, below which there was a soft tissue, and upon sectioning the tissue it was found to be lipomatous.

### Extradural Abscess and Sinus Thrombosis.

Dr. Samuel Salinger presented a pathologic specimen from a case of extradural abscess and extensive sinus thrombosis. He had removed a large clot extending from the knee to the bulb and tied the jugular. The boy got along well for a week, but the jugular wound became infected with what proved to be a diphtheroid organism. On the tenth day the dressings over the neck wound were found to be saturated with blood. The patient was put on the operating table and removal of the dressings was followed by an enormous gush of blood. The common carotid was tied but the patient expired shortly afterward. The specimen presented showed an erosion of the common carotid from without about the size of a small pea. Dr. Salinger was not sure whether the rupture was due to infection, to the rubbing of the ligature on the artery, or whether Dakin's solution, with which the wound had been irrigated, had anything to do with it. He asked for an expression of opinion.

## DISCUSSION.

Dr. J. Holinger stated that he read a paper a year ago on sinus thrombosis and mentioned the report of a case in which the erosion of the carotid artery by the ligature on the jugular vein caused the death of the patient. There is no way of avoiding such accidents after ligature of the vein because the artery and vein are so close together in the same sheath. The movement of the pulsating artery will produce erosion.

Dr. Joseph C. Beck did not agree with Dr. Holinger as to the cause of the rupture. He had seen a similar rupture in a case of suspected carcinoma, which, however, was a healed out Bezold abscess. In that case they made a complete dissection of the common carotid, both external and internal, and the jugular vein. These were protected with dressings and the next day upon dressing the patient, who was a physician, they found an enormous bullae formation over the side of the neck. Upon puncturing these bullae they found a pure culture of a diplococcus. The wound was left exposed for subsequent X-ray treatment and in four or five days they found a small white spot on the external portion of the carotid artery. The next day it was slightly larger, with a little bulging, and on the sixth or seventh day they were compelled to do a temporary compression of the common carotid, thinking that by reducing the amount of blood going through they would get a granulation of the wall of the artery. On the same day Dr. Pollock was called in a hurry because the patient had a sudden gush of blood from the neck wound and he succeeded in grasping the bleeding point with an artery forcep. In the afternoon they made a complete ligation with tape and were able to take off the artery forceps, as there was no bleeding. The patient developed a hemiplegia during the night and died two or three days later. They should not have made the dissection, but the case was sent in as carcinoma. Subsequent examination showed that it was simply inflammatory, and the patient had carried the infection around for years.

In his opinion the case reported by Dr. Salinger was a similar one, the organism producing an arteritis from the exterior and causing a rupture. If it had been exposed earlier and tied they might have been able to save the patient.

Dr. Salinger (closing the discussion) said he did not think the ligature had eroded the artery by friction in this case. The erosion was not directly opposite the ligature and in his opinion it was due rather to infection from the exterior. He had seen one case where carcinoma had eroded the common carotid, and another similar to the one reported by Dr. Beck, but this was the first case of this kind that had come to his notice.

### Bead in the Bronchus.

Dr. George W. Boot reported a case of a small boy who had been left in his father's care and was taken with a severe coughing spell. The father did not know what the child had inhaled, but supposed it was a bead, as a broken string of beads varying in size was found. Roentgen examination show nothing, as the bead was transparent to X-rays. Upon listening to the child's chest the bead could be heard flying up and down the trachea with each inspiration and expiration. Dr. Boot did upper bronchoscopy and tried to get the bead but the forceps would not hold it and in the effort to grasp it the bead was pushed into the left bronchus where it was firmly lodged. It was smooth and hard and forceps always slipped off. A probe could not be insinuated past it. He finally evolved the instrument which he presented for inspection. The problem was to have an instrument small enough to pass through a small bronchoscopic tube and yet permit enough light to pass so that the instrument could be passed into the hole in the bead under direct visual guidance and at the same time hold firmly enough to dislodge the head. With this little appliance which V. Mueller and Company made for him, he was able to remove the bead.

Dr. Clark W. Hawley (by invitation) presented a paper entitled "Abnormalities of the Mastoid in Reference to the Facial Nerve," and exhibited specimens of the temporal bone showing anomalies of the nerve.

A number of specimens were shown showing the abnormal position of the lateral sinus.

Also two specimens where the facial nerve passed down the center of the mastoid bone instead of in the base of the posterior wall of the ear. The nerves were situated in the path of the operation and would be injured unless the operator was on the lookout for the malposition. Such abnormalities may account for some of the facial paralyses that occur. The knowledge of their occurrence will be useful to the expert witness in malpractice cases.

### DISCUSSION.

Dr. George E. Shambaugh stated that it was not easy to judge of the exact relation of the facial nerve to the surrounding parts by a dissection of this sort that works in from the surface. Students who are attempting to visualize the anatomic relations of the temporal bone do not accomplish this successfully by performing the operation on the mastoid and observing the relations as they are uncovered in the course of this procedure. The reason for this is that one important relation after another is destroyed in making an opening into the mastoid. It is necessary to make a series of anatomic sections, each one devised to bring out an important anatomic relation in order to study definitely the exact relation of the facial nerve as it courses through the temporal bone. The best type of preparation is made by a section which passes through the tympanum in the perpendicular plane and lays open the facial canal from the point where it turns downward just in front of the horizontal semicircular canal until it leaves the stylomastoid opening. A section made in this way leaves no chance for deception in measuring the relation of the facial canal. The impression Dr. Shambaugh gathered from an examination of the preparations presented was, that the facial nerve was entirely in its normal position. He has seen only one anomalous variation in the course of the facial nerve. This was in the preparation exhibited by Dr. Behrens.

There are several facts in connection with the course of the facial nerve that should always be kept in mind when operating on the temporal bone: First, that the nerve enters the tympanum in front and above the oval window. Second, the relation which the nerve bears to the posterior wall of the exterior auditory meatus. This relation at the upper part of the typmpanum is quite different from what it is at the floor of the tympanum. In the former location the nerve lies close to the posterior wall of the tympanum and on a level with the inner wall of this cavity. As the nerve runs downward toward the stylomastoid opening, two alterations take place in relation to the tympanum. The first is, that it lies farther and farther away from the posterior wall of this cavity until it reaches the floor of the tympanum. At this point it is separated usually by one-quarter inch from the tympanum cavity. The second alteration is that as the canal extends downward from the knee instead of lying at a depth parallel with the inner wall of the tympanum, it extends out farther and farther along the postmeatal wall. This latter fact has been responsible for injury to the facial nerve when operators have attempted to flatten out the posterior wall of the meatus.

Dr. Joseph C. Beck stated that his purpose in asking Dr. Hawley to present this subject before the Society was that thus far there was only one specimen, to which Dr. Shambaugh had referred, and it occurred to him in mentioning this fact not less than eight times as a witness in defending a physician against malpractice suits, by bringing this fact to the attention of the judge and jury and having it save the doctor in summing up the evidence, that if it could occur once it might occur again, and this case of Dr. Hawley's was probably one of those cases. When Dr. Hawley showed Dr. Beck the specimens he had the same impression that Dr. Shambaugh had—that the facial canals were no different from others he had seen. When one considered Cheatle's collection of temporal bones and remembered that in not a single case was there a repetition of the specimen shown by Dr. Behrens, one realized that the course of the facial nerve was very definite and constant and in the course of an ordinary mastoid operation this injury does not occur. Dr. Beck wished there was another case on record like Dr. Behrens' because one case was not enough.

Dr. Beck added one point to those brought out by Dr. Shambaugh: That the facial nerve does not extend external to the prominence of the horizontal semicircular canal, and if one keeps external to that when taking off the posterior lower wall there will not be much trouble. This point had helped him greatly. They very seldom had any facial paralysis, but it does occasionally occur in the hands of the best operators.

Dr. Hawley had not yet proven the point that he made when he showed the same specimens at the Illinois State meeting. Dr. Beck had expected him to make sections and cross sections of the specimens and present them in detail, but this unfortunately had not been done.

Dr. J. Holinger said the question of the course of the facial nerve was especially important when in a case of Bezold's mastoiditis, the cell causing the perforation into the neck is to be sought. This cell was often very deep, and unless it be drained, the operation could not be considered completed. Dr. Holinger thought that one could never see too much of the individual variations of the anatomy of these parts.

Dr. George W. Boot agreed with Dr. Shambaugh that the upper part of the nerve was very definite in its course. The lower part always emerges at the stylomastoid foramen. If these two points are connected a pretty good idea of the course the nerve runs with respect to the parts operated on can be had. At birth the nerve emerges on the outer surface of the temporal bone for the mastoid apophysis has not yet been formed. The reason the course of the nerve seems to vary is because of the varying amount of development of the mastoid apophysis. Its relation to the drum membrane and middle ear is quite constant.

Dr. Clark W. Hawley said he never had a discussion of any kind without somebody getting up and questioning the truth of what they saw. He believed that if Dr. Shambaugh had carefully examined the specimens he would have recognized that the nerve in the specimen, which had not been disturbed at all, was not in the posterior wall but ran down almost exactly on the center of the canal. In the one it was two-thirds away from the posterior wall of the ear. If he had not put the paint in he thought it would be a little more evident, but he had thought the paint would bring it out better. He had made three hundred dissections and had never found another case like these, although they did the radical dissection on all of them, and they had not touched the facial nerve at any time. On the specimens he had presented the nerve was very plainly shown. In teaching he always shows the students the course of the nerve as it travels in the petrous portion and also in the mastoid. He had found one or two instances where the facial nerve did not travel as Dr. Shambaugh had said and anyone who attempted to scrape away granulations from the mastoid antrum would have injured the nerve, for it did not go along the base of the middle ear but at the upper portion. It must also be remembered that the specimens were not intended to demonstrate the anatomic relation, but simply to show the students how to do a mastoid operation. In the specimens both posterior walls were preserved and the mastoid tip was not disturbed at all. Dr. Hawley thought that if these nerves were not displaced he would certainly have found the same position in many of the other operations done on the cadaver.

Dr. Howard C. Ballenger read a paper on

### "Acute Hemorrhagic Otitis Media."*

### DISCUSSION.

Dr. George W. Boot stated that when he saw the child whose case was reported by Dr. Ballenger, Dr. Ballenger favored operation while Dr. Boot opposed it. The following day he reluctantly gave his consent and had the child sent to the hospital because Dr. Ballenger could not be reached. Before the following morning set for the operation the child apparently had improved so no operation was done and the patient was returned to Dr. Ballenger's care. In another case Dr. Boot had operated on a man of 80 years under local anesthesia because of a streptococcus infection in a patient who had chronic interstitial nephritis. The mastoid cells were found filled with clotted blood. Unfortunately the patient developed facial erysipelas on the side of the wound. This cleared up only to be followed by erysipelas on the opposite side and this in turn by erysipelas of the leg with multiple abscess formation and the patient finally died of the erysipelatous infection.

Dr. Samuel Salinger thought it would be interesting to know in what condition the mastoid cells were found—whether there was a hemorrhagic mastoiditis as well, and also the condition of the bone.

Dr. Harry L. Pollock said that during the epidemic last year they had several cases in which there was bleeding from the ear. The examination of patients who came in with pain, swelling and redness of the membrane showed on close inspection with the otoscope that this appeared in the form of a blister. They had severe pain and temperature and in opening these blisters they got a bloody exudate which persisted for several days. Dr. Pollock's little son had a light attack of grip and about ten days later suddenly developed an earache and within a few minutes his ear drum was apparently bulging. This condition persisted for two days. Dr. Beck saw the patient and opposed doing a paracentesis. The thing ruptured spontaneously during the night and there was a discharge of bloody serum for several days, but there was no perforation in the middle ear. In none of the cases did they find it necessary to do any mastoid operation or paracentesis. Several of the cases looked like a mastoiditis, but after a few days the symptoms subsided very rapidly. One lady, who had a most excruciating pain for twenty-four hours, had complete relief from the pain when the little bleb ruptured, but the discharge continued. Had they performed a paracentesis they might have set up an otitis media, as there was pain all over the side of the head.

Dr. Pollock pointed out that Dr. Ballenger had not mentioned the X-ray pictures. If X-ray pictures were taken in these cases no mastoid involvement would have been shown.

As to indications for operating on the mastoid, the principal one was the hearing and in these cases, while the hearing was affected it was not so markedly as in the mastoid with involvement of the

---

*See page 539.

middle ear. The hearing recovered very quickly. In the otitis media cases, if the picture showed the mastoid to be cloudy, and they waited several days and then took another in order to see whether the condition was breaking down or clearing up, was one indication. If the hearing continued to grow less acute it was an indication to do a mastoid operation.

In their cases all the organisms found were streptococci.

Dr. J. Holinger asked whether in the case of hemorrhagic nephritis any carbolated glycerin had been used as eardrops. He knew that several cases of hemorrhagic nephritis had been reported in which carbolated glycerin had been used. In his practice he never advised the use of carbolated glycerin.

Dr. Harry Kahn said the subject was discussed in Pollitzer's book rather fully. The whispered voice test was a differential test between the myringitis and an abscess of the middle ear. In the epidemic last year many of these cases of sudden onset ruptured in a short time and hemorrhage from the ear was met with in many of the cases. He thought that this was nothing unusual in an influenzal epidemic, and that nothing new had been brought out. So far as he knew all the cases were of streptococcal origin and were probably entirely due to the influenza.

Dr. Robert Sonnenschein felt that even with very slight exudate in the middle ear, as proven by a paracentesis afterward, the hearing for the whispered voice was often as good as two or three meters for the high tones.

In reference to the differential diagnosis between an otitis media and a myringitis, aside from the other tests there are the tuning fork tests. While the Weber reaction is often unreliable, still in the case of an otitis media it is usually lateralized to the affected side, not so where a simple myringitis is present. The Rinne is usually negative with middle ear involvement and is usually positive in myringitis.

Dr. Joseph C. Beck thought that Dr. Ballenger's paper was very opportune. The point he brought out, which should be remembered, was not to operate on many of these cases. In the epidemics of the last couple of years they had seen quite a large number of such cases that had been operated upon less on the mastoid than on the drum membrane—a repeated sticking of the drum. In one case the ear had been jabbed fourteen times by an otologist in this city (not much of an otologist). The patient would not submit to further paracentesis and recovered simply when the ear was left alone.

As to the lateralization, they made the test and it did lateralize to that side where one found these blood blisters. There was no history of this. The Weber does lateralize and he thought Dr. Sonnenschein was mistaken.

Dr. Alfred Lewy thought an important point in Dr. Ballenger's paper was that apparently the less manipulation aside from paracentesis, in these cases, the better they got along. He also called attention to the fact that Dr. Ballenger's cases had marked mastoid tenderness, as well as persistent bleeding and later purulent discharge, so they were evidently not merely myringitis. He remembered reading a report by an Eastern otologist who boasted that out of one hundred middle ear suppurations he only had thirty mastoids. Compared to this man, Dr. Ballenger would certainly classify as a conservative, and his results appear to justify his position.

Dr. Lewy had recently had an interesting experience with an early mastoid operation. He was generally opposed to operating within so short a time from the onset, but this child developed suddenly a swelling mostly in the zygomatic area which extended over the face. The patient had had measles six weeks previously, with an occasional earache since, without discharge, but had apparently been well two weeks when the swelling referred to suddenly appeared. The drum membrane was thickened, there was no discharge and no sinking in of the canal wall. There was headache, temperature over 102° and a white cell count of 12,000. Paracentesis was done, resulting in bloody discharge which became purulent within a few hours, but after two days no relief of symptoms. X-ray showed a clouding of the mastoid area, but no definite breaking down of cell walls. With pain, tenderness, swelling and a histroy of a possible six weeks' infection, dating back to the measles, instead of a four day affair, it was decided to do the mastoid operation. The cortex was found unaltered, but the region of the antrum and the tip cell were softened so that the curette alone was sufficient. White cell count ordered before the operation for some reason was not done until three hours afterward, and was 27,000, which suggests that in doing the operation for the purpose of establishing drainage, we are at the same time opening up avenues of extension for the infection. This always happens to a greater or less degree, but Dr. Lewy believes that there is a greater probability of such spread in early operation before nature has had time to establish her defenses.

Dr. Ballenger (closing) said that in this series it was necessary to operate on only two cases and they were done for the persistent otorrhea. Both mastoids were broken down. The cases that he knew about which were operated early showed a blood filled or negative mastoid. Most of these cases had mastoid tenderness to some degree, usually rather severe, and there was great prostration. The X-ray examination was not made in any of these cases in early stages as the patients were too sick to go to the hospital, but where the radiograph was taken later, after the formation of the pus, the shadows were dark.

In reply to Dr. Holinger's question, in regard to carbolated glycerin, he did not believe the carbolated glycerin would cause hemorrhagic nephritis before rupture or incision of the ear drum. Drs. Wall and Aldrich saw the case with the bloody urine and made the diagnosis of hemorrhagic nephritis.

# INDEX OF THE LITERATURE.

## SECTION 1.—LARYNGOLOGY AND OTOLOGY—GENERAL AND HISTORICAL.

**Adeodato, J.** Medical terms in otology.
Brazil med., Rio de Jan., 1920—XXXIV—511.

**Brühl.** Otologic hints for the general practitioner.
Deutsch. med. Wchnschr., Berl., 1920—XLVI—973, 1000, 1030, 1117, 1145.

**Foster, J. H.** Need of systematized postgraduate teaching of ophthalmology and otolaryngology.
Texas State J. M., Fort Worth, 1920—XVI—285.

**Hays, H., Palmer, A., and Winslow, T. S.** Vaccine therapy vs. tonsillectomy in systemic disease of tonsillar origin.
Med. Rec., N. Y., 1921—XCIX—301.

**Henke, F.** Status lymphaticus and its relations to other diseases.
Deutsch. med. Wchnschr., Berl., 1920—XLVI—1257.

**Irons, E. E.** Chronic systemic infections and their sources.
J. Am. M. Ass., Chicago, 1921—LXXVI—627.

**Loeb, H. W., and Wiener, M.** The borderland of otolaryngology and ophthalmology.
Ann. Ohol., Rhinol. and Laryngol., St. Louis, 1921—XXX—74.

**Machado, Renato.** Otorhinolaryngology lecture.
Brazil méd., Rio de Jan., 1920—XXXIV—637.

**Maier, M.** Diseases of the ear.
Therap. Monatsh., Berl., 1920—XXXIV—493.

**Mullin, W. V., and Ryder, C. T.** Experimental lesions of lungs produced by inhalation of fluids from nose and throat.
Am. Rev. Tuberc., Baltimore, 1920—IV—683.

**Popper, J.** Case of acute articular rheumatism complicating otitis media.
Med. Rec., N. Y., 1921—XCIX—270.

**Ryland, A.** Assessment of aural disability resulting from military service.
J. Laryngol., etc., London, 1920—XXXV—354.

**Shambaugh, G. E.** Popular fallacies in practice of otology.
Laryngoscope, St. Louis, 1920—XXX—683.

**Smith, Ferris.** Plastic surgery: Its interest to the otolaryngologist.
J. Am. M. Ass., Chicago, 1920—LXXV—1554.

## SECTION 2.—RESPIRATORY SYSTEM, EXCLUSIVE OF THE EAR, NOSE AND THROAT.

**Jesberg, S.** Study of nasal conditions occurring in bronchial asthma.
Calif. State J. M., San Francisco, 1921—XIX—33.

Mullin, W. V., and Ryder, C. T. Experimental lesions of lungs produced by inhalation of fluids from nose and throat.
Am. Rev. Tuberc., Baltimore, 1920—IV—683.

Park, W. H., Williams, A. W., and Krumwiede, C. Microbic studies of acute respiratory infections with special consideration of immunologic types.
J. Immunol., Baltimore, 1921—VI—1.

Shambaugh, G. E. Nasal cavities and asthma.
Illinois M. J., Oak Park, 1921—XXXIX—10.

Von Sholly, A. I., and Park, W. H. Report on prophylactic vaccination of 1,536 persons against acute respiratory disease, 1919—1920.
J. Immunol., Baltimore, 1921—VI—103.

Zahorsky, J. Resistance of acute disease of the respiratory tract in children.
Am. J. Dis. Child., Chicago, 1921—XXI—183.

## SECTION 3.—ACUTE GENERAL INFECTIONS, INCLUDING DIPHTHERIA, SCARLET FEVER AND MEASLES. THE EAR, NOSE AND THROAT.

Albert, H. Classification of diphtheria bacilli based on toluidin blue-iodin method of staining.
Am. J. Pub. Health, Boston, 1920—X—936.

Allen, J., and Wood, D. R. Diphtheria carriers of unusual type.
Brit. M. J., Lond., 1920—II—818.

Bears, E. Diphtheria from standpoint of school nurse.
Kentucky M. J., Louisville, 1920—XVIII—409.

Beatti, M. Influenza.
Semana méd., Buenos Aires, 1920—XXXIV—58.

Bell, H. H. Relation of different strains of influenza bacilli as shown by cross agglutination and absorption tests.
J. Infect. Dis., Chicago, 1920—XXVII—464.

Bieber, W. Tests with diphtheria tonin-antitoxin mixture.
Deutsch. med. Wchnschr., Berlin, 1920—XLVI—1184.

Bieling, R., and Weichbrodt, R. Serodiagnosis in influenza and epidemic encephalitis.
Deutsch. med. Wchnschr., Berlin, 1920—XLVI—1183.

Boecker, W. Metastatic paranephritis after influenza.
München. med. Wchnschr., 1920—LVII—1149.

Bonnamour, S., and Bardin, J. Diphtheria antitoxin in prevention of orchitis and mumps.
Presse méd., Paris, 1920—XXVIII—929.

Brandies, F. Diphtheria from standpoint of family physician.
Kentucky M. J., Louisville, 1920—XVIII—408.

Buchholtz. Influenza epidemic in 1920.
Ugesk. f. Laeger. Kjovenh., 1921—LXXXIII—147.

Coca, A. F., and Kelley, M. F. Serologic study of Pfeiffer bacillus.
J. Immunol., Baltimore, 1921—VI—87.

Colard, A. Duration of immunity to influenza.
Arch. med. belg., Liége, 1920—LXXIII—835.

**Cooke, J. V.** Complement fixation in influenza with B. influenzae antigens.
J. Infect. Dis., Chicago, 1920—XXVII—476.

**Dopter, C.** Proofs of acquired immunity to influenza.
Paris méd., 1920—X—289.

**Fitzgerald, J. G.** Analysis of diphtheria deaths in Ontario.
Public Health J., Toronto, 1920—XI—485.

**Fraser, A. R., and Duncan, A. G. B.** Treatment of diphtheria carriers with detoxicated Klebs-Löffler vaccine.
Lancet, London, 1920—II—994.

**Frost, W. D., Charlton, Alice M., Little, Mary F.**—A rapid cultural method of diagnosing diphtheria.
J. Am. M. Ass., Chicago, 1921—LXXVI—30.

**Gelien, J., Moss, W. L., and Guthrie, C. G.** Effect of diphtheria antitoxin in preventing lodgment and growth of diphtheria bacillus in nasal passages of animals.
Johns Hopkins Hosp. Bull., Balt., 1920—XXXI—381.

**Gilbert, R. B.** Diphtheria therapeutic comparisons.
Kentucky M. J., Louisville, 1920—XVIII—406.

**Glenny, A. T., and Allen, K.** Testing diphtheria toxin and antitoxin by intracutaneous injections into guinea pigs.
J. Path. and Bacteriol., Edinburgh, 1921—XXIV—91.

**Guthrie, C. G., Gelien, J., and Moss, W. L.** Diphtheria bacillus carriers.
Johns Hopkins Hosp. Bull., Balt., 1920—XXXI—388.

**Hachen, David S., and Isaacs, Raphael.** The alkali reserve in epidemic influenza and bronchopneumonia.
J. Am. M. Ass., Chicago, 1920—LXXV—1624.

**Hall, J. C.** Influenza studies: A search for obligate anaerobes in respiratory infections. An anaerobic micrococcus.
J. Infect. Dis., Chicago, 1921—XXVIII—127.

**Harry, F.** Hematology of influenza.
Deutsch. Arch. f. klin. Med., Leipzig, 1921—CXXXIII—237.

**Henry, Jonathan E.** Milk-borne diphtheria: An outbreak traced to infection of a milk handler's finger with B. diphtheriae.
J. Am. M. Ass., Chicago, 1920—LXXV—1715.

**Hermann, Elise.** Diphtheria in young infants.
Jahrb. f. Kinderh., Berl., 1920—XCVIII—273.

**Hildebrandt, W.** Chronic influenza.
München. med. Wchnschr., 1920—LXVII—1008.

**Howes, J. B.** Tuberculosis and influenza.
Boston M. & S. J., 1920—CLXXXIII—596.

**Irons, E. E.** Chronic systemic infections and their sources.
J. Am. M. Ass., Chicago, 1921—LXXVI—627.

**Logan, W. R.** Study of pneumococcus and streptococcus groups in their relation to influenza.
Brit. M. J., Lond., 1921—I—189.

**McCullough.** Administration of digitalis to children with diphtheria.
South. M. J., Birmingham, 1921—XIV—110.

602     INDEX OF THE LITERATURE.

**Messerschmidt.** Occurrence and staining of influenza bacilli.
Deutsche med. Wchnschr., Berl., 1920—XLVI—1023.

**Michiels, J.** The diphtherin skin reaction.
Arch. méd. belges, Liege. 1920—LXXIII—506.

**Much et al.** Diagnosis and treatment of influenza.
München. med. Wchnschr., 1920—LXVII—1057.

**Moss, W. L., Guthrie, C. G., and Marshall, B. C.** Experimental inoculation of human throats with a virulent diphtheria
bacilli.
Johns Hopkins Hosp. Bull., Balti., 1921—XXXII—37.

**Morgan, J. W.** Why diphtheria? Reasons and remedies.
Colorado Med., Denver, 1920—XVII—285.

**Murphy, W. E.** Acute mastoiditis following influenza.
Ohio M. J., 1921—XVII—18.

**Neufeld, F.** The causative agent in influenza.
Deutsche med. Wchnschr., Berl., 1920—XLVI—957.

**Neven.** Treatment of influenza.
Médicine, Paris, 1920—II—215.

**Olitsky, P. K., and Gates, F. L.** Experimental studies of nasopharyngeal secretions from influenza patients. Transmission experiments with nasopharyngeal washings.
J. Exper. Med., Baltimore, 1921—XXXIII—125.

**Olitsky, P. K., and Gates, F. L.** Studies of the nasopharyngeal
secretions from influenza patients. Preliminary report on
cultivation experiments.
J. Am. M. Ass., Chicago, 1921—LXXVI—640.

**Paludino, F.** Medicinal treatment of influenza.
Rev. med. Uruguay, Montevideo, 1921—XXIII—381.

**Park, William H.** The use of antitoxin in the treatment of diphtheria.
J. Am. M. Ass., Chicago, 1921—LXXVI—109.

**Park, W. H., and Cooper, G.** Accidental inoculation of influenza
bacillus on mucous membranes of healthy persons, with
the development of infection in at least one. Persistence of type characteristics of bacilli.
J. Immunol., Baltimore, 1921—VI—81.

**Park, W. H., Williams, A. W., and Krumwiede, C.** Microbic studies
of acute respiratory infections with special consideration
of immunologic types.
J. Immunol., Baltimore, 1921—VI—1.

**Pirkey, B. E.** Indications for intubation in diphtheria.
Kentucky M. J., Louisville, 1920—XVIII—408.

**Povitzky, O. R., and Denny, H. T.** Grouping of influenza bacilli with
special reference to permanence of type in carrier.
J. Immunol., Baltimore, 1921—VI—65.

**Robbins, V.** Diagnostic methods of city health othce in diphtheria.
Kentucky M. J., Louisville, 1920—XVIII—410.

**Sajous, C. E. de M.** Newer interpretation of pathogenesis, prophylaxis and treatment of influenza.
Indian M. Gaz., Calcutta, 1920—LV—361.

Sante, L. R. Study of influenzal pneumonia by serial roentgen. ray examination.
Missouri M. Ass. J., St. Louis, 1921—XVIII—43.

Schmidt, P. Etiology of colds and influenza.
Deutsch. med. Wchnschr., Berlin, 1920—XLVI—1181.

Small, W. D. D. Influenza.
Edin. M. J., 1920—XXV—375.

Strassberg, M. Relation of influenza and syphilis.
Wien. klin. Wchnschr., 1920—XXXIII—797.

Tanon, L. The Shick reaction.
Médicine, Paris, 1920—II—229.

Treupel, G. Chronic influenza.
Deutsch. med. Wchnschr., 1920—XLVI—1159.

Tuley, H. E. Value of Schick test.
Kentucky M. J., Louisville, 1920—XVIII—412.

Utheim, K. Agglutination in influenza.
J. Infect. Dis., Chicago, 1920—XXVII—460.

Van Horn, Alfred F. Report of a case of round cell sarcoma of the epipharynx and a case of primary diphtheria of the middle ear.
J. Am. M. Ass., Chicago, 1921—LXXVI—32.

Von Sholly, A. I., and Park, W. H. Report on prophylactic vaccination of 1,536 persons against acute respiratory disease, 1919—1920.
J. Immunol., Baltimore, 1921—VI—103.

Weaver, G. H. Diphtheria carriers.
J. Am. M. Ass., Chicago, 1921—LXXVI—831.

## SECTION 4.—SYPHILIS.

Brown, W. H., and Pearce, L. Experimental syphilis in rabbit. V. Syphilitic affections of mucous membranes and mucocutaneous borders.
J. Exper. M., Maltimore, 1920—XXXII—497.

Bruggone, C., and Vecchia, E. Intratrachael injection of neoarsphenamin.
Policlin., Roma, 1920—XXVII—1384.

Gerber. Latent syphilis of the throat.
Deutsche med. Wchnschr., Berl., 1920—XLVI—1110.

Lund, R. Syphilis of the outer ear.
Ugesk. f. Laeger, Kjbenh., 1920—LXXXII—1335.

Strassberg, M. Relation of influenza and syphilis.
Wien. klin. Wchnschr., 1920—XXXIII—797.

## SECTION 5.—TUBERCULOSIS.

Berry, M. Roentgen ray treatment of tuberculous glands.
Brit. J. Tuber., London, 1921—XV—13.

Howes, J. B. Tuberculosis and influenza.
Boston M. & S. J., 1920—CLXXXIII—596.

McBrayer, R. Differential diagnosis of tuberculosis and hyperthyroidism: Study of Goetsch test.
South. M. J., Birmingham, Ala., 1920—XIII—783.

**Oppikofer, E.** Cholesteatoma with tuberculous otitis media.
Schwdeiz. med. Wchnschr., Basel, 1920—L—993.

**Zeisler, E. P.** Tuberculosis of lip.
Arch. Dermat. and Syph., Chicago, 1921—III—14.

## SECTION 6.—ANATOMY, PHYSIOLOGY AND PATHOLOGY.

**Harper, J.** Tonsil and its function.
Glasgow M. J., 1920—XII—344.

**Kahn, A.** Logical cause, pathology and treatment of brain lesions.
Laryngoscope, St. Louis, 1920—XXX—809.

**Logan, W. R.** Study of pneumococcus and streptococcus groups in
their relation to influenza.
Brit. M. J., Lond., 1921—I—189.

**Mudd, S., Grant, S. B., and Goldman, A.** The etiology of acute in-
flammations of the nose, pharynx and tonsils.
Ann. Otol., Rhinol. and Laryngol., St. Louis, 1921—XXX—1;
Also, J. Lab. and Clin. Med., St. Louis, 1921—VI—175.

**Rogers, L.** · Observations on the developmental anatomy of the
temporal bone.
Ann. Otol., Rhinol. and Laryngol., St. Louis, 1921—XXX—103.

**Spielberg, W.** Etiology of deviations of the nasal septum: anatomic
theory.
J. Am. M. Ass., Chicago, 1920—LXXV—1646.

**Wernstedt, W.** Pathologic anatomy of congenital stridor.
Hygiea, Stockholm, 1920—LXXXII—609.

## SECTION 7.—EXTERNAL NOSE.

**Dufourmentel.** Cartilage support for sunken-in nose.
Paris méd., 1920—X—272.

**Graham, H. B.** Nasal plastic surgery.
Calif. State J. M., San Fran., 1920—XVIII—383.

**Hajek, M.** Rhinogenous origin of retrobulbar neuritis.
Wien. klin. Wchnschr., 1920—XXXIII—267.

**Hanrahan, E. M.** Surgical treatment of rhinophyma; report of a
case.
Johns Hopkins Hosp. Bull., Balti., 1921—XXXII—49.

**Lannois and Sargnon.** Radium therapy of tumors in ears, nose or
throat.
Lyon méd., 1920—CXXIX—807.

**Oertel, T. E.** Submucous replacement for external deviation.
Ann. Otol., Rhinol. and Laryngol., St. Louis, 1921—XXX—147.

**Oppenheimer, S.** Development of cosmetic rhinoplasty.
N. York State J. M., N. Y., 1920—XX—355.

**Wolf, G. D.** Round cell sarcoma of the nasal vestibule.
Med. Rec., N. York, 1921—XCIX—178.

## SECTION 8.—NASAL CAVITIES.

**Alikham, M.** Reflex neurosis of nasal origin.
Rev. med de la Suisshe Rom., Geneva, 1920—XL—813.

**Bonner, W. H.** Nasal and aural conditions associated with flying.
Delaware State M. J., Wilmington, 1920—X—17.

**Bookwalter, C. F.** Intranasal dacryocystostomy.
Arch. Ophth., N. Y., 1920—XLIX—568.

**Borras y Torres, P.** Imaginary pharyngitis and rhinitis.
Rev. Espan. de med. y cir., Barcelona, 1920—III—591.

**Cronk, H. L.** Renal complications of acute lacunar tonsillitis.
Practitioner, London, 1920—CV—351.

**De Levie.** Treatment of ozena.
Nederl. Tijdsch. v. Geneesk., Amst,. 1920—II—2656.

**Dufourmentel.** Cartilage support for sunken-in nose.
Paris méd., 1920—X—272.

**Dunlap, L. G.** Perforations of the nasal septum due to inhalation of
arsenous oxid.
J. Am. M. Ass., Chicago, 1921—LXXVI—368.

**Gelien, J., Moss, W. L., and Guthrie, C. G.** Effect of diphtheria antitoxin in preventing lodgment and growth of diphtheria
bacillus in nasal passages of animals.
Johns Hopkins Hosp. Bull., Balt., 1920—XXXI—381.

**Graham, H. B.** Nasal plastic surgery.
Calif. State J. M., San Fran., 1920—XVIII—383.

**Green, John, Jr.** Chronic dacryocystitis treated by curettage and
rapid dilatation.
J. Missouri M. Ass., St. Louis, 1920—XVII—480.

**Hajek, M.** Rhinogenous origin of retrobulbar neuritis.
Wien. klin. Wchnschr., 1920—XXXIII—267.

**Jesberg, S.** Study of nasal conditions occurring in bronchial
asthma.
Calif. State J. M., San Francisco, 1921—XIX—33.

**Lannois and Sargnon.** Radium· therapy of tumors in ears, nose or
throat.
Lyon méd., 1920—CXXIX—807.

**Lemere, H. B.** Antrum as main source of nasal catarrh.
Neb. State M. J., Norfolk, 1920—V—326.

**Mudd, S., Grant, S. B., and Goldman, A.** The etiology of acute in-
flammations of the nose, pharynx and tonsils.
Ann. Otol., Rhinol. and Laryngol., St. Louis, 1921—XXX—1;
Also, J. Lab. and Clin. Med., St. Louis, 1921—VI—175.

**Oertel, T. E.** Submucous replacement for external deviation.
Ann. Otol., Rhinol. and Laryngol., St. Louis, 1921—XXX—147.

**Pierce, H. W.** Conservative nasal surgery.
J. Mich'. M. Soc., Grand Rapids, 1920—XIX—507.

**Phelan, C. A.** Nasal catarrh.
Calif. State J. M., San Fran., 1921—XIX—81.

**Reitter, George S.** Rhamdomyoma of the nose: Report of·a case.
J. Am. M. Ass., Chicago, 1921—LXXVI—22.

**Reynolds, J. S.** Chronic atrophic catarrh or fetid ozena.
Laryngoscope, St. Louis, 1921—XXXI—31.

**Schmidt, P.** Etiology of colds and influenza.
Deutsch. med. Wchnschr., Berlin, 1920—XLVI—1181.

**Selfridge, G.**  Vasomotor disturbances of nose, with special reference to hay fever; report for 1919.
Laryngoscope, St. Louis, 1920—XXX—611.

**Shambaugh, G. E.**  Nasal cavities and asthma.
Illinois M. J., Oak Park, 1921—XXXIX—10.

**Sonnenschein, R.**  Headaches, with special reference to those of nasal origin.
Illinois M. J., Oak Park, 1920—XXXVIII—315.

**Spielberg, W.**  Etiology of deviations of the nasal septum: anatomic theory.
J. Am. M. Ass., Chicago, 1920—LXXV—1646.

**Tydings, O.**  The eye in relation to diseases of the nose, throat and teeth.
Illinois M. J., Oak Park, 1921—XXXIX—59.

**Unger, M.**  Intranasal drainage of frontal sinus through natural opening.
N. York State J. M., N. Y., 1920—XX—351.

**Walker, C. B.**  Nasolacrimal surgery in ophthalmic perspective.
Arch. Ophth., N. Y., 1920—XLIX—585.

**Walker, C. B.**  New devices combining dissection and suction for use in septum, tonsil and other operations.
J. Am. M. Ass., Chicago, 1921—LXXVI—793.

**Walter, F. J.**  Hay fever: "rose cold."
J. Florida M. Ass., Jacksonville, 1920—VII—61.

**Whale, H. L.**  Intranasal dacryocystostomy.
Brit. M. J., Lond., 1920—II—701.

**Wheeler, J. M.**  Extirpation of lacrimal sac in trauamtic dacryocystitis.
Texas State J. M., Ft. Worth, 1920—XVI—286.

**Wilkinson, O.**  Local anesthesia in nasal and throat surgery.
Laryngoscope, St. Louis, 1921—XXXI—27.

**Wolf, G. D.**  Round cell sarcoma of the nasal vestibule.
Med. Rec., N. York, 1921—XCIX—178.

## SECTION 9.—ACCESSORY SINUSES.

**Barnes, H. A.**  Combined operative and radium treatment of malignant disease of nasal accessory sinuses.
Boston M. & S. J., 1920—CLXXXIII—648; also Laryngoscope, 1920—XXX—646.

**Bonner, W. H.**  Nasal and aural conditions associated with flying.
Delaware State M. J., Wilmington, 1920—X—17.

**Brandao, P.**  Flushing of the maxillary sinus.
Brazil méd., Rio de Jan., 1920—XXXIV—491.

**Bryan, J. H.**  Case of extradural and subdural abscess following suppurating frontal sinusitis and osteomyelitis of frontal bone.
Am. J. M. Sc., Phila., 1920—CX—687.

**Cavanaugh, J. A.**  Sphenoid sinuses.
Illinois M. J., Oak Park, 1920—XXXVIII—521.

Jobson, G. B. Sinus disease and ocular involvement.
Penn. M. J., 1921—XXIV—205.

Lemere, H. B. Antrum as main source of nasal catarrh.
Neb. State M. J., Norfolk, 1920—V—326.

Lynch, R. C. Technic of radical frontal sinus operation which has given me the best results.
Laryngoscope, St. Louis, 1921—XXXI—1.

Paunz, M. Complications of sinusitis in children.
Jahrb. f. Kinderh., Berl., 1920—XCIII—313.

Pierce, H. W. Conservative nasal surgery.
J. Mich. M. Soc., Grand Rapids, 1920—XIX—507.

Schlittler, E. Sinusitis.
Schweiz. med. Wchnschr., Basel, 1920—L—1142.

Skillern, R. H. Ethmoidal problem.
Laryngoscope, St. Louis, 1920—XXX—687.

Theobald, W. H. A radical treatment for chronic suppuration of the antrum with modification of the Canfield technic.
Ann. Otol., Rhinol. and Laryngol., St. Louis, 1921—XXX—131.

Thomson, S. Treatment of acute nasal sinusitis.
Practitioner, London, 1921—CVI—1.

Tilley, H. Inflammatory lesions of the nasal accessory sinuses.
Brit. M. J., London, 1920—II—963.

Unger, M. Intranasal drainage of frontal sinus through natural opening.
N. York State J. M., N. Y., 1920—XX—351.

Webb, G. B., and Gilbert, G. B. Bronchiectasis and bronchitis associated with accessory sinus disease.
J. Am. M. Ass., Chicago, 1921—LXXVI—714.

White, F. W. Pathologic nasal accessory sinusitis in children.
Ann. Otol., Rhinol. and Laryngol., St. Louis, 1921—XXX—221.

Wilkinson, O. Local anesthesia in nasal and throat surgery.
Laryngoscope, St. Louis, 1921—XXXI—27.

## SECTION 10.—PHARYNX, INCLUDING TONSILS AND ADENOIDS.

Abadal, L. V. Postoperative mishaps with tonsillectomy.
Rev. espan. de med. y cirurg., Barcelona, 1920—III—530.

Amersbach. Treatment of carcinoma of the larynx and pharynx.
Deutsch. med. Wchnschr., 1920—XLVI—1269.

Armand-Delille, Marie and Dujarier. Gangrene of the pharynx.
Bull. soc. méd. d. hop., Paris, 1920—XLIV—1468.

Bloomfield, A. L. Significance of bacteria found in the throats of healthy people.
Johns Hopkins Hosp. Bull., Balti., 1921—XXXII—33.

Borello, F. P. Treatment of Vincent's angina.
Pediatria, Napoli, 1920—XXVIII—1039.

Borras y Torres, P. Imaginary pharyngitis and rhinitis.
Rev. Espan. de med. y cir., Barcelona, 1920—III—591.

**Carmack, J. W.**   Local indications for tonsillectomy and adenoidectomy.
J. Indiana M. Ass., Ft. Wayne, 1920—XIII—376.

**Castex, A.**   Spurious adenoid disturbances.
Bull. Acad. de méd., Paris, 1920—LXXXIV—278.

**Cronk, H. L.**   Renal complications of acute lacunar tonsillitis.
Practitioner, London, 1920—CV—351.

**Davis, E. D. D.**   Early diagnosis of carcinoma of oro- and laryngopharynx.
J. Laryngol., Lond., 1920—XXXV—321.

**Davis. E. D. D.**   Malignant growths of upper jaw and antrum; a survey of notes of thirty-nine cases.
Lancet, London, 1920—II—1090.

**Feliciangeli, G.**   Case of Ludwig's angina in a hemophiliac.
Policlin., Roma, 1921—XXVIII—8.

**Fuller, T. E.**   Tonsillar hemorrhage.
Ann. Otol., Rhinol. and Laryngol., St. Louis, 1921—XXX—205.

**Fulton, J. A.**   New method of tonsillectomy.
Northwest. Med., Seattle, 1921—XXI—44.

**Gerber.**   Latent syphilis of the throat.
Deutsche med. Wchnschr., Berl., 1920—XLVI—1110.

**Goddard, H. M.**   Tonsils considered from viewpoint of specialist and general practitioner.
Penn. M. J., Harrisburg, 1920—XXIV—153.

**Goheen, R. H. H.**   Tonsillectomy: A simple method used in 840 cases.
Indian M. Gaz., Calcutta, 1920—LV—411.

**Harper, J.**   Tonsil and its function.
Glasgow M. J., 1920—XII—344.

**Hays, H., Palmer, A., and Winslow, T. S.**   Vaccine therapy vs. tonsillectomy in systemic disease of tonsillar origin.
Med. Rec., N. Y., 1921—XCIX—301.

**Holinger, J.**   The removal of the tonsils in the presence of a peritonsillar abscess.
Ann. Otol., Rhinol. and Laryngol., St. Louis, 1921—XXX—195.

**Jervey, J. W.**   Surgical requirements of nasopharyngeal adenoid.
Laryngoscope, St. Louis, 1920—XXX—697.

**Kunz, H.**   Infections following operations of nose and throat.
Laryngoscope, St. Louis, 1920—XXX—717.

**La Force, B. D.**   Technic of closing sinus tonsillaris by suturing the pillars of the fauces with the aid of La Force's hollow suture needle and ligature knot fastener.
Laryngoscope, St. Louis, 1921—XXXI—42.

**Lannois and Sargnon.**   Radium therapy of tumors in ears, nose or throat.
Lyon méd., 1920—CXXIX—807.

**Mudd, S., Grant, S. B., and Goldman, A.**   The etiology of acute inflammations of the nose, pharynx and tonsils.
Ann. Otol., Rhinol. and Laryngol., St. Louis, 1921—XXX—1;
Also, J. Lab. and Clin. Med., St. Louis, 1921—VI—175.

**Moss, W. L., Guthrie, C. G., and Marshall, B. C.** Experimental inoculation of human throats with a virulent diphtheria bacilli.
Johns Hopkins Hosp. Bull., Balti., 1921—XXXII—37.

**Morris, W.** Dissection of the faucial tonsils under local anesthesia. .
Lancet, London, 1921—I—169.

**O'Conor, J.** Simple method of tonsillectomy.
Lancet, London, 1920—II—998.

**Olitsky, P. K., and Gates, F. L.** Experimental studies of nasopharyngeal secretions from influenza patients. Transmission experiments with nasopharyngeal washings.
J. Exper. Med., Baltimore, 1921—XXXIII—125.

**Olitsky, P. K., and Gates, F. L.** Studies of the nasopharyngeal secretions from influenza patients. Preliminary report on cultivation experiments.
J. Am. M. Ass., Chicago, 1921—LXXVI—640.

**Ostrom, L.** Peritonsillar abscess and its radical treatment.
Illinois M. J., Oak Park, 1920—XXXVIII—325.

**Packard, M., and Flood, E. P.** Pathogenesis of acute leukemia: report of a case of acute mycloblastic leukemia, with the association or complication of Vincent's angina.
Am. J. M. Sc., Phila., 1920—CLX—883.

**Park, W. H., and Cooper, G.** Accidental inoculation of influenza bacillus on mucous membranes of healthy persons, with the development of infection in at least one. Persistence of type characteristics of bacilli.
J. Immunol., Baltimore, 1921—VI—81.

**Portmann, G.** Subacute hypertrophy of the tonsils.
Ann. méd., Par., 1920—VIII—185.

**Reckord, F. D., and Baker, M. C.** Vincent's angina infection: Its prevalence, manifestations, bacteriology and treatment: Report of fifty-six cases.
J. Am. M. Ass., Chicago, 1920—LXXV—1620.

**Roberts, J. B.** Treatment of complicated cleft palate.
Penn. M. J., Harrisburg, 1920—XXIV—64.

**Sanger, F. D.** Semisuspension in the treatment of tonsil infections.
South. M. J., Birmingham, 1921—XIV—54.

**Schmerz, H.** Retropharyngeal goiters.
Beitr. z. klin. Chir., Tübing., 1920—CXX—483.

**Sleight, R. D., and Haughey, W.** Tonsillectomy for focal infections.
J. Mich. M. Soc., Grand Rapids, 1920—XIX—503.

**Stewart, T. M.** Tonsil facts.
Laryngoscope, St. Louis, 1920—XXX—706.

**Thompson, J. A.** Simple bloodless tonsillectomy with simple, safe local aneshthesia.
Laryngoscope, St. Louis, 1921—XXXI—26.

**Tixier, L.** Gangrenous sore throat rapidly cured with antigangrenous serum.
Bull. Soc. méd. d. hop., Paris, 1920—XLIV—1323.

**Tod, H.** Removal of adenoids in infancy.
Practitioner, London, 1920—CV—335.

**Tydings, O.** The eye in relation to diseases of the nose, throat and teeth.
Illinois M. J., Oak Park, 1921—XXXIX—59.

**Van Horn, Alfred F.** Report of a case of round cell sarcoma of the epipharynx and a case of primary diphtheria of the middle ear.
J. Am. M. Ass., Chicago, 1921—LXXVI—32.

**Vilches, J. M. Barajas de.** Congenital cyst in neck infected from throat.
Siglo méd., Madrid, 1920—LXVII—608.

**Vlasto, M.** Indications for removing tonsils by dissection or by reverse guillotine.
Lancet, London, 1921—I—169.

**Walker, C. B.** Control of lung abscess following tonsillectomy and retropharyngeal abscess. The suction dissector.
Laryngoscope, St. Louis, 1920—XXX—701.

**Walker, C. B.** New devices combining dissection and suction for use in septum, tonsil and other operations.
J. Am. M. Ass., Chicago, 1921—LXXVI—793.

**Watson, E. E.** Mouth breathing.
Virginia M. Month., Richmond, 1920—XLVII—407.

**Williams, E. W.** Risks after operation for tonsils and adenoids in outdoor clinics.
Brit. M. J., Lond., 1920—II—887.

**Wilkinson, O.** Local anesthesia in nasal and throat surgery.
Laryngoscope, St. Louis, 1921—XXXI—27.

**Witherbee, W. D.** Roentgen ray treatment of tonsils and adenoids.
Am. J. Roentgenol., N. York, 1921—VIII—25.

**Woodman, G. S.** Case of tonsillar calculus of unusual size.
Brit. J. Surg., Brixton, 1921—VIII—375.

**Zahorsky, J.** Does removal of adenoid vegetations prevent acute disease of the middle ear?
Laryngoscope, St. Louis, 1921—XXXI—22.

## SECTION 11.—LARYNX.

**Amersbach.** Treatment of carcinoma of the larynx and pharynx.
Deutsch. med. Wchnschr., 1920—XLVI—1269.

**Bana, F. D.** Functional aphonia in case of homicidal cut throat.
Indian M. Gaz., Calcutta, 1920—LV—373.

**Calderin, A. Martin.** Pathogenesis of laryngospasm in children.
Arch. Espan. de ped., Madrid, 1920—IV—513.

**Denegri, J.** Laryngoscopic signs of aortic aneurysm.
Cron. méd., Lima, 1920—XXXVII—312.

**Garel, J., and Gignoux, A.** Fracture and contusion of the larynx.
Lyon méd., 1920—CXXIX—969.

**Gerber.** Latent syphilis of the throat.
Deutsche med. Wchnschr., Berl., 1920—XLVI—1110.

**Johnson, J. S.** Case of postaural hoarseness.
Dublin J. M. Sc., 1920—IV—416.

**Kelly, A. B.** Chorditis fibrinosa.
J. Laryngology, etc., Edinburgh, 1921—XXXVI—5.

**Lannois and Sargnon.** Radium therapy of tumors in ears, nose or throat.
Lyon méd., 1920—CXXIX—807.

**Moore, I.** Angioma of the larynx.
J. Laryngol., etc., Edinburgh, 1921—XXXVI—11, 49.

**Moore, I.** Endolaryngeal hemorrhage during or after thyrofissure in removal of vocal cord for intrinsic cancer of larynx; chief vessel concerned, and its control.
J. Laryngol., Lond., 1920—XXXV—326.

**Pirkey, B. E.** Indications for intubation in diphtheria.
Kentucky M. J., Louisville, 1920—XVIII—408.

**Plum, A.** Recurring papillomas in larynx of children.
Hosp.-Tid., Kjbenh., 1920—LXII—1405.

**Sarkies, M.** Case of persistent hiccough, complicated with spasm of the larynx.
Lancet, London, 1921—I—171.

**Tydings, O.** The eye in relation to diseases of the nose, throat and teeth.
Illinois M. J., Oak Park, 1921—XXXIX—59.

**Wernstedt, W.** Pathologic anatomy of congenital stridor.
Hygiea, Stockholm, 1920—LXXXII—609.

**Wilkinson, O.** Local anesthesia in nasal and throat surgery.
Laryngoscope, St. Louis, 1921—XXXI—27.

## SECTION 12.—TRACHEA AND BRONCHI.

**Bruggone, C., and Vecchia, E.** Intratrachael injection of neoarsphenamin.
Policlin., Roma, 1920—XXVII—1384.

**Chamberlin, W. B.** Difficulties encountered in removing a peanut from a bronchus.
Laryngoscope, St. Louis, 1920—XXX—719.

**Goodloe, A. E.** New bronchoscope.
Larynogscope, St. Louis, 1920—XXX—723.

**Jensen, F.** Scrap of bacon aspirated into trachea.
Ugesk. f. Laeger, Kjbenh., 1920—LXXXII—1290.

**Lynch, R. C.** Fluoroscopic bronchoscopy, esophagoscopy and gastroscopy.
Laryngoscope, St. Louis, 1920—XXX—714.

**Marcondes, F. C.** Removal of foreign body from bronchus of boy of ten.
Brazil méd., Rio de Jan., 1920—XXXIV—703, 777.

**Odermatt, W.** Intratracheal struma.
Deutsche Zeit. f. Chir., Leipzig, 1920—CLVII—279.

**Pennington, C. L.** Extraction of foreign bodies from trachea, bronchi and esophagus.
Georgia Med. Ass. J., Atlanta, 1921—X—235.

**Ribadeau-Dumas.** Importance of roentgenoscopy in diagnosis of disease in tracheobronchial glands.
Paris méd., 1920—X—419.

**Teschendorf.** Esophageal cancer perforating into trachea.
Deutsche. med. Wchnschr., Berl., 1920—XLVI—1249.

**Webb, G. B., and Gilbert, G. B.** Bronchiectasis and bronchitis associated with accessory sinus disease.
J. Am. M. Ass., Chicago, 1921—LXXVI—714.

**Werelius, A.** Removal of nail from left bronchus by aid of fluoroscope.
Illinois M. J., Oak Park, 1920—XXXVIII—335.

**Wood, H.** Twenty cases of foreign body in trachea and esophagus.
J. Tenn. M. Ass., Nashville, 1920—XIII—295.

## SECTION 13.—VOICE AND SPEECH.

**Bana, F. D.** Functional aphonia in case of homicidal cut throat.
Indian M. Gaz., Calcutta, 1920—LV—373.

**Green, J. S.** Falsetto voice in the male; four cured cases.
Laryngoscope, St. Louis, 1921—XXXI—33.

**Levbarg, J. J.** Voice and speech: A neglected medical study.
Laryngoscope, St. Louis, 1920—XXX—711.

**Mourgue, R.** Aphasia and psychology of thinking.
Encephale, Paris, 1921—XVI—26.

**Scripture, E. W.** Inscriptions of speech.
Brit. M. J., Lond., 1920—II—783.

## SECTION 14.—ESOPHAGUS.

**Ayer, G. D., and Buff, J. H.** Removal of foreign bodies from esophagus and bronchial tree.
Georgia Med. Ass. J., Atlanta, 1921—X—230.

**Bevan, Arthur Dean.** Diverticula of the esophagus.
J. Am. M. Ass., Chicago, 1921—LXXVI—285.

**Bohmansson, G.** Successful antethoracic esophageal plastic operation.
Acta chir., Scand., Stockholm, 1920—LIII—91.

**Chabrol, E., and Dumont, J.** Primary dilatation of esophagus.
Paris méd., 1920—X—226.

**Freeman, E. B.** Value of esophagoscopy in diagnosis of diseases of esophagus.
Ann. Med., Hagerstown, Md., 1920—I—.

**Guisez, J.** Incomplete valvular stenosis of the esophagus.
Bull. acad. de med., Paris, 1921—LXXXV—61.

**Hartmann, H.** Diverticula of the esophagus.
J. de chir., Paris, 1920—XVI—481.

**Jackson, C., and Spencer, W. H.** Safety pins in the stomach; peroral gastroscopic removal without anesthesia.
J. Am. M. Ass., Chicago, 1921—LXXIV—577.

**Kirschner.** Reconstruction of esophagus without tube.
Arch. f. klin. Chir., Berl., 1920—CXIV—606.

**Kreuter, E.** Technic of antethoracic esophagoplasty.
Zentralbl. f. Chir., Leipzig, 1920—XLVII—1266.

**Lund, F. B., and Foley, J. A.** Hemorrhage from the stomach and esophagus.
Boston M. & S. J., 1921—CLXXXIV—163.

**Lynah, H. L.** Borderline diseases of the esophagus.
Ann. Otol., Rhinol. and Laryngol., St. Louis, 1921—XXX—164.

**Lynch, R. C.** Fluoroscopic bronchoscopy, esophagoscopy and gastroscopy.
Laryngoscope. St. Louis, 1920—XXX—714.

**Mostajo, J. J.** Endless dilatation for stenosis of the esophagus.
Cron. méd., Lima, 1920—XXXVII—313.

**Pennington, C. L.** Extraction of foreign bodies from trachea, bronchi and esophagus.
Georgia Med. Ass. J., Atlanta, 1921—X—235.

**Roy, J. N.** A case of foreign body in the esophagus, removed by external esophagotomy; cure.
Ann. Otol., Rhinol. and Laryngol., St. Louis, 1921—XXX—159.

**Schröder, A.** Dilatation of esophageal stricture.
Zentralb. f. Chir., Leipz., 1920—XLVII—1102.

**Téschendorf.** Esophageal cancer perforating into trachea.
Deutsche. med. Wchnschr., Berl., 1920—XLVI—1249.

**Wood, H.** Twenty cases of foreign body in trachea and esophagus.
J. Tenn. M. Ass., Nashville, 1920—XIII—295.

## SECTION 15.—ENDOSCOPY.

**Ayer, G. D., and Buff, J. H.** Removal of foreign bodies from esophagus and bronchial tree.
Georgia Med. Ass. J., Atlanta, 1921—X—230.

**Chamberlin, W. B.** Difficulties encountered in removing a peanut from a bronchus.
Laryngoscope, St. Louis, 1920—XXX—719.

**Freeman, E. B.** Value of esophagoscopy in diagnosis of diseases of esophagus.
Ann. Med., Hagerstown, Md., 1920—I—.

**Goodloe, A. E.** New bronchoscope.
Larynogscope, St. Louis, 1920—XXX—723.

**Jackson, C., and Spencer, W. H.** Safety pins in the stomach; peroral gastroscopic removal without anesthesia.
J. Am. M. Ass., Chicago, 1921—LXXIV—577.

**Lynch, R. C.** Fluoroscopic bronchoscopy, esophagoscopy and gastroscopy.
Laryngoscope, St. Louis, 1920—XXX—714.

**Marcondes, F. C.** Removal of foreign body from bronchus of boy of ten.
Brazil méd., Rio de Jan., 1920—XXXIV—703, 777.

**Pennington, C. L.** Extraction of foreign bodies from trachea, bronchi and esophagus.
Georgia Med. Ass. J., Atlanta, 1921—X—235.

**Werelius, A.** Removal of nail from left bronchus by aid of fluoroscope.
Illinois M. J., Oak Park, 1920—XXXVIII—335.

**Wood, H.** Twenty cases of foreign body in trachea and esophagus.
J. Tenn. M. Ass., Nashville, 1920—XIII—295.

## SECTION 16.—EXTERNAL EAR AND CANAL.

**Albright, G. C.** Some aural complications of acute epidemic parotitis.
Iowa M. J., Des Moines, 1921—XI—38.

**Bonner, W. H.** Nasal and aural conditions associated with flying.
Delaware State M. J., Wilmington, 1920—X—17.

**Broom, R.** Spinose ear tick (ornithodorus megnini duges) in human ear in South Agrica.
J. Laryngol., etc., London, 1920—XXXV—362.

**Brühl.** Otologic hints for the general practitioner.
Deutsch. med. Wchnschr., Berl., 1920—XLVI—973, 1000, 1030, 1117, 1145.

**Curtis, H.** Plastic operation to restore part of ear, using a silver wire frame.
Lancet, London, 1920—II—1094.

**Hays, H. M.** Hemorrhage from the ear.
Laryngoscope, St. Louis, 1921—XXXI—20.

**Lannois and Sargnon.** Radium therapy of tumors in ears, nose or throat.
Lyon méd., 1920—CXXIX—807.

**Lund, R.** Syphilis of the outer ear.
Ugesk. f. Laeger, Kjbenh., 1920—LXXXII—1335.

**Maier, M.** Diseases of the ear.
Therap. Monatsh., Berl., 1920—XXXIV—493.

**Maier, M.** Treatment of diseases of the ear.
Therap. Halbmonatsh., Berl., 1920—XXXIV—557.

**Rosenbluth, M.** Serious ear conditions and complications in ambulatory patients.
N. York M. J., 1921—CXIII—54.

**Ryland, A.** Assessment of aural disability resulting from military service.
J. Laryngol., etc., London, 1920—XXXV—354.

**Wingrave, W., and Ryland A.** Infection of middle ear and external auditory meatus with Vincent's organism.
J. Laryngol., etc., Edinburgh, 1921—XXXVI—27.

**Zahorsky, J.** Herpetic sore throat.
South. M. J., Birmingham, Ala., 1920—XIII—871.

## SECTION 17.—MIDDLE EAR, INCLUDING TYMPANIC MEMBRANE AND EUSTACHIAN TUBE.

**Albright, G. C.** Some aural complications of acute epidemic parotitis.
Iowa M. J., Des Moines, 1921—XI—38.

**Andrew, F.** Suppurative middle ear.
Med. J. Australia, Sidney, 1920—II—376.

**Bane, W. C.** Mastoiditis in acute otitis media.
Colorado Med., Denver, 1921—XVIII—38.

**Baylor, J. W.** Restoration of hearing in case of gunshot injury of eustachian tubes.
Johns Hopkins Hosp. Bull., Balti., 1920—XXXI—454.

**Bonner, W. H.** Nasal and aural conditions associated with flying.
Delaware State M. J., Wilmington, 1920—X—17.

**Brannon, W. H.** Chronic suppurative otitis media.
South M. J., Birmingham, Ala., 1920—XIII—824.

**Brühl.** Otologic hints for the general practitioner.
Deutsch. med. Wchnschr., Berl., 1920—XLVI—973, 1000, 1030, 1117, 1145.

**Callison, J. G.** Acute purulent otitis media in children.
Med. Rec., N. Y., 1921—XCIX—386.

**Emerson, F. P.** Minor role of conduction apparatus in slowly progressive deafness.
Boston M. & S. J., 1920—CLXXXIII—736.

**Friedman, J., and Greenfield, S. D.** Middle ear disease in children.
N. York M. J., 1920—CXII—1024.

**Guttman, J.** Case of carcinoma of middle ear.
Laryngoscope, St. Louis, 1920—XXX—727.

**Hays, H. M.** Hemorrhage from the ear.
Laryngoscope, St. Louis, 1921—XXXI—20.

**Kopetsky, S. J.** Systemic infections in relation to acute middle ear diseases.
N. York State J. M., N. Y., 1920—XX—353.

**Lannois and Sargnon.** Radium therapy of tumors in ears, nose or throat.
Lyon méd., 1920—CXXIX—807.

**Maier, M.** Diseases of the ear.
Therap. Monatsh., Berl., 1920—XXXIV—493.

**Maier, M.** Treatment of diseases of the ear.
Therap. Halbmonatsh., Berl., 1920—XXXIV—557.

**Marx, H.** Ear changes in gout.
München. med. Wchnschr., 1920—LXVII—1283.

**McKenzie, D.** Aqueduct of fallopius and facial paralysis.
J. Laryngol., Lond., 1920—XXXV—335.

**Milligan, W.** Chronic catarrhal otitis media.
Practitioner, London, 1921—CVI—9.

**Oppikofer, E.** Cholesteatoma with tuberculous otitis media.
Schwdeiz. med. Wchnschr., Basel, 1920—L—993.

**Perkins, C. E.** Sixth nerve involvement in purulent otitis media.
Laryngoscope, St. Louis, 1920—XXX—666.

**Popper. J.** Case of acute articular rheumatism complicating otitis
media.
Med. Rec., N. Y., 1921--XCIX—270.

**Rogers, L.** Observations on the developmental anatomy of the
temporal bone.
Ann. Otol., Rhinol. and Laryngol., St. Louis, 1921—XXX—103.

**Rosenbluth, M.** Serious ear conditions and complications in ambulatory patients.
N. York M. J., 1921—CXIII—54.

**Ryland, A.** Assessment of aural disability resulting from military
service.
J. Laryngol., etc., London, 1920—XXXV—354.

**Sautter, C. M.** Brain abscess of otitic origin with epileptiform
attacks; decompression; recovery.
J. Am. M. Ass., Chicago, 1921—LXXVI—378.
Laryngoscope, St. Louis, 1920—XXX—823.

**Scheibe, A.** Deafness in gout.
Muenchen med. Wchnschr., 1920—LXVII—1282.

**Shapiro, I. F.** Ear massage with Politzer diagnostic tube.
Laryngoscope, St. Louis, 1921—XXXI—32.

**Strauss, J. F.** Accidents in aural paracentesis.
Ann. Otol., Rhinol. and Laryngol., St. Louis, 1921—XXX—232.

**Van Horn, Alfred F.** Report of a case of round cell sarcoma of the
epipharynx and a case of primary diphtheria of the middle
ear.
J. Am. M. Ass., Chicago, 1921—LXXVI—32.

**Wingrave, W., and Ryland A.** Infection of middle ear and external
auditory meatus with Vincent's organism.
J. Laryngol., etc., Edinburgh, 1921—XXXVI—27.

**Zahorsky, J.** Does removal of adenoid vegetations prevent acute
disease of the middle ear?
Laryngoscope, St. Louis, 1921—XXXI—22.

## SECTION 18.—MASTOID PROCESS.

**Albright, G. C.** Some aural complications of acute epidemic parotitis.
Iowa M. J., Des Moines, 1921—XI—38.

**Brühl.** Otologic hints for the general practitioner.
Deutsch. med. Wchnschr., Berl., 1920—XLVI—973, 1000, 1030,
1117, 1145.

**Clark, J. S.** Some complications in cases of acute mastoiditis.
Illinois M. J., Oak Park, 1920—XXXVIII—536.

**Collet, F. J.** Hysteric pains in the mastoid.
Lyon méd., 1920—CXXIX—847.

**Cook, A. H.** Three cases of mastoiditis with severe complications and recovery.
Laryngoscope, St. Louis, 1921—XXXI—12.

**Encina, Cristobal Jimenez.** Invasion of the mastoid in children.
Arch. Espan. de ped., Madrid, 1920—IV—534.

**Gill, E.** Atypical mastoiditis with report of three cases.
Ann. Otol., Rhinol, and Laryngol., St. Louis, 1921—XXX—228.

**Hammond, P.** Healing processes following mastoid operations.
Laryngoscope, St. Louis, 1920—XXX—662.

**Krauss, F.** Mastoiditis in children.
Penn. M. J., Harrisburg, 1920—XXIV—147.

**Maier, M.** Diseases of the ear.
Therap. Monatsh., Berl., 1920—XXXIV—493.

**Maier, M.** Treatment of diseases of the ear.
Therap. Halbmonatsh., Berl., 1920—XXXIV—557.

**Murphy, W. E.** Acute mastoiditis following influenza.
Ohio M. J., 1921—XVII—18.

**Peabody, J. R.** Lateral sinus thrombosis with a case report.
Kentucky M. J., Louisville, 1920—XVIII—428.

**Peterson, R. A.** Postoperative complications of acute mastoiditis.
Nebraska State M. J., Norfolk, 1921—VI—23.

**Robinson, J. A.** Cavernous sinus thrombosis following a secondary mastoidectomy.
Laryngoscope, St. Louis, 1920—XXX—695.

**Rogers, L.** Observations on the developmental anatomy of the temporal bone.
Ann. Otol., Rhinol. and Laryngol., St. Louis, 1921—XXX—103.

**Rosenbluth, M.** Serious ear conditions and complications in ambulatory patients.
N. York M. J., 1921—CXIII—54.

**Roy, D.** Paralysis of the external rectus, in the right eye, following mastoiditis in the left ear.
Ann. Otol., Rhinol. and Laryngol., St. Louis, 1921—XXX—244.

**Ryland, A.** Assessment of aural disability resulting from military service.
J. Laryngol., etc., London, 1920—XXXV—354.

**Siegelstein, M. J.** Encephalitis lethargica as a postoperative complication of acute mastoiditis, with report of a case.
Ann. Otol., Rhinol. and Laryngol., St. Louis, 1921—XXX—201.

**Taylor, H. M.** Atypical mastoiditis following staphylococcemia.
South. M. J., Birmingham, 1921—XIV—167.

**White, J. W.** Report of cases: 1. Simple mastoidectomy on man 81 years old. 2. Infected sigmoid sinus thrombosis; a positive blood culture with streptococcus mucosus capsulatus present.
Ann. Otol., Rhinol. and Laryngol., St. Louis, 1921—XXX—199.

## SECTION 19.—INTERNAL EAR.

**Albright, G. C.** Some aural complications of acute epidemic parotitis.
Iowa M. J., Des Moines, 1921—XI—38.

**Bane, W. C.** Mastoiditis in acute otitis media.
Colorado Med., Denver, 1921—XVIII—38.

**Bonner, W. H.** Nasal and aural conditions associated with flying.
Delaware State M. J., Wilmington, 1920—X—17.

**Borries, G. V. T.** Head nystagmus in man.
Hos. tid., Kpenh., 1920—LXIII—569.

**Broca, A.** The semicircular canals.
Bull. acad. de méd., Paris, 1921—LXXXV—141.

**Brühl.** Otologic hints for the general practitioner.
Deutsch. med. Wchnschr., Berl., 1920—XLVI—973, 1000, 1030.
1117, 1145.

**Hulburt, H. S.** Case of unilateral auditory hallucinosis.
Med. Rec., N. Y., 1921—XCIX—267.

**Jamison, S. C.** Vertigo or dizziness.
N. Orl. M. & S. J., 1921—LXXIII—313.

**Kerrison, P. D.** Vestibular vertigo of nonsuppurative origin: factors bearing on prognosis; reports of cases.
Laryngoscope, St. Louis, 1920—XXX—626.

**Leegaard, F.** Diagnosis of disease of internal ear.
Norsk Mag. f. Laegevidensk., Kristiania, 1920—LXXXI—961.

**Lundborg, H.** Heredity of dreafmutism, and Mendel's laws.
Svens. Läk.-Sällsk. Handl., Stockholm, 1920—XLVI—88.

**Maier, M.** Diseases of the ear.
Therap. Monatsh., Berl., 1920—XXXIV—493.

**Maier, M.** Treatment of diseases of the ear.
Therap. Halbmonatsh., Berl., 1920—XXXIV—557.

**Marx, H.** Ear changes in gout.
München. med. Wchnschr., 1920—LXVII—1283.

**Maxwell, S. S.** Labyrinth and equilibrium. III. Mechanism of static functions of labyrinth.
J. Gen. Physiol., Baltimore, 1920—III—157.

**McKenzie, D.** Aqueduct of fallopius and facial paralysis.
J. Laryngol., Lond., 1920—XXXV—335.

**Mygind, S. H.** Head nystagmus of human beings.
J. Laryngol., etc., Edinburgh, 1921—XXXVI—72.

**Poulton, E. P., and Mollison, W. M.** Tumor of acoustic nerve; operation; recovery; subsequent death.
J. Laryngol., Lond., 1920—XXXV—333.

**Rogers, L.** Observations on the developmental anatomy of the temporal bone.
Ann. Otol., Rhinol. and Laryngol., St. Louis, 1921—XXX—103.

**Rosenbluth, M.** Serious ear conditions and complications in ambulatory patients.
N. York M. J., 1921—CXIII—54.

**Ruggles, W. G.** Education of the vestibular sense.
Laryngoscope, St. Louis, 1921—XXXI—6.

**Ryland, A.** Assessment of aural disability resulting from military service.
J. Laryngol, etc., London, 1920—XXXV—354.

**Scheibe, A.** Deafness in gout.
Muenchen med. Wchnschr., 1920—LXVII—1282.

**Stenvers, H. W.** Diagnosis of cerebellopontine tumors.
Nederl. Tijdsch. Geneesk., Amst., 1920—II—1871.

**Weve and Sonnen.** Vestibular tests with ocular paralysis.
Nederl. Tijdschr. v. Geneesk., Amst., 1920—II—1528.

## SECTION 20.—DEAFNESS AND DEAFMUTISM, AND TESTS FOR HEARING.

**Baylor, J. W.** Restoration of hearing in case of gunshot injury of eustachian tubes.
Johns Hopkins Hosp. Bull., Balti., 1920—XXXI—454.

**Emerson, F. P.** Minor role of conduction apparatus in slowly progressive deafness.
Boston M. & S. J., 1920—CLXXXIII—736.

**Harrison, S.** Care of blind and deaf children.
Med. J. Australia, Sidney, 1920—II—393.

**Inglis, H. J.** Asthenic hypoacousis.
Ann. Otol., Rhinol. and Laryngol., St. Louis, 1921—XXX—237.

**Marx, H.** Ear changes in gout.
München. med. Wchnschr., 1920—LXVII—1283.

**Podesta, E.** War deafmutism.
Policlin., Roma, 1920—XXVII—1139.

**Rennie, G. E.** Deafness in children.
Med. J. Australia, Sidney, 1920—II—391.

**Scheibe, A.** Deafness in gout.
Muenchen med. Wchnschr., 1920—LXVII—1282.

## SECTION 21.—FOREIGN BODIES IN THE NOSE, THROAT AND EAR.

**Ayer, G. D., and Buff, J. H.** Removal of foreign bodies from esophagus and bronchial tree.
Georgia Med. Ass. J., Atlanta, 1921—X—230.

**Chamberlin, W. B.** Difficulties encountered in removing a peanut from a bronchus.
Laryngoscope, St. Louis, 1920—XXX—719.

**Jackson, C., and Spencer, W. H.** Safety pins in the stomach; peroral gastroscopic removal without anesthesia.
J. Am. M. Ass., Chicago, 1921—LXXIV—577.

**Jensen, F.** Scrap of bacon aspirated into trachea.
Ugesk. f. Laeger, Kjbenh., 1920—LXXXII—1290.

**Marcondes, F. C.** Removal of foreign body from bronchus of boy
of ten.
Brazil méd., Rio de Jan., 1920—XXXIV—703, 777.

**Pennington, C. L.** Extraction of foreign bodies from trachea,
bronchi and esophagus.
Georgia Med. Ass. J., Atlanta, 1921—X—235.

**Roy, J. N.** A case of foreign body in the esophagus, removed by
external esophagotomy; cure.
Ann. Otol., Rhinol. and Laryngol., St. Louis, 1921—XXX—159.

**Sundelöf, E. M.** Foreign body in the jaw; report of a case.
J. Am. M. Ass., Chicago, 1921—LXXVI—790.
**Werelius, A.** Removal of nail from left bronchus by aid of fluoro-
scope.

Illinois M. J., Oak Park, 1920—XXXVIII—335.
**Wood, H.** Twenty cases of foreign body in trachea and esophagus.
J. Tenn. M. Ass., Nashville, 1920—XIII—295.

## SECTION 22.—ORAL CAVITY, INCLUDING TONGUE, PALATE AND INFERIOR MAXILLARY.

**Abels, H.** The role of infections in scurvy.
Wien. klin. Wchnschr., 1920—XXXIII—899.

**Albright, G. C.** Some aural complications of acute epidemic parotitis.
Iowa M. J., Des Moines, 1921—XI—38.

**Benedict, W. L.** Value of dental examination in treatment of ocular disorders.
Am. J. Ophth., Chicago, 1920—III—860.

**Bonnamour, S., and Bardin, J.** Diphtheria antitoxin in prevention
of orchitis and mumps.
Presse méd., Paris, 1920—XXVIII—929.

**Cavazzutti, A. M.** Chronic osteitis of upper jaw.
Semana méd., Buenos Aires, 1920—XXVII—17.

**Cevario, L.** Tumors of the salivary glands.
Policlin., Roma, 1920—XXVII—381.

**Chick, Harriette, and Dalyell, E. J.** Epidemic of scurvy in school
children.
Ztschr. f. Kinderh., Berl., 1920—XXVI—257.

**Coughlin, W. T.** Immobilization of proximal fragment in fracture
of jaw above angle.
Surg., Gynec. and Obst., Chicago, 1920—XXXI—574.

**Conghlin, W. T.** Reconstruction of hard palate with cartilage
transplant.
J. Am. M. Ass., Chicago, 1920—LXXV—1781.

**Crip, W. H.** Relationship between ocular and dental disease.
Colorado Med., Denver, 1921—XVIII—37.

**Dalche, P.** Excessive functioning of the parotids.
Presse méd., Paris, 1920—XXVIII—785.

**Dallenbach, J. C.** Abscess of tongue.
Illinois M. J., Oak Park, 1920—XXXVIII—522.

**Davis. E. D. D.** Malignant growths of upper jaw and antrum; a survey of notes of thirty-nine cases.
Lancet, London, 1920—II—1090.

**Escher, T.** Improved technic for operation on harelip.
Zentralb. f. Chir., Leipz., 1920—XLVII—1169.

**Fargin-Fayolle, P.** Dental caries in the tuberculous.
Presse méd., Paris, 1921—XXIX—44.

**Fineman, B. C.** Study of thrush parasite.
J. Infect. Dis., Chicago, 1921—XXVIII—185.

**Gardner, B. S.** Roentgenology in disease of the teeth.
Am. J. Roentgenol., N. York, 1920—VII—587.

**Giorgi, E.** Epidemic scurvy.
Pediatria, Napoli, 1921—XXIX—66.

**Goldring, Morris.** Thrush complicated by acute polyarthritis in an infant.
J. Am. M. Ass., Chicago, 1921—LXXVI—724.

**Grizzard, R. W.** Dentigerous cyst of mandible.
J. Tenn. M. Ass., Nashville, 1920—XIII—308.

**Hämmerli, A.** Hyperplasia of salivary glands with endocrine disease.
Deutsch. Arch. f. klin. Med., Leipzig, 1920—CXXXIII—111.

**Helliwell, J. P.** Teeth in recruits.
Brit. M. J., London, 1920—II—968.

**Hess, A. F.** Scurvy in world war.
Internat. J. Public Health, Geneva, 1920—I—302.

**Ivy, R. H.** War surgery of face and jaws as applied to injuries and deformities of civil life.
Penn. M. J., Harrisburg, 1920—XXIV—69.

**Kouindjy, P.** Treatment of salivary fistulas by massage and hot air.
N. York M. J., 1920—CXIII—8.

**Lanz, O.** Furuncles of the lip.
Nederl. Tijdschr. v. Geneesk. Amst., 1920—II—2475.

**Laroyenne, L., and Wertheimer, P.** Multilocular cyst of the lower jaw.
Lyon chirurg., 1920—XVII—713.

**Moreau, L.** Large mixed tumor of the soft palate.
Lyon chirurg., 1920—XVII—721.

**Payne, M. J.** Removal of parotid gland for malignant growth.
South. M. J., Birmingham, Ala., 1920—XIII—813.

**Pierquin, J., and Blanc, L.** Radiodiagnosis in dentistry.
Paris méd., 1921—XI—116.

**Richard, W. J., and Mackinnon, W. D.**  Scurvy among adults in Glasgow.
Glasgow M. J, 1920—XII.—336.

**Roger, H.**  Pigmentation in the mouth.
Bull. Soc., méd. d. hop., Paris, 1920—XLIV—1580.

**Sartori, S.**  Unerupted teeth in the upper jaw.
Rev. méd. d. Uruguay, Montevideo, 1920—XXIII—551.

**Sjollema, B.**  Relation between diet and scurvy.
Nederl. Tijdschr. v. Geneesk., Amst., 1921—I—34.

**Smith, E. T.**  Retrobulbar neuritis and dental sepsis.
Med. J. Australia, Sydney, 1921—I—25.

**Stevens, P. A.**  Epithelioma of lip.
Med. J. Australia, Sydney, 1920—II—472.

**Sundelöf, E. M.**  Foreign body in the jaw; report of a case.
J. Am. M. Ass., Chicago, 1921—LXXVI—790.

**Tellier, J.**  .Oral sepsis and systemic disease.
Lyon méd., 1920—CXXIX—813.

**Thoma, K. H.**  Cysts of jaws.
Boston M. & S. J., 1920—CLXXXIII—730.

**Tydings, O.**  The eye in relation to diseases of the nose, throat and teeth.
Illinois M. J., Oak Park, 1921—XXXIX—59.

**Vecchis, B. de.**  Cancer of the mouth.
Rifroma méd., Naples, 1920—XXXVI—987.

**Vetri, A.**  Anesthesia for operations in mouth.
Policlin., Roma, 1921—XXVIII—77.

**Watson, E. E.**  Mouth breathing.
Virginia M. Month., Richmond, 1920—XLVII—407.

**Watson, W. B.**  Oral sepsis.
Lancet, London, 1921—I—11.

**Woodroffe, J. H.**  Oral sepsis and its radiographic diagnosis.
Arch. radiol. and electro., London, 1920—XXV—217.

**Zeisler, E. P.**  Tuberculosis of lip.
Arch. Dermat. and Syph., Chicago, 1921—III—14.

## SECTION 23.—FACE.

**Cevario, L.**  Tumors of the salivary glands.
Policlin., Roma, 1920—XXVII—381.

**Escher, T.**  Improved technic for operation on harelip.
Zentralb. f. Chir., Leipz., 1920—XLVII—1169.

**Ivy, R. H.**  War surgery of face and jaws as applied to injuries and deformities of civil life.
Penn. M. J., Harrisburg, 1920—XXIV—69.

**Kouindjy, P.**  Treatment of salivary fistulas by massage and hot air.
N. York M. J., 1920—CXIII—8.

**Lanz, O.** Furuncles of the lip.
Nederl. Tijdschr. v. Geneesk. Amst., 1920—II—2475.

**Payne, M. J.** Removal of parotid gland for malignant growth.
South. M. J., Birmingham, Ala., 1920—XIII—813.

**Stevens, P. A.** Epithelioma of lip.
Med. J. Australia, Sydney, 1920—II—472.

**Zeisler, E. P.** Tuberculosis of lip.
Arch. Dermat. and Syph., Chicago, 1921—III—14.

## SECTION 24.—CERVICAL GLANDS AND DEEPER NECK STRUCTURES.

**Berry, M.** Roentgen ray treatment of tuberculous glands.
Brit. J. Tuber., London, 1921—XV—13.

**Vilches, J. M. Barajas de.** Congenital cyst in neck infected from throat.
Siglo méd., Madrid, 1920—LXVII—608.

## SECTION 25.—THYROID AND THYMUS.

**Antunez.** Endemic goiter in Ancash region of Peru.
Cron. méd. Lima, 1920—XXXVII—371.

**Armand-Delille, P. F.** Dwarf growth and infantilism of thyroid.
Bull. soc. méd. d. hop., Paris, 1920—XLIV—1392.

**Baker, W. C.** Roentgen ray therapy in hyperthyroidism.
N. York M. J., 1921—CXIII—273.

**Belot, J.** Radiotherapy of exophthalmic goiter.
Bull. méd., Paris, 1920—XXXIV—1063.

**Boitel, W.** Etiology of goiter.
Rev. méd. de la Suisse Rom., Geneva, 1920—XL—717.

**Boothby, W. M.** Adenoma of thyroid with hyperthyroidism; history of recognition of this disease as a clinical entity.
Endocrinol., Los Angeles, 1921—V—1.

**Bram, I.** Exophthalmic goiter and surgery.
N. York M. J., 1921—CXIII—330-366.

**Brenizer, A.** Goiter: A clinical study.
South. M. J., Birmingham, Ala., 1920—XIII—815.

**Brown, Herbert R.** Malignant adenopathy of bones of foot, probably of thyroid gland origin.
J. Am. M. Ass., Chicago, 1920—LXXV—1780.

**Brown, N. W.** Determination of relative activity of thyroid lobes.
Endocrinol., Los Angeles, 1921—V—29.

**Callison, J. C.** Thyroid deficiency in otolaryngology.
N. York M. J., 1921—CXIII—283, 326.

**Canelli, A. F.** The thymus.
Pediatria, Napoli, 1920—XXVIII—1056.

**Canelli, A. F.** The thymus in young children.
Pediatria, Naples, 1920—XXVIII—1002, 1108.

**Cauchoix, A.** Operative treatment of exophthalmic goiter.
Bull méd., Paris, 1920—XXXIV—1060.

**Chewer, D.** Are there reliable criteria of operability in exophthalmic goiter?
Arch. Surg., Chicago, 1921—II—21.

**Clagett, A. N.·** Treatment of goiter with radium.
Illinois M. J., Oak Park, 1920—XXXVIII—318.

**Cordua, R.** Basedow's disease and myxedema.
Mitt. a. d. Grenzgeb. d. Med. u. Chir., Jena, 1920—XXXII—288.

**Couland, E.** Medical treatment of goiter.
Bull. méd., Paris, 1920—XXXIV—1066.

**Couland.** The thyroid in the tuberculous.
Bull. soc. méd. d. hop., Paris, 1920—XLIV—1551.

**Couland.** Tuberculosis in the region of endemic goiter.
Bull. soc. méd. de hop., Paris, 1921—XLV—5.

**Crile, G. W.** Relation of thyroid and of suprarenals to electric conductivity of other tissues.
Endocrinol., Los Angeles, 1920—IV—523.

**Deaver, J. B.** Surgical aspect of hyperthyroidism.
N. York M. J., 1921—CXIII—265.

**Dubs, J.** Suturing of the musculature to goiter stump.
Zentralbl. f. chir., Leipzig, XLVII—1294.

**Edwards, C. R.** Acute infection of the thyroid gland.
J. Am. M. Ass., Chicago, 1921—LXXVI—637.

**Elsesser, O. J.** Laboratory as aid in diagnosis and treatment of diseases of thyroid.
Illinois M. J., Oak Park, 1920—XXXVIII—328.

**Frantz, M. H.** Hyperthyroidism in the child.
N. York M. J., 1921—CXIII—275.

**Friedman, G. A.** Possible relation of suprarenal cortex to exophthalmic goiter and to myxedema.
Med. Rec., N. Y., 1921—XCIX—295.

**Garibaldi, A.** Influence of thyroidectomy on formation of immune antibodies in the dog.
Cron. méd., Lima, 1920—XXXVII—315.

**Haberer.** Goiter and thymus.
Mitt. a. d. Grenzgeb. d. Med. u. Chir., Jena, 1920—XXXII—329.

**Hammer, A. W.** Thyroid gland and thyrotoxicosis.
N. York M. J., 1921—CXIII—245.

**Hardenbergh, D. B.** Hypothyroidism; twenty-six years' supplemental thyroid feeding.
Med. Rec., N. Y., 1920—XCVIII—1054.

**Harrower, H. R.** Hyperthyroidism, infiltration and hypertension.
Med. Rec., N. Y., 1920—XCVIII—854.

**Hunziker, H.** Thrree years' measurements of the thyroid.
Schweiz. med. Wchnschr., Basel, 1920—L—1009.

**Ives, G.** Pathology of the thyroid.
Missouri M. Ass. J., St. Louis, 1921—XVIII—37.

**Jelliffe, S. E.** Parathyroid and convulsive states.
N. York M. J., 1920—CXII—877.

**Klewitz.** Exophthalmic goiter.
Deutsche med. Wchnschr., Berl., 1920—XLVI—971.

**Kreuter, E.** Ligation of arteries in goiter operations.
Zentralbl. f. Chir., Leipzig, 1920—XLVII—1317.

**Lahey, F. H.** Goiter.
J. Maine M. Ass., Portland, 1920—XI—145.

**Lobenhofer, W.** Ligation of arteries in goiter operations.
Zentralbl. f. Chir., Leipzig, 1920—XLVII—1319.

**McBrayer, R.** Differential diagnosis of tuberculosis and hyperthyroidism: Study of Goetsch test.
South. M. J., Birmingham, Ala., 1920—XIII—783.

**McLean, A.** Thyroid glands: metastasizing effects.
J. Mich. M. Soc., Grand Rapids, 1920—XIX—558.

**McKay, W. J. S.** Role played by physician and surgeon in treatment of exophthalmic goiter.
Med. J. Australia, Sidney, 1920—II—357.

**Monge, C.** Endemic goiter in Urubamba district of Peru.
Cron. méd., Lima, 1920—XXXVII—394.

**Morris, M. F.** Hyperthyroidism.
Med. Rec., N. York, 1921—XCIX—133.

**Northrup, H. L.** Goiter.
N. York M. J., 1921—CXIII—277.

**Odermatt, W.** Intratracheal struma.
Deutsche Zeit. f. Chir., Leipzig, 1920—CLVII—279.

**Parhon and Stocker.** The thyroid in a case of melancholia.
Encephale, Paris, 1921—XVI—13.

**Pemberton, J. de J.** Surgery of substernal and intrathoracic
goiters.
Arch. Surg., Chicago, 1921—II—1.

**Rhodes, R. L.** Toxic goiter: Diagnosis.
J. Georgia Med. Ass., Atlanta, 1920—X—198.

**Roeder, C. A.** Squamous cell epithelioma of the thyroid.
Ann. Surg., Phila., 1921—LXIII—23.

**Roth, N.** Parathyroid grafts in pregnancy tetany; recovery.
Wiener. klin. Wchnschr., 1920—XXXIII—886.

**Roussy, G.** Basal metabolism in exophthalmic goiter.
Paris méd., 1920—X—245.

**Roussy, G., and Cornil, L.** Emotions and exophthalmic goiter.
Presse méd., Paris, 1920—XXVIII—753.

**Roussy, G., and Cornil, L.** Exophthalmic goiter.
Bull. méd., Paris, 1920—XXXIV—1057.

**Schmerz, H.** Retropharyngeal goiters.
Beitr. z. klin. Chir., Tübing., 1920—CXX—483.

**Sebileau, P.** Removal of goiter.
Paris méd., 1921—XI—49.

**Sebileau.** Thyroidectomy.
Paris méd., 1921—XI—33.

**Siegel, A. E.** Thymic disease.
N. York M. J., 1921—CXIII—290.

**Stevens, J. T.**  Management of toxic goiter with radiation.
   N. York M. J., 1921—CXIII—247.

**Udaondo, C. Bonorino.**  Somnolency from thyroid insufficiency.
   Rev. Asoc. méd. argent., Buenos Aires, 1920—XXXIII—413.

**Williams, C.**  Classification of goiter: Analysis of 100 cases.
   Am. J. Med. Sc., Phila., 1921—CLXI—223.

**Wilson, C. M., and Wilson, D.**  Determination of basal metabolic
   rate; Its value in diseases of thyroid.
   Lancet, London, 1920—II—1042.

## SECTION 26.—PITUITARY.

**Duffy, W. C.**  Hypophysial duct tumors.
   Ann. Surg., Phila., 1920—LXXVII—537.

**Duffy, W. C.**  Three cases of hypophysial duct tumors and a fourth
   case of cyst of Rathke's pouch.
   Ann. Surg., Phila., 1920—LXXII—725.

**Lacouture, Charbonnel and Lafargue.**  Surgery of the pituitary.
   J. de chir., Paris, 1920—XVI—491.

**Motzfeldt, K.**  Pituitary body and its disorders.
   Norsk. Mag. f. Laegevidensk, Kristiania, 1920—LXXXI—1194.

**Otrich, G. C.**  Pituitary extract in conjunction with local anesthesia.
   J. Am. M. Ass., Chicago, 1921—LXXVI—591.

**Pribram, B. O.**  Hypophysis and Raynaud's disease.
   München med. Wchnschr., 1920—LXVII—1284.

**Rasmussen, A. T.**  Hypophysis cerebri of woodchuck with special
   reference to hibernation and inanition.
   Endocrinol., Los Angeles, 1921—V—33.

## SECTION 27.—ENDOCRANIAL AFFECTIONS AND LUM-
## BAR PUNCTURE.

**Barré, J. A., and Schraf, R.**  Pressure of the cerebrospinal fluid.
   Bull. méd., Paris, 1921—XXXV—63.

**Bryan, J. H.**  Case of extradural and subdural abscess following
   suppurating frontal sinusitis and osteomyelitis of frontal
   bone.
   Am. J. M. Se., Phila., 1920—CX—687.

**Frazier, Charles H.**  A refinement in the radical operation for trigeminal neuralgia.
   J. Am. M. Ass., Chicago, 1921—LXXVI—107.

**Kahn, A.**  Logical cause, pathology and treatment of brain lesions.
   Laryngoscope, St. Louis, 1920—XXX—809.

**Kopetzky, S. J.**  Six cases of septic sinus thrombosis in children.
   Laryngoscope, St. Louis, 1920—XXX—763.

**Martin, H. H., and Crowe, S. J.**  Lateral sinus disease.
   Laryngoscope, St. Louis, 1920—XXX—817.

**Noguchi, H.**  Test for changes in the protein content of the cerebrospinal fluid based on flocculation of lipoids.
   J. Am. M. Ass., Chicago, 1921—LXXVI—632.

**Peabody, J. R.** Lateral sinus thrombosis with a case report.
Kentncky M. J., Louisville, 1920—XVIII—428.

**Perkins, C. E.** Sixth nerve involvement in purulent otitis media.
Laryngoscope, St. Louis, 1920—XXX—666.

**Poulton, E. P., and .Mollison, W. M.** Tumor of acoustic nerve;
operation; recovery; subsequent death.
J. Laryngol., Lond., 1920—XXXV—333.

**Robinson, J. A.** Cavernous sinus thrombosis following a secondary
mastoidectomy.
Laryngoscope, St. Louis, 1920—XXX—695.

**Sautter, C. M.** Brain abscess of otitic origin with epileptiform
attacks; decompression; recovery.
J. Am. M. Ass., Chicago, 1921—LXXVI—378.
Laryngoscope, St. Louis, 1920—XXX—823.

**Schutt, W.** Infectious thrombosis.
Muenchen. med. Wchnschr., 1920—LXVII—1292.

**Stenvers, H. W.** Diagnosis of cerebellopontine tumors.
Nederl. Tijdsch. Geneesk., Amst., 1920—II—1871.

**Webster, R.** Lumbar puncture and meningitis.
Med. J. Australia, Sydney, 1920—II—487.

**White, J. W.** Report of cases: 1. Simple mastoidectomy on man 81
years old. 2. Infected sigmoid sinus thrombosis; a positive blood culture with streptococcus mucosus capsulatus
present.
Ann. Otol., Rhinol. and Laryngol., St. Louis, 1921—XXX—199.

## SECTION 28.—CRANIAL NERVES.

**Hajek, M.** Rhinogenous origin of retrobulbar neuritis.
Wien. klin. Wchnschr., 1920—XXXIII—267.

**McKenzie, D.** Aqueduct of fallopius and facial paralysis.
J. Laryngol., Lond., 1920—XXXV—335.

**Payr, E.** Access to maxillary nerve.
Zentralbl. f. Chir., Leipzig, 1920—XLVII—1226.

**Poulton, E. P., and Mollison, W. M.** Tumor of acoustic nerve;
operation; recovery; subsequent death.
J. Laryngol., Lond., 1920—XXXV—333.

**Roy, D.** Paralysis of the external rectus, in the right eye, following
mastoiditis in the left ear.
Ann. Otol., Rhinol. and Laryngol., St. Louis, 1921—XXX—244.

**Smith, E. T.** Retrobulbar neuritis and dental sepsis.
Med. J. Australia, Sydney, 1921—I—25.

## SECTION 29.—PLASTIC SURGERY.

**Bohmansson, G.** Successful antethoracic esophageal plastic operation.
Acta chir., Scand., Stockholm, 1920—LIII—91.

**Curtis, H.** Plastic operation to restore part of ear, using a silver
wire frame.
Lancet, London, 1920—II—1094.

**Graham, H. B.**  Nasal plastic surgery.
Calif. State J. M., San Fran., 1920—XVIII—383.

**Oppenheimer, S.**  Development of cosmetic rhinoplasty.
N. York State J. M., N. Y., 1920—XX—355.

**Smith, Ferris.**  Plastic surgery: Its interest to·the otolaryngologist.
J. Am. M. Ass., Chicago, 1920—LXXV—1554.

## SECTION 30.—INSTRUMENTS.

**Godwin, D. E.**  Boilable tip and connection for Politzer bag.
Laryngoscope, St. Louis, 1921—XXXI—41.

**Goodloe, A. E.**  New bronchoscope.
Larynogscope, St. Louis, 1920—XXX—723.

**La Force, B. D.**  Technic of closing sinus tonsillaris by suturing
the pillars of the fauces with the aid of La Force's hollow
suture needle and ligature knot fastener.
Laryngoscope, St. Louis, 1921—XXXI—42.

**Shapiro, I. F.**  Sterilization for atomizers, etc.
Laryngoscope, St. Louis, 1920—XXX—726.

**Walker, C. B.**  New devices combining dissection and suction for
use in septum, tonsil and other operations.
J. Am. M. Ass., Chicago, 1921—LXXVI—793.

## SECTION 31.—RADIOLOGY.

**Baker, W. C.**  Roentgen ray therapy in hyperthyroidism.
N. York M. J., 1921—CXIII—273.

**Barnes, H. A.**  Combined operative and radium treatment of malignant disease of nasal accessory sinuses.
Boston M. & S. J., 1920—CLXXXIII—648; also Laryngoscope,
1920—XXX—646.

**Beclere, A.**  Radiotherapy of the ductless glands.
Paris méd., 1921—XI—97.

**Belot, J.**  Radiotherapy of exophthalmic goiter.
Bull. méd., Paris, 1920—XXXIV—1063.

**Berry, M.**  Roentgen ray treatment of tuberculous glands.
·    Brit. J. Tuber., London, 1921—XV—13.

**Clagett, A. N.**  Treatment of goiter with radium.
Illinois M. J., Oak Park, 1920—XXXVIII—318.

**Gardner, B. S.**  Roentgenology in disease of the teeth.
Am. J. Roentgenol., N. York, 1920—VII—587.

**Lannois and Sargnon.**  Radium therapy of tumors in ears, nose or
throat.
Lyon méd., 1920—CXXIX—807.

**Pierquin, J., and Blanc, L.**  Radiodiagnosis in dentistry.
Paris méd., 1921—XI—116.

**Ribadeau-Dumas.**  Importance of roentgenoscopy in diagnosis of
disease in tracheobronchial glands.
Paris méd. 1920—X—419.

**Stevens, J. T.**  Management of toxic goiter with radiation.
N. York M. J., 1921—CXIII—247.

**Werelius, A.** Removal of nail from left bronchus by aid of fluoroscope.
Illinois M. J., Oak Park, 1920—XXXVIII—335.

**Witherbee, W. D.** Roentgen ray treatment of tonsils and adenoids.
Am. J. Roentgenol., N. York, 1921—VIII—25.

**Woodroffe, J. H.** Oral sepsis and its radiographic diagnosis.
Arch. radiol. and electro., London, 1920—XXV—217.

## SECTION 34.—EYE.

**Belot, J.** Radiotherapy of exophthalmic goiter.
Bull. méd., Paris, 1920—XXXIV—1063.

**Benedict, W. L.** Value of dental examination in treatment of ocular disorders.
Am. J. Ophth., Chicago, 1920—III—860.

**Bookwalter, C. F.** Intranasal dacryocystostomy.
Arch. Ophth., N. Y., 1920—XLIX—568.

**Bram, I.** Exophthalmic goiter and surgery.
N. York M. J., 1921—CXIII—330-366.

**Cauchoix, A.** Operative treatment of exophthalmic goiter.
Bull méd., Paris, 1920—XXXIV—1060.

**Chewer, D.** Are there reliable criteria of operability in exophthalmic goiter?
Arch. Surg., Chicago, 1921—II—21.

**Crip, W. H.** Relationship between ocular and dental disease.
Colorado Med., Denver, 1921—XVIII—37.

**Foster, J. H.** Need of systematized postgraduate teaching of ophthalmology and otolaryngology.
Texas State J. M., Fort Worth, 1920—XVI—285.

**Friedman, G. A.** Possible relation of suprarenal cortex to exophthalmic goiter and to myxedema.
Med. Rec., N. Y., 1921—XCIX—295.

**Green, John, Jr.** Chronic dacryocystitis treated by curettage and rapid dilatation.
J. Missouri M. Ass., St. Louis, 1920—XVII—480.

**Hajek, M.** Rhinogenous origin of retrobulbar neuritis.
Wien. klin. Wchnschr., 1920—XXXIII—267.

**Jobson, G. B.** Sinus disease and ocular involvement.
Penn. M. J., 1921—XXIV—205.

**Klewitz.** Exophthalmic goiter.
Deutsche med. Wchnschr., Berl., 1920—XLVI—971.

**Loeb, H. W., and Wiener, M.** The borderland of otolaryngology and ophthalmology.
Ann. Otol., Rhinol. and Laryngol., St. Louis, 1921—XXX—74.

**McKay, W. J. S.** Role played by physician and surgeon in treatment of exophthalmic goiter.
Med. J. Australia, Sidney, 1920—II—357.

**Roussy, G.**  Basal metabolism in exophthalmic goiter.
Paris méd., 1920—X—245.

**Roussy, G., and Cornil, L.**  Emotions and exophthalmic goiter.
Presse méd., Paris, 1920—XXVIII—753.

**Roussy, G., and Cornil, L.**  Exophthalmic goiter.
Bull. méd., Paris, 1920—XXXIV—1057.

**Smith, E. T.**  Retrobulbar neuritis and dental sepsis.
Med. J. Australia, Sydney, 1921—I—25.

**Tydings, O.**  The eye in relation to diseases of the nose, throat and teeth.
Illinois M. J., Oak Park, 1921—XXXIX—59.

**Walker, C. B.**  Nasolacrimal surgery in ophthalmic perspective.
Arch. Ophth., N. Y., 1920—XLIX—585.

**Weve and Sonnen.**  Vestibular tests with ocular paralysis.
Nederl. Tijdschr. v. Geneesk., Amst., 1920—II—1528.

**Whale, H. L.**  Intranasal dacryocystostomy.
Brit. M. J., Lond., 1920—II—701.

**Wheeler, J. M.**  Extirpation of lacrimal sac in trauamtic dacryocystitis.
Texas State J. M., Ft. Worth, 1920—XVI—286.

# ANNALS

OF

# OTOLOGY, RHINOLOGY

AND

# LARYNGOLOGY

INCORPORATING THE INDEX OF OTOLARYNGOLOGY.

| VOL. XXX. | SEPTEMBER, 1921. | No. 3. |

### XXXIII.

## TREATMENT OF MULTIPLE PAPILLOMAS OF THE LARYNX IN CHILDREN.*

GORDON B. NEW, M. D.,

SECTION ON LARYNGOLOGY, ORAL AND PLASTIC SURGERY,

MAYO CLINIC,

ROCHESTER, MINNESOTA.

The treatment of multiple papillomas of the larynx in children has always been difficult because of the tendency to recurrence. Many methods have been employed, such as tracheotomy, thyrotomy and cautery, endoscopic operative measures, fulguration, the application of various medicines locally, and X-ray and radium. The lack of uniformity of methods employed in the treatment of this condition emphasizes the fact that results have not always been good. During the last six years I have treated the condition by radium inside

---

*Presented before the American Radium Society, Boston, June 6, 1921.

the larynx and the outside of the neck, and the results have been much more satisfactory than with any previous methods.

In 1901, McKenzie established the fact that in many cases multiple papillomas of the larynx in children disappear of themselves if a tracheotomy is performed; he advocated tracheotomy instead of treating the papillomas. Clark, in 1905, and Smith, in 1914, stated that they believed tracheotomy to be the most efficient method of treating these cases. While the value of tracheotomy is well known, cases are reported in which the patients have worn tubes for years without any improvement of the condition. I examined a woman, aged 22, who had worn a tracheotomy tube since she was two and her larynx was filled with papillomas. Polyak, in 1911, discussed the treatment of three patients by radium, two adults and one child. He believes that radium will take the place of operative measures in these cases. Abbe, in 1898, was the first in this country to treat multiple papillomas of the larynx with radium. The patient was a woman aged 30. In 1912 he treated a girl aged 16 with papillomas of the larynx with complete clearing up of the condition. Harris, in 1913 and 1914, reported thirteen collected cases which included Abbe's, Polyak's, and Freudenthal's cases. Cohen told of a child aged 5, treated by Bernham, in whom the results were exceedingly good. Plum, in 1920, reported sixteen cases of multiple papillomas; four of the patients were treated by radium, two with good results, and one with a fair result. Plum believes that the results are encouraging. Several observers report poor results by the use of radium. Hopkins, in 1914, reported a case in which radium was used, and was followed by adhesions of the anterior three-fourths of the larynx, and brought up the question of whether or not the scarring was due to the radium treatment. Iglauer, in discussing Smith's article, spoke of the scarring in the larynx following the treatment by 50 mm. radium for seven or eight hours. Jones reported a case of multiple papillomas unsuccessfully treated with radium, but the dosage was not given. Duffey, in 1919, reported a case of a child, aged 3, who developed diffuse thyroiditis and died, following the application of radium inside and outside the larynx. Lynch has perfected the suspension apparatus that is now used and which has added a great deal to the efficient care of these patients.   His results in removing the papillomas by operative measures have been superior to any others on record in this country.   He, however, now believes that the dissection of multiple papillomas from the larynx is an unsuccessful procedure and that the best method for treating these conditions is by fulguration or by acid nitrate of mercury.

During the years from 1914 to 1920, I have examined at the Mayo Clinic twenty-six children under 12 with multiple papillomas of the larynx.   The youngest child was ten months; and the oldest was twelve years.   Such patients are usually brought to the Clinic because of hoarseness and shortness of breath, which may have started at the age of two or three months, as a slight wheezing or crowing cough, or the condition may not have been noticed until the child began to talk. Sometimes the first symptoms are not observed until the child is three or four years of age.   He may later become unable to speak above a whisper, and may get blue when crying and require emergency tracheotomy.   Frequently parents state that the hoarseness came on after whooping-cough, measles, or a cold, which they believe is the cause of the trouble.

Multiple papillomas of the larynx are often diagnosed as laryngismus, stridulus, asthma, and enlarged thymus, but these conditions are readily ruled out by careful history taking. The diagnosis can be made only by laryngoscopic examination, by means of which the typical picture is seen.

Many of the patients in my series had been operated on by endoscopic methods.   One patient had had six thyrotomies and cauteries performed by a general surgeon and was wearing a tracheotomy tube.   The glottis was so badly scarred that a small probe only could be passed through it.   One patient had had six suspensions and the removal of the papillomas, but when he came to the Clinic a large papillomatous mass stood up from the larynx and almost filled the laryngopharynx. The upper margin of the mass was on a level with the tip of the uvula.   The conditions of the other patients were not unusual; the larynx was usually filled with a varying amount of papillomatous tissue.   Nineteen of the patients had had tracheotomies previously or tracheotomy was performed for marked dyspnea shortly after their arrival.   Tracheotomy was not performed unless obstruction made it necessary.   One patient not included in the group of twenty-six died on the train coming to Rochester from laryngeal obstruction (Fig. 1).

### TREATMENT.

The treatment in this series of cases was given under ether, by means of a Lynch suspension apparatus. Except in a few of the early cases no attempt was made to remove the papillomas. A small tube, containing the emanations or the radium salt, was inserted into the glottis and held there by means of forceps. The tube was kept moving under direct observation so that no particular area was overtreated and so that the part needing treatment received it (Fig. 2). The patient was kept asleep during the entire treatment, and from 75 mg. to 150 mg., or millicuries, of radium were used for from twenty minutes to thirty-five minutes, and occasionally longer if indicated by the particular condition. No screening was used except the silver tube which contained the salt, or the emanation, and is less than 1 mm. thick. Patients were treated, as a rule, about once in six weeks or two months. If recurrence was noted, further treatment was given before the recurrence became marked. Parents are always told that unless the child can be brought back at definite intervals it is of little use to begin treatment. The most suspensions given in one case were six, and the least one. Besides these suspension treatments, radium was applied outside the larynx; as a rule about 3,000 mg. hours were given, using 2.5 cm. of wood and 2 mm. of lead screening. These external applications were frequently given between the suspension treatments.

### RESULTS.

Of the twenty-six cases, nine cannot be considered in the results. One patient died about twelve hours after an emergency tracheotomy. One patient died at home between treatments for the want of a tracheotomy, after having had dyspnea for a week. Four patients did not remain for treatment since they could not return at definite intervals. Two patients received one or two treatments and were unable to return. One patient could not be traced, but at the last examination was remarkably improved.

Of the seventeen patients of whom definite information was obtained, eleven are entirely free from papillomas; nine of these had had tracheotomies and the tracheotomy tube had been removed. The tube is always left in place at least six months after the larynx is free from papillomas. One child, on whom a tracheotomy was performed at the age of two and one-half years, had worn the tube for one year and seven months and it could not be removed after the larynx was entirely free from papillomas because of the apparent collapse of the trachea above the tracheotomy opening. A two-way tube was inserted in place of the old tube, and later this was removed, and the trachael opening closed. This was the only instance in which any difficulty occurred in removing the tracheotomy tube. Two of the eleven patients did not have tracheotomies and were not suspended; they received treatment entirely outside the larynx because they had colds at the time of their examination and it was thought inadvisable to give ether. Six of the seventeen patients are still under treatment, but five during the last year only. The larynx of four of the six patients is almost entirely cleared up; possibly there may be an occasional papilloma, but the voice is fairly good. Three of these four had tracheotomies and they can cork their tracheotomy tube. One of the six is much improved but papillomas are present and the voice is hoarse. This patient is wearing a tracheotomy tube and can cork it. One of the six patients, the one referred to as having had so much operative work before coming to the Clinic, is so remarkably improved that the papillomatous mass is now intralaryngeal. In the entire group I have not seen any bad results follow the use of radium, but I believe that this is undoubtedly owing to the fact the radium was under direct observation and was kept moving while in the glottis (Fig. 3).

## BIBLIOGRAPHY.

1. Abbe, R.: Papilloma of the Vocal Cords Cured by Radium. Med. Rec., 1912, xxxi, 703-705.

2. Clark, J. P.: Papilloma of the Larynx in Children. Boston Med. and Surg. Jour., 1905, cliii, 377-381.

3. Cohen, L.: Treatment of Multiple Papillomas of the Larynx in Children. Sect. Laryngol., Rhinol. and Otol., Am. Med. Assn., 1916, 244-245.

4. Duffey, W. C.:  Papilloma of the Larynx.  Report of a Case
Treated with Radium With Resultant Chronic Diffuse Thyroiditis.
Johns Hopkins Hosp. Rep., 1919, xviii, 417-438.

5. Freudenthal:  Quoted by Harris.

6. Harris, T. J.: Radium in the Treatment of Multiple Papillomata of the Larynx.  Tr. Internat. Cong. Med., 1913-1914, Sect.,
Rhinol., Laryngol., pt. 2, 93-96.

7. Hopkins, F. E.:  A Case of Papilloma of the Larynx Treated
by Radium.  Ann. Otol., Rhinol. and Laryngol., 1914, xxiii, 878-880.

8. Iglauer, S.:  Discussion.  Jour. Am. Med. Assn., 1914, lxiii,
2211.

9. Jones, S.:  Cases Illustrative of the Value of Treatment of
Papilloma of the Larynx by Radium and by X-rays. Jour. Laryngol.,
Rhinol. and Otol., 1920, xxxv, 113-114.

10. Lynch, R. C.:  Suspension Laryngoscopy as a Means of
Diagnostic and Operative Approach to the Larynx.  Ann. Otol.,
Rhinol. and Laryngol., 1920, xxix, 416-421.

11. McKenzie, G. H.:  The Treatment of Laryngeal Growths in
Children.  Brit. Med. Jour., 1901, ii., 883-885.

12. Plum, A.: Les papillomes du larynx chez l'enfant.  Acta
otolaryngol., 1920, ii, 119-143.

13. Polyak, L.:  (Radiumtherapy of Multiple Papilloma of the
Larynx).  Orvosi hetil., 1911, lv, 828-830.

14. Smith, H.:  Papilloma of the Larynx.  Jour. Am. Med. Assn.,
1914, lxiii, 2207-2211.

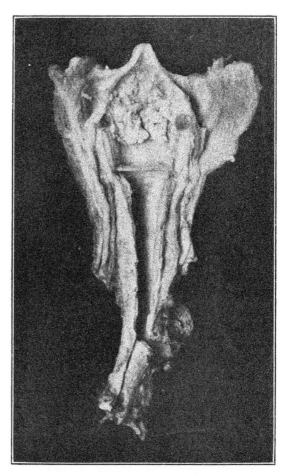

Fig. 1. Specimen taken at necropsy of a multiple papilloma of the larynx in a child who died on the train on the way to Rochester for an examination.

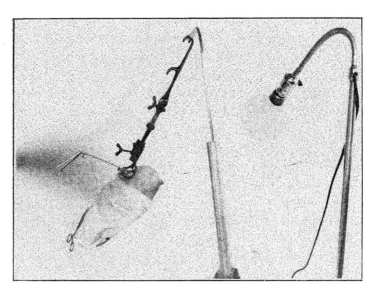

Fig. 2. A child under suspension. The forceps in the mouth holds a tube of radium directly in the glottis. The radium tube is kept moving during the application.

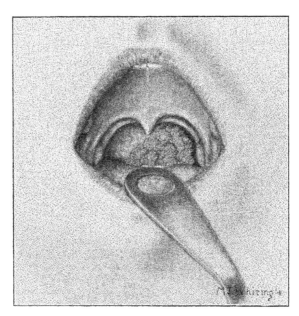

Fig. 3. An extensive papilloma of the larynx which has extended up into the pharynx from the glottis, the result of repeated operative treatment. The condition has now almost entirely disappeared under radium treatment.

# XXXIV

## THE ENDONASAL OPERATION OF THE LACRIMAL SAC.

By William B. Chamberlin, M. D.,

Cleveland, Ohio.

In 1917, the writer had the honor to present a paper on the foregoing subject before the section on ophthalmology of.the American Medical Association, reporting at that time some eight cases, with one failure. Since that time ten cases have been operated upon, with no failures, as far as restoration of physiologic function was concerned, though not all were free from pus. As in the previous series, secondary operations were performed on three cases. Such a series is not large in number, but is sufficient from which to draw certain conclusions.

Anatomy.—A detailed description of the anatomy of the canaliculus, sac and duct may be gained from the better textbooks. To those less familiar with the anatomy the accompanying illustrations may be helpful. The anatomic essentials, from a point of view of disturbance of function, are that the passageway for the tears presents two constrictions, one where the sac joins the duct and another where the duct enters the nose. This latter constriction is increased by the presence of a distinct valve, the socalled valve of Heister.

Indications.—Briefly, the endonasal operation may be said to be indicated whenever the normal passageway for the tears has become obstructed, and the ordinary conservative measures for restoration, such as probing and irrigation, have been unsuccessful.

External Operation.—This operation, revived by Berlin in 1863 and subsequently by Toti in 1904, presents certain decided disadvantages. The external operation, even if successful in so far as the cure of the abscess was concerned, did not cure the epiphora. This condition so annoyed and inconvenienced the patient that the subsequent removal of the gland become necessary. The resulting scar and its subsequent contrácture was frequently unsightly. Occasionally, too, a fistula remained. These disadvantages prompted West in 1908 to attempt the operation from within the nose, rather than from without, and to thus restore the normal and physiologic drainage into the nasal cavity.

Endonasal Operation.—The advantages of this over the previous methods, to quote from West, are as follows:

"1· The physiologic function of the path for the tears is again restored, so that not only a suppuration of the sac, a lacrimal fistula or a phlegmon is healed, but also the tears flow normally through the nose. A later epiphora is accordingly avoided.

"2· A socalled cure by probing is rendered unnecessary.

"3. The lacrimal gland is spared.

"4. A skin incision or a curetting from without, with eventual scar foundation, is avoided."

The disadvantages seem to be two only. Certain persons, it is true, by sharply blowing the nose, can force air out through the canaliculus. This objection would seem to be theoretical rather than practical, as West asserts that this condition was never complained of by his patients.

My attention has been called to another disadvantage by Dr. William E. Bruner, by whom most of my cases have been referred. In certain cases where there was a complete restoration of physiologic function, it was still possible to express slight traces of pus through the punctum on milking the sac. Such a condition would of course render a cataract operation impossible, on account of the danger of infection.

Operation.—The most popular methods of operation at the present time are four—those of West, Yankauer and Mosher, and more recently the operation of Wiener and Sauer, reported and described by them before the last meeting of the section on ophthalmology of the American Medical Association. The operation of Yankauer I have performed on the cadaver and once upon the living. It is both ingenious and difficult. The objection would seem to be that it confines itself rather to the duct than the sac, in an endeavor to restore the passageway into the inferior meatus. It seems to carry too great a danger of subsequent stenosis at the junction of the sac and duct.

The operation of Mosher I have performed only on the cadaver. With the operation of Sauer and Wiener I am not familiar.

My operation of choice is that of West, with slight modifications, too unimportant to possess any merit as to originality. After preliminary cocainization and infiltration of $\frac{1}{2}$ per cent novocain, to the dram of which two minims of adrenalin have been added, a three sided incision is made. The first two incisions are parallel with the floor of the nose and extend as far forward as possible from two points, the upper from the point of attachment of the middle turbinal and the lower from a point opposite the free border of the middle turbinal. For these incisions the right angled knife of Freer is exceedingly well adapted. The anterior ends of these incisions are then joined by a vertical incision made as for forward as possible and carried well down to the bone. This flap is now elevated submucously, the periosteum being of course included, and is deflected backward, as on a hinge, between the middle turbinal and the septum, where it is held out of the field during the remainder of the operation by a small pledget of cotton. The posterior lip of the dense ascending process of the superior maxilla is now attacked with chisel and gouge until the nasal wall of the sac is presented to view. This is easily recognized by palpation with a probe. Sufficient bone should be removed to uncover the sac freely in almost its entire nasal aspect. At this point I have found it of advantage to insert a probe through the canaliculus into the sac, thus pushing its nasal surface, tentlike, well over toward the septum. A thin scalpel is then inserted between the probe and the lateral nasal wall, the outer or free end of the probe being held by an assistant or fastened to the forehead by a strip of adhesive. By so doing it is possible to resect a larger portion of the sac. Loose pieces may subsequently be removed by means of the smallest sized forceps of Gruenwald. West's dictum, that at the completion of the operation the probe introduced through the canaliculus into the sac must pass horizontally into the nose should be strictly adhered to. The submucous flap is now replaced, its upper half covering the sac resected and the lower portion held in position for twenty-four hours by light packing. Subsequently the nose should be kept free from crusts until healing takes place. If desired, the sac may be irrigated through the canaliculus. I have not always found it necessary. I have sometimes wondered if the replacement of the lower portion of the flap might not be dispensed with.

My results from this operation, as far as restorations of the physiologic pathway is concerned, have been uniformly good. As before mentioned, it has occasionally been possible to express a slight amount of pus from the canaliculus. So far I have not operated upon any cases of acute abscess. West has performed this operation on all possible types of cases and in 1913 reported 130 operations with 90 per cent of cures.

One of my most interesting cases was a fourth year medical student, who had suffered from suppuration of the sac and constant epiphora. He had developed a habit spasm and would unconsciously squeeze out the secretion from the sac every few minutes during his waking hours. Subsequent to the operation this habit disappeared.

Difficulties.—That the endonasal operation presents certain decided technical difficulties is undoubtedly true. My feeling is that it is performed by comparatively few rhinologists for two reasons: (1) On account of the fancied difficulty, and (2) because of the unwillingness of the ophthalmologist to refer appropriate cases. As regards the first, the operation, to my mind, is no more difficult than the average submucous resection. The operation should be performed at first upon the cadaver until a proper technic is attained. As regards the second, the operation is, or should be, an example of team work on the part of the ophthalmologist and rhinologist, just as the correction of mouth breathing is, in many cases, the result of team work on the part of the rhinologist and orthodontist. Each is essential to the success of the other. Fortunately, the man who embraces all four specialties in his domain is becoming the exception, rather than the rule, so it is only by the courtesy of the ophthalmologist that the rhinologist may obtain cases.

The purpose of this paper is not to describe any original technic, but to present a record of my own successes and failures, in the hobe of stimulating interest in an operation which may bring relief to many and which, it would seem, should have a wider popularity than it at present enjoys.

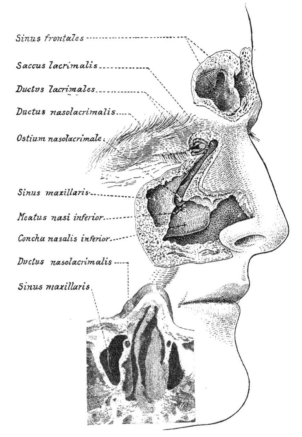

Fig. 1. A dissection showing the nasolacrimal passageways and the relations of the nasolacrimal duct to the maxillary sinus and the inferior nasal meatus. The inset is a transection of the nasal fossae, the maxillary sinuses and the nasolacrimal ducts. By courtesy of P. Blakiston & Co. Schaeffer: The Nose and Olfactory Organ.

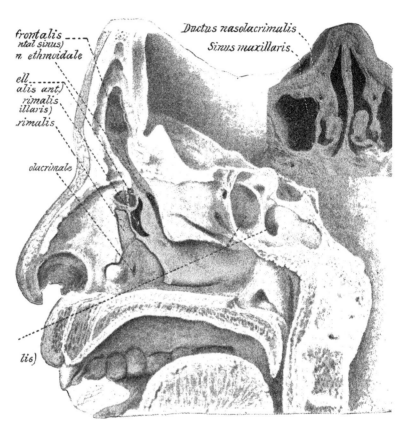

Fig. 2. A dissection of the lateral nasal wall with especial reference to the nasolacrimal sac (indicated by dotted outline in white), the agger cell, the prelacrimal recess of the sinus maxillaris. The insert is a transection showing the relations of the nasolacrimal duct. By courtesy of P. Blakiston's Son & Co. Schaeffer: The Nose and Olfactory Organ.

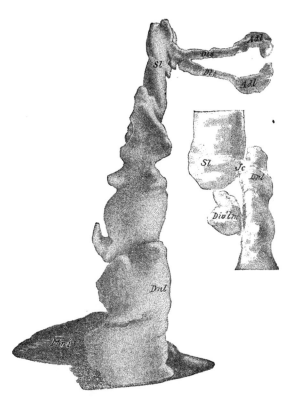

Fig. 3. Reconstruction of the nasolacrimal passageways of an adult aged 65 years; medial view. Especially note the irregularity and the diverticula of the nasolacrimal duct. The insert shows the details of the side to side union of the lacrimal sac and the nasolacrimal duct; moreover, illustrates the large bud-like diverticulum from the nasolacrimal duct. By courtesy of P. Blakiston's Son & Co. Schaeffer: The Nose and Olfactory Organ.

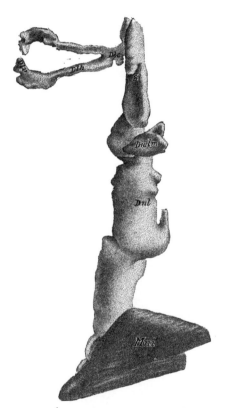

Fig. 4. Reconstruction of the nasolacrimal passageways of an adult aged 65 years; lateral view. By courtesy of P. Blakiston Son & Co. Schaeffer: The Nose and Olfactory Organ.

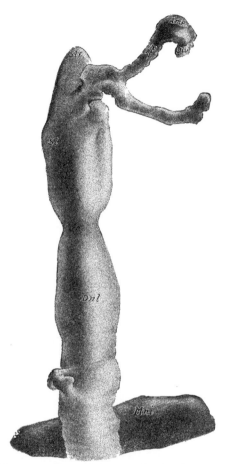

Fig. 5. Reconstruction of the nasolacrimal passageways of an adult aged 60 years. Note the regularity of the nasal duct and the gradual mergence of the lacrimal sac into the nasolacrimal duct at the constriction of the isthmus. By courtesy of P. Blakiston's Son & So. Schaeffer: The Nose and Olfactory Organ.

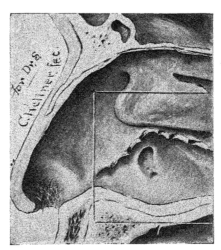

Fig. 6.   Finished operation.

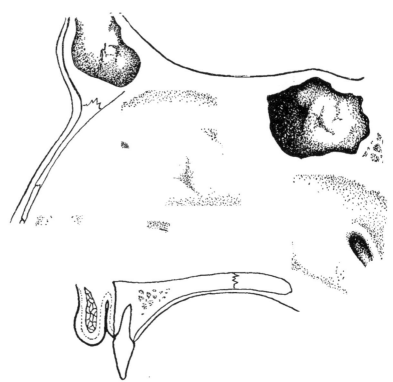

Fig. 7.   Flap turned back and incision being made through the bone.

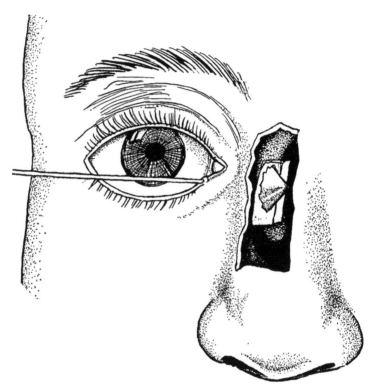

Fig. 8. Showing sac bared and probe passing horizontally into the nose.

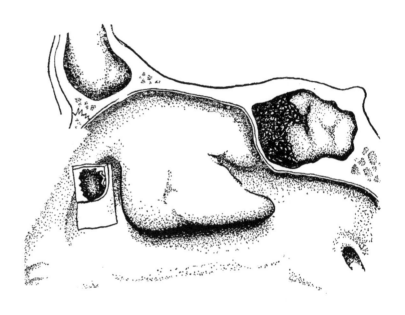

Fig. 9. Lacrimal sac bared above. Flap replaced; the flap cut
away above to show this.

SOME

AI

Lung
are cat
sibly a
organis

The
three c
develop
secretic

The
followi
should
emboli:
in a d
of Mec
respira
toward
cases a

Reg:
a discr
some c
ciation

The
in Bell

---

*Rea
Laryng

## XXXV.

## SO𝔸E OBSERVATIONS ON LOCALIZED PUL𝔸ON-ARY SUPPURATION, TREATED BY ENDO-BRONCHIAL IRRIGATION.*

By CHARLES J. IMPERATORI, M. D.,

NEW YORK CITY.

Lung abscesses may be divided into three classes, those that are caused by aspiration, by embolism and another type, possibly a tubercular cavitation with a secreting lining of infecting organisms.

The aspiration type of cases have been known to occur in three days; this, however, is exceptional; the abscess usually developing from thirteen to fifteen days after the inhalation of secretions or foreign bodies.

The embolic type usually occurs within three to five days following some operative procedure. It would seem that there should be more cases of lung abscesses, especially of the embolic type, following tonsillectomy, as has been suggested in a discussion by Coakley before the New York Academy of Medicine. The movement of the pharyngeal muscles, the respiratory efforts and the open veins would seem to tend toward embolism; however, from clinical observation these cases are very rare.

Regarding the third type, I am not prepared to enter into a discussion of their etiology at present, but it is hoped at some early future date that I can present before the association further studies.

The following observations have been conducted on patients in Bellevue Hospital on the service of Dr. Coakley, and while

*Read at the Forty-third Annual Congress of the American Laryngological Association, May 30th, 1921, at Atlantic City, N. J.

not a great number, still some conclusions may be drawn from them:

There are seven cases, two being alive and still under treatment. Of the five deaths, one died from a carcinoma of the bronchus and was reported at the February meeting of the Eastern Section of the American Laryngological, Rhinological and Otological Society. One was operated elsewhere, that is, a pneumectomy was done, but the patient succumbed on the table and the other three cases died from an intercurrent pneumonia.

The family history in all these cases, in so far as it concerns our observations, is negative.

The past history averaged about four to six months duration of cough, profuse expectoration and accompanied by more or less pain in the chest.

In two of the cases there was considerable loss of weight.

None of these cases followed tonsil operation, all of them came on insidiously.

The age of the patients ranged from 26 to 52 years and there were six males and one female.

Sinuses and tonsils negative.

All of these cases had varying degrees of pyorrhea alveolaris.

Temperature in most of the cases never ranged over 100 to 101, excepting in one case, that was of the septic type.

They were all ambulant cases, excepting toward the end.

There was no special amount of dyspnea and never any stridor.

Six of these cases showed marked clubbing of the fingers and one of the toes.

Blood examinations, that is differential leukocyte and total leukocyte count, varied so that they were inconclusive.

Bacteriology showed so many different varied bacteria that no definite conclusions can be drawn from this observation.

The diagnosis of all these cases was confirmed by radiographs.

The average size of these lung abscesses was from three to four inches in diameter, and of an irregular outline.

Location in four cases was in the right middle lobe, two in the left lower lobe and one in the right lower lobe.

Repeated sputum analyses were all negative in these cases for tubercle bacilli and yet in the four cases autopsied four showed marked evidences of tubercle.

The amount of sputum was remarkably controlled by bronchial irrigations. General well being and the amount of appetite usually much improved. Less cough. Sleeping much better. Fewer pains in the chest, although, as a rule, following the bronchial irrigations, there would be some chest pains. All of these cases appeared to do well for a time.

The longest time that any one case was under treatment was nine months.

Patients having from three to four cupfuls of sputum a day, that is material raised from the lung and saliva amounting to a pint, could by these bronchial irrigations be reduced to less than a cupful. The number of irrigations given was from one to thirty, average twenty. Starting in with one a week, and as the patients became accustomed to the passing of the bronchoscope which, of course, was done under local anesthesia, they were irrigated every five days.

The apparatus used was usually a 7 mm. Jackson bronchoscope passed through a Mosher laryngoscope and two ordinary bronchial aspirating tubes, one for the injection of the saline and the other for its withdrawal. In the first few cases the Yankauer apparatus, suction and injecting tube, was used but it was too delicate an instrument for hard usage. However, the method is entirely that of Yankauer.

From eight to ten ounces of normal saline solution would be injected into the bronchiole, from which the maximum amount of pus was coming and that had been previously determined at the original bronchoscopy. This would be immediately aspirated through the aspirating tube, some would be ejected through the bronchoscope. When the washings came through clear, a bismuth-oil mixture was injected; this consisted of 30 grains to the ounce of bismuth-subnitrate in one ounce of olive oil; in latter cases, bismuth-subcarbonate was used. This was properly sterilized before use. As a rule, most of this bismuth mixture would be coughed up before the patient left the table. Bismuth-sulphide was noted in the first washings, at subsequent irrigations, in most of the cases that were irrigated every five days. In some few cases the bismuth remained in the neighborhood of the abscess or in the bronchi. The odor of the sputum was considerably lessened and the extremely fetid characteristic was not so marked. On stopping the irrigations and injections the odor returned and the amount would be markedly increased.

### CONCLUSIONS.

Of the five cases that died, four were autopsied and proven, beyond doubt, to be tubercular; one being a carcinoma with a tuberculosis. All of these cases were repeatedly examined, careful sputum analyses made, fluoroscoped, radiographed and decided that they were probably not tubercular and referred from either the medical, surgical or tubercular wards as cases suitable for treatment. The remaining two cases, clinically, have the same characteristics that the other five have.

Simple bronchial irrigations, in the writer's opinion, in the control and treatment of lung abscesses of this type are of little use, except as noted above. It is very possible, with the use of the spiral irrigating tubes of Lynah, better results may be obtained and this method shall be pursued in subsequent cases.

Various medicaments were used in some of the early treatments of these cases, such as iodoform emulsion, iodine in olive oil, tincture iodine, weak Dakin solution—one and ten, and boric acid solution. All with negative results. Warm saline solution and the injection of olive oil, impregnated with the 5 per cent bismuth, seemed to be as efficacious as anything.

Idiopathic lung abscess, and by that is meant that type of abscess other than that directly traceable to aspiration or trauma of some foreign substance, or the embolic abscess following some surgical procedure, is possibly a tubercular cavitation with a lining area of pyogenic organisms. This cannot be given as a definite conclusion and is merely sugges‐ tive from these personal observations, and must be proven by a larger series of cases.

## XXXVI.

## AN INVISIBLE SCAR METHOD IN COSMETIC NASAL SURGERY.

By Ira Frank, M. D., and Jerome F. Strauss, M. D.,

Chicago.

We have for some years been rather dissatisfied with the usual methods of approach in cosmetic plastic surgery of the nose. This dissatisfaction we have felt most keenly in those cases where medium degrees of deformity are presented for correction, such cases carrying with them especially serious hazzards for the conscientious surgeon. The failure of an operator to produce desirable results in extreme plastic cases such as old third degree burns, gunshot wounds of the face, and crushing injuries of the nasal bridge, may be countenanced by the patient, and by surgical colleagues—the condition is at least not likely to be worse after operation than before. But in the plastic operations of less degree a far greater responsibility rests with the surgeon; in these cases the patient must be submitted to the minimum amount of risk of cosmetic injury and infection to the end that no disfigurement shall be added to, or substituted for, the original deformity.

The operations of modern plastic surgery of the nose may be classified into two main divisions:

1. Serious malformations, not only of supporting structures but also involving the cutaneous covering of the nose, such as may be produced by crushing injuries, lacerating wounds, cured malignant new growths, granulomas, etc., with marked destruction of the organ and loss of tissue.

These cases have been treated for years with varying satisfaction by the old Italian and the Indian flap methods, and have no place in this discussion.

2. The second group (by far the most numerous in our experience in civil practice) consists of defects of milder degree—moderate deformities of the supporting structures which go to make up the nasal bridge and not involving the skin

of the nose. These are the saddle noses, the humped or hooked noses, and the abnormally broad noses, possessors of which may suffer embarrassment and mental anguish in business life and social intercourse. It is in this type of case that a special responsibility is presented to the rhinologist, in that a correction must be made with the least possible risk to the patient in the matter of finished result, and that the offending feature be made an asset instead of a liability.

The intranasal operations (of continental origin) have been largely used for the correction of these milder deformities. The method consists of an incision made through the mucous membrane of the nose above the superior edge of the triangular cartilage, or at the junction of the frontal processes of the maxillae with the lateral nasal cartilages. Through this incision the periosteum of the nasal bridge is elevated in the midline; humps are reduced to becoming contour with suitable rasps; and for broad noses, by specially constructed saws, the frontal processes of the maxillary bone are sawed through, fractured, and held in proper place by external and internal splints.

The external method, used in America among plastic surgeons, consists of a small horizontal incision over the bridge of the nose at the level of the inner canthi, through which the periosteum of the midline is elevated downwards to the tip. With the field thus prepared, humps are removed, or, in the case of saddle noses, suitably shaped bone or cartilage grafts or plates of inert rigid substance (French ivory) are inserted.

The chief disadvantage of the first or internal method is, of course, the inability of the surgeon to sterilize properly the operative field; and for this reason above all others we have hesitated to subject our patients to such a risk, a risk seemingly out of proportion to the end in view. Further, in our earlier work, when this method was used, we were in many instances unable to gain a satisfactory breadth of operative field on the nasal ridge without running an additional risk by making a similar incision on the other side.

This method may be used in the three principal types of deformities, but is most successful in the hooked nose which is reduced by saw, rasp, or spokeshave. The broad nose requires a bilateral intranasal incision in order to reach both frontal processes with the saw, which doubles the risk of infection; while in the depressed or saddle nose the suitable graft is passed through the questionably sterilized nostril to the bridge of the nose. This operation we have attempted with subsequent regret.

The external or intercanthal operation is a vast improvement upon the foregoing method and seems now to be gaining in popularity throughout the country, though it is applicable only in humped and saddle noses. It offers a sterile field and a more direct approach to the nasal bridge. In our own experience, however, we have had one regrettable infection of unknown origin, which seriously threatened the final result and terminated in an embarrassing scar on which a secondary plastic operation was indicated. We have also had occasion to regret the resulting scar in a number of other postoperatives by this method.

This unreliability of the result so far as scars are concerned, even though the majority of the cases operated on were satisfactory, offered us a problem of some importance, and our inability to remedy the broad nose through the intercanthal opening gave added significance to our problem.

We have, therefore, modified the external method of operation in a manner which has proved exceedingly satisfactory in our hands. We claim no striking originality in either the method or the technic, and we present it merely as the solution to our problem. We have found that we are able now to operate successfully upon either of the three types of bridge deformity through an incision made in a field readily sterilized and in a location sufficiently hidden to relieve us of all anxiety should malunion, infection, or pigmented scar persist.

### TECHNIC.

Before entering the operating room the patient's face and forehead is thoroughly washed with soap and water. With an indelible pencil a line one-quarter inch in length is drawn on the horizontal axis of the left eyebrow, as close to its median extremity as it is possible to approach without extending beyond the hair line. The brow is then partly or wholly removed with scissors, leaving the pencil marked location of the incision plainly visible on the skin. On the operating table the eyes are covered individually with sterile cotton pads pressed with sterile water, and the remainder of the skin of the face is thoroughly sponged with alcohol-ether. The patient is then put to sleep with ether through a sterile mask, which is discarded for the ethervapor machine as soon as narcosis is reached.

The incision is made one-quarter inch in length, down to the frontal bone (superciliary ridge) through the periosteum. A periosteal elevator with a slightly curved shank (Fig. 1, A) is introduced and the skin and subcutaneous tissues are elevated from the bone and cartilage along the median line of the bridge of the nose down to the tip, the instrument being guided in its subcutaneous course by the operator's hand. (Fig. 2.)

Into the pocket thus formed a slightly curved rasp (Fig. 1, B) may be introduced and humps removed; or in the case of depressed nose, a properly prepared transplant of bone or cartilage may be inserted. For the broad nose, two incisions are required: the usual one in the left eyebrow, and one similarly placed on the right side (Fig. 3). Through these openings the periosteum covering the frontal processes of the superior maxillae is elevated and a small, specially designed saw (Fig. 4) is inserted. The processes are then sawn through at the base of the nasal bridge (Fig. 3) and the walls of the nose are pressed inward to a position cosmetically satisfactory and retained with an external splint of padded heavy sheet copper.

The incisions are closed with interrupted horse hair and sealed with tincture of benzoin over a thin wisp of cotton.

The skin of the nose and the lower forehead lends itself admirably to this operative procedure. It is loosely attached to the subjacent areolar tissue, and consequently is very freely movable. Indeed in some individuals it is possible to use the straight rasps and elevators of the intercanthal operation through the eyebrow incision which can actually be moved inwrad until it lies in the midline.

The wound heals very rapidly owing partly to adequate blood supply and partly to the fact that there is practically no tension to the skin. The scar is usually invisible through the regrowing hair of the eyebrow by the time the stitches are removed.

The accompanying illustrations show the few instruments necessary for this type of operation. The rasp and elevator are simple modifications of those used in the intranasal and intercanthal methods. They have been curved to the left to permit their use in the left eyebrow, as the leftsided operation is the one of choice for the righthanded operator. The frontal process saw is merely a segment of a small circular bone saw, attached to a straight shank and handle.

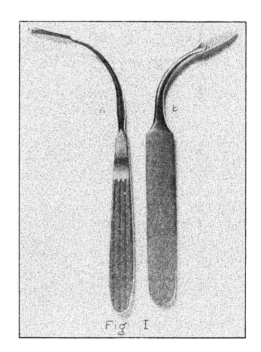

Fig. 1.

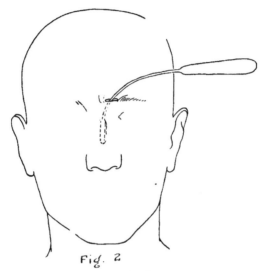

Fig. 2

Fig. 2.

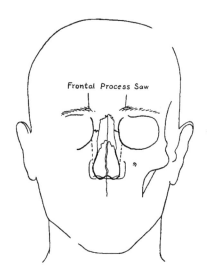

Fig 3

Fig. 3.

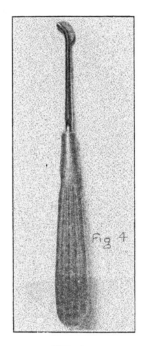

Fig. 4

# THE ACCESSORY SINUSES AS AN ETIOLOGIC FACTOR IN BRONCHIECTASIS.*

By W. V. Mullin, M. D.,

Colorado Springs, Colo.

I intend in this paper to discuss the etiologic relationship of disease of the accessory nasal sinuses to diseases of the bronchi, with the subsequent development of bronchiectasis, and I will begin by stating my own position as I have done previously.

Patients with bronchiectasis will usually be found to have a well-marked sinusitis, and the degree of the bronchial infection is usually in proportion to the amount of sinus involvement present, the well-advanced cases of bronchiectasis having a pansinusitis, as the lantern slides shown later will demonstrate. In going over some of the authoritative literature on bronchiectasis we have not noted such an association mentioned. There have been observations on the nasal cavities as the cause of nontuberculous pulmonary disease—as, for example, those of Rist, Sergeant and Saylor, cited by Gilbert in a former discussion of this subject. But nowhere do we find any emphasis on an etiologic relationship or on the possible pathways of infection linking the upper and lower respiratory fields. Even very recent works, such as the Oxford System of Medicine and Nelson's System of Medicine, make no mention of the sinuses in connection with bronchiectasis. It is of interest to note that McPherson in Osler's System of Medicine mentions brain abscess as a relatively frequent complication of bronchiectasis. The question immediately arises in our mind that since brain abscess is also a frequent complication of sinus disease, do not the bronchiectatic subjects in whom this complication is found develop it not from their bronchi but from an unrecognized sinusitis? While this paper is meant to deal entirely with the sinuses as an etiologic cause, I feel that to

*Read before the Western Section of the American Laryngological, Rinological and Otological Society, Los Angeles, California, Jan. 29, 1921.

avoid confusion and make myself understood I should mention that a digest of the views expressed by McPhedrin, Stengel, Powell and Hartley and by MacCallum, permitted us to make the following classification:

1. Bronchiectasis due to mechanical obstruction.
    a. Foreign bodies in bronchi.
    b. Tumors, including aneurism.
2. Cases of general "bronchiolectasis" in young children after acute bronchitis.
3. Cases, especially in infants, where there is bronchial dilatation to compensate for atelectasis.
4. Cases associated with fibroid tuberculosis, or other extensive fibrosis, as after empyema or organizing pneumonia, where there is contraction and compensatory bronchial dilatation.

These four groups of known or partially known etiology comprise a minority of the cases of bronchiectasis, and leave a majority to be classed as:

5. Cases attributed to chronic bronchitis or to an acute bronchitis or bronchopneumonia which has left sequelae.

This fifth group of cases includes all not included in the first four. That is, all the obscure cases. In them the history is often vague and the real cause distinctly hypothetical.

Let me here review briefly some experimental work on animals which I have carried on with the help of Dr. Ryder during the last four years. The work falls into two divisions. The first, on the lymph drainage of the accessory nasal sinuses, was reported two years ago. In it we proved, by the use of carbon suspensions and tubercle bacillus emulsions, that the lymph drainage of the antrum is by way of the submaxillary and deep cervical nodes. These latter in the rabbit are long nodes which take the place of the entire deep chain in man, including the retropharyngeal. From these nodes drainage passes onward by the cervical lymph ducts, the great veins, the right side of the heart and the pulmonary artery, to the lungs. The frontal sinuses appear to drain by the same route. We believe this to be the first complete demonstration of this path. Schaeffer, in his recent book on the nose, follows Most, and carries the drainage of the accessory sinuses only as far as the retropharyngeals, and this dubiously. André, working on the cadaver, concluded that drainage was to the retropharyngeal and cervical nodes, but did not completely demonstrate it. New has noted metastasis of malignant tumors from the antrum to the parotid submaxillary and cervical nodes.

In our first series we also inoculated a few rabbits in the antrum with pneumococci from a human antrum and produced inflammation of the antrum, phlegmon of the neck, an intense tracheitis and bronchitis, and pneumonia.

In the course of the first series we became interested in the question of pulmonary involvement by inhalation. We, therefore, carried out another series, completed last year and in part published, in part about to be. In this second series we found that if india ink or baterial suspensions were injected into the nasal fossae, or into the antrum in such amount that a good deal escaped into the nasal fossae, they were readily inhaled. In the latter case lesions or pigmentations of the antrum and lung were produced simultaneously.

Thus we have demonstrated the two routes which connect the accessory sinuses with the lungs and bronchi—the lymphatic or circulatory route, which can function even in the case of an antrum which does not discharge at all into the nose; and the inhalation or bronchial route, which is open to any substance reaching the nasal fossae from the accessory sinuses or elsewhere, provided it be converted into droplets or aspirated by sudden inspiration.

Here, then, is the situation: A condition, bronchiectasis, develops inexplicably in a certain number of cases, often with the history of acute bronchitis—a disease nearly everybody has at some time—or of bronchopneumonia, followed by chronic cough. Acute bronchitis and bronchopneumonia as well, though to a less degree, are usually phases of an infection which involves the whole upper respiratory mucous membrane, often including the sinuses.

That sinus infection and acute bronchitis may develop simultaneously is hardly to be questioned. Bronchiectasis does not occur in the majority of the cases of chronic bronchitis, and the tendency is to get well unless fostered and fed by a chronic sinus infection.

I have already demonstrated two routes in which this infection may take place, add to this lowered bodily resistance due to chronic infection and I believe you have the solution. The theory that sinus disease may develop secondary to the bronchial may be put forth, but this is extremely improbable since there is no ready route from the bronchi to the sinuses. The number of cases with cough, moist rales at the bases, particularly in children, who get well after early diagnosis and proper treatment of the sinuses, also disapproves it, as the case of R. L., age 10, will demonstrate when shown.

To those who are inclined to say that the large quantities of secretion coughed up from the bronchi might readily infect the sinuses I might only cite the similar instance in pulmonary tuberculosis without the same coincidence existing.

The coexistence of bronchiectasis and chronic sinus infection in a large number of cases surely must be explained on other grounds than coincidence.

I asked my friends doing chest work to endeavor to find me a case of nonobstructive bronchiectasis without sinue disease. The one case coming without demonstrable sinus disease had the following history which is self explanatory:

John O. Referred by Gilbert, Age 39. Came to Colorado Springs for pulmonary tuberculosis. History: Always well and never had cough until six years ago or at the age of 33. Seven years ago had difficulty with stomach which proved to be an ulcer. He was operated upon for this under ether anesthesia. Began to cough immediately after and has coughed ever since. Now raises quantities of foul smelling greenish material. You will see this case cannot be put in class five.

The slides I am about to show do not represent my whole series, but rather were picked to bring out points that should be emphasized.

1. Many of these cases are mistaken and treated for pulmonary tuberculosis, and the majority of them consult the internist and chest man first. If the patient's history of "no nose trouble" alone is accepted without a most thorough investigation of the sinuses, then the diagnosis will not be made nor the best interests of the patient served.

2. A careful search for sinus disease in the early stages of a persistent bronchitis, especially in children, will clear many cases, while it is very evident that treatment of the infected sinuses in well developed bronchiectasis will not effect a cure.

Every means has been carried out by competent chest men to rule out pulmonary tuberculosis and establish a diagnosis of bronchiectasis.

While this paper deals with the etiologic cause of bronchiectasis, it is because it is the final sequela, and the relationship of the two existing conditions can more easily be demonstrated by slides. But mention might be made of numbers of cases of chronic coughs and bronchitis where a roentgenogram would show nothing, and only a careful auscultation would reveal the true condition.

Careful attention to the histories of this series will show:

1. That the majority of them started with nose trouble and cough when children.

2. That the advanced cases have pansinusitis.

3. That the bacterial flora from the sinuses and the sputa is the same.

4. That those who have only slight sinus involvement, thereby lessening their absorption, do get results by treatment.

5. That a goodly number had no symptom or clinical evidence of sinus disease such as is usually manifested by discharge and headache, especially where the maxillaries were involved.

Because of the lack of appreciation of sinus-bronchus disease as a common clinical entity, it seems desirable to pile up emphasis on this point. For this reason I have recently compiled and reported a series of 14 cases, showing lantern slides of the radiographs of the sinuses and chest. Here I will give in full two cases selected because of their special interest and will summarize the rest.

Case 1.—Miss G. H., is not one of the bronchiectasis, but of pulmonary tuberculosis, and is chosen in order to demonstrate the lymphatic pathway from the upper air passages to the thorax. Radiograph showed calcification of the cervical glands and a continuous chain leading down into the mediastinum. The tonsils were most likely the portal of infection in this case. They were removed under local anesthesia, and a pathologic examination revealed extensive scars, suggesting healed and fibrosed tuberculosis.

Case 2.—Master R. L., aged 10, I report in detail, because I believe it shows clearly the process of development in these cases and what treatment will do if the diagnosis is made early. Family history negative. Past history: measles at three; tonsils and adenoids removed at four. First seen by the present writer at the age of six because of cervical adenitis. Stumps of tonsils and remnant of adenoid were removed at that time. Good recovery and disappearance of glands. Next seen in June, 1919, three years later, when he was nine years old. Mother brought him because he was having so much catarrhal dropping from nasopharynx. Was seen several times then and not seen again until six months later. This time he was brought in for frontal headaches of such severity that he could not remain in school. Double maxillary sinusitis was ssuspected and a radiographic plate was made. Report was as follows: "Frontals not well developed or clear; ethmoids not definitely clear; right and left maxillaries decidedly clouded—in fact, it would be impossible to tell from the plate whether maxillary cavities are present or not."

Exploratory puncture, under general anesthesia, of both maxillary sinuses was advised but this was not accomplished, and the boy was not seen until eight months later when he was referred to me in October, 1920, by Dr. H. C. G. with the following report: "A poorly nourished and anemic looking boy. Examination of the lungs shows rales after cough in both bases and some fine rales in the apex of the right lung after expiratory cough. Von Pirquet test—slightly positive. Urine has been examined on five different occasions and albumin, varying from slight trace to a double positive, was found each time. Hyaline and granular casts were found on various occasions. Examination of sputum negative." On October 25, 1920, under ether anesthesia, both maxillary sinuses were opened under the inferior turbinate and the nasoantral floor removed with the bone drill. No pus was found, but on exploring with the probe the mucous membrane appeared to be soft and thick. A piece was removed from the wall of each sinus for pathologic examination. The pathologic report was as follows: "Antrum curettings: Masses of very loose edematous and congested vascular connective tissue showing marked infiltration with leucocytes both monos and polys. Several hyperplastic lymph follicles present. Surface covered with antral epithelium showing marked papillary overgrowth. No free pus on surface." Another physical examination on November 15th showed the chest free from rales. There was no cough, and the boy has remained well ever since (April 1, 1921).

The following is a summary of the remaining cases of the series. One patient was sixteen years of age, one thirty-four and one forty-eight; the other nine ranged between twenty and twenty-eight years; the youngest patient was the one reported in full, who was ten.

Eight patients gave a history of headaches and nasal discharge from childhood, and the diagnosis of combined sinus and bronchial disease could readily have been made if the possibility had been duly borne in mind. Three had no symptoms of sinus disease and gave no history suggesting it. On the contrary, they were absolutely unconscious of it until the sinuses were radiographed and the pus washed out. One had very slight headache and nasal discharge, but had never associated it with her cough.

Six of the patients had actually gone to sanatoria and had been treated for tuberculosis.

Only one of the series had bronchial asthma, and this was associated with bronchiectasis. He had been thoroughly tested with proteins with negative results, and his asthma was quite certainly due to his nasal disease.

Seven cases were definitely helped by suitable treatment of the sinus condition, plus postural drainage.

In ten cases bacteriologic examinations were made and the same organisms found in the sputum and the discharge from the sinuses. In two cases of hyperplastic type pathologic examinations were made of the tissues removed and these showed chronic inflammatory changes.

# XXXVIII.

## THE MANAGEMENT OF RECENT FRACTURES OF THE NOSE.

By Lee Cohen, M. D.,

Baltimore.

It is not my intention to present a lengthy dissertation on a subject which to some may appear too trivial to engage the attention of this august body.  I wish simply to place before you a method of treatment which has yielded uniformly excellent results, both as to the external appearance of the nose and prevention of obstructive conditions within, which only too often follow fractures.  At the same time I feel also constrained to mention my deep conviction that the rhinologist should apply himself seriously in the matter of impressing upon the general medical profession the importance of early and prompt treatment of nasal fractures, lest the same chaotic state of mismanagement which has heretofore prevailed continue.

Only recently an instance was brought to my attention where the nose of a boy of fifteen was badly broken by a baseball. When seen by the family physician a few hours afterwards he was advised to wait a month before having the "bones set"; a month later, on returning, he was told that it would be best to wait one year before attempting to correct the *now* existing marked external and internal deformity.  This may be an extreme instance of the indifference of the general man to the need of seeking expert advice, in such cases, but other instances are constantly being brought to the notice of many of us wherein the patient is dismissed with a simple strip of adhesive over the nose, or told that with the disappearance of swelling all will be well.

However, since most cases are first seen by the general man when the extent of the injury is frequently masked by the enormity of the swelling, it is not surprising that one untrained in this work should fall into such error.  Besides, in a survey of the literature appearing in the past twenty-five years, one is amazed at the small space allotted to the discussion of this subject in most textbooks, and at the utter lack of unanimity in the methods of treatment. All do agree that the constituent parts of the nose should be set in their proper anatomical position—some say immediately, while others advise waiting four or five days for swelling to disappear.

To retain the nose in position the methods mentioned are so varied and often so ambiguous as to leave one beginning the study of the subject largely at sea. Transfixing the nose with pins just beneath the lower ends of the nasal bones, the use of internal metal splints, made fast to the teeth by complicated dental appliances, the placing of Simpson's sponge splints, or the perforated hard rubber splints of Ashe within the nose, and finally packing the nasal vestibule with gauze, may be mentioned as the types of internal support advocated. As to the use of an external support, many contend that none is necessary; that the nose once placed in proper position tends to remain there, supported only from within. This is certainly at variance with my own experience, and likewise with that of others who have given much thought to this matter. Plaster casts, hard rubber splints and other types of stiff plaster molds have been employed. None with which I am familiar, however, are so easily made and applied, or so effective, as the simple copper splints, held in place by adhesive. This type was first used by Dr. John O. Roe in his work on nasal deformities.

The advantages of this splint are manifold. The equal pressure exerted by it over the entire nose holds all fragments in absolute alignment, and prevents their outward displacement, thus diminishing callus formation along the lines of fracture to a minimum. Ridges, offsets and other irregularities in the contour of the nose, so prone to follow fractures, and due to such callus, are thereby prevented. This splint also hastens the disappearance of swelling, and gives to the nose a uniformly good shape not to be obtained by any other which I have tried. Held in place securely with adhesive, trauma and possible refracture during the process of healing are prevented, and lateral deviation of the nose from the middle line of the face so frequently observed after these injuries is obviated.

An experience of some years in corrective rhinoplasty convinces me that the majority of acquired external nasal deformities and a vast number of septal deflections are the end results of fractures faultily treated. The effects of these nasal obstructions in the production of serious local and systemic disturbances are too well known to dwell upon here.

What, then, should be done to impress upon the general medical men the seriousness of treating lightly injuries of this character? My feeling is that the rhinologist should go before the medical societies in his locality and there emphasize the importance of the same prompt expert treatment of fractured bones of the nose as that accorded fractures of other bones; that such cases should be directed to someone able to ascertain the extent of the injury inside the nose as well as outside, and who has been trained to afford the necessary relief. For correction immediately following the injury is a simple matter, as you know, compared with the extensive operative procedure required at a later period.

It has been said that fractures of the nose are infrequent in comparison with other bones of the body. P. Bruns stated some years ago that in over 40,000 patients treated in the clinics and hospitals of Berlin only 1.1 per cent had fracture of the nose. Gurlts estimated that only 1 per cent of all fractures applying for treatment were of the nasal bones. These estimates, it must be apparent to all, are ridiculously low in this country, where football, baseball, basketball and other sports are a regular part of the school life, and where automobile accidents and boxing also furnish a liberal quota.

No time need be spent before this society in general anatomical consideration, but it is well to bear in mind that the nasal bones are quite thin at the lower extremity; hence fracture is most prone to occur at their lower third, and it often requires only a slight blow from the side to cause a break. Also the extent of articulation between the perpendicular plate of the ethmoid and the nasal bones is variable. Zukerkandl found in a large number of skulls that the bony septum extended as far down as the middle of the nasal bones in 40 per cent, to the junction of the lower and middle thirds in 38 per cent, only to the junction of the upper and middle thirds in 10 per cent, and finally in 3 per cent the bony septum did not reach the nasal bones at all.  In isolated instances, therefore, extensive fractures of the nose may occur without involving the bony septum.  In such cases, the cartilaginous septum is always broken or displaced, and this makes retention of the nose in the middle line of the face at the time of correction a more difficult task.

Detection of fracture is on the whole easily accomplished. A careful comparison of the relationship of the middle line of the forehead and of the chin with the tip of the nose is often sufficient to convince one of the existence of fracture.  Palpation enables us to ascertain whether the break involves one or both nasal bones, and to detect any displacement or irregularity in the contour of the nasal arch.  Crepitus may in most instances be elicited.  X-ray may show the extent of the fracture, but is by no means essential in making a diagnosis.  Inspection of the interior of the nose discloses the extent of septal injury.

Treatment should, in my opinion, be instituted as soon after injury as possible, without awaiting the disappearance of swelling, no matter how great this may be.  Even in compound fractures, where suturing of a wound was found necessary, this principal has been followed with the utmost satisfaction. At times it has been deemed wise to give a preventive dose of tetanus serum.  The administration of ether has been found best in all cases for the actual operation.  After the patient is asleep the extent of the injury and amount of displacement can be better ascertained.  A postnasal tampon is introduced to prevent blood finding its way into the nasopharynx.

In young subjects, where organic matter in the bones preponderates, a tendency to lateral deviation of the nose after reduction often exists.  This has been especially true where a blow from the side results in a complete fracture of one nasal bone and only a partial fracture of the other—so-called *green-stick fracture*.  Satisfactory reduction in such cases cannot be accomplished until all resiliency of the partially fractured bone has been removed by making the fracture a complete one.  In other words, in all cases when the nose fails to remain in the proper position after being so placed, it must be so thoroughly mobilized by such further fracture that the flail nose can be molded to suit oneself.  For this purpose the Adams forceps generally serves, but at times the hammer must be called into requisition.

In other cases where the nasal bones can be placed in absolute alignment, there may still exist a tendency to lateral deviation of the entire nose from the middle line of the face, on account of septal displacement. Moreover, there may also exist a depression along the dorsum nasi from the same cause. Replacement of the septal fragments and elevation of the dorsum to the proper plane often requires considerable force. This can best be supplied also by the Adams forceps or one of its modifications. With one blade on each side of the septum, parallel with and just beneath the bridge, the entire nose is, as it were, lifted forcibly forward and upward, moderate pressure being simultaneously exerted on the septum Generally during this manipulation the slipping of the bones into place can be felt.

Mobilization once accomplished, the replacement of fragments, with a small rubber covered elevator held in the right hand and manipulated from the inside of the nose, while the left hand of the operator remains over the outside, presents little difficulty.

Reduction satisfactorily completed, the anterior portion of both nasal fossae and vestibules are packed with half-inch iodoform gauze tape. No other form of internal support can be applied with such precision, so that greater or lesser pressure may be placed where required; not only is the septum kept in place but the fragments of the nasal bones, no matter how badly comminuted, are prevented from falling inward out of alignment. The fingers of the left hand held over the nose during this process prevents forcing of the fragments outward by too tight a packing.

The external splint should now be applied. Since the publication of the monograph, "The Necessity for Prompt Management of Fractures of the Nose," in The Military Surgeon of November, 1918, a number of inquiries have been received as to the splint there mentioned, and its mode of application. One of our leading instrument makers recently wrote asking directions for making it, saying he had orders for same, but as each splint must be made for the individual case as it presents itself, such blanket instructions would be useless. I shall, therefore, endeavor by means of the motion picture to show the procedure of making and applying the splint.

We first proceed to make a paper pattern. A strip of paper is held across the nose, extending from the frontal notch to tip. A pentil dot on each side of the nose, just above the inner canthi, indicates the limit of the edges of the pattern above, while a dot on each side, in the nasolabial crease, indicates the limit of the edges below. This pattern is then folded down the center, so that the dots on one side of the nose appose the corresponding ones on the other side. Thus folded the pattern is cut in rounded form from one dot to the other. When completed this paper pattern furnishes a true model from which the splint is made. It is now laid on a sheet of 20 gauge copper and its outline marked, after which the metal is cut out with a small pair of tinner's shears, and covered on both sides with adhesive. It is then bent over a piece of iron pipe—in this instance the screen frame answered the purpose. Thus bent a perfect mold is formed to fit over the nose like a saddle. The splint is now lined with surgeon's lint, on the smooth side of which adhesive plaster has been stuck to give it body and prevent wrinkling.

The splint so made is held in place by a 1¼ inch strip of adhesive applied in the following manner: One inch from its end a notch, to be placed beneath the right ear, is cut in the upper edge, and the strip made fast to the right cheek, which is pulled forward, as the adhesive is drawn snugly over the top of splint. The left cheek is now held 'forward and the adhesive made fast thereto,.passing beneath the left ear where a similar notch is cut in the upper edge. The cheeks thus pulled forward furnish the elasticity necessary for even and continuous pressure of the splint. Bands of garter elastic and other materials first tried were discarded, for two reasons: firstly, they had a tendency to slip, and secondly, in passing around the nape of neck interference with the return circulation caused headaches. While applying adhesive strip, splint must be firmly held with left hand of operator to prevent displacement of nose. The eyes are completely covered with adhesive when first applied; subsequently the upper half of the strip, extending from one outer canthus to the other, is cut away to make space for vision. The strip is now too low down on the splint, and unless placed on a higher level so that pressure is brought to bear about the middle of the bony arch, depression of the nasal tip is likely to result. Likewise the tension of the adhesive on each side of strip must be equalized, lest lateral deviation of the nose follow. Palpation of strip, with one index finger on each side, will detect the slightest inequality.

Balancing tension and placing adhesive strip on a higher plane is accomplished by means of a small elevator made for this purpose, heated quite hot over a spirit lamp to prevent adhesive sticking to it. This hot elevator is passed from below upward, between splint and adhesive, and the strip raised clear of the splint. Thus held the plaster may be shifted to any desired position. A pencil dot in center of upper edge of splint, and one directly below it on upper edge of strip, aid much in judging the extent of change made in shifting the adhesive.

Last, an additional strip of adhesive half-inch wide is placed vertically from the lower end of splint over the middle of forehead to the hair line. This strip, reinforced with two cross strips on the forehead and two over the splint itself, prevents it from slipping downward.

Perforations in the splint, made by a small dental punch, add greatly to the comfort of the patient and lessens masceration of the skin during hot weather.

The external splint is worn over a period of four weeks, but changed every fourth day, at which time the skin beneath is cleansed with alcohol. Packing within, while changed every third day, is discontinued after the tenth day.

Photographs here shown are of a 16-year-old boy, struck on the nose with a baseball. He was discharged only a few days ago, having worn the splint one month.

1820 Eutaw Place.

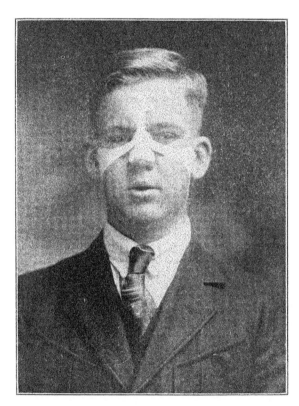

Fig. 1—Type of splint employed.

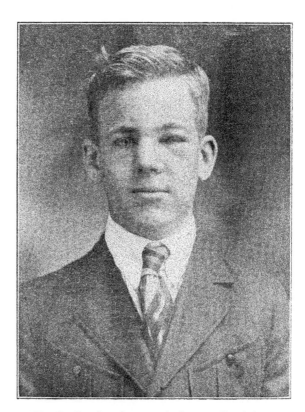

Fig. 2—Fractured nose, six hours after injury.

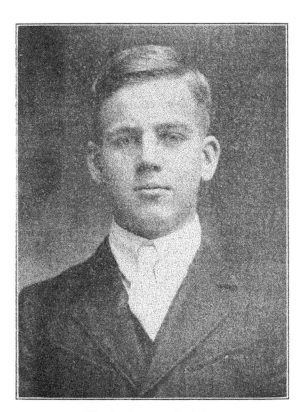

Fig. 3—Four weeks later.

## XXXIX.

## RESONATORS AS POSSIBLE AID IN TUNING FORK TESTS—A PRELIMINARY REPORT.

By Robert Sonnenschein, M. D.,

Chicago, Ill.

On November 19, 1912, I read before this society a paper entitled "Resonators, with Special Reference to the Schaefer Apparatus." It will, perhaps, best serve our purpose at this time to quote largely from that article a number of selections:

"To properly appreciate and intelligently apply a subject like otology, and particularly the functional testing of the ear, requires, it would seem, some knowledge of acoustics which embraces among other topics, the subject about to be discussed.

"In the consideration and application of resonance and resonators, we have a most interesting and important field bearing on the appreciation of many phenomena connected with hearing and with the voice, besides offering those who are concerned with the study of acoustics per se a splendid opportunity of solving many different questions. Resonators have been used in various ways, for instance: by Helmholtz and others, for the analysis of tones, particularly of the different vowels; by Wien for the determination of tone intensities; by Abraham and Schaefer for the purpose of solving the difficult problem of 'interference tones;" by Schaefer and later by Waetzmann to furnish proof of the existence of objective physical combination-tones in the sounds produced by vibration of membranes or diaphragms. It seems that a useful application of resonators would consist in testing therewith the various forks which we buy in order to be certain of their pitch should any doubt exist and no other accurate forks be at hand with which to compare. A few years ago Edelmann constructed and introduced a continuous series of resonators evidently intended to supplement the Bezold tuning forks. This will, perhaps, lead to the former becoming a part of the otologist's armamentarium.

"Resonators, be it said, are instruments capable of and used for selecting out special sounds for reinforcement. Resonance, or sympathetic vibration, which is the reinforcement or intensification of sound due to the union of direct and reflected waves, depends upon the principle that a number of slight impulses properly applied will finally create a considerable momentum, as seen in the well-known fact of giving impulse to a swing or a pendulum at the proper phase of the oscillation. When, therefore, a vibrating body is brought near the corresponding resonator the latter is caused to vibrate in its fundamental tone. To induce a rigid body like a tuning fork to respond to or resonate with another fork, or other sounding body, requires that both objects have exactly the same number of vibrations per second, or that the vibration number of one is a simple multiple of the other. When, however, a more elastic substance such as a column of water or air is used as a resonator, the two sounds need not be absolutely in unison, but should be nearly so. In most resonators a column of air is employed, as is also the case in the Schaefer apparatus.

"To produce a resonator for any one tone is a comparatively simple procedure. A lamp chimney, a tube of cardboard or a bottle may do. By placing in water a cylindrical glass or metal tube open at both ends, and having a length of approximately a meter, and a diameter of a few centimeters, it can be made to resonate for tones ranging from about 100 to 3,000 vibrations per second, depending upon the depth of the immersion. The disadvantage, however, of these water resonators lies in the fact that the ear of the person to be examined cannot easily be connected with the node of the air wave which is formed at the surface of the water column. For this purpose the spherical resonators of Helmholtz are very serviceable in that they have opposite the sound opening a small funnel-shaped open tip or prolongation which can easily be inserted into the ear.

"A resonator open at both ends reinforces better a higher tone that one open only at one end. In other words, resonators of this type are of higher pitch than those in which one end is closed. On the other hand, a resonator is of deeper pitch: (1) the larger the air containing area, and (2) the narrower the sound opening (Schalloch) happens to be.

"Schaefer advises using resonators in the analysis of sound without insertion into the ear because the instruments are caused to vibrate by very slight disturbances, such as faint noises or sounds. The fundamental tone of the respective resonator is thus produced, giving confusing results. But this very sensitiveness of resonators can be utilized in otology, for the introduction of the apparatus into the ear will serve as a last resort in the hearing of an otherwise inappreciable sound. Therefore, perhaps, the diagnosis of total deafness should not be made until a fairly loud sound intensified by the corresponding resonator fails of perception.

"Tones of medium pitch are the ones most intensely reinforced, the very low and the very high ones much less so. Schaefer, Koenig and Helmholtz maintain that there is no practical value in producing resonators with less than a hundred double vibrations, that is, about A (108 v. d.).

"Each Koenig or Helmholtz resonator gives a maximum reinforcement for one certain tone, but less for sounds just above or below this one. There are certain tones, therefore, lying between succeeding resonators which are not reinforced to their maximum.

"Schaefer claims that the ideal instrument is a 'continuous or universal resonator apparatus, adjustable for any desired tone between at least c (128 v. d.) and c3 (1024 v. d.), one producing maximum reinforcement of every tone, easily manipulated, compact and comparatively cheap.' These qualities are held to be embodied in his apparatus.

"These resonators are four in number, of different lengths but the same diameter, cylindrical in shape, and made of brass. One end is open, the other closed by a plate having a central aperture. Over the latter is a conical extension intended to be placed in the meatus auditorius or to be connected with a tubing for introduction into the ear. For occluding the small opening when the resonators are not to be inserted in the ear, rubber plugs are provided.

"Each resonator tube fits accurately into another cylinder but can be moved in and out. The inner tube is graduated in millimeters, so that the length of the resonators, depending on the amount that the inner tube is withdrawn, can at a glance be read. At the same time the tones for which the resonator acts at different lengths are indicated by letters giving the notes of the scale. As is customary in Germany, H is used to designate the b of our scales. The resonators are graduated to correspond to the tones of the temperate scale, based on the tone of $a^1$ (435 v. d.) at a temperature of 18° C. (about 64.4° F.). Experiments have shown, however, that at ordinary room-temperature varying somewhat from 18° C., no correction in reading is necessary. The range of these resonators is from about A (108 v. d.) to a little above $c^3$ (1024 v. d.).

"The graduation is also based on the assumption that the smaller opening is closed when the resonators are used. When applied in the ear the drum acts as obturator, but when used outside the ear the smaller aperture should be occluded with a rubber plug or the end of a finger. Otherwise inaccurate result swill be had, for a resonator open at both ends is of higher pitch than one in which only a single end is open, as was previously pointed out. Judging by a few experiments, this difference in pitch amounts in most cases to about one-half of a tone. It has been shown that the freely movable membrana tympani acts just as well in closing one end of the resonator as does the rubber plug. It will be interesting to see what effect the presence of a perforation in the drum membrane has as regards the pitch of the resonator used.

"There has been considerable dispute regarding the advantage of spherical over cylindrical resonators, Helmholtz supported by Watson and others claiming that the former give a purer tone and a more powerful resonance. Schaefer, on the other hand, disputes this statement, and claims that even granting it for the lowest and highest tones only, the difference is so slight as not to count from a practical standpoint.

"Resonators can therefore be used for various purposes: (1) In physical research in the analysis of tones, etc.; (2) in testing tuning forks to see if the actual tone is the one claimed to be present; (3) for determining the pitch of unmarked forks, or that of any other sounding body whose tone comes within the range of the resonators used: (4) and last, but not least, for testing the absolute duration of hearing. With the corresponding resonator inserted in the ear, a tuning fork, no longer heard alone, will still be appreciated; but when its sound ceases to be heard despite reinforcement the limit of hearing has been reached.  To determine actual deafness forks not at all heard alone can thus be used with resonators to establish the diagnosis."

The present paper covers examination of fifty unselected consecutive cases, and is only preliminary in character.  It is our intention to use the resonator for a considerable time in order to see what findings may be had in a large series and then to report more definite conclusions, if possible.

At this time I desire to express my thanks and deep appreciation to my Associate, Dr. S. J. Pearlman, for the great aid he has given in the examination of the patients.

The tests were made in this manner.  The $a^1$ fork (435 v. d.) was excited in a uniform manner by holding it at right angles to the body and allowing a small rubber pleximeter to fall of its own height and weight from a perpendicular position directly upon one of the prongs.  When the fork was no longer heard by air conduction the time was noted, the tip at the end of the tubing connected with the resonator attuned to the tone of $a^1$ was then inserted into the ear, the fork held near the resonator and the fact noted, either that the sound was not again appreciated by the patient, or if heard, for how long a period.

In order to facilitate the handling of the resonator we had a frame or cradle constructed in which it lies so that the tubing could be inserted into the ear without disturbing the resonator.

We have used the $a^1$ fork (435 v. d.) since its pitch lies in the speech area designated by Bezold, and if not heard by air, usually means that all hearing for speech is lost.

The use of the resonator is better than increasing excitation of the fork by again striking it when the patient no longer hears it, as we cannot then get uniform increase in intensity of vibration such as a resonator set at the same point always produces.  It is true that holding the resonator to the normal ear often gives a sound like that of a sea shell, due to the reinforcement by the resonator of any sound in the surrounding air which has the same pitch as that to which the resonator is attuned, or which is an overtone of that sound.  This is often confusing to the person under examination, as he cannot then very well distinguish between that adventitious sound

and the tone of the tuning fork of the same pitch, especially
when the intensity of vibration has already greatly diminished
after a certain length of time. This may to a large extent
account for the discrepancies in findings with the resonator,
especially in those cases with good hearing where the tuning
fork is heard for a long time via air, and then when no longer
perceived is held near the resonator now connected with the
ear. That the noise in the downtown district, where most
of us have offices, may have a bearing on this fact is, perhaps,
shown by the results obtained in those persons (Nos. 2, 3,
4, 5, 6, 7, 8, 9 10, 11, 12, 13) who were tested in a quiet room
in the residential section, and in everyone of whom there was
a distinct and often very marked increase of hearing of forks
by the resonator when no longer heard via air.

At the same time, this very fact of the resonator producing
a reinforcement of the sound in the surrounding atmosphere
corresponding to its fundamental tone may prove of assistance
in determining the pitch of a tinnitus aurium. By changing
the length of the resonator the patient may be able to tell when
the pitch approaches or coincides with his own head noises.
The pitch of the latter, as we know, varies often, depending
on whether a nerve degeneration or a middle ear lesion is
present, being high in the former and usually low in the latter.

The degree of the person's intelligence is also a factor as
indeed it is in all hearing tests, for they are, in the main,
subjective ones and we are dependent upon the patient's own
statements. It is therefore necessary to show him exactly what
is desired so that he may closely observe and give reliable
statements.

Where the resonator no longer caused the fork to be heard
after the patient stated it had stopped sounding by air (for
instance, 40 seconds), it was possible that the fork had actually
ceased vibrating and therefore its tone could, of course, no
longer be accentuated by the resonator. To check this the
fork was again excited in the usual manner and held near the
resonator connected with the ear, and the time noted during
which the fork was heard to see whether the actual duration
of hearing was now the same as before. It was rather surprising to note how long a good fork like the Edelman a[1]
vibrates beyond the time usually detected by the unaided ear.

The otologist may use any resonator he desires which is attuned to the fork to be employed, but we have used the Schaefer apparatus because it is accurate, compact and easily adjusted.

The greatest value of the resonators probably lies in the ability to test absolute duration of hearing for those forks especially whose pitch lies in the speech area. It is unfortunate that many cases of far advanced impairment of hearing do not appear in our series, but as previously pointed out, those reported were unselected. At a future time we hope to have results in a large number of defective ears. It will also be interesting to note in a larger series what effect perforations of the drum membrane may have in altering the pitch of the resonators.

So far as I am aware, resonators, while used very extensively in purely physical research, have not been employed in clinical work. While we cannot in this paper propound or prove any startling fundamental principles, we do feel that it is much worth while for all of us to utilize any means at our command to study phenomena of hearing in order that some benefits in the way of aids to diagnosis or treatment may be evolved. An appliance which at first sight does not offer much prospect of improving our technic may on closer investigation add at least a small contribution to the refinement of our methods of functional testing of the ears. I trust this thought will justify my inflicting this paper upon you this evening.

Following are the tables showing the findings in the fifty cases examined:

| Name Sex Age | Diagnosis | Weber | Schwabach | Rinne r. l. | Drum Membranes r. l. | Suppuration r. l. | n'fork via air r. l. | Resonator in seconds r. l. | Whispered voice r. l. |
|---|---|---|---|---|---|---|---|---|---|
| No. 1 A. V. M., 57 | Auditory nerve degeneration. | Not Lat. | Much shortened (25 secs) | + + | Both dull and retracted. | 0 0 | 15 sec 18 sec | 45 40 Inc. | Not heard. |
| No. 2 J. H. M., 22 | Recurrent otitis media. (Now dry.) | " | Slightly lengthened | + + | Dull Dull | 0 0 | 50 37 | 65 60 Inc. | 7 8 Meters |
| No. 3 H. T. M., 23 | Normal ears. | " | Normal | + + | Neg. Neg. | 0 0 | 50 40 | 65 60 Inc. | " |
| No. 4 A. R. M., 23 | " " | " | " | + + | " " | 0 0 | 47 45 | 75 65 Inc. | " |
| No. 5 E. Z. M., 23 | " " | " | " | + + | " " | 0 0 | 45 44 | 73 70 Inc. | " |
| No. 6 A. L. M., 23 | " " | " | " | + + | " " | 0 0 | 48 58 | 75 100 Inc. | " |
| No. 7 J. R. M., 25 | " " | " | " | + + | " " | 0 0 | 40 50 | 83 90 Inc. | " |
| No. 8 S. L. M., 28 | Cerumen left. Otherwise normal. | " | " | + + | " " | 0 0 | 55 45 | 92 82 Inc. | " |
| No. 9 L. L. M., 25 | Normal ears. | " | " | + + | " " | 0 0 | 50 35 | 76 70 Inc. | " |
| No. 10 S. F. M., 22 | " " | " | " | + + | " " | 0 0 | 35 45 | 62 68 Inc. | " |
| No. 11 J. S. M., 25 | " " | " | " | + + | " " | 0 0 | 55 54 | 83 105 Inc. | " |
| No. 12 I. R. M., 23 | Cerumen bilat. Drums normal. | " | " | + + | " " | 0 0 | 54 60 | 75 76 Inc. | " |
| No. 13 W. R. M., 25 | Some cerumen bilat. Drum normal. | " | " | + + | " " | 0 0 | 43 44 | 55 80 Inc. | " |
| No. 14 M. L. F., 26 | Otitis media acuta sinistra. | Lat. to left. | " | + + | " red | 0 + After paracentesis. | 35 0 | 50 10 Inc. | 6M. 0.3M. |
| No. 15 S. F. M., 26 | Large cerumen plugs. | Not lat. | " | + + | Both slightly retracted | 0 0 | 40 40 | 45 40 Inc. Some | 5M. 5M. |

| No. | Patient | Sex, Age | Diagnosis | Lateralization | Bone conduction | ± | Otoscopy | | | | | Readings | | |
|---|---|---|---|---|---|---|---|---|---|---|---|---|---|---|
| 16 | J. A. | F., 38 | Otitis media chronica sinistra. | Lat. to left. | Lengthened slightly | + | Neg. Moderate perforation | 0 | + | 30 | 30 | 40 30 Inc. | 7M. | 4M. |
| 17 | C. S. | F., 21 | Otitis media chronica dextra. | Lat. to right. | Slightly lengthened | − | Large perforation. Neg. | + | 30 | 60 | | 30 60 Same | | 1M. | 6M. |
| 18 | M. S. | M., 7 | Otitis media acuta dextra. | " | " | − | Small perf. Neg. | + | 20 | 50 | | 25 50 Inc. Same | | 0.5M. | 6M. |
| 19 | S. M. | M., 29 | Auditory nerve degeneration left. | " | Normal | + | Neg. Slight retraction at time of test | 0 | 40 | 24 | | 75 40 Inc. Inc. | | 7M. | 10Cm. |
| 20 | A. Z. | M., 42 | Lateral ot. media acuta. Auditory nerve degeneration. | Not lat. | Diminished | − | Neg. Dull | 0 | 15 | 15 | | 30 25 Inc. Inc. | | 20Cm. | 20Cm. |
| 21 | J. G. | F., 40 | Auditory nerve degeneration. | Lat. to right. | " | + | Neg. | 0 | 40 | 40 | | 40 40 Same | | 6M. | 6M. |
| 22 | H. H. | M., 9 | Tubal catarrh. Begining nerve degeneration. | Lat. to left. | Increased | + | Neg. Red. Bulging | 0 + After paru. | 38 | 38 | | 38 30 Same | | 6M. | 10Cm. |
| 23 | M.T.H. | M., 25 | Otitis media acuta dextra. | Lat. to left. | Normal | + | Both retracted | 0 | 35 | 22 | | 45 45 Inc. | | 4M. | 4M. |
| 24 | A. J. | M., 15 | Chr. tubal catarrh. | Lat. to right. | Diminished | + | Neg. Neg. | 0 | 55 | 25 | | 60 50 Inc. | | 7M. | 20Cm. |
| 25 | F. K. | F., 25 | Auditory nerve degeneration left. | Not lat. | Much Increased | − | Dull. Dull | 0 | 18 | 12 | | 19 12 Same | | 20Cm. | 0 |
| 26 | R.J.K. | M., 30 | Otosclerosis. | Not lat. | Normal | + | Dull " | 0 | 30 | 30 | | 30 20 Same | | 0.6M. | Ad.C. |
| 27 | M. K. | F., 30 | Chr. tubal catarrh with nerve degeneration left. | Lat. to right. | A little increased | + | Slight dullness | 0 | 25 | 25 | | 25 30 Same Inc. | | 10Cm. | 10Cm. |
| 28 | M. L. | M., 62 | A typical otosclerosis with nerve degeneration. | Lat. to left. | A little short | + | Dry perforation. Dull. After removing cerumen from both ears, resonator heard 8 to 10 seconds longer. | 0 0 | 20 | 20 | | 25 35 Inc. Inc. | | 20Cm. | 1M. |
| 29 | H. P. | M., 18 | Dry perforation left. Auditory nerve degeneration right. | Lat. to right. | Prolonged | + + | Some dullness. Hearing much improved by catheter. | 0 0 | 48 | 48 | | 48 43 Same | | 1M. | 5.0Cm. |
| 30 | R. R. | F., 26 | Severe tubal catarrh. Otosclerosis with nerve degeneration. | " | Normal | − | Normal | 0 | 15 | 15 | | 15 20 Same | | 20Cm. | 20Cm. |

| Name, Sex, Age | Diagnosis | Weber | Schwabach | Rinne (r. l.) | Drum Membranes (r. l.) | Suppuration (r. l.) | a'fork via air (r. l.) | Resonator in seconds (r. l.) | Whispered voice (r. l.) |
|---|---|---|---|---|---|---|---|---|---|
| No. 31, M. S. | Cerumen. | Not lat. | " | + + | After cerumen removed. | 0 0 | 33 55 | 33 55 / 42 55 | GM. GM. |
| No. 32, R. S., M., 30 | Nerve degeneration left. | Not lat. | Shortened | + + | Neg. Neg. | 0 0 | 30 30 | 38 30 / Inc. Same | 7M. 15Cm. |
| No. 33, S. T., F., 39 | Tubal catarrh left. | " | Normal | + + | Slight retraction | 0 0 | 35 32 | 35 32 / Same | GM. GM. |
| No. 34, E. S., M., 61 | Otitis media acuta dextra. | Lat. to right | Moderately shortened | − + | Injection / Neg. | After para. 0 | 10 45 | 22 45 / Inc. Same | Ad.C. 5M. |
| No. 35, L.R.C., F., 30 | Tubal catarrh with auditory nerve degeneration left. | Lat. to left | Shortened | + − | Neg. / Slight retraction | 0 0 | 30 20 | 45 38 / Inc. | GM. 1.5M. |
| No. 36, E. C., F., 14 | Cerumen especially right. | Lat. to right | Normal | + + | Neg. / Some dullness | 0 0 | 38 38 | 38 38 / Same | GM. 4M. |
| No. 37, G. C., F., 28 | Acute tubal catarrh left. | Lat. to left | " | + + | Neg. / Some dullness | 0 0 | 40 45 | 40 43 / Same | GM. GM. |
| No. 38, O. C., M., 37 | Some nerve degeneration and tubal catarrh left. | Not lat. | " | + − | Cloudy | 0 0 | 40 25 | 40 25 / Same | GM. 1M. |
| No. 39, W.J.D., M., 26 | Auditory nerve degeneration left. | Lat. to right | Shortened | + + | Neg. Neg. | 0 0 | 55 35 | 55 35 / Same | GM. 1M. |
| No. 40, M. F., M., 7 | Severe nerve degeneration left following parotiditis. | Lat. to left | | + − | Dull, slight retraction | 0 0 | 48 12 | 48 12 / Same | GM. 0.3M. |
| No. 41, J. F., M., 25 | Otitis media acuta sinistra. | Lat. to left | Lengthened | + + | Neg. / Red & perforated | 0 + | 50 18 | 50 30 / Same Inc. | GM. 1M. |
| No. 42, E. S., F., 50 | Normal ears. | Not lat. | Somewhat shortened | + + | Neg. | 0 0 | 40 35 | 40 45 / Same Inc. | GM. GM. |
| No. 43, E. B., F., 40 | " | " | " | + + | " | 0 0 | 40 35 | 50 40 / Inc. | GM. 6M. |
| No. 44, F. C., F., 20 | " | " | " | + + | " | 0 0 | 35 35 | 45 40 / Inc. | GM. GM. |

| No. / Initials / Age | Diagnosis | Lat. | Membrane | | Appearance | | | | | | | |
|---|---|---|---|---|---|---|---|---|---|---|---|---|
| No. 45 S. P. M., 29 | | " | Normal | + | Cloudy | Neg. | | 45 | 35 | 70 75 Inc. | GM. | GM. |
| No. 46 S. G. F., 52 | Otitis externa and otitis media non-suppurativa dextra. | Lat. to right | Normal | + | Neg. | Neg. | | 25 | 35 | 30 35 Inc. Same | 1M. | 6M. |
| No. 47 S. A. M., 28 | Cerumen right, otherwise normal. | Not lat. | | + | Dull | Neg. | | 40 | 45 | 45 50 Inc. | 7M. | 7M. |
| No. 48 S. G. M., 23 | Otalgia probably from teeth. Ears normal. | " | | + | | | | 35 | 35 | 48 40 Inc. | 7M. | 7M. |
| No. 49 M. G. F., 17 | Otitis media chronica bilat. Dry on left side. | " | Longthened | − | Large perforations | Dry | + | 30 | 25 | 45 40 Inc. | 1.5M. | 5M. |
| No. 50 R. X. F., 27 | Auditory nerve degeneration. | Lat. to left | Much shortened | + | tions Some dullness | | 0 | 35 | 28 | 35 28 Same | 0.5M. | 15Cm. |

### ANALYSIS.

Series I.—Cases in which the fork was heard by *both ears* with resonator when no longer appreciated by air conduction:

| | Diagnosis | Increases in Seconds | Pct. of Increase |
|---|---|---|---|
| No. 1. | Auditory nerve degeneration | r. 15 to 45=30 | 200 |
| | | l. 18 " 40=22 | 22 |
| No. 2. | Recurrent otitis media (now healed) | r. 50 " 65=15 | 30 |
| | | l. 37 " 60=23 | 62 |
| No. 3. | Normal ears | r. 50 " 65=15 | 30 |
| | | l. 40 " 60=20 | 50 |
| No. 4. | Normal ears | r. 47 " 75=28 | 59 |
| | | l. 45 " 65=20 | 44 |
| No. 5. | Normal ears | r. 45 " 73=28 | 62 |
| | | l. 44 " 70=26 | 59 |
| No. 6. | Normal ears (Musician) | r. 48 " 75=27 | 56 |
| | | l. 58 " 100=42 | 72 |
| No. 7. | Normal ears | r. 40 " 83=43 | 107 |
| | | l. 50 " 90=40 | 80 |
| No. 8. | Normal ears | r. 55 " 92=37 | 67 |
| | | l. 45 " 82=37 | 82 |
| No. 9. | Normal ears | r. 50 " 76=26 | 50 |
| | | l. 35 " 70=35 | 100 |
| No. 10. | Normal ears | r. 35 " 62=27 | 77 |
| | | l. 45 " 68=23 | 51 |
| No. 11. | Normal ears | r. 55 " 83=28 | 50 |
| | | l. 54 " 105=51 | 94 |
| No. 12. | Normal ears | r. 54 " 75=21 | 38 |
| | | l. 60 " 76=16 | 26 |
| No. 13. | Normal ears | r. 43 " 55=12 | 28 |
| | | l. 44 " 80=36 | 82 |
| No. 14. | Otitis media acuta sin. Right ear normal | r. 35 " 50=15 | 43 |
| | | l. 0 " 10=10 | .... |
| No. 16. | Otitis media chronica sin. | r. 30 " 40=10 | 33 |
| | | l. 25 " 30= 5 | 20 |
| No. 19. | Aud. nerve degen. left, with later otitis media acuta | r. 40 " 75=35 | 87 |
| | | l. 24 " 40=16 | 67 |
| No. 20. | Auditory nerve degeneration | r 15 " 30=15 | 100 |
| | | l. 15 " 25=10 | 67 |
| No. 23. | Chronic tubal catarrh | r. 35 " 45=10 | 28 |
| | | l. 22 " 45=23 | 105 |
| No. 24. | Auditory nerve degeneration left | r. 55 " 60= 5 | 9 |
| | | l. 25 " 50=25 | 100 |
| No. 28. | Dry perforation left drum membrane. Nerve degeneration right. Cerumen | r. 20 " 25= 5 | 25 |
| | | l. 30 " 35= 5 | 16 |

(After removal of cerumen, resonator heard 8 to 10 seconds longer.)

| | Diagnosis | Increases in Seconds | Pct. of Increase |
|---|---|---|---|
| No. 35. | Tubal catarrh with nerve degen. left............ | r. 30 to 45=15<br>l. 20 " 38=18 | 50<br>90 |
| No. 43. | Normal ears.................. | r. 40 " 50=10<br>l. 35 " 40= 5 | 25<br>15 |
| No. 44. | Normal ears.................. | r. 35 " 45=10<br>l. 35 " 40= 5 | 28<br>15 |
| No. 45. | Normal ears................:. | r. 45 " 70=25<br>l. 35 " 70=40 | 56<br>115 |
| No. 47. | Cerumen right. Otherwise normal ears.......... | r. 40 " 45= 5<br>l. 45 " 50= 5 | 12<br>11 |
| No. 84. | Ears normal. Otalgia probably from teeth.... | r. 35 " 48=13<br>l. 35 " 40= 5 | 37<br>15 |
| No. 49. | Otitis media chron. bilat.; dry on left side | r. 30 " 45=15<br>l. 25 " 40=60 | 50<br>60 |

TOTAL: 27 cases.

Average seconds **increase** for 54 ears 20.4 second.

Average percentage of increase......................................... 54.7

Series II.—Cases in which hearing in *one* ear *increased* with resonator and *not* increased in other ear:

| | | | | |
|---|---|---|---|---|
| No. 15. | Cerumen. Otherwise negative ...................... | r. 40 to 45 Inc. 5 sec.<br>l. 40 " 40 No change | | 12 |
| No. 18. | Otitis media acuta dextra ........................ | r. 20 " 25 Inc. 5 sec.<br>l. 50 " 50 Same | | 25 |
| No. 27. | A typical otosclerosis with nerve degenerat'n | r. 25 " 25 Same<br>l. 18 " 30 Inc. 12 sec. | | 67 |
| No. 32. | N e r v e degeneration left ........................ | r. 30 " 30 Inc. 8 sec.<br>l. 30 " 30 Same | | 27 |
| No. 34. | Otitis media acuta dextra ........................ | r. 10 " 22 Inc. 12 sec.<br>l. 45 " 45 Same | | 120 |
| No. 41. | Otitis media acuta sinistra ...................... | r. 50 " 50 Same<br>l. 18 " 30 Inc. 12 sec. | | 67 |
| No. 42. | Normal ears.................. | r. 40 " 40<br>l. 35 " 45 Inc. 10 sec. | | 29 |
| No. 46. | Otitis externa and otitis media non-suppurativa dextra............. | r. 25 " 30 Inc. 5 sec.<br>l. 35 " 35 Same | | 20 |

TOTAL: 8 cases showing increase with resonator.

Average increase in 8 ears..................................................... 8.5 second
Average percentage of increase......................................... 45.9

### GRAND TOTAL AVERAGES:

SERIES I, 54 ears and
SERIES II, 8 ears

Increase ........................................................................... 18 7
Percentage of increase..................................................... 53.5

Series III.—Cases in which hearing is not increased in ear with resonator after being no longer appreciated by air:

No. 17. Otitis media chronica dextra.............................. r. 30　　l. 60
No. 21. Tubal catarrh with beginning nerve degen-
　　　　eration (?) ........................................................... r. 40　　l. 40
No. 22. Otitis media acuta sinistra.............................. r. 38　　l. 30
No. 25. Otosclerosis ..................................................... r. 18=　l. 12
No. 26. Chr. tubal catarrh with nerve degen. left........ r. 30　　l. 20
No. 29. Severe tubal catarrh....................................... r. 48　　l. 43
No. 30. Otosclerosis with nerve degeneration............ r. 15　　l. 20
No. 31. Cerumen ......................................................... r. 33　　l. 55
N. B. After cerumen removed resonator heard............. r. 42　　l. 55
No. 33. Acute tubal catarrh left................................... r. 35　　l. 32
No. 36. Cerumen especially right................................ r. 38　　l. 38
No. 37. Acute tubal catarrh left................................... r. 40　　l. 45
No. 38. Some nerve degen. and tubal catarrh left...... r. 40　　l. 25
No. 39. Auditory nerve degeneration left.................... r. 55　　l. 35
No. 40. Severe nerve degeneration left following
　　　　parotiditis ......................................................... r. 48　　l. 12
No. 50. Auditory nerve degeneration.......................... r. 35　　l. 28

TOTAL: 15 cases.　　=

### RESU  E OF ANALYSIS.

With reference to their response to the resonator, the cases studied fall into two main groups.

1. Thirty-five cases in which one or both ears show increased hearing of the $a^1$ fork on using the resonator.

2. Fifteen cases in which the resonator failed to increase the hearing at all.

Group I. Hearing of the fork was increased by the resonator in 18 cases (Nos. 3, 4, 5, 6, 7, 8, 9, 10, 11, 12, 13, 43, 44, 45, 47, 48, 15 and 42), representing 34 normal ears (in cases 15 and 42 only one ear was influenced by the resonator), the average increase being 23 seconds, and the average percentage of increase being 52.

There were seven cases showing auditory nerve degeneration; of these, both ears involved in 2 cases (Nos. 1 and 20), only one ear in 5 cases (19, 24, 27, 28, 35), representing altogether 9 ears thus affected, and the latter showed an average increase of 17 seconds and an average percentage of increase of 82.

There were 5 cases of otitis media (Nos. 14, 18, 34, 41, 46), acuta unilateralis, i. e., 5 ears showing an average increase of 8.4 seconds, and a percentage of increase of 66.

(N. B.—In case 14 the percentage value is arbitrarily set at 100 for convenience.) Two cases of otitis media chronica (Nos. 16 and 49), representing 3 ears, wtih an average increase of 11.6 seconds and an average percentage of increase of 43.3. Two cases of chronic tubal catarrh (Nos. 23 and 35), representing 3 ears with an average increase of 16 seconds and average percentage of increase of 61. There was one ear (No. 28) with dry perforation showing an increase in hearing of 5 seconds or a percentage of 16. There was also one case of healed bilateral recurrent otitis media acuta (No. 2) which showed an average in both ears of 19 seconds increase and a percentage of 46.

Group 2. Among the 15 cases in which hearing was not increased by the resonator were otosclerosis (Nos. 25 and 30), otitis media acuta (No. 22), otitis media chronica (No. 17), acute tubal catarrh (Nos. 33 and 37), chronic tubal catarrh (Nos. 21, 26 and 29), auditory nerve degeneration (Nos. 38, 39, 40 and 50), and cerumen (Nos. 31 and 36). In case (31) after removal of the cerumen the resonator caused an increase in hearing of 10 seconds.

From this resumé it will be seen that in all of the normal cases the hearing was considerably increased by means of the resonator, namely, 23 seconds or a percentage of increase of 52. It seems strange, however, that some cases of auditory nerve degeneration show improvement with the resonator and others do not; this fact is also noted with reference to acute and chronic otitis media, as well as chronic tubal catarrh. Is it possible that the degree of involvement determines the phenomena or is it some other factor? Only the study of many cases may throw light upon this question, for we find among the nerve cases some with very marked degeneration, others with only moderate involvement, and yet the reaction to the resonator is about the same.

The cases of otosclerosis showed no improvement with the resonator. One instance of cerumen (No. 31), in which the hearing was influenced by the resonator, showed considerable increase after the cerumen was removed. In two other cases (Nos. 15 and 28), in which the resonator improved the hearing despite the cerumen, the improvement was still greater after cleaning the external auditory canals.

### CONCLUSIONS.

1. The hearing by air conduction of the $a^1$ fork (435 v. d.) was considerably increased by means of the properly attuned resonator, at least in all the normal ears examined.

2. Cases of auditory nerve degeneration, or of certain middle ear affections showed in some instances an increase in hearing, and in some no change, with the resonator.

3. It is easy with the resonator to test the actual duration of vibration of various forks.

4. In determining the presence of complete deafness for certain tones resonators will be of great aid. When a fork, especially one whose pitch lies in the "speech area," is not heard at all when reinforced by the resonator, the hearing for that tone can be said to be entirely absent.

5. It may be possible to determine the pitch of a tinnitus aurium from the patient's own observations when the resonator is attuned to various sounds in the surrounding air.

6. While tests with the resonator indicate that its use may have some significance, to really decide its actual clinical value, if any, in otology such as an aid to diagnosis, etc., will require extensive further investigation.

### BIBLIOGRAPHY.

1. Helmholtz: Lehre der Tonempfindungen.
2. Wien: Annal d. Phys., Vol. 56, 1896.
3. K. L. Schaefer: Beiträ zur. Anat. Phys. d. Ohres, etc., Bd. 3.
4. Millikan and Gale: Text-book of Physics.
5. Waetzmann: Resonanz Theorie d. Hörens.
6. Zellner: Vorträge über Akustik.
7. Watson: Text-book of Physics.
8. Sonnenschein: The Laryngoscope, May, 1913.

29 EAST MADISON STREET.

# XL

# NONSUPPURATIVE NEUROLABYRINTHITIS, WITH SPECIAL REFERENCE TO FOCAL INFECTION AND SYPHILIS AS CAUSATIVE FACTORS.*

By J. L. Maybaum, M. D.,

New York.

The tremendous advance, during the past decade, in our knowledge of functional examination of the labyrinth, has been of inestimable value in the diagnosis of obscure pathologic conditions arising from this important organ. At the start our attention was largely focused upon suppurative labyrinthine diseases and their complications. More recently, however, increasing thought and attention have been directed to the study and investigation of the nonsuppurative types of disease, conditions for which the term nonsuppurative neurolabyrinthitis is more applicable. By means of a thorough functional examination, a study of a series of those cases which present the most common problem—that is, cases of chronic middle ear catarrh, will almost invariably elicit findings diagnostic of otitis interna or neurolabyrinthitis, in not a small proportion of the total. A diagnosis of neurolabyrinthitis having been established, the problem with which we are next confronted, before appropriate therapeutic measures can be instituted and a reasonable prognosis given, is to determine the etiologic factor or factors which are the basis for the diseased condition.

In this article I shall confine myself to the cases of neurolabyrinthitis due to syphilis and those cases the origin of which is obscure and often difficult to determine—that is, those for which, in all probability, some form of focal infection can be assigned. In order to obtain an insight as to the extent of the possible causative factors of nonsuppurative neurolabyrinthitis, I shall give the comprehensive classification of G. Alexander.

---

*Candidate's Thesis to the American Laryngological, Rhinological and Otological Society, 1921.

Consideration of syphilitic neurolabyrinthitis is purposely omitted by Alexander in his splendid paper, and no reference whatever is made by him directly to focal infection as a factor.

According to Alexander, nonsuppurative labyrinthitis embraces the following:

A. Congenital labyrinthine anomalies and diseased conditions arising during embryonal development.

B. Postembryonal labyrinthine disease.

      Group A includes:

      1. Congenital labyrinthine deafness.

      2. Congenital labyrinthine deafness involving the static labyrinth (rare).

      3. Progressive labyrinthine deafness occurring in juveniles.

      4. Congenital deafmutism.

      5. Congenital labyrinthine diseases occurring in cretins.

      Group B includes:

I. Primary cases (those affecting inner ear directly, either from external conditions or general diseases).

II. Secondary cases includes those which follow middle ear affections.

I. Primary cases:

      1. Traumatic diseases of inner ear (acute).

      2. Traumatic diseases of inner ear (chronic), occupational.

      3. Metabolic and constitutional diseases causing inner ear disease, such as gout, diabetes, rachitis, endemic cretinism.

      4. Diseases of the blood or blood forming organs— anemia, chlorosis, pernicious anemia, hemorrhagic diatheses.

      5. Diseases of the arterial system.

      6. Nephritis.

      7. Toxic conditions: quinin, salicylates, arsenic, alcohol, nicotin, radium.

      8. The infections (nonsuppurative) diseases of the inner ear—scarlet, measles, diphtheria, cerebrospinal

meningitis, pertussis, mumps, typhoid, erysipelas, rheumatism.

·9· Chronic infectious diseases: syphilis and tuberculosis.

10. Disease of the brain and spinal cord: acoustic tumor, dural tumors, brain tumors, acute and chronic hydrocephalus, tabes, multiple sclerosis.

II.   Secondary: Nonsuppurative inner ear disease following
      1. Chronic middle ear suppuration.
      2. Chronic adhesive process in middle ear.
      3. Otosclerosis.

This classification, while thorough and comprehensive, may in a measure be considered rather didactic, in parts at least, because of the extreme rarity and problematical nature of some of the conditions referred to as causes for the disease in question.

Considered from a practical standpoint, in a larger majority of instances the disease is due to syphilis in the secondary or tertiary stages or as early evidence of a parasyphilitic condition. Hereditary cases are not common. In taking a history of the cause of noninflammatory labyrinthine disease some damaging influence can be discovered, often dating back a considerable time.

The first manifestations may be preceded by a history of continued abuse of alcohol or tobacco, ptomaine poisoning, long and persistent use of quinin and salicylates, or there may be a history of occupation exposing the patient to loud noises. A general infectious disease, as syphilis, influenza or typhoid, may be the etiologic factor. I. Friesner has recently seen a series of atypical cases of lethargic encephalitis in which the acoustic and static functions were decidedly impaired. In a number of these cases the vestibular function was more markedly involved. He has, as yet, not published these cases. Infectious diseases of childhood are often mentioned, and of these mumps is the most is the most common. Secondary degenerative changes in the labyrinth not uucommonly occur durin gthe course of chronic middle ear suppuration, chronic adhesive process in the middle ear and otosclerosis.

According to observations of Shambaugh and others, a group of cases of labyrinthine disease can be recognized in patients who are free from middle ear disease and no history of general disease to account for the labyrinth involvement.

According to I. H. Jones, the toxemia affecting the inner ear may be grouped into two classes:

A. Evanescent toxemias, which had produced no degeneration in the inner ear and its intracranial pathways.

B. Toxemias which produced definite impairment in the ear and its pathways. These toxemias result from such powerful toxins as those of mumps or syphilis, and milder toxins, such as those from the gastrointestinal tract or from focal infection.

These toxemias may result either in slow degenerative changes within the labyrinth or eighth nerve, producing attacks of vertigo from time to time, with gradual impairment of hearing. In some of these cases symptoms are limited to disturbances in the cochlea or to vestibular apparatus alone, while in many cases there is complete interference with the labyrinthine function.

F. P. Emerson similarly regards these cases of nerve deafness of nonspecific origin as due to toxemia or low grade infection from a definite focus; and that the primary focus in such cases is usually constant for the individual, as indicated by the location of exacerbations. Billings, Hunter and many other investigators have shown bacteriologically that focal processes in the teeth, tonsils or sinuses are responsible for a low grade of infection of adjacent tissues, and that during acute exacerbations this might extend by continuity or directly by way of the blood stream or lymphatics to neighboring or remote organs. In many cases, where the tonsils are the active cause of deafness, free pus can be demonstrated on one or both sides, especially in cases showing toxemia. This is really an enclosed abscess of streptococcic origin and subject to repeated acute exacerabation. The toxemia is marked and probably the cause of chronic degenerative change in the auditory nerve and its ending in the organ of Corti.

Méniéré was first to associate attacks of vertigo, when combined with deafness and tinnitus, with diseases of the inner ear. He believed that the disturbance was the result of hemorrhage into the labyrinth. The assumption was that where distinct periodic attacks occurred, repeated hemorrhages into the labyrinth was the cause of the condition. It is now known that such an occurrence is rather uncommon, most of the cases of genuine Méniéré's disease reported being associated with leukemia. A single hemorrhage into the labyrinth is responsible for the labyrinthine symptoms occurring during this comparatively rare disease.

Recent investigations have shown that chronic arthritis and neuritis, chronic cardiovascular degeneration and chronic nephritis are frequently the result of chronic latent foci of infection. According to Shambaugh, the course of these diseases gives evidence of a chronic progressive character, punctuated, as a rule, from time to time, by acute exacerbations, which are accounted for by a fresh shower of bacteria discharged from time to time into the circulation from the infected focus.

To account for the phenomena observed in many of these cases of internal ear disease as a result of focal infection, we have only to assume that the ending of the eighth nerve may be the structure peculiarly susceptible to bacteria liberated from the infected focus. With each acute exacerbation of inflammatory reaction in the focus, a sudden depression of function results either in the cochlea or vestibular nerve ending, separately or, if both are simultaneously affected, there results a complete picture of Méniéré's symptom complex—that is, deafness and tinnitus with vertigo.

As a rule only partial suppression of function results from a single attack, so that deafness as well as tinnitus are most marked immediately following that attack. The vertigo usually disappears rather promptly after a few days or weeks. In these cases of partial suppression of function, there will very likely be subsequent attacks, provided the focus of infection persists. In some cases the attacks of Méniéré's symptom complex persists at irregular intervals over several years, associated with an increasing loss of function, the attacks ceasing only after the function of the labyrinth has been entirely destroyed. Occasionally a single attack or a few attacks may be followed by one severe enough to produce total permanent suppression of function in the affected labyrinth.

The vertigo in such cases will be very severe because of the complete unilateral suppression of labyrinthine function, but it will gradually disappear as the normal labyrinth adapts itself to the changed condition and as soon as other special organs are called into play. No further attacks occur unless the other ear should later become involved. Shambaugh very correctly states the problem in the following manner: "With the conception that the internal ear may be the target for systemic infection of focal origin, we have at once a plausible explanation not alone for the chronic progressive character of the nerve degeneration going on in the labyrinth, but also for the apoplectiform attacks with which these degenerative changes are prone to be punctuated."

That labyrinth cases of obscure origin may be caused by focal infection cannot be denied. It is, therefore, necessary in examining such cases to make a careful search for foci of infection just as we are in the habit of doing in cases of rheumatism and allied conditions.

In recent years an extensive literature has sprung up upon the subject of auditory neuritis of syphilitic origin. Interest in the subject has been especially intensified by the assertion of not a few prominent aurists, here and abroad, that the advent of salvarsan was responsible for the large number of cases reported. The reports of marked increase in frequency of the cases which is claimed to have resulted from the use of salvarsan has undoubtedly been exaggerated, as demonstrated by a study of the literature of cases of acoustic nerve paralysis before the use of salvarsan. O. Mayer reported 55 cases of auditory neuritis due to syphilis, 30 occurring within the first year in the secondary stage and 10 cases within three weeks of the primary lesion.

Wintermute reported observations of Benario, who had collected a series of 210 cases of general neuritis following the use of salvarsan and 121 following the use of mercury. Of the 210 cases, 79 were of the acoustic nerve, and of the 121 the acoustic was involved 46 times. From this observation he concluded that the frequency of auditory neuritis was no greater from the use of salvarsan than from mercury. In 17 cases other cranial nerves were affected besides the eighth.

Gerber distinguished the effect of salvarsan upon the eighth nerve which occurs within a few hours or days after infection from that due to true neurorecurrences, which ordinarily do not appear before two or three months after the injection of salvarsan, the former being regarded similar to the Herxhimer skin reaction. These early changes following salvarsan injection are due to pressure upon the eighth nerve from its swollen sheath, such swelling being caused by the sudden liberation of syphilitic toxins. The present attitude of otologists is that most of the suspected cases of arsenic toxemia are really neurorecurrences of syphilis due to the administration of a dose of salvarsan insufficient to completely destroy the spirochete.

Cases have been frequently reported of neurorecidives following the use of salvarsan which disappeared completely upon repeated injection of the remedy. Mackenzie very properly states the importance to the otologist of this subject in that "the otologist in recognizing the clinical picture of syphilis of the inner ear and eighth nerve bears the same relation to the internist as does the ophthalmologist who recognizes the characteristic retinal changes in nephritis."

The onset of a sudden or rapidly progressive bilateral deafness in a syphilitic patient is not uncommon. The importance of not regarding and treating the condition as an isolated affection of the auditory apparatus becomes apparent, when we realize that the aural disturbance is in reality an early manifestation of an extremely serious condition, syphilitic involvement of the central nervous system. According to Fraser, one-third of the cases of nerve deafness of unexplained origin have a plus Wassermann. When the disease has become latent, the reaction may be negative in about 50 per cent of cases, so that a negative Wassermann cannot be taken as complete proof of the absence of syphilis.

Many cases of deafmutism are in reality due to intrauterine syphilis or the syphilitic changes in the ear occurring before the child has learned to talk. In the absence of any other assignable cause, a primary bilateral labyrinthine or nerve deafness should be regarded with suspicion as due to syphilis and investigated accordingly. In the case of primary unilateral labyrinthine or nerve deafness the contrary holds true, syphilis being rather the exceptional cause.

Because of the insidious character of the infection and the usually somewhat casual nature of the aural examination, the condition is not infrequently overlooked, so the frequency with which auditory disturbance complicates constitutional syphilis cannot be estimated accurtely. In Politzer's book the vague statement is made that from 7 to 48 per cent of cases of syphilis show aural lesions; the latter figure is undoubtedly high.   V. Dabney regards 5 per cent as sufficiently near the proper proportion to serve as a guide for study and investigation.

The pathologic data relating to this subject are meager. Considerable discussion has arisen as to the exact location of the lesion in auditory apparatus.   The earlier writers were of the opinion that the lesion is in the labyrinth.   Gradenigo was the first to differ in this view, his contention being that the lesion was oftener a neuritis of the auditory nerve rather than an affection of the labyrinth.   At the present time the concensus of opinion inclines to the view that in the majority of cases of deafness from syphilis the nerve is affected before the labyrinth; that not infrequently the labyrinth does become involved but to a lesser degree.   Exceptionally the labyrinth may become involved, while the nerve escapes; such findings are extremely rare.

The pathologic diagnosis has been questioned in such instances because of carelessness on the part of the investigator in failure to report nerve findings and in depending entirely on microscopic appearances.   Microscopically the auditory nerve shows degenerative changes of neuritis with atrophy of its end organ; in some instances there is a concomitant involvement of othe other cranial nerves, particularly the second, fifth and seventh.   M. Nonne was first to draw attention to this coincidence.   The all-important statement of Ellis and Swift, convincingly indicated that deafness occurring in the course jof syphilis was rarely due to an isolated infection of the eighth nerve or labyrinth, but is generally a manifestation of an involvement of the cerebrospinal system.   This view further enlarged our conception of the extent of the disease process. In their opinion the eighth nerve involvement is associated 'with a basal meningitis, a fact which they emphasized by means of their reference to lumbar puncture findings.   They refer to nine cases reported by Knick and Zolozieki, seven of which had a positive Wassermann of spinal fluid, one was negative and in one case no report was given.   Cytologic and chemical findings of the spinal fluid characteristic of meningeal irritation were present.

The prognosis of syphilitic deafness, formerly regarded bad, has been greatly improved by the intraspinal injection of salvarsanized serum suggested by Ellis and Swift. Many early cases of marked impairment of hearing due to syphilis have been decidedly improved by this treatment.

Of all the cranial nerves, none is so vulnerable to the syphilitic infection as the eighth nerve. For this reason it frequently happens that the eighth nerve is first to feel its influence and the otologist is thereby afforded an opportunity to recognize the general character of the disease from the start. In a majority of cases the cochlear branch is affected to a far greater degree than the vestibular. The cochlear and vestibular branches may be simultaneously affected, but as a rule the cochlear branch is first to be involved. While recovery from vestibular symptoms is complete under appropriate treatment, the symptoms due to cochlear involvement, tinnitus and impairment of hearing, are likely to be more or less permanent; a few cases of neuritis of the vestibular nerve alone have been reported. Some patients do not complain of ear symptoms, though it is not difficult to demonstrate the associated aural involvement. A larger number present predominant ear disturbances and in less frequent instances examination of the ear leads to the diagnosis of cerebrospinal disease. It must be remembered that though the cochlear nerve is considered most frequently attacked, a complete examination of these cases shows interference with both cochlear and vestibular functions.

In the majority of cases the first symptom to attract the attention of the patient in whom the cochlear branch is involved is an abrupt onset of tinnitus—usually bilateral—which soon becomes constant, diminising only as the pathologic changes in the nerve progresses or as the patient responds to thorough treatment. Following this, sudden impairment of hearing, usually very profound in degree, is noticed. No assistance is obtained from the drum picture as it is not affected in any characteristic way, whereas a coincident suppuration or a pre-existing chronic middle ear catarrh may actually obscure the etiology. That mixed conditions, syphilitic involvement of the inner ear and eighth nerve, combined with chronic catarrhal or suppurative otitis media do exist is accepted by otologists everywhere.

Where reliance is placed mainly upon the history and otoscopic picture pointing to chronic middle ear catarrh, rather than upon functional test findings, the otologist is apt to overlook the inner ear and eighth nerve condition and satisfy himself with a diagnosis merely of the middle ear lesion. In most cases little can be expected of a patient's history. In those cases where the hearing and equilibrium tests show involvement of the inner ear or eighth nerve the Wassermann test should be made. This also obtains in all those cases of middle ear affection where the hearing is found to be reduced below that allowable for uncomplicated middle ear disease and where the suspicion of complications in the inner ear and nerve has been confirmed by tuning fork and vestibular tests. Where the blood Wassermann is negative, in strongly suspicious cases, Wassermann test upon spinal fluid should be made.

If, in addition to cochlear involvement, the vestibular branch is affected, the symptoms to which it gives rise are far more distressing to the patient. Attacks of vertigo, disturbance of equilibrium and sometimes vomiting result. The vertigo is characteristic of the labyrinthine variety, causing subjective sensations of objects revolving about the patient. These attacks, lasting two or three days, are not infrequently varied by intermissions, during which the patient is entirely free from symptoms. Neuritis of the seventh nerve as a concomitant involvement, may be present, manifesting itself as a facial paresis, complete paralysis seldom occurring. At times the facial nerves involvement preceded that of the eighth nerve, in contradiction to inflammatory affections of the labyrinth, in which the paralysis follows or is concomitant with labyrinth symptoms. The extrinsic eye muscles are next in frequency involved. The fifth nerve, seldom affected, produces characteristic parasthesias and anesthesias in the areas of its distribution.

In tabes, Haberman found almost complete degeneration of the cochlear and partial degeneration of the vestibular nerve. The nerves were replaced with connective tissue and here and there were found distinct signs of neuritis still present. These changes indicate secondary atrophy following a primary neuritis.

The characteristic and diagnostic findings in cases of inner ear or nerve deafness are, as regards the cochlear apparatus, as follows:

Conversation may be heard fairly well, while the watch, acumeter, and especially the Galton whistle, will elicit little if any response. Weber is referred to the better ear. In a unilateral case of pure internal ear disease we observed, in the milder grades, a Rinné positive, but as the deafness increases the character gradually changes until it becomes plusminus eventually, with absolute deafness, the Rinné becomes negative (infinitive). The reason for the negative Rinné is that the bone conduction is transferred from the sound ear. Usually both ears are affected in syphilis, so that the positive character of the Rinné is accentuated. In testing the complete range of hearing with tuning forks, islands of hearing may be demonstrated. There is a decided shortening of bone conduction. These findings point to a lesion located in the inner ear or its nerve.

In the marked shortening of bone conduction we have one of the most reliable and striking evidences of luetic infection, as it is perhaps a most striking sign, occurring in 95 per cent of cases. A deafness without apparent middle ear trouble showing a positive Rinné should at once arrest the attention of the aurist. There is a marked lowering of the upper tone limits so that high pitched tones are badly heard, low pitched tones are better heard than the high pitched. O. Beck of Vienna is of the opinion that the prolonged bone conduction present in middle ear disease of nonsyphilitic is absent in syphilitic cases. In his opinion, shortening of bone conduction is cases of syphilitic auditory neuritis is present in a large number of cases even in the primary stage before the appearance of general symptoms.

In the opinion of Berens, Friesner, Mackenzie, Jones, Dabney and others the vestibular findings may be of even greater importance in the diagnosis of syphilitic neurolabyrinthitis than the auditory tests. Especially characteristic of these findings are the apparent inconsistency and irregularity of the reactions and the confused and variable findings from day to day. Among the vestibular findings especially suggestive of syphilis are a progressive reduction of vestibular irritability, or a reduction remaining constant in presence of other evidence of syphilis.

I. H. Jones regards the recognition of progressive impairment of vestibular function from day to day, as demonstrated by repeated tests, evidence of an active toxemia. This strongly suggests syphilis, especially in the presence of a suspicious initial lesion which cannot be accounted for definitely. In such affections as mumps, scarlet fever, diphtheria, gastrointestinal toxemias, etc., where the inner ear or eighth nerve had been previously involved, the resulting impairment is constant. Graham and others regard the absence of turning reaction with caloric reaction present or vice versa, quite characteristic. The same may be said of irregularities in reaction between the vertical and horizontal canals and the presence of vertigo without nystagmus, or exaggerated after-turning or caloric nystagmus without vertigo.

The presence of a psontaneous rhythmic nystagmus when looking straight ahead is more than presumptive evidence of a lesion in the static labyrinth or vestibular nerve. Characteristic of inner ear or eighth nerve lesion involving the vestibular branch, there occurs a rhythmic nystagmus to the side opposite the lesion if one side alone is affected, or to the side of the lesser loss if both sides are involved. Alexander and Barany have observed a characteristic fistula symptom at times in cases of auditory neuritis of syphilitic origin, particularly in the hereditary form. They ascribe this to an extreme static irritability in the earlier stages.

It has long been recognized that when the inner ear is destroyed from any cause, the eighth nerve continues to react to electrical stimulation; if the eighth nerve is destroyed no amount of current strength, even up to 20 ma., will produce nystagmus. The galvanic test is applied as follows: With the cathode in contact with the tragus of the tested ear and the anode held in the patient's hand, there results a rotary nystagmus towards the tested ear. When the anode or positive pole is in contact with the tested ear, a rotary nystagmus in the direction of the opposite ear follows. A current strength of

4 ma. should induce the reaction if the nerve and its ending are intact. Alexander and Mackenzie regard a current strength of more than 4 ma., i. e., 6 to 15 ma., to induce a reaction evidence of diminished vestibular irritability. With complete degeneration of the nerve the reaction is entirely absent. Mackenzie, in the Laryngoscope of June, 1916, reported a case of specific auditory neuritis in which, by means of repeated galvanic tests, he was able to note the difference in intensity of the pathologic process in the auditory nerve, from hypersensitiveness in the first test (3.5 ma.) to diminution and almost complete suppression of function in a later test (8 ma.).

In hereditary tertiary lues, defective hearing is frequent. The onset is usually rapid and bilateral, with or without vertigo. The condition develops most frequently in the second or third year of life, less frequently later and only exceptionally after the twentieth year. There are the accompanying signs constituting Hutchinson's triad—keratitis and Hutchinson's teeth. Ulcerations or scars of the nose, throat and skin may be present. The keratitis nearly always precedes the ear lesions by weeks or days, though it may develop simultaneously with it. The presence of a beginning keratitis is, therefore, not only diagnostic of an aural condition impending or actually active, but a warning as well that treatment started at this time may heal, partially at least, an aural lesion. The prognosis of hereditary luetic deafness is bad, despite the use of specific treatment; complete deafness results as a rule. Autopsy findings in a number of these cases have disclosed destruction and replacement of the labyrinth and the internal auditory meatus with bone.

Of a series of forty-five cases of otitis interna recently studied by me, most of them in the service of Dr. T. P. Berens, Manhattan Eye, Ear and Throat Hospital, ten were definitely classified as of syphilitic origin. Many presented themselves with no other complaint than impaired hearing and tinnitus. Some, at various times, had had attacks of vertigo. Particularly instructive is the fact that the diagnosis of neurolabyrinthinitis would have been overlooked if careful tuning fork tests, labyrinthine examination and Wassermann reactions had not previously been made. In many of our crowded clinics these cases are not infrequently diagnosed chronic catarrhal otitis media from otoscopic findings and the history of impaired hearing. In one case (No. 1) further physical examination—reflexes, pupillary reaction, etc.—established a diagnosis of early tabes. Mild attacks of dizziness and slightly impaired hearing had been the only complaint in this case, the real condition having been unrecognized. He had been treated for O M. C. C. for a period of two years. Of the thirty-five non-specific cases the causes discovered in a majority were: long continued use of quinin, noisy occupation, mumps, trauma, cerebrospinal meningitis and advanced middle ear catarrh. In quite a number no definite cause could be assigned. The question of latent syphilis must still be considered and the possibility of focal infection or some metabolic disturbance in the light of our present knowledge, is not to be overlooked.

Tuning forks used in these tests: C (64 D. V.), C (128), C₄ (2048). A—air conduction. M—mastoid.

Case I.—J. 'V. V., Male, age 48 years, came to the Manhattan Eye, Ear and Throat Hospital, complaining of constant tinnitus of long duration and defective hearing. During the past year he has had repeated mild attacks of vertigo and nausea. The only treatment he had received was catheterization of the eustachian tube. History of syphilitic infection 26 years ago. Thorough antisyphilitic treatment for a few years. Had received five injections of salvarsan one year ago.

Otoscopic picture: Slight retraction and dullness both drums. Eustachian tubes patent.

| Right ear 10 ft. | | Left ear 5 ft. |
|---|---|---|
| Lateralizes | Whisper to the right | |
| cA—11 sec. | | cA—5 sec. |
| cM— 4 sec. | | cM—3 sec. |
| c4—A—3 sec. | | c4—A—3 sec. |
| 64 D. V. Plus | | 64 D. V. Plus |

Turning to the right==Nystagmus (horizontal) to the left 10 sec. Turning to the left==Nystagmus (horizontal) to right 16 sec.

Caloric (cold water) right ear==Nystagmus (rotary) to the left after 1½ min. Caloric (cold water) left ear==Nystagmus (rotary) to the right after 4 min.

Pupils: Unequal. Right pupil Argyle-Robertson. Left

pupil only slight reaction to light. Reacts to accommodation. Knee-kerks diminished.

Romberg present. Wasserman (blood) 4+.

The patient went to the Neurological Institution for treatment. This case of tabes had been treated at various clinics during a period of two years for chronic middle ear catarrh.

The tuning forks used in testing these cases were the following: C (64D.V.), C (128), C₄ (2048). A=air. M= mastoid.

Case II.—P. W., Female, 40 years, admitted to the clinic complaining of impaired hearing and tinnitus in both ears for one year. No family history of deafness. Frequent attacks of dizziness lasting a few minutes. No symptoms or signs referable to syphilitic infection. Otoscopic picture that of chronic middle ear catarrh. Wassermann 4 +.

Functional examination:

| Right ear | Voice | Left ear |
|---|---|---|
| No hearing | | 15 ft. |
| cA = 0 | Lateralizes | cA = 10 |
| cM = 4 sec. | | cM = 6 |
| c4 = 0 | | c4A = 4 sec. |
| 64 D. V.  Minus | | 64 D. V. minus |

Noise apparatus in left ear; does not hear loud shouting in right.

Caloric right ear=Fine rotary nystagmus to left after 4 min. Caloric left ear=Coarse rotary nystagmus after 2 min.

Case III.—S. I.—Male, age 50 years, came to me complaining of tinnitus and defective hearing extending over many years. During this time his treatment had consisted of catheterization of eustachian tubes. Complained also of attacks of dizziness. History of syphilitic infection 25 years ago for which he had received two years of careful treatment. Wassermann negative.

Otoscopic examination—Drums, dull and retracted; short processes and posterior folds prominent; light reflexes incomplete.

| Right ear | | Left ear |
|---|---|---|
| 12 ft. | | 5 ft. |
| cA = 7 | Does not lateralize | cA = 5 |
| cM = 3 | Whisper | cM = 3 |
| c4 = 4 | | c4 = 5 |
| 64 D. V.  Plus | | 64 D. V.  Plus |

Turning to the right=(horizontal) nystagmus to left 15 sec. Turning to the left==(horizontal) nystagmus to right 10 sec.

Caloric (left)=rotary nystagmus to the right after 5 min. Caloric (right)==rotary nystagmus to the left after 4 min.

Pupils: Knee jerks, normal. No Romberg.

Under specific treatment attacks of dizziness and tinnitus lessened and finally ceased. Hearing, practically no change; tuning fork tests about same as above.

Case IV.—Traumatic labyrinthitis (unilateral).

D. S., Male, age 24 years, came to the hospital complaining of defective hearing, left ear; two years duration. No tinnitus. History of fracture of skull three years ago; hearing defective since then. Discharge of blood from the left ear at the time of injury. No history of syphilis. Otoscopic examination negative.

| Right ear 20 ft. | Whisper Lateralizes | Left ear 0 |
|---|---|---|

Noise apparatus in right ear; hearing absent in left ear on loud shouting. Normal hearing left ear.

Caloric (cold water)—Left ear negative as to nystagmus after 5 min. Caloric (cold water)—Right ear, rotary nystagmus after 40 min.

Case V.—M. L., age 40 years. History of defective hearing, tinnitus and fullness left ear. Condition began during a severe influenza attack four months ago.

Otoscopic examination both ears, appearance associated with middle ear catarrh.

Functional ear examination:

| Right 20 ft. 20 ft. | Acoumeter Spoken voice Lateralizes | Left 0 0 |
|---|---|---|

Noise apparatus right ear; does not hear loud shouting left ear.

| cA = 25 sec. cM = 12 sec. c4 = A. 14 sec. 64 D. V. Plus | | cA = 0 cM = 7 sec. c4 = A 0 64 D. V. Negative |
|---|---|---|

Turning to right (horizontal)—Nystagmus (rotary) to the left 10 sec. Turning to left (horizontal)—Nystagmus (rotary) to the right 18 sec.

Caloric (cold water) left ear negative after 5 min. Caloric (cold water) right ear after 1 min. fine nystagmus (rotary) to the left.

Base jointing and falling reactions normal.

Wassermann (blood) negative. Spinal Wassermann had not been made.

Case VI.—This case is one of unilateral complete suppression of labyrinthin function following an unusually severe attack of influenza.

M. L., Male. Defective hearing and tinnitus of four months' duration, following influenza. History negative otherwise. Otoscopic examination, minor changes of middle ear catarrh, both ears.

Functional ear examination:

| Right 20 ft. | | Left 0 |
|---|---|---|
| cA = 22 | Voice | cA = 0 |
| cM = 12 | Lateralizes | cM = 7 sec. |
| c4A = 12 sec. | | c4A = 0 |
| 64 D. V.— | | 64 D. V.— |

Noise apparatus in right ear does not hear loudly spoken noise in left ear.

Right ear caloric (cold water)—Fine nystagmus after 1 min. Left ear (caloric)—No nystagmus after 5 min. irrigation.

Wassermann (blood) negative. Patient refused lumbar puncture for spinal Wassermann.

Case VIII.—A. M., age 28 years, male. Initial lesion, August, 1914. One month after receiving injection of salvarsan from his physician, patient informed me that his hearing became decidedly impaired. Patient believes that hearing in the left ear had improved, but condition of right ear had shown no change. Had severe attacks of vertigo and nausea at time of sudden impairment of hearing.

Otoscopic picture negative. Does not lateralize.

Noise apparatus in left ear—Does not hear loudly spoken voice. Raised his voice to a high pitch when asked to read while noise apparatus is used in left ear. Acoustic function normal in left ear.

Caloric (cold water) right ear, head 30 deg. forward—Nystagmus (rotary) to left after 3 min. Head backward 60 deg., horizontal nystagmus to the left after 4 min.

Caloric (cold water) left ear, head 30 deg. forward—Nystagmus (rotary) to the right after 2½ min., head backward 60 deg. (horizontal)—Nystagmus to the right after 3 min.

Turning to the right (horizontal)—Nystagmus to the left 18 sec. Turning to the left (horizontal)—Nystagmus to the right 16 sec.

Past pointing and falling normal.

Case VIII.—J. H., referred to me by his physician.

Male, age 45 years, complained of tinnitus and impaired hearing left ear of three months' duration. Occasional attacks of vertigo. No history of syphilis.

Otoscopic examination—Negative.

Functional examination (left ear) showed rinne positive shortened bone conduction. Lowering of upper tone limits. Lateralizes to the right.

Caloric (cold water) head forward 30 deg.—(Rotary) nystagmus to the opposite side in 1 to 1½ min. Caloric (cold water) head backward 60 deg.—Nystagmus (horizontal) to the opposite side in 2 to 2½ min.

Pointing and falling react normal. Despite negative history of syphilis, a Wassermann test was advised. Report returned by Wassermann 4 +. Case was referred back to her physician for treatment. Five injections of salvarsan and 25 injections of mercury were administered. Examination after four months' treatment hearing decidedly improved. Tinnitus still present. Attacks of vertigo have ceased. Two Wassermann reports negative.

Case IX.—Congenital syphilitic neurolabyrinthitis.

L. R., female, age 13 years. Deafness four years and attacks of vertigo. Bilateral keratitis six years. Wassermann 3 +.

Functional ear examination:

| | |
|---|---|
| cA = 2 | cA = 3 |
| cB = 5 | cB = 6 |
| c4 = 0 | c4 = 0 |
| 64 D. V.— | 64 D. V.— |
| Does not lateralize | |

The vestibular test showed considerable reduction in after nystagmus after turning to right and left (10; 15 respectively) for horizontal and vertical canals.

Right ear—Caloric (cold water) head forward 30 deg. (rotary) nystagmus to the left after 2½ min.

Left ear—Caloric (cold water) (rotary) nystagmus to right after 3 min.

This case of hereditary neurolabyrinthitis passed from observation.

Case X.—Congenital syphilitic neurolabyrinthitis.

E. T., age 18, male, referred to me June 25th, 1920, by his family physician. Mother infected with syphilis third month of her pregnancy. Physician informed me that child was born with all evidences of syphilis; had hydrocephalus. Antiluetic treatment administered to mother and child. Later sent to an institution and treatment indifferently followed. Had usual diseases of childhood. Mother informed me that until five years ago patient had fairly good hearing. Indefinite history of attacks of vertigo and falling few years ago.

Examination: Well developed young man, rather more robust than those of his age usually are. Marked defect of speech; patient difficult to understand. Hearing for conversation, absent. Markedly impaired vision. Bilateral keratitis and external squint. Hutchinson teeth. Romberg absent; knee jerks diminished.

Left ear drum dull; handle of malleus retracted; short process prominent. Right ear, large perforation of drum; anterior two-thirds defect and suppurating; noise apparatus in right ear, does not hear loudly spoken voices in left. Noise apparatus in left ear, hears loud shouting in right. Patient hears tuning forks 128, 256, in right ear but insufficient to record air or bone conduction. No spontaneous nystagmus. Caloric (cold water) left ear, head erect, to right—Nystagmus after 4 minutes. Head to back 60 degrees—(Horizontal nystagmus) to right after 3 minutes. Caloric (cold water) right ear—(Rotary) nystagmus to the left after 2½ minutes. Head back 60 degrees—(Horizontal) nystagmus to the left after 1 minute. Past pointing and falling normal.

No Romberg; reflexes normal; Wassermann negative. Patient is still under antiluetic treatment by family physician.

### SUMMARY.

1. Impaired hearing with apparent middle ear disease showing a positive Rinné should at once arrest the attention of the aurist.

2. Shortening of bone conduction is one of the most constant, reliable and striking evidences of luetic infection. This shortening of bone conduction and, at times, gradual daily impairment of vestibular function, is one of the earliest signs of constitutional syphilis.

3. Recognition of syphlitic auditory neuritis is of paramount importance, as this may be evidence of an incipient cerebrospinal syphilis.

4. Salvarsan, far from causing the continuance or recurrence of syphilitic auditory neuritis, is a means of curing the condition.

5. Prognosis of acquired syphilitic auditory neuritis, while fairly good as to improvement of hearing, should be guarded. Prognosis of the hereditary type is bad.

6. Nonsuppurative neurolabyrinthitis, as a cause of Ménière's symptom complex, may be associated with chronic middle ear catarrh or suppuration. Reliance should, therefore, not be placed upon the history or otoscopic findings, but upon functional ear examinations and laboratory findings.

7. Focal infection or metabolic disorders may be the causative factor in obscure cases of Ménière's symptom complex.

### BIBLIOGRAPHY.

Mackenzie, G. W.: American Journal of Syphilis, 2:241, April, 1918.

Shambaugh, G. E.: Annals of Otol., Rhin. and Laryngol., Sept., 1915, p. 479.

Alexander, G.: Wien. klin. Wchnsch. No. 37, 43, 47, 49, 1913.

Emerson, F. P.: Annals of Otol., Rhin. and Larynol., Dec., 1917, p. 1007.

Mayer, O.: Wien. klin. Wchnsch., Mar. 16, 1911, XXIV, p. 381.

Jones, I. H.: Equilibrium and Vertigo.

Willicutt, M. H.: Journal A. M. A., Aug. 14, 1915.

Wintermute, G. P.: Journal A. M. A., Aug. 14, 1915, p. 608.

Dabney, V.:   American Journal of Syphilis, 1918, p. 26.
Nonne, M.:   Lehr. der Ohrenheil., 1918.
Ellis and Swift:   Journal A. M. A., May 1, 1915.
Knick and Zolozecki:   Berlin klin. Wchnsch., 1912, XLIX, 639.
Graham, H. B.:   American Journal of Syphilis, 3:26, Jan., 1919.
Beck, O.:   Annals Otol., Rhin. and Laryngol., 1913, XXII, 1099.
Pollitzer:   Lehr. der Ohrenheil, 1908.
Fraser:   Glasgow Med. Journal, 1916, 5.
Haberman:   Arch. f. Ohrenh., LXIX, 120.
Billings, F.:   Focal Infection (Lane Medical Lectures), 1917.

# XLI

# A CASE OF LABYRINTHITIS AND CEREBELLAR ABSCESS.

CHAS. E. PERKINS,

NEW YORK.

R. F., male, nine years old, had suppuration of the right ear since infancy. Entered Dr. Dench's service at St. Luke's Hospital July 20, 1920.

Tests showed hearing in diseased ear for loud whisper 6 ft. Lower tone limit, 90; upper tone limit, normal; vestibular mechanism, active; spinal fluid, normal. No history or symptoms of brain involvement.

On July 22nd I performed the radical mastoid operation with primary skin graft. Thirty-six hours later the patient developed vertigo, marked nystagmus to sound side, vomited and complained of headache. Temperature 101°. Total deafness of operated ear, tested with dressings removed. Douching the ear with cold water did not increase the nystagmus or vertigo, with hot water did not produce nystagmus to the diseased side. Spinal fluid contained 350 cells to the millimeter with high polymorphonuclear percentage. Globulin test strongly positive. Right pupil dilated. Eye grounds practically normal.

Labyrinth operation was done after the Neumann method. There was free flow of cerebrospinal fluid from the internal auditory meatus, also from the cochlear region after the removal of the mediolus.

Improvement took place after this operation and convalescence was apparently becoming established. Headache and fever subsided, nystagmus and vertigo became progressively less. This continued for ten days, when a free purulent discharge from the region of the internal auditory meatus developed. The patient became drowsy, complained of headache and vomited. His spinal fluid contained 20 cells to the cubic millimeter. Globulin test mildly positive, overpointed with right hand indiscriminately.  As I was off service, the subsequent care of the case fell to Dr. Bowers.

Operation August 6th.  Sequestrum of bone removed from the region of the internal auditory meatus.  This opened an abscess in the cerebellum from which a considerable quantity of pus escaped.  Culture of this pus grew the pyocyaneous. An attempt was made to tie off the sinus, in order to obtain more room to evacuate and drain the abscess, but it was unsuccessful on account of hemorrhage, which was controlled with difficulty by packing.  The patient showed much improvement after this operation.  This continued for eighteen days.  Then there was an attack of projectile vomiting. Headache, nystagmus to both sides; overpointed to left with right hand; inequality of pupils, right the larger.  These symptoms continued for about a week, when a further attempt was made to locate and drain an intracranial abscess.  The temporosphenoidal lobe was explored with negative results. Cerebellum exposed posterior to the sinus and explored with the grooved director.  Upon passing this instrument rather deeply into the upper part of the cerebellum, a hard resisting wall was encountered, which at the time was interpreted as the tentorium, but which at autopsy was found to be the thick capsule of an abscess.  After this operation there was no improvement.  The patient died eight days later.

Autopsy showed meningitis at the base, and "A large abscess, with thick wall, occupying a large portion of the upper two-thirds of the right cerebellar hemisphere, extending to within two centimeters of the posterior pole."  Cultures of pus from this abscess grew the pyocyaneus.

This case raises several points to which I will allude briefly:

1.  Upon opening the dura at the internal auditory meatus there was a free flow of cerebrospinal fluid.  I have come to regard this occurrence as an omen of good augury.  It doubtless means that the cerebellopontine cysterna has been opened and when it occurs the active process seems more likely to be localized in this region.  At any rate the meningitis in this patient began to improve as shown by the subsidence of the temperature and headache and clearing up of the spinal fluid. The next specimen, taken twelve days later, after cerebellar

symptoms had developed, showed a cell count of 20 with practical disappearance of the globulins.

2.    The question arises as to the time of the cerebellar infection.    Whether it occurred previous to the radical operation or if after it. Was it present at the time of the labyrinth operation, or did it take place some ten days later when wound infection became evident with pus discharging from the internal auditory meatus?    The importance of fixing this date arises from the fact that it gives the length of time during which a brain abscess may form a thick hard capsule.    Dr. Bowers, who performed the later operations and was present at the autopsy, believes that it would have been impossible for such an abscess and capsule to form in the forty-eight days intervening between the radical operation and death, but that it was present in a latent form when the patient entered the hospital.    However, it seems improbable that an abscess of such size should occupy and more or less destroy a large part of one cerebellar hemisphere and yet produce no symptoms. More likely the cerebellar infection occurred between the labyrinthitis and meningitis and the wound infection.    That is, between the 39 and 29 days before capsule was discovered upon exploration.    So this would be the length of time in which abscess developed and formed a thick, dense capsule. The part played by the pyocyaneus infection in producing a capsule is to be noted.    The pneumococcus is perhaps found more often than any other germ in abscesses with capsules. This observation shows that in so far as the germ determines this condition the pyocyaneus is effective.

3.    The inadequacy of the grooved director as an exploring instrument is strikingly shown in this case.    The resistance of the capsule was so great that it was believed to be the tentorium.    Perhaps a sharp knife would have evacuted the pus. It would seem that a procedure advocated by Ballance, which largely has fallen into disuse in this country, might have resulted in locating the abscess.    I refer to digital exploration The finger surely would have succeeded in making out such a large, firm abscess.

4.    Finally, the difficulty of using the sinus area as an approach is shown.    The attempt to tie off the sinus as advised by Ballance and independently by Friesner, failed on account

of free hemorrhage, which required packing. There are two objections to this procedure. First, one hesitates to inflict sufficient traumatism to the cerebellum properly to insert the ligatures. Second, the resistance of the dura would interfere with their being tied sufficiently tight to occlude the sinus lumen unless they tear their way through, when bleeding would be very likely to occur. So, while approach through the sinus area is ideal in those cerebellar abscesses following sinus thrombosis and has been utilized by McKernon and others, it is not liable to be of very much use when the blood is freely flowing through a patent sinus.

# XLII.

## PULSATING SPHENOIDITIS.

Harry L. Pollock, M. D.,

Chicago.

In 1916 we had referred to us by an oculist of Milwaukee, a patient in whom a diagnosis of retrobulbar tumor, probably sarcoma, had been made. Inasmuch as this condition is not connected with the subject under discussion this evening, I will not go into details concerning his ocular findings, except to state that we did a Kroenlein operation and found no tumor but a marked cellulitis, which resolved after long continued suppuration. He also had a pansinuitis on the same side (left) as his exophthalmos. An ethmoid exenteration was done and the sphenoid opened. As soon as the postoperative reaction had subsided, we noticed a thick, profuse, yellowish discharge from the sphenoid, which persisted for a long time, notwithstanding the usual treatment for this condition. At various times a slight pulsation was noted in the sphenoid. *i.e.*, there was pulsation transmitted to the pus in the cavity. Not having noticed this condition previously, we began to discuss the probable reason for this pulsation. Being synchronous with the heart beat, only one assumption was possible, but just how, why and wherefrom this pulsation arose, was somewhat a conjecture. It could not come direct from the internal carotid, or it would be present all the time. It might possibly be transmitted through the cavernous sinus, and if this were the case, it certainly could be exaggerated by dilating the sinus or causing an increased blood pressure within the cavernous. This, we knew, could be brought about by compressing the return venous flow from the cranial cavity. We compressed both internal jugulars by pressing deeply with both thumbs, and found that the pulsation became more marked and continued as long as the compression ensued and disappeared as promptly as the pressure was removed. After irrigating the sphenoid and allowing some fluid to remain in the cavity, pulsation could be brought about by again compressing the jugulars. We were very much interested in the probable size of the sphenoid and removed the anterior wall and parsethmoidalis down to the floor. To our great surprise, the curved probe could be passed for at least two and one-quarter inches below the opening, the direction being downwards and backwards. On the right side, the probe could be passed only about one-half inch. With a long probe in the sphenoid, no pulsation could be felt, but immediately upon compressing the jugulars, there was a pulsation of the probe which could be observed on the portion extending out of the nose. The Wassermann, which had been made before the Kroenlin operation, proved to be positive. The patient was given intensive antiluetic treatment and kept under observation, and after several months' treatment, the pus discharge abated and finally stopped.

We have had several more cases, almost identical of the above case, and found that they ran about the same course.

That the pulsation was transmitted through the cavernous sinus from the carotid, there can be no doubt, but why in only these few cases and not in all cases of sphenoid suppuration?

We know that the floor of the sphenoid sinus lies just over the body of the sphenoid and that the latter is composed of cancellous bone. There is no doubt that the solid floor of this cavity is necrosed, most probably due to the lues, and the infection thereby affects the cancellous portion of the body of the sphenoid, accounting for the immense depth of this sinus. It is also possible that the carotid takes an anomalous position and passes directly through the sphenoid cavity. My associate, Dr. J. Beck, has a photograph of a specimen which shows the carotid in this position.

Fortunately, all of our patients recovered, so that we were not able to prove postmortem that our deductions were correct. We also know that dehiscences occur in the sphenoid cavity just as in the frontal sinus or other bony cavities, and these might also account for this peculiar and interesting phenomena.

There are other etiologic conditions which may produce pulsation in and around the sphenoid cavity. Aneurysm of the internal carotid and in this region may cause pulsation. We have also had another case in which distinct pulsation could be observed very nicely in the sphenoid. This was in a man whom a diagnosis of hypopituitarism or Froehlich's disease had been made, in which we suspected a tumor of the hypophysis. We operated transphenoidally and removed the floor of the sella turcica and found a large cyst, which was opened and drained. The patient made an uneventful recovery and has remained well now about seven years. After all postoperative reaction disappeared, we could observe this distinct pulsation, which was the pulsation of the brain. In this case, however, there was no infection or suppuration of the sinus. At that time we did not observe whether a compression of the jugulars would increase the pulsation or not.

Let us study the anatomic relations of the cavernous sinus and the sphenoid and see how easily this phenomena may occur. The following is taken from Gray's Anatomy: "The cavernous sinus is named from presenting a reticulated structure, due to being traversed by numerous interlacing filaments. There are two cavernous sinuses of irregular form, larger behind than in front, and placed one on each side of the sella turcica, extending from the sphenoidal fissure and opening behind into the petrosal sinuses. On the inner wall of each sinus is found the internal carotid artery, accompanied by filaments of the carotid plexus and by the sixth nerve. On its outer wall, by the third, fourth and ophthalmic division of the fifth nerve. These parts are separated from the blood flowing along the sinus by the lining membrane, which is continuous with the inner coat of the veins. The cavernous sinus receives some of the cerebral veins, and also the sphenoparietal sinuses. They communicate with the lateral sinuses by means of the superior and inferior petrosal sinuses, and with the facial veins through the ophthalmic vein. They also communicate with each other by means of the circular sinus."

Thus, we see the upper portion of the sphenoid sinus is practically surrounded by this network of bloody sinuses and in very close proximity of the internal carotid artery. Furthermore, Loeb and others have brought to our attention the various formations and irregularities in the size and position of the sphenoid sinus. It is often prolonged downwards into the pterygoid process and base of the greater wings of the bone. Occasionally they extend into the basilar process of the occipital bone, nearly as far as the foramen magnum. Thus we see that a dehiscence or a necrosis of the posterior or upper wall of the sphenoidal cavity can easily give rise to a pulsation within the sinus. Naturally, any engorgement of the large blood vessels would bring about this exaggeration of the pulsation, and this is easily done by compressing the internal jugulars.

In our experience the prognosis of this form of sphenoiditis is much graver, especially as to the length of time, than an ordinary suppurative case. The etiology is based upon a luetic infection and leads us to believe that there is an actual necrosing osteitis, which causes a greater destruction than the ordinary sphenoiditis in which the pathologic lesion is limited to the lining mucous membrane or a superficial osteitis. The treatment, besides the ordinary local routine one, is directed to the underlying cause, viz., lues, and a long intensified anti-luetic treatment must be undertaken. In these cases one must be cautious in probing and curetting, as it would be quite easy to lacerate the cavernous sinus or even the carotid, and the ensuing hemorrhage would be severe and probably fatal.

The points which I desire to emphasize in this condition of pulsating sphenoiditis are: (1) there is a necrosing osteitis which destroys a portion of the bony wall of the solid cavity or there may be the congenital dehiscences, thereby permitting the pulsation to be transmitted from the carotids through the cavernous tissue to the sphenoid. (2) The underlying etiologic factor is lues and often this must be carefully searched for, as none of our cases gave a positive history. (3) The duration of the sphenoiditis is unusually long, most of our cases lasting from eighteen to twenty-four months. (4) The treatment is (a) surgical, *i e.,* at least seeing that the opening is sufficiently large to permit drainage and (b) intensive anti-luetic treatment, both by salvarsan or similar products and by mercury and potassium iodid.

# XLIII

## CASE OF INTRANASAL EPITHELIOMA.—CURED BY EXCISION AND RADIUM.—LITERATURE.

DUNBAR ROY, M. D.,

ATLANTA, GA.

Mrs. S. B. R. (white), age 42 of Toccoa, Ga. Patient consulted the writer on account of some soreness and stopping of the left nasal cavity which had been present for several months.

History. Patient was of an unusually strong and healthy looking physique. Weight 160 pounds. Had never had any severe illness nor chronic complaints which necessitated the consultation of a physician. No history of any malignant disease in her family. Her only complaint was susceptibility to colds in the head. '

Present History. For the last three months has had some irritation and some stopping of the left nasal cavity. This was accompanied by scabby condition and an occasional bloody discharge. She had been able to see a small growth just within the external opening on the outer side which was evidently increasing in size.

Examination. No external swelling or congestion. No enlargement of the cervical or submaxillary glands. On inspection just within the left nasal cavity could be seen a small growth at the anterior end of the inferior turbinate close to the mucocutaneous margin. It was dry and about the size of a bean, slightly scabby, sessile in form with a slight tendency to bleed if touched. The patient gave no history of nose bleed. To all appearances the growth gave every indication of being a fibrous papilloma. Under cocaine anesthesia the growth was very easily removed with the cold wire snare and the raw surface cauterized with the electrocautery. There was very little hemorrhage.

The growth was submitted to Dr. John Funke, pathologist, who gave the following report:

"Specimen consists of a reniform mass 1.2 by 0.6 by 0.4 cm. which is reddish grey in color and rather firm.

Microscopic Examination. The sections are surrounded by a stratified layer of squamous epithelium which at one point is clearly destroyed by a very small ulcerated area. Extending from this area for a short distance the superficial portion of the epithelial stratum is undermined. The structures underlying the ulcerated and undermined area are infiltrated with cells which for the most part are arranged in plugs, but some are in long strings. These cells are polyhedral in shape, are about the size of the cells occupying the lowermost portion of the epithelial stratum. They stain well, especially the nucleus. The protoplasm is granular and rather scanty.

The stroma is abundant, stains rather feebly and contains a few blood vessels.

Diagnosis. "Basil cell epithelioma."

Subsequent History. The patient returned in one week's time, showing no signs of reaction and nothing more upon the surface than would be expected from the removal of a benign growth. A sedative ointment had been given to be used in the nasal cavity.

Nov. 16th, 1919. Three weeks later the patient was again seen. There was considerable irritation inside the nose, accompanied by scabbing and bleeding. The patient said she felt very uncomfortable. She was then referred to Dr. O. D. Hall for radium treatment. I saw the patient at intervals during the radium treatment, but only for observation. The radium was used as follows, being placed just inside the nasal cavity and properly screened.

Nov. 15th, 1919. 50 milligrams. Time 2 hours.

Dec. 15th, 1919. Same amount. Time 4½ hours.

Feb. 11th, 1920. Same amount. Time 2½ hours, making a total of 450 milligram hours.

Jan. 15th. Examination shows a complete disappearance of the growth, smooth surface, and only slightly scabby condition.

Oct. 22nd, 1920. Nasal cavity looks normal and patient told to report at the slightest indication of discomfort in the nose.

A letter from the patient May 15th, now 19 months since operation indicates there is no further trouble.

Contrary to the opinion of several observers, my own experience leads me to conclude that radium is much more effective in epitheliomata than in other forms of malignant growths.

In 1919, before the American Ophthalmological Society, I reported two cases of epithelioma of the eyeball, where exenteration of the orbit followed by the use of radium produced a complete cure up to the present, six years in one and eleven years in the other.

In 1916, the writer reported a case of epithelioma of the pharyngeal wall treated by complete excision with the electric cautery, and which has remained cured up to the present date. Radium was not used, but in epitheliomata accessible for complete excision, especially by electrocautery, results will nearly always be favorable. This has been frequently demonstrated in the removal of skin epitheliomas in the region of the face or from skin surfaces.

The cure of epitheliomata is entirely a different proposition, however, when they are located in a vascular region like the ethmoid or have their origin in a closed cavity like the antrum maxillary. Thorough eradication is practically impossible, but it is in just such cases that radium does its best work.

The splendid results shown in Boston last year by Drs. Barnes and Greene in the combined use of surgery and radium in malignant growths of the head certainly leads us to be far more optimistic in our views than has heretofore been the case.

I take the liberty of presenting a bibliography of the literature bearing on the treatment of nasal epitheliomata, especially in regard to the results obtained by the use of radium. No doubt this is far from being complete, but if other observers will add to this series, we may begin to have more exact statistics.

### RADIUM IN THE TREATMENT OF EPITHELIOMA OF THE NASAL CAVITIES.

#### CASE REPORTS.

Adam[2] reports a case of endothelioma in which the tumor filled the right half of the nasopharynx, appearing to grow from the eustachian orifice. Two radium applications were made on November 29, 1915, and January 12, 1916; 50 mg. of radium screened by 1 mgm. of gold was applied for twenty-three hours at the first treatment, and for eleven hours at the second. At the time of the report, August, 1916, the parts seemed normal. Sufficient time has not elapsed to establish a permanent cure, but the result is certainly better than could have been obtained by surgical interference. (Sonnenschein refers to this case as epithelioma.)

Botey[5] treated two cases of endonasal epithelioma with radium with poor results. In both the growth progressed and the patients died.

Delavan[6] in his report on radium in the treatment of the growths of the upper air passages, at the Memorial Hospital, includes three tumors of the "nasal mucosa," treated by radium. Two of these had advanced recurrent lesions. (The nature of these tumors is not indicated.) In the third case, a recurrent epidermoid carcinoma of the posterior portion of the nasal septum, occluding both nasal passages, an excellent result was obtained by removing the growths with a snare and treating their bases with radium. There was no recurrence in three months.

"The difficulties of making accurate applications of radium to the nose are very great, unless the lesion is an early one and situated low down." These cases are also reported by Janeway in his book.[11]

Hill[9] reports one case of epithelioma originating in the left antrum, extending into the nasal cavity, the ethmoid cells and nasopharynx, treated by radium; 100 mgm. of radiobromide was inserted through a breaking down area over the hard palate into the antrum; 50 mg. into the same cavity by the inferior nasal route; a small tube of 20 mg. in the ethmoid region; a fourth tube of 50 mg. in the nasopharynx. A 48 hour exposure was made, as the growth was fungating. The growth cleared up within a few days, but apparently had invaded the cranial cavity, as the patient died "shortly afterwards" from intracranial pressure.

In general, Hill says that radium is worth trying in any malignant growth of the nose and throat "which is considered hopelessly outside the range of radical excision by the knife, provided always that an adequate amount is available,

and that the primary growth is accessible and not too far advanced and extensive, that the secondary adjacent growths and
more remote metastases are not a contraindication, and provided also that the general health of the patient is fairly good."
If an extensive growth is treated and reacts well, a massive
dose of toxins may cause not only general malaise and fever,
but "a very definite toxemia."

Generally speaking, round cell sarcomas and most endotheliomas react rapidly and consistently well to radium; spindle
celled sarcomas and fibrosarcomas react fairly; squamous epitheliomas and carcinomas "are far more uncertain in the way
they react to radium. It may be asserted, however, that some
epitheliomas in the nose, throat and gullet do react beneficially
to radium, in striking contrast to those of the tongue and of
the vulva."

In the case reported the author calls attention to the fact
that the tumor—through an epithelioma—reacted immediately
"after the manner of a round celled sarcoma." There is usually, he says, a longer latent period in carcinoma.

Kelly[12] reports one case of epithelioma of the nasopharynx,
the tumor being attached to the roof and resting on the palate,
hiding the entire right posterior nares and all but the outer segment of the left posterior nares. Nasal fossæ normal. It
caused nasal obstruction and a severe hemorrhage. On January 27, 1915, 50 mg. of radium was screened with 2 mm. of
silver and covered with 2 mm. of rubber was applied for twenty-four hours. This caused ulceration of the palate and fauces
for a week. On March 10th, the tumor had shrunk so that
the nose was free, but a small rounded mass was still present
on the roof of the nasopharynx. Radium was again applied
in the same dosage as before. On May 14th and June 2d there
was no sign of the growth, but the site of origin was covered by an adherent crust of mucus. Underneath was an
apparently healthy surface. A third radium treatment was
given on June 2d. Last examinaiton on February 22, 1916.
Still crusting behind the right choanal arch, but the underlying surface was healthy, and there was no sign of recurrence.

Kofler[13] reports on the treatment by radium of three lymphosarcoma and eleven carcinoma of the nose, mouth and throat.

The results were better in the carcinoma than in the sarcoma. One of these was a basal cell carcinoma filling the right side of the nose, originating from the region of the infundibulum. Operation of Langenbeck, followed by application of radium. Patient in good health and free from recurrence at last report. (Operation in October, 1912; report published early part of 1913, exact date not given.)

New[16] reports results from the use of radium in 211 neoplasms of the nose, throat and mouth at the Mayo Clinic.

In cases suitable for surgical treatment, radium alone is not used, he says.

Of the 211 tumors, 9 were intranasal epitheliomas and 5 epithelioma of the nasopharynx. In regard to the results, New says, "it is too soon to report end results in this group."

Of the results in nasal epithelioma he says that: "Operative measures in the treatment of epithelioma of the nose are usually of little value. Radium frequently clears up the ulceration and discharge and scars down the growth, giving the patient much relief, and sometimes accomplishing more than this." No further detail in regard to results is given.

The author's general conclusion is: "The immediate results of the treatment of neoplasms of the nose, throat and mouth with radium are, as a whole, very encouraging. Many patients previously operated on with a recurrence following are now treated with radium and the neoplasm disappears, giving months or years of relief, with no surgical mortality. The patients are made much more comfortable than they would be with an operation. The number of patients that will be permanently cured of a true malignancy with radium is probably very small relatively, but the number of inoperable cases that are markedly relieved and receive months or years of comfort is quite large. We do not, however, recommend the treatment by radium of any neoplasm that is surgical. In such cases the patient should have the benefit of both surgery and radium. The use of radium has entirely changed the prognosis in neoplasms of the nose, throat and mouth."

Schmeigelow[20] reports twelve cases of malignant tumors of the nose, pharynx and oral cavity treated by radium in 1918 and 1919. Three patients died; one (epithelioma of the right tonsil) from metastasis in the liver; one (cancer of the left tonsil) from recurrence in the pharynx with ulceration and hemorrhage; one (nasopharyngeal sarcoma) from septic abscess without recurrence or metastasis of the tumor. In one case (epithelioma of the soft palate and left tonsil), the tumor disappeared, but the patient suffered from a radium burn, probably due to a faulty radium tube. In another case (cancer of the tonsils) the tumor did not recur, but the glands were involved and continued painful in spite of both radium and Roentgen treatment.

In the other patients of this series, results were excellent, without recurrence in a year or over. One of these cases was an epithelioma of the nasopharynx in a woman 70 years old. The tumor was located on the posterior wall of the nasopharynx. Three radium tubes (30 mg.) of radium were applied through the nose for 24 hours on June 26, 1919; this was followed by immediate improvement, but two subsequent treatments were given as a preventive on July 31st and October 11th, although the tumor had entirely disappeared, and the tissue appeared entirely normal. Clinically the cure was complete at the time of the report (June, 1920).

Schmeigelow says that Lederman and Kuznitzky[15] report one case of advanced squamous celled epithelioma of the nasopharynx which improved under Roentgen treatment, but was entirely cured by mesothorium and radium. Their original report is not available.

## II.—CASES OPERATED.

(Including only a few cases operated. See also notes with reference for results with operation.)

Beck[3] includes in his report on malignant disease of the upper respiratory tract, 7 cases of intranasal carcinoma, including the accessory sinuses; 3 cases operated; 5 followed up to recent date. All died.

Dougherty[7] reports two cases of epithelioma of the frontal sinus, both operated. One patient died several weeks after the operation from purulent meningitis; the other died two months after operation from extension and ulceration of the growth.

Ferreri[8] states that epithelioma of the nasal fossæ is undoubtedly rare. His table of cases shows 1 epithelioma of the antrum of Highmore, cured by operation; 1 case of rhino-

pharyngeal epithelioma inoperable, death; 5 cases of epithelioma of the nasal fossæ and diffuse epithelioma of the nose,
of which one was cured by operation, the others were inoperable; 1 epithelioma of the left maxillary sinus, not operated.
One epithelioma of the roof of the mouth was treated by radium; the patient died. This is the only case of epithelioma
included in the report in which radium was used.

Thomson[23] reports two cases operated, using Moure's operation. Case 1. Endothelioma of the ethmoid and antrum:
Moure's operation; no recurrence in 5½ years. Case 2. Epithelioma of the left maxillary antrum; Moure's operation; no
recurrence after 3½ years.

### III.—GENERAL CONCLUSIONS IN REGARD TO THE VALUE OF RADIUM IN THE TREATMENT OF EPITHELIOMA.

Boggs[4] makes no mention of epithelioma of the nasal cavities specifically, but says in regard to radium treatment of epithelioma in general:

"Primarily epithelioma is not a surgical disease, because, in
order to remove all the cancerous cells, it is nearly always
necessary to remove too much healthy tissue. The permanency of the end-results, in the past few years in many thousands of cases, has shown that radiation far surpasses any
other method.

"Radium is the best form of radiation locally on the lesion
and in regions where glandular metastases are likely to take
place. Radium used over glandular centers or junctions with
complete roentgen treatment over the tributaries, is far superior to the most complete and often unnecessary dissection."

"Each year," he says, "there is a smaller percentage of
surgeons removing epitheliomas. I do not mean to say that
surgery is never indicated, but I believe that it is seldom, if
ever, indicated in primary cases."

Janeway[10] in his 1918 article says that at the Memorial Hospital they "have been encouraged to treat a rather large number of operable cancers of the mucous membranes" with radium. "The remarkable improvement in some of the cases
treated palliatively has not alone stimulated this attempt, but
more especially the favorable result obtained on many early
cancers in patients refusing operation, or in whom operation
was contraindicated for other reasons. Two facts have been

demonstrated by this experience; first, within the time limits in which we have been working, single applications were often sufficient to cause apparent complete retrogressions; and second, in the larger lesions, where this favorable result was not obtained, the lesion has become more of an operable one than it was before treatment."

The cases reported by Janeway in this article do not include any malignant growth of the nasal cavities. See report under Delavan's name in section on case reports.

Lannois, Saignon and Moutet,[14] in their report on radium therapy in tumors in otorhinolaryngology, report 13 cases treated by radium. These include six tumors of the nose and sinuses, and four tumors of the nasopharynx, but all of these were sarcoma, none epithelioma.

In general, they say that nonepithelial tumors are much improved, often completely cured by radium, but that results are not so good in epithelioma, especially ectodermic epitheliomas containing epithelial pearls (globe corné) are very slightly influenced by radium.

Pancoast[18] reports several cases of sarcoma and carcinoma of the tonsil and one case of sarcoma of the left turbinates and antrum. No case of epithelioma of the nose or nasopharynx.

His general conclusions are:

"In the treatment of inoperable malignant growth, originating in cavities such as the mouth, throat and ear, radium therapy is an extremely valuable adjunct, for the reason that it can usually be applied directly to the growth, which is more or less inaccessible to direct roentgen ray exposure. This alone is not sufficient, and the growth should also be attacked from every possible direction by cross firing, either by radium or roentgen rays or both. Any near by area in which metastasis is likely to occur should also be exposed.

"Sarcomatous growths, especially in the tonsillar region, are more amenable to treatment than carcinomas.

"It would be best to continue treatment for some time after the apparent complete disappearance of the growth."

Sonnenschein[22] in his paper on radium in the treatment of malignant tumors of the nose and throat says little definite in regard to epithelioma of the nasal cavities as distinguished from other malignant tumors. The specific cases mentioned by him are reviewed elsewhere in this report under the authors' names.

In his table he includes 41 malignant tumors of the nose and sinuses in which radium was "the main form of treatment employed"; of these 13 were apparently cured, 2 were free from recurrence for one year or more, 14 were improved, 12 unimproved. Of 12 cases of malignant tumors of the nasopharynx treated by radium all were apparently cured. This table does not differentiate between carcinomas or sarcomas. Some writers, Sonnenschein says, "merely speak of 'malignant disease' of certain tissues or structures so that it is impossible to differentiate in the table."

From the study of the subject presented in this article he comes to the conclusion that:

"The future of radium therapy seems very bright, particularly in reference to applications in tumors of the nose and throat; but great caution is advisable in statements regarding actual cures. It is important to watch for recurrences during a period of from two to five years.

"Radium is probably of great value before, and certainly after operations. It is very efficient in relieving pain, hemorrhage. discharge, etc., in many inoperable cases.

"Sarcomas are especially responsive to radiation; the carcinomas yield much less readily, and the squamous type of epithelioma is scarcely amenable to radium at all.

"Radium has many advantages as compared with roentgen rays, especially for application in the nose and throat.

"The diagnosis of the malignant cases should be made by a competent laryngologist, and the radium applied either by him or in cooperation with a radiologist. Only in this way will correct statistics and reliable results be obtained, with greatest benefit to the patient and the safest guide to the profession."

Wickham and DeGrais[24] say that "the value of radium in malignant tumor of the mucous membrane is incontestable, but varies according to the region and the nature of the tumor —sarcoma being by far the most amenable to treatment."

Their cases reported do not include any malignant tumors of nasal cavities.

Barnes reports a series of malignant tumors of the nasal accessory sinus treated by operation and radium. For the operation the Moure incision is made in the cheek, and "every particle of tumor tissue, all necrotic or soft bone" removed. Wherever possible, it is desirable to remove a small margin of normal tissue. A triangular flap of integument, "having its base in the upper incision and its apex at the lower limits of the antrum," is removed from the cheek, leaving a permanent opening into the operative cavity, so that any tendency to recurrence may be observed. The deformity following this is not great. The cavity is lightly packed with gauze, in the center of which a radium emanation tube "of appropriate strength" is placed. The tube remains in place about two weeks, being reinserted at each dressing. As the tube loses one-sixth of its radiating strength every 24 hours, it is practically inert at the end of convalescence. Three or four later radium treatments are given at weekly intervals as a preventive measure. Marked reaction of the tissues should be avoided in these treatments.

In the series reported by the author there were six carcinomas, one small round celled sarcoma and one fibrosarcoma. With the exception of the last named, all were of long standing and involved both the ethmoid and the sphenoid. Three (all carcinomas) were operations for recurrences, and one (sarcoma) had had an enucleation of the eye one year before, further operation being abandoned on account of the extent of the growth. Neither sarcoma shows any sign of recurrence (14 and 26 months after operation). Of the carcinomas, three patients have died, one has extensive recurrences, two are well with no sign of recurrence 25 and 17 months after operation respectively. One of the deaths was postoperative, due to septic meningitis. The carcinoma in this case involved all the sinuses except the frontal.

The author believes that in these massive tumors of the sinuses "radium without operation is useless." However, "thorough operation combined with immediate radiation through a wide opening in the face which for purposes of observation is allowed to remain permanently, will give, I believe, better results than we have been accustomed to consider possible."

Guichard reports two cases of epithelioma of the nasal fossa that invaded the sinuses, the orbit and, in one case, the cranial cavity. No treatment is reported in one case. The other case was operated and given several X-ray treatments. The treatment was successful and the patient remained in good health. (Operation in August, 1919; report published March, 1920.)

In a later article (October 10, 1920) Lannois and Saignon review their work on radium treatment of tumors of the ear, throat and nose, but report no new cases. In their work they employ Dominci radium tubes; they use doses of 25 to 160 mg., left in place for 6 to 24 hours, occasionally for 36 hours, exceptionally for 48 hours.

### REFERENCES.

1. Aboulker, H.: Contribution à l' étude des tumeurs malignes du nasopharynx. Bull. d'oto-rhino-laryngol. 15:115, 1912.
Recommends surgery for treatment of malignant tumors of the nasopharynx. Merely mentions possibility of the use of radium.
2. Adam, J.: Endothelioma of Nasopharynx Apparently Cured by Radium. J. Laryngol., Rhinol. & Otol. 31:346, 1916.
3. Beck, J. C.: Management of Malignant Diseases of Upper Respiratory Tract. Illinois M. J. 32:194, 1917.
4. Boggs, R. H.: Treatment of Epithelioma with Radium. Am. J. M. Sc., 158:87, 1919.
5. Botey, R.: (Radium in Cancer of Upper Passages.) Rev. Española de med. y cir. 1:275, 1918.
6. Delavan, D. B.: Radium in the Treatment of Growths of the Upper Air Passages. Am. Laryngol. Ass. Tr. 35:21, 1917.
7. Dougherty, D. S.: Primary Epithelioma of Frontal Sinus. Laryngoscope 27:37, 1917.
8. Ferreri, G.: Trattamento e prognosi dei tumori maligni dellé fosse nasali e dell epifaringe. Internat. Cong. Med. 1913 Trans. Sect. 15:149. See also: Arch. internat. de larygol. 35:337, 1913; 36:733; 37:77; 414, 1914.
9. Hill, W.: Treatment of Inoperable Growths of the Nose and Throat by Radium. J. Laryngol. 29:487, 1916.
10. Janeway, H. H.: Treatment by Radium of Cancerous Mucous Membrane. Ab. J. Roentgol. n.s. 5:414, 1918.
11. Janeway, H. H.: Radium Therapy in Cancer. New York, P. B. Hoeber, 1917.
12. Kelly, A. B.: Nasopharyngeal Neoplasm Dispelled by Radium. J. Laryngol., Rhinol. & Otol. 31:345, 1916.
13. Kofler, K.: Erfahrunged mit der Radiumbehandlung. Monatschr. f. Ohrenheilk. 47:244, 1913.
14. Lannois, Sargnon, A. and Moutet: La radiumthérapie des tumeurs en oto-rhino-laryngologie. Bull. Acad. de Méd. 81:638, 1919.

15. Lederman, P. and Kutzsnitzky, E.: Ueber die radiologische Behandlung von Nasenrachenraumgeschwülsten. Strahlentherapie 8:1917.

16. New, G. B.: Value of Radium in the Treatment of Neoplasms of the Nose, Throat and Mouth. Mayo Clinic Collected Papers. 10:809, 1918.

17. Oppikofer, E.: Ueber die primären malignen Geschwülste des Nasenrachenraumes. Arch. f. Laryngol. u. Rhinol. 27:526, 1913. Twenty-one cases reported, none in which radium was used. All fatal except two lymphosarcoma.

18. Pancoast, H. R.: Malignant Disease of the Throat and Sinuses. J. A. M. A. 69:980, 1917.

19. Safrank, J.: Ueber primäre, bösartige Geschwülste der Nasenhöhle und der Nasennebenhölen. Beitr. z. klin. Chir. 84: 126, 1913. Advises operation whenever possible in malignant tumors of the nose and nasal sinuses.

20. Schmiegelow, E.: Einige Beobachtungen hinsichtlich der Wirkung des Radiums auf inoperable maligne Neubildungen im Munde, Rachen und in der Nase. Arch. f. Laryngol. u. Rhinol. 33:1, 1920.

21. Sendziak, J.: Les tumeurs malignes des sinus du nex et de la cavité nasopharyngienne. Arch. internat. de laryngol. 35:371, 1913. Nothing of interest.

22. Sonnenschein, R.: Radium in the Treatment of Malignant Tumors of the Nose and Throat. J. A. M. A. 75:860, Sept. 25, 1920.

23. Thomson, St. C.: Malignant Disease of the Nose or Accessory Sinuses. Lancet, 1916, 1:987.

24. Wickham, L. and De Grais, P.: Radium as Employed in the Treatment of Cancer and Other Affections. London, 1913.

The following references are to periodicals that were still at the binder's when this report was made:

Earnes, H. A.: Combined Operative and Radium Treatment of Malignant Disease of the Nasal Accessory Sinuses. Laryngoscope, 30:646, 1920.

Dubreuilh, W.: Roentgen-Ray Treatment of Epitheliomas with Massive Doses. Paris Med. 10:265, Oct. 9, 1920.

Guichard, P.: Epitheliomas des fosses nasales. Rev. de Laryngol. 41:137, 1920.

Lannois and Saignon: Radium Therapy in Tumors of Ears, Nose and Throat. Lyon med. 129:807, Oct. 10, 1920.

BIBLIOGRAPHY.

Barnes, H. A.: Combined Operative and Radium Treatment of Malignant Diseases of the Nasal Accessory Sinuses. Laryngoscope, 30:646, 1920.

Dubreuilh, W.: Roentgen-Roy Treatment of Epitheliomas with Massive Doses. Paris Med. 10:265, Oct. 9, 1920. (Skin epitheliomas only.)

Guichard, P.: Epitheliomas des fosse nasales. Rev. de laryngol. 41:137, 1920.

Lannois and Saignon: Radium Therapy in Tumors of Ears, Nose or Throat. Lyon med. 129:807, Oct. 10, 1920.

## XLIV.

## CANCER OF THE LARYNX.

By N. B. Carson, M. D.,

St. Louis.

In treating the subject of cancer of the larynx it seems like ancient history to go back to 1887, when I did my first laryngectomy. Since that time I have had four other cases, with three operative deaths. This is a very high mortality and would seem to make the operation of laryngectomy unjustifiable were it not for the fact that others have been more successful and had the mortality not steadily decreased from 40 odd per cent at that time to about 10 per cent at present. This change has resulted from improved technic in operative methods, but principally from the introduction of intratracheal and especially local anesthesia.

This mortality was due in part, if not entirely, to the fact that the cases were not selected, as I do not believe the comfort of the patient should be sacrificed for the benefit of statistics. I have seen many apparently hopeless cases of cancer relieved of their sufferings—very materially relieved—and their lives made decidedly more endurable and sometimes saved by operation. In a case that I call to mind, a patient had an apparently hopeless cancer of the breast and I did what I intended to be a palliative operation, making it as complete as possible; it was so complete that the patient is still alive, with no signs of return of the disease, after more than thirty years.

Of the malignant diseases affecting the larynx we have both sarcoma, which is very rare, and carcinoma, but I shall consider carcinoma only, as I have never seen a case of sarcoma.

Jacobson (Operations of Surgery, 5th Edition, 1908, Vol. I, page 657), referring to the subject of extreme disease of the larynx, says: "The question as to how far operations in these cases are justifiable arises. Interference here is one of those instances in which the surgeon may have a difficulty in deciding where to stop owing to the extent of the disease. Where the

pharynx, epiglottis and surrounding soft parts have been extensively extirpated the patient usually gains a prolongation of
life, rarely a cure, at the cost, to put the matter moderately,
of great discomfort."

Jacobson then quotes Cohen, who says "it is most important
to distinguish between recovery and mere survival after operation in these cases." Continuing, Jacobson refers to Prof.
Gluck's article (British Med. Jour., Oct. 21, 1903, page 1122),
doing so only to condemn his views. He says: "To enable my
readers to form an opinion for themselves in this matter, I
will refer them to the illustrations in Prof. Gluck's article
above referred to, wherein the results demonstrate what
especial experience may achieve with especial operative skill,
but this is only half the picture. Such figures as those, showing
the steps in the technic by which such results may be attained,
show also inevitable mutilations by which the patient's future
must be rendered a sad one."

Just here I would ask, can the patient's future be made
more sad by operation than it is before operation, in advanced
cases?

Quoting Prof. Gluck's words in the article referred to in
the British Medical Journal, where he says "first save and
prolong the life of your patient, and do not trouble yourself
too much about the post-operative state; the restitution of
function will be a secondary care, the imminent danger once
dissipated." Jacobson says these remarks are justified, as far
as they go, but they do not go far enough, and he claims,
without the least exaggeration, the fact remains that, of all
the mutilations inflicted by surgery, that for extrinsic malignant
disease of the larynx is the most terrible." Jacobson and
others who oppose operations for extrinsic cancer of the
larynx and, for that matter, cancer in other parts of the body,
seem to forget that the parts are already destroyed beyond
redemptation and that the surgeon is not causing a mutilation
but that by removing the already destroyed parts he is doing
the patient a great kindness in taking away the source of the
foul odor and discharges which are the cause of this toxemia
which results, and at the same time this removal sometimes
ends in a cure.

Further on, in the same connection, Jacobson acknowledges

that if the patient survives he will be free from pain, especially pain in the ears, and much of his cough from toxemia, and he will put on flesh. How far he can follow any occupation must depend upon the nature of this, and how far it requires the ordinary voice, which of course the patient has lost.

Professor Chiari of Vienna, in an address on cancer delivered before the Laryngological, Rhinological and Otological Societies in 1909, states that "it is remarkable how long, comparatively, these patients may remain in this stage without being delivered from their terrible suffering by an inflammation of the lung or a toxic condition of the blood. They generally succumb to the ever increasing weakness from disturbed nutrition and frequently recurring hemorrhages. On this account any effort to cure cancer of the larynx is a real blessing to humanity, and a surgeon is likewise obliged to undertake serious operations if there is merely a prospect for radical cure." To this statement I will add that if there is a chance to relieve the sufferer for even a short time he should have the benefit of that chance, regardless of statistics.

There are two methods adopted for the relief of cancer of the larynx. One is palliative and employs so-called cancer cures, which include injections into the blood, into the muscles and under the skin, and also X-ray, radium, etc. If cures come from these methods, I have never seen them, but I have seen bad results follow their employment. I have in mind one particular case of an intrinsic cancer, a most favorable case for removal, where the patient was persuaded to submit to injections into the blood, and died in a comparatively short time and in much suffering.

The other method—surgery—has up to the present time been the only successful method of cure, and I must here join the large army of surgeons who treat cancer and who believe that in order to be successful the removal must be early and thorough.

Of the four surgical methods employed for the removal of cancer the internal method would not be considered if it were not that some operators claim that with the aid of the suspension apparatus growths in the larynx can be diagnosticated early, their limits clearly defined and in some cases satisfactorily removed. This may be true in the hands of a few experts provided with the suspension apparatus, but the procedure itself must necessarily be in most cases not only unsatisfactory but dangerous.

While I have seen cases of tumors, supposed to be malignant, removed from the inside that have recovered and remained well, I cannot help believing that the procedure is unjustifiable for the reason that we cannot be sure that the removal is complete, and if not complete new avenues for infection would be open. In this connection I wish to enter my very decided protest against the custom of taking pieces for examination, unless the patient's full consent has previously been obtained to proceed immediately with the operation if it should be deemed necessary. I believe there is danger of a spread of the disease from the opening up of avenues by incomplete removal. I fully agree with Dr. John Mackenzie when he says "the removal of a piece for microscopic examination too often means the beginning of the end." Chiari claims this statement to be incorrect, as he says many operators, including himself, have never seen such a result, but he goes on to say, almost in the same breath, "that he does not wish to deny that any incomplete removal of a carcinoma may increase its growth." He then, as proof of the last part of his assertion, cites a case of Knight's in which a growth on the vocal band, held to be a singer's node, was removed by the cold wire snare and recognized to be cancer, whereupon a rapid growth of the carcinoma resulted, and he says "there, as I have long claimed, the external operation is not to be postponed longer than a few days, or at most two weeks after the removal of the piece for examination if the carcinoma has been determined histologically. In this way the intralaryngeal operation can do no harm."

I cannot agree that the incomplete removal of the growth, under any circumstances, is free from danger of a spreading of the disease, even for a few days, and I think, as I have said above, that this incomplete removal should never be undertaken unless there is a perfect understanding with the patient beforehand. In this opinion, I think, I will be supported by most surgeons who have much experience in the treatment of cancer.

Quoting from Jacobson again, who says Newman of Glasgow sounded the following note of warning: "Intralaryngeal excision for microscopic purposes exposes the patient to very serious danger by increasing the rapidity of secondary new formations. The incision of a cancerous growth, or its partial removal, has justly been regarded as a most dangerous procedure, probably because the absorption of the infected material takes place rapidly from a wounded surface. While conscious of the propriety of removing portions of a laryngeal neoplasm for diagnostic purposes, I desire to express my strong conviction that it should not be resorted to unless the patient is willing to have a radical operation performed immediately after the diagnosis is completed."

In proof of the statement that a section of cancerous growth taken for any purpose is dangerous unless followed immediately by a radical operation, I will cite two cases: First, one by Cobb of Boston (Annals of Surgery, Feb., 1905), who reports a case where an interscapular thoracic amputation was to be done and where the patient insisted that a diagnostic incision be made. This step showed that the deltoid was infiltrated. Very sharp reaction followed and eight days later, when the major operation was performed, numerous thrombi were found in the subscapular vein.

The second case was that of a young doctor who came to me, referred by the surgeon who had operated on him three weeks before but had not succeeded in removing the growth entirely, because the periostium and bone were involved. When I saw him the infiltration had already reached the shoulder and, as in Cobb's case, the disease had spread through the incised veins. Three weeks after I saw the patient I did an interscapular thoracic amputation. Microscopic examination proved the tumor to be a mixed celled sarcoma, thus confirming the diagnosis made of the section at the time of the first operation. This patient is still alive and practicing his profession after the lapse of fourteen years.

Thyrotomy as a means of removal of cancer of the larynx is very highly extolled by Butlin, Semon and others, who claim most brilliant results in small freely movable growths involving the front part of the larynx and in persons over forty-five years of age.

E. J. Moure of Bordeaux (Revue de laryngol., d'otologie et de rhinol., Jan. 15, 1920) claims that "in persons under forty-five cancer is very malignant and is more likely to return than in old persons and therefore laryngectomy should always be done in these cases."

In confirmation of this assertion I can cite a case of a friend of mine who had a small growth removed from his larynx before he was forty-five years old only to have it return in a comparatively short time. He then had it removed by hemilaryngectomy, but again it rèturned and further operation was denied him and he was condemned to X-ray, much suffering and death, which fortunately soon followed.

Thyrotomy has one great advantage and that is that it exposes the growth and enables the operator to get a correct idea of its limits, something that is impossible when depending upon the laryngoscope. This proved to be true in all the cases that I have operated upon, as the disease was found to be far more extensive in some of them than the laryngoscopic picture· showed it to be.

A careful study of the literature on this operation convinces me that it should be limited to a comparatively few favorable cases, and that when so limited the results are more than favorable, while on the other hand a complete extirpation, if it had been done on a number of cases unfavorable for this operation, would have saved a number of lives.

The operation for removal of half of the larynx for cancer should not be considered justifiable as when the disease has gone beyond the reach of thyrotomy it, without doubt, has advanced beyond the reach of hemilaryngectomy. It is a much more dangerous operation and one more difficult to perform than laryngectomy and should never even be considered after a return of the disease, following any other attempt to ,remoᵥe the cancer, as a complete laryngectomy—very complete—is the only procedure to be undertaken in these cases.

From my personal experience with cancer of the larynx, and from the cases of others that I have been privileged to see, I feel safe in affirming that laryngectomy, as done at the present time, is the operation of choice in all but a comparatively few cases. With the present technic it is a fairly safe procedure, and when done early there will be fewer returns than by any other method. In my second case, during the consultation, the question arose whether on account of the high

mortality and on account of the mutilation that would necessarily result, and which was likely to destroy his usefulness,
it would not be better to postpone the operation until such a
time as he would be compelled to give up his work on account
of the advance of the disease, especially as he was then earning
good wages as a bricklayer. To that I would not consent and,
fortunately, the patient agreed with me that if he were operated
on at once his chances of recovery would be decidedly better
and he would in the meantime be saved much suffering and
would probably be able to earn his "good wages" much longer
than if he were to wait for a "last resort" operation.

The wisdom of this conclusion is evidenced by the fact that
he recovered and was back at his work in less than three
months and that now, after seventeen years, he is still well
and is earning the wages of a bricklayer and, moreover, he is
able without artificial means to make himself understood not
only by his fellow workmen but by almost anyone he may come
in contact with.

My first operation for laryngectomy was done on a woman,
the only woman that I have ever seen with cancer of the
larynx. In this case, in order to confirm the diagnosis of
cancer, we gave her large doses of iodid of potash, which
resulted in edema of the larynx, which necessitated tracheotomy. The opening in the trachea had to be made very low
and the tracheal tube used proved to be too short so that it was
with much difficulty that it was kept in position during the
night. In spite of all our efforts it came out the next day,
but in the meantime it had accomplished its purpose, the edema
having subsided sufficiently to allow the patient to breathe with
comparative comfort. No effort was made to return the tube,
and when the laryngectomy was done the tracheal wound had
entirely closed.

It had been my intention to remove the larynx without the
aid of a preliminary tracheotomy, a step in the operation which
was thought by most operators at that time to be the best
method, but this forced tracheotomy did not cause me to make
a change in my technic. The larynx was removed after a
complete separation of the soft parts, including large cervical
glands, through a "T" incision, and the trachea was then
divided, cocainized and lifted out of the way and the anesthetic

tube inserted. The larynx was then removed from below upwards with very little loss of blood and scarcely any shock. After the larynx had been completely removed I noticed that the mucous membranes from the larynx and pharynx fell together in such a way as to shut off the pharynx from the field of operation. Recognizing the advantage of this condition, I introduced sufficient sutures to hold the parts together. The patient made a rapid recovery and a year later died from a heat stroke without any evidence of a return of the disease. I saw her several months after the operation and she expressed herself as being comfortable and as well satisfied with her condition as one could be without a larynx. She was able to make those about her understand her wants without much difficulty.

My third case was also one of special interest. In the first place because it was associated with a latent tuberculosis of the left lung. Although tubercle bacilli were present in the sputum, it was not thought of sufficient seriousness to contraindicate an operation to relieve him of his suffering. In the second place, on account of the fact that two pieces removed from the larynx at different times by the same operator (Dr. H. Loeb) brought two different opinions from two pathologists who examined them. Here we have an example of how little reliance is to be placed in examination of sections taken by the intralaryngeal method. If we had not been satisfied from the appearance of the growth presented by the laryngoscope we would have allowed the patient's suffering to increase with the disease without an effort to relieve it. This patient died on the eighth day after the operation. Cause unknown.

The above cases were reported in the Interstate Medical Journal, July, 1904.

The fourth case was a male, fifty-two years of age, and was one of extrinsic cancer involving the larynx, the epiglottis, part of the pharynx and part of the esophagus. When he entered the hospital he was suffering intensely and was literally starving to death. In order to nourish him and diminish the pain a gastrostomy was done, after which his condition was very materially improved and his suffering relieved somewhat.

Gastrostomy is now often done as a step in laryngectomy and it is claimed that it lessens the danger of bronchopneumonia by diverting the food from the mucous membrane closing the pharynx, as this membrane is often infected by the food passing over it and by the pressure of the permanent feeding tube. This operation also prevents the mucous membrane closing the pharynx from being torn by the introduction of the tube for the purpose of feeding the patient.

When this patient was operated upon the parts involved proved to be more extensive than they had been thought to be before the operation. He lived several days and died of bronchopneumonia.

The fifth case was also done to relieve the patient of his sufferings. He was operated on July 23rd and died August 1st from bronchopneumonia. I regret that I did not do a gastrostomy in this case, as the sutures in the mucous membrane closing the pharynx gave way, allowing the field of operation to become infected, this infection extending to the lungs caused the bronchopneumonia which caused his death.

The last two cases have not been reported before and are not as complete as I would like to make them, as the records were either lost or destroyed while changes were being made in the hospital.

In conclusion, I would like to make a prediction that the plastic operations which are being done at present to close defects left by the extensive removal of parts destroyed by the disease and for the restoration of the part of the esophagus necessarily taken away, will be further extended and by the use of cartilage grafts, aided by skin flaps and skin grafts, a very good imitation of the larynx will be made which will overcome one of the objections to laryngectomy.

# XLV

# ROENTGENOLOGY OF THE MASTOIDS WITH CON-CLUSIONS BASED ON ONE HUNDRED CASES.*

### By Frank R. Spencer, M. D.,

#### Boulder, Colorado.

The difficulties of obtaining accurate radiographic knowledge of the mastoids have been many. However, these have been largely overcome in the past few years by improved positions for both the patient and the tube, so that the work of the roentgenologists have greatly facilitated an accurate diagnosis. In fact, almost every case should be submitted to an X-ray examination of the right and left mastoid prior to operation.

Any study of radiograms of the mastoids is of very little value unless one realizes what should be seen not only in the normal but in the abnormal. Iglauer,[1] Lange,[2] Birkett,[3] Pirie[4] and others have all been pioneers in this field of otology and have worked with the roentgenologist. It has been their untiring efforts which have made this work of practical value in the diagnosis of mastoiditis, especially of the acute type. More recently a very valuable article has appeared by Bigelow[5] from which I shall quote freely.

Whiting[6] has emphasized the importance of looking for the lateral sinus well forward in a long, narrow mastoid process while operating. Conversely it lies far back, as a rule, in a wide process. The pneumatic and diploic types have long been recognized anatomically and surgically, as well as a combination of these two. Theoretically a pneumatic mastoid should be the easiest to examine by X-ray. However, a very thick cortex over all or most of the cells may increase the difficulty of recognizing the individual cell structure, thus making the process look a trifle cloudy, when in reality it is clear. Conversely a thin cortex may give a rather clear radiogram when the cells are at least slightly diseased. It is almost

---

*Read before the Mid-Western Section meeting of the American Laryngological, Rhinological and Otological Society, Colorado Springs, February 26th, 1921.

needless to state that with extensive necrosis, granulations and
pus throughout the mastoid there should be very little difficulty
in obtaining a radiogram which will show the extensive
destruction.   However, it is not a case, with such marked
involvement, in which the X-ray is most needed as an aid in
diagnosis but a case in which the clinical evidences are less
pronounced.                                    .

The diploetic type of thick cortex is almost certain to
give a slight suggestion of haziness even when the cells are
normal.   Therefore, the roentgenologist can state only what
he finds and his report, like those from the other laboratories,
must be weighed and compared with all the rest of the clinical
evidence before deciding for or against operation.   In spite of
this fact, Bigelow[5] very properly says, "The X-ray is our best
consultant," or words to that effect; and, "When in doubt,
radiograph; if still in doubt, operate."   If his advice is followed there will be fewer exploratory mastoidectomies
required, because the X-ray affords one of the best means of
determining what changes are taking place in the mastoid
process.

If the lateral sinus is well forward, where it may be uninten-
tionally opened, the radiogram will usually show this.   However, if well covered with dense cortex, necrotic cells, granulations and pus it is almost impossible to detect its bony groove.
The X-ray differentiates densities, so that if all is very dense
in the mastoid process the details are lost.

Cheatle[7] [8] [9] [10] has written extensively upon the mastoid
anatomically and he has the following to say:  "I apply the
term 'infantile' to those bones which retain throughout life the
characteristics of the outer antral wall and the mastoid mass
as seen in infancy.   On making a lateral vertical section
through the antrum and the mastoid mass in infancy it will
be seen that the outer wall of the antrum is composed of two
layers; a thin outer layer of compact bone and an inner layer
of fine cells.   These cells are formed before birth, therefore
I call them the 'fetal cells' to distinguish them from any which
may form in later life and from which they can be differentiated always by their fineness and inward direction.   The
mastoid mass is, as a rule, diploetic, but it may be formed of
dense bone.   If the mass is diploetic, a thin layer of compact

bone, which can be easily demonstrated by scraping away the diploe, separates it from the antral cavity. There are, therefore, two types in infancy: one in which the mastoid mass is diploetic, and one in which the mastoid mass is dense. Each type may persist all through life but, of course, on an exaggerated scale."

Type 1.—"The diploetic type in the adult. In this type the thin outer compact layer of the antral wall has increased in thickness from the periosteal side and is of extreme density; the inner layer of 'fetal cells' is still seen; the mastoid mass is entirely diploetic and the separating layer between the diploe and the cavity of the antrum is much increased in thickness. Whenever the mastoid process is entirely diploetic the outer antral wall is always formed of dense bone. This type is seen in about twenty per cent of all bones, and it can be seen at all ages.

Type 2.—"The dense form in the adult. In this type the dense mastoid mass persists all through life, but the outer antral wall remains the same as in the diploetic type, the outer layer being very much increased in thickness and of extreme density, while the inner layer of 'fetal cells' is still seen. This form is seen in only about one or two per cent of all bones.

"The outer antral wall is often of great thickness as well as density in these infantile types. The greatest depth of antrum from the surface is seen in them and it may measure three-quarters of an inch (19 m. m.). A forward lateral sinus is usual and is found much more frequently and to a much greater extent than in the cellular types. The sinus often comes well forward below the level of the antrum and may reach the posterior meatal wall, or it may even dip in between the cavity of the antrum and the surface. The antrum may be large or small; if large, the posterior wall may be of extreme thinness and translucency, and may have either the cerebellum or lateral sinus, or both, lying against it In some specimens the posterior antral wall is pushed in by the cerebellum thus narrowing the antral cavity from before backward. As in all types, the antrum may be highly placed, or the middle fossa may dip down either between the antral cavity and the surface or external to the superior semicircular canal, causing a low, flat antrum."

If the otologist will bear in mind Cheatle's classification while studying the radiogram and while operating there will be less opportunity for errors in interpretation."

Iglauer,[1] in 1909, advocated taking the radiogram at an oblique angle in order to avoid the dense bone at the base of the skull, which in the horizontal plane would be superimposed. To quote him exactly, he has the following to say: "The radiograms were taken in an oblique profile, i. e., the rays coming from the target were made to center just below the parietal eminence on one side of the skull and were directed through the cranium in the direction of the temporal bone on the opposite side of the skull. At this angle the best skiagrams were obtained. In this position Dr. Lange found that the axis of the X-ray diaphragm was tilted upward at an angle of 25 degrees from the base of the skull (Reid's line) and that it was inclined backward 20 degrees from the vertical plane passing through both external auditory canals."

While Iglauer's technic is a very desirable one to follow, this position can be varied slightly by different technicians and yet give satisfactory results. The important things to remember are as follows:

1. The dense bones at the base of the skull are not superimposed upon the mastoid.

2. The mastoid rests directly against the film or negative when the exposure is made, thus insuring more accurate detail in the radiogram.

I believe the method described and advocated by Iglauer in 1909, or some modification of this, will probably give the best exposure with the least likelihood of faulty interpretation. However, this does not permit the taking of stereoscopic plates.

I have often noticed a very good picture of the tip cells in stereoscopic radiograms of the accessory sinuses taken antero-posteriorly, especially in certain types of wide skulls. However, this exposes only a very limited portion of the mastoids. This position was utilized by Kuhne[11] and Plagemann[12] in 1908 in their efforts to secure a satisfactory exposure. Voss[13] and Winkler[14] used the transverse position in 1907.

Stereoscopic radiograms of the accessory sinuses, taken laterally, often show the mastoids very clearly. However, I cannot recommend this method in preference to Iglauer's.

Ingersoll[15] has emphasized the differentiation, which a good mastoid radiogram gives, between slight involvement of the cells and areas of necrosis with destruction of bone and also the absence of involvement of the tip cells in a sclerosed mastoid prior to a radical operation. Hence the necessity of not opening the tip. He believes, in acute cases of the pneumatic type, with areas of necrosis showing, we should operate early and bases this opinion on the radiographic findings.

Bigelow[5] believes a radiogram will, in most instances, help us at least to detect what the Harvard otologists call a "double decked" mastoid, which consists of two strata of cells separated by a bony partition more or less completely dividing the process into two parts. With a well taken radiogram the deeper cells are less apt to be overlooked at the time of operation.

One is usually able to recognize the following: The external auditory meatus, the mastoid antrum, the internal auditory meatus, the lower boundary of the middle cranial fossa, and sometimes the groove for the lateral sinus as well as the boundary of the posterior cranial fossa. If the tip cells are large these can be more easily seen than the smaller and higher cells.

As otologists we are especially anxious to know in what per cent of the cases the roentgenographic findings are corroborated at the time of operation. With this question in mind I examined the X-ray reports of 100 cases of mastoiditis in the Ear, Nose and Throat Clinic at the Base Hospital, Camp Lewis, Washington. Of this number fully 80 per cent confirmed the X-ray findings at the time of operation. In many of the case records either the X-ray or operative findings or both were very briefly or even incompletely written down. All of these indefinite or doubtful cases are included in the 20 per cent. I believe if the notes had been complete for all of the 100 cases that the X-ray findings would have been confirmed by operation in more than 80 per cent.

Are not these figures conclusive evidence of the value of an accurately taken radiogram? Are other lines of laboratory diagnosis apt to yield a higher percentage of aid in making the complete diagnosis? I am not advocating too great dependence upon roentgenographic findings, especially to the exclusion of other methods of diagnosis, but I do believe the

X-rays are a valuable aid and as such I expect to use them in the future more than in the past.

## BIBLIOGRAPHY.

1. Iglauer, S.: The Clinical Value of Radiography of the Mastoid. J. A. M. A., Chicago, 1909, liii, 1005.

2. Lange, S.: Stereoscopic Mastoid Radiograms. Laryngoscope, St. Louis, 1910, xx, 437.

3. Birkett, H. S.: Exhibition of Radiograms Illustrating the Pathology of Mastoiditis. Ann. Otol., Rhin. and Lar., St. Louis, 1913, vvii, 649.

4. Pirie, A. Howard: Radiography in the Diagnosis of Mastoid Disease. Arch. Roentg. Ray, 1912-13 xvii, 126.

5. Bigelow, F. Nolton: Types of Mastoid Structure with Special Reference to Their Differentiation by Means of Stereoradiography. Ann, Otol., Rhin. and Lar., xxvii, 887, 1918, St. Louis.

6. Whiting, Frederick: The Modern Mastoid Operation. Text Book Pub., by Blakiston, 1905.

7. Cheatle, A. H.: The Infantile Type of Mastoid With Ninety-six Specimens. Jour. Lar., London, 1907, xxii, 256.

8. Cheatle, A. H.: Twenty Specimens of Chronic Middle Ear Suppuration and Its Sequelae, Eighteen of the Bones Being of the Infantile Type and Two Cellular. Proc. Roy. Med. Soc., Lond., 1909-10, iii, Otol., Sec. 41.

9. Cheatle, A. H.: The Infantile Types of Mastoid and Their Surgical Importance. Lancet, London, 1910, 491.

10. Cheatle, A. H.: Three Specimens of Chronic Middle Ear Suppuration in each of which the Opposite Side Was Normal the Six Bones being All of the Diploetic Infantile Type. Proc. Roy Soc. Med., London; 1911, Vol. v, iv, Otol., Sec. 112.

11. Cheatle, A. H.: The Report of an Examination of Both Temporal Bones From a Hundred and Twenty Individuals in Reference to the Question of Symmetry in Health and Disease. Ann. Otol., Rhinol. and Lar., St. Louis, 1913, v, xxii, p. 19.

11. Kuhne and Plagemann: Fortsch, a. d. Geb. d. Roentgenstr. Sept. 1, 1908, xii, No. 1.

12. Plagemann: Verhandl, d. Deutsch. Roentgen-Gesellsch., Sept., 1908, iv.

13. Voss, O.: Verhandl. d. Deutsch. Otol Gessellsch., May, 1907.

14. Winkler: Abstr. Ztsch. f: Chrenh: July, 1907, liv, 208.

15. Ingersoll: Trans. Amer. Acad. Ophth. and Oto-Lar., 1916, p. 241.

## XLVI.

## A REVIEW OF THE MEDICAL ASPECT OF AVIATION.

By Charles Moore Robertson, M. D.,

Chicago.

During the past few years aviation has passed from the experimental to a stabilized form of science. It is now a business just the same as railroading, motoring or sailing the seas. Before the recent world war very little attention was given aviation from a medical viewpoint. Although some thought had been given to this branch of the science as early as 1911, at the outbreak of the German invasion it became a means of hostility and thus it became an important matter for each nation to develop its aerial resources to the maximum extent. In our own country we did nothing unusual until two years after the opening of hostilities in Europe.

You are probably all conversant with the work done by the author during the latter part of 1917 and the beginning of 1918. In February of 1918 I read a paper before this society giving the results of experiments conducted upon accepted aviation cadets.

It was in March, 1918, that the Medical Research Laboratory was opened at Mineola, and the real experimental work of the Government began. Up to this time work done by other countries was individual, some doing more, while others did less in trying to solve the medical problems pertaining to flying or the flier.

The history of the work done by the Government is published in a book from the Surgeon General's office entitled "Medical Air Service," and in this book very much valuable information realtive to flying may be found.

At the suggestion of the Surgeon General's office, Professors Henderson and Schaefer of Harvard and Yale universities were placed in charge of the Research Laboratory of our Government, and it was their ideas which formulated most of the investigations which were carried on at the Mineola Laboratory.

Several years ago these two gentlemen, together with two eminent physiologists from Cambridge and Oxford, had done some experiments on Pike's Peak in Colorado to determine the effects of low oxygen tension on humans subjected to an altitude of 14,000 feet.

The thought advanced by Henderson and Schaefer was that being on Pike's Peak and at an altitude of 14,000 feet in a vertical dimension at any other place would be the same and if they tested for low oxygen tension on a mountain they would get the same result as would obtain in a flight in an airplane at that altitude at any place over a level country or at the sea level.

I called the attention of the Surgeon General's office to the fact that there was a marked difference in air conditions on mountains and at an altitude attained on level country by rising through the different strata of air such as we would experience over a flat country.

The observers failed to grasp the fact that the atmosphere flows over mountains like a blanket, while ascending through air on level territory an entirely different condition is experienced in passing through successive strata of air.

I cited the fact that fliers could not cross mountains easily from the fact that they could sail a plane up one side of a mountain with ease, while after they had reached the summit, it was impossible to fly on the level on the far side of the mountain.

As a fact, the plane going over a mountain experiences a downward current of air the moment it passes the summit, and this will surely cause the plane to fall from non-support, and the aviator can only save himself from a crash by sailing around the peak till he meets the upward flow of air as it mounts toward the peak from the direction he approached the elevation.

For example, if the flier is sailing from east to west he can easily climb the eastern side of the mountain till he reaches the top, when the down current will be so great he must veer to the north or south around the mountain once more to pick up the east to west current of air or he will crash on the west side of the mountain.

This phenomenon proves that air flows up and over mountains and therefore results found at the top of mountains will not be the same as conditions at a like altitude straight up in the air over flat territory.

In other words mountains do not, strictly speaking, stick up through the air.

As a result of their theory of low oxygen, the Harvard and Yale professors carried on their work at the Research Laboratory on this one thought, as they felt that this low oxygen was the one and only problem to be met in aviation. It appeared to me that the test instituted was not a test for the fitness of a man to become an aviator, but was rather a test to ascertain how long a man could resist anesthesia, for that is all the test amounted to, as he was fed nitrogen gas in increasing quantity until he collapsed and his endurance was measured by the length of time he could withstand the poison and the result was registered in the low limit of the oxygen of his breathing mixture at the time he collapsed.

I have witnessed strong men who were alert and desirable fail in this test, while others who were thin, sickly looking fellows, could go much further, and yet appeared to me to be inferior subjects for flying.

I do not wish to say the test has not good points, but rather to say it was one-sided, and if the flier were supplied with oxygen tanks, as all should be, they would not have to come in contact with the requirements of any such condition in actual work in a plane.

There is, of course, oxygen loss at great altitudes, and if a man were kept in this medium without a supply of oxygen, he would be under the same condition as is represented in this rebreather test, but it was a common practice before the war ended to supply oxygen through the Dreyer or Clark mask, which fed the gas automatically as the altitude was increased, and which shut off the supply as the altitude was lessened.

This machine did the same thing for the carburetor of the ship also, as it is necessary to have more oxygen for complete combustion of the fuel gas at great altitudes.

Men doing low flying do not require oxygen and where the aviator was doing high flying, the oxygen made him able to do more work without fatigue.

The test for a simulated flight, which was used at Mineola, was a very poor substitute for a flight, as the tank was large and the journey into space was too slow, while the descent was in no way similar to the descent made by fliers in machines. Then, too, they provided oxygen tubes so the man might or might not use oxygen during the test at any time and in any quantity, great or little, as he chose, which amount was not measured at all, so each individual tested obtained a different air mixture. This made the test of no scientific value at all.

I had expressed to the Surgeon General's office that as there was a mask to obtain oxygen at the different levels automatically, the test for oxygen want might be dispensed with, as there were other things which happened in flying which they should consider, such as the change in blood pressure and the loss of carbon dioxid from the body.

This suggestion fell upon deaf ears and, in my opinion, they missed the main medical question pertaining to aviation.

As it appears to me, the aviator should be tested as follows:

He must be found physically sound, which means he must have—

A. A sound body.

B. He must have good eyesight without glasses.

C. He must have a functioning labyrinth.

D. He must be put through a vacuum test for—

1. Heart and blood pressure changes.

2. Changes due to labyrinth stimulation.

3. Changes in muscle tone for fatigue.

A. It is not necessary to go into details concerning a sound body.

B. Good eyesight should mean 20/20 vision for the one eye and not less than 20/30 for the other.

Imbalance of muscles must not be sufficient to produce diplopia.

C. The functional labyrinth should not be less than 8 seconds of nystagmus unless the man has been made immune by reason of practice, nor should his nystagmus be more than 35 seconds.

It has been found that the man who has a labyrinth with a low nystagmus finding is less liable to vertigo than one with a more sensitive ear. This was brought out in my original paper, which the Government would not accept at that time. The one will not experience vertigo while the more sensitive ear may produce bewilderment in the aviator and cause him to end in a crash from his confusion.

D. He should be subjected to a vacuum test which simulates an actual flight. That is, he should ascend at the rate of 1000 feet a minute and descend at the rate of 5000 feet in thirty or forty-five seconds, which is a fair average flight. He should be examined before and after the test for—

1. The pressure of his blood, both diastolic and systolic, the character and rate of pulse to determine if the blood stream is elevated or depressed, the pulse accelerated or retarded, or whether they remain unchanged.

2. The labyrinth should be examined after the test to find whether or not the ear is stimulated or depressed or remains the same.

3. The muscle fatigue as measured by the manometer or by measuring the accommodative power to determine how much fatigue is felt.

This will give us a key to the expected deportment of the flier and can be given from time to time to show the condition of the man as to staleness. Many of the rules formulated at Mineola were found to be incorrect, as men were observed after training, and this was particularly true of the labyrinthian tests as expressed by vertigo.

Some of the earlier men at Mineola found that where men were turned repeatedly they developed an immunity to vertigo and when this fact was made known, the work was stopped at once.

In actual practice with troops it was determined that vertigo could be lessened and the observations by Griffith at the University of Illinois showed that the vertigo as expressed by nystagmus could be reduced 50 to 100 per cent in many instances and the immunity lasts for weeks and months. Where the immunity gradually lessened, the subject did not return to the original degree of vertigo on returning after a lapse of months.

In the work by Dr. Mosher and myself, in which men were subjected to the vacuum test, it was shown that vertigo was reduced in nearly all of our cases and in many instances to a degree of 50 per cent with the one test of a few minutes. We noticed the direct relation of nystagmus to blood pressure changes. We found that not only were nystagmus and blood pressure altered, but fatigue as represented by muscle strength occurred in 80 per cent of the cases examined. The material we had to pass upon was the same as that which was used by the Government, and thus our findings should represent the personnel of the aviator as he is.

Time will not permit of my detailing, as might be done, but I wish to ask your consideration of the following points.

1. It is definitely proven that men who have normal nystagmus can by repeated turnings decrease the nystagmus time more than 75 per cent and in some cases to 100 per cent, and this immunity, once attained, will continue for several weeks or months.

That cadets trained in the orientator will obtain immunity quicker and can learn to disregard the labyrinth stimulation in 10 to 20 days with a practice of 10 or 15 minutes daily.

That nystagmus is cut in most cases to one-half by a vacuum flight in a few minutes.

That the man who has a functionating labyrinth with the least amount of nystagmus makes the best aviator and this man can soon reduce his nystagmus to zero.

2. That the pulse and blood pressure are affected in practically all during the vacuum test and that where the blood pressure is elevated to a moderate degree the man is most fit to fly.

That when it is greatly depressed the man is liable to shock and syncope and is the worst possible risk as a flier.

That those whose pulse and pressure remain the same or nearly the same are considered fair risks as fliers.

3. That when muscle fatigue is more than 50 per cent after the vacuum test the man is a bad risk, while the man who remains the same or the muscle force is elevated would be the very best risk as a flier.

It has been noted that many men have fallen to death.

These accidents are due to one of two causes: either from a fault of the machine or a fault in the aviator.

Under the latter head would come men who become unfit as I have outlined above. It was determined in the German Army that many aviators fell and in cases where they were not killed by impact with the earth that many of the planes were covered with blood.

On post mortem examination it was found that the lungs were torn or the aorta was ruptured, which proved the great elevation of the arterial pressure which may occur in rapid descent.

When an aviator ascends he is traveling slowly upward at not over 1000 feet per minute, and is going from a denser medium into a less dense atmosphere, due to less dense air tension.

The surface pressure is removed from the external surface of the body, including the lung tissue.

Therefore, the peripheral pressure is removed from the heart and the pulse beat is quickened, the heart is less filled with blood, which lowers the blood pressure. This has been proven in actual flight by taking readings of the heart in actual flight.

In descent the man is coming down at the rate of a couple of hundred miles an hour, and in the instance of the faster planes he touches the ground at the rate of one hundred miles per hour.

He is traveling from a rare air into a denser medium and the body is subjected to a sudden application of external pressure.

This causes a back pressure upon the heart, which becomes filled fuller with blood, the beat becomes slower and more powerful, which elevates the pressure to a great degree with the attendant rupture of the lung tissue or the aorta or some other vessel in the body, if the blood vessel is unable to take the additional strain placed upon it.

Thus we account for the sudden deaths as found by the German examinations.

We thus may have an apoplexy in the brain or in the labyrinth, producing vertigo or paralysis of some vital area.

This was shown in my former paper in citing the case of aviators who fell to a certain distance in full control of their ship to succumb at a short distance from the earth's surface, and who crashed to death while already unconscious.

Many aviators who have done much high flying show distinct changes in the dimension of the heart, it being hypertrophied and exhibiting pathologic sounds or irregular contractions, as evidenced by premature systolic sounds.

Many men during the war were found to grow stale.

Many of these were neurotic types, while some of them showed distinct yellow streaks, while others were unfitted by too much drinking and social excesses.

Most of our fliers had had less than 300 hours in the air, so that they were not unfitted by actual flying.

I showed in my tests that of the first 50 men examined, that 26 per cent were not able to qualify according to the vacuum test, while in the second series of 50 there were 33 per cent which failed to come up to the standard test

This just about tallies with the percentage of men in actual work who failed as aviators and it showed to me that had they been selected by the vacuum test they might never have been accepted.

As aviation has come to be a fixed and routine business with a large number of men, and as it will be but a short while when we will have great transportation companies carrying thousands of persons through the air, it is of the utmost importance that we study the necessary qualifications of the flier and adopt some sort of laws by which we may standardize applicants for positions as aviators or employees in aerial transport service.

It is a great responsibility to be a pilot when we realize that he cannot fail in his efficiency for even a half a second or the ship he is sailing may crash to earth, killing all who are in his charge.

You have read of the new Italian airship, which is equipped to carry one hundred passengers, and the day is here when this mode of travel will become commonplace. It is, therefore, our duty as otologists to do our part in making traveling as safe as possible in this new mode of locomotion.

# SOCIETY PROCEEDINGS.

## CHICAGO LARYNGOLOGICAL AND OTOLOGICAL SOCIETY.

*Meeting of Monday Evening, March 7, 1921.*

THE PRESIDENT, DR. ALFRED LEWY, PRESIDING.

### Facial Paralysis.

Dr. Joseph C. Beck presented a soldier who had received a bullet wound in the forehead, the bullet passing through the ear and coming out of the scalenous region. The rotation test gave a mild response to the labyrinth. Radical mastoid operation was performed, namely a neuroplastic, employing the facial, spinal accessory and descending hypoglossal nerves. The end of the facial nerve, which was drawn out of the facial canal at the styloforamen, was joined to the severed spinal accessory where it enters the trapezius muscle. Then the descending hypoglossal was severed as low down as possible and joined to the distal (muscular end) of the spinal accessory. The united nerves were surrounded by small collars of fascia obtained in the neck region. This operation was performed in July and the patient now has some action in the lower part of the face.

Dr. Beck pointed out that it was of some interest to note that even if there was complete paralysis of the upper portion, still it was possible to secure considerable action, as was shown by the application of a deep sinusoidal current. The operation was not a difficult one, only made up of details.

The second patient was a little girl, who had an acute mastoiditis in 1920 during an attack of influenza, and had suffered a recurrence this year. The hearing was now good; there was no trouble with the labyrinth. There had developed at the end of the third week, facial paralysis due to disturbance at the tip of the mastoid process. She was operated on (simple mastoidectomy especially at the tip) at 11 o'clock one morning, and at 3 o'clock the same afternoon she had full control of all facial movements, which had remained since the day of the operation. There was a profuse discharge from the ear and great tenderness preceding the operation. The preservation of function of the chorda tympani, demonstrated that the pressure was at the tip of the mastoid. This case was presented on account of the rapid recovery of the complete facial paralysis following operation on the mastoid process.

The third patient had recently had two radical mastoid operations performed by a general surgeon. She was first seen by Dr. Beck one week previously, when suppuration still persisted and there was present complete facial paralysis of the left side. At the time of presentation, in spite of the fact that there had been a complete facial paralysis, deafness and no reaction to the labyrinth, the patient was beginning to get some action in the lower portion of the face. The paralysis was no longer complete and Dr. Beck would not operate as long as there was a chance of further improvement. Some cases had finally recovered as late as a year after a mastoid operation. This patient was first operated in June, 1919, and again in January, 1920.

The fourth patient was a man who had been in the Balkan military service for five years as a gunner. Both ear drums were ruptured and one labyrinth was markedly involved. An acute facial paralysis had recently come on during an acute otitis in the left, chronically discharging ear. There was no doubt a real connection with the chronic suppurative condition to which attention had been called by Moure (Bordeaux) who had seen many of these cases, and mentioned the dehiscence of the fallopian canal in which acute attacks were liable to set up acute facial paralysis.

Dr. Beck next reported a case of double facial paralysis of a girl six years old, who was now under his care, but too ill to be presented. There was a history of otitis media and the subsequent development of facial diplegia. The face was completely immovable, it being impossible to close the eyes or mouth, for some time, but at present there was a slight movement of some of the muscles of the face. The radiographic examination revealed nothing and the ear was healed, although there was bilateral suppuration in connection with an attack of measles a short time previously. Dr. Beck had seen three such cases, two of them being syphilitic and described as basal meningitis. He illustrated the above case by a number of stereoptographs.

### Paraffinoma.

Dr. Beck presented a woman with redness and broadening of the nose, who had been operated ten years previously, at which time paraffin was injected in the region of the inferior turbinate for the relief of atrophic rhinitis. The patient was not seen for several years but recently returned. Her family physician had noticed some swelling about the nose and applied the rays of a solar lamp, and immediately following the use of the light there was increase in the swelling. It was the first case Dr. Beck had seen of a paraffinoma arising from injections within the nose, but he had had three cases of paraffinoma resulting from injections outside of the nose. This patient, in contradistinction, had no pain, and the peripheral nerves were not involved, and it was hoped that this complication could be prevented by treatment. A placebo of a mercury plaster was being used and a histologic study of the mass would be made.

Another case demonstrated was a patient from whom paraffinoma had been removed. The removal relieved the pain but the growth was recurring in spite of all treatment. In this case the nose had been injected by a charlatan in this city, who is still performing the same operations. Dr. Beck thought it would be well for the Society to take some action regarding this work and keep the advertising out of the newspapers, if possible. He was convinced that paraffin should not be used in these cases.

### Bilateral Otitis Externa and Media.

The last case shown was that of a boy with bilateral otitis media and externa, which did not respond to any treatment, local or general. Both tympanic membranes were perforated and there was present a bilateral suppuration from the middle ear. Diabetes was suspected but repeated examinations of the urine showed no sugar. Two weeks previously the patient developed a large carbuncle on his back, which convinced Dr. Beck that it was a diabetic affair and the patient was referred to Dr. Sutton for a basal metabolism test and blood test and blood sugar was found in excess. He asked the Chairman to give Dr. Sutton, who was present, the privilege of saying a few words about this end of the examination.

Dr. Don C. Sutton stated that he considered the case interesting on account of the blood sugar. After the boy had fasted all night and until about 10 o'clock in the morning, the blood sugar was .166 grams per 100 c. c. The normal was usually considered between .09 and .10 grams per c. c. blood. In a normal person the blood sugar rarely rises above .15 after ingestion of 100 grams of glucose. Along with the .166, the boy showed a basal metabolism of +16, which was probably to be accounted for in the increase of the blood sugar concentration. For years it has been recognized that furunculosis and other skin infections very frequently show increased blood sugar, and this is also found in chronic arthritis. Frequently when the local infection and arthritis clear up, the blood sugar returns to normal, but if the arthritis does not clear up the blood sugar remains high, even though the focal infection is removed. In this case the speaker thought that one of the factors of the continued infection was the high blood sugar. On a full diet the patient did not show sugar in the urine, but in spite of that the blood sugar remained high all the time. In cases of hypothyroidism the blood sugar remains high and hyperpituitarism usually shows an increase also, following ingestion of adrenalin. In his opinion, part of the treatment should consist of a low carbohydrate diet in an effort to reduce the blood sugar within the normal range, and the patient had shown marked improvement on such diet.

Dr. Robert Sonnenschein briefly reported a case of

### Facial Paralysis.

which occurred at the Durand Hospital two months ago. The patient was a boy aged eleven years, who was suffering with scarlatina. He had had an acute otitis media for ten days and suddenly showed complete paralysis of all branches of the facial nerve on the left side. The speaker realized that this was an urgent indication for operation, and did a simple mastoid operation. Within twenty-four hours there was a very slight improvement, which gradually increased, and within three and a half or four weeks function was restored, and the patient made a complete recovery.

Dr. Charles H. Long presented the following report of

## Two Interesting Sphenoid Cases.

The cases which he presented belonged to the ordinary chronic suppurative variety of sphenoids, the diagnosis of which is easy, compared with those termed the closed or non-suppurative type, but not so the treatment, which is wholly surgical and often disappointing. Among the causes may be mentioned:

1. Anatomic anomalies of the sinuses.
2. Complications, local and general.
3. Sinus habit.
4. Refusal of operative procedure by patient.
5. Faulty surgical technic.

Since he had had the good fortune to familiarize himself with these anomalies by the examination of more than a hundred cadavers, he could account for the failures. Every conceivable variation may be present even to the absence of the sphenoids altogether.

Fortunately the X-ray is of considerable service in demonstrating the size and relationship of the sphenoid cells, especially when they can be filled with a solution of barium in buttermilk, as suggested by Dr. John A. Cavanaugh of Chicago, Dr. B. C. Cushway, also of Chicago, by following the method of Bond of St. Louis, has been able to give a fairly clear picture, but it is of limited assistance in diagnosing the pathology.

Local complications, such as the suppuration of adjacent cells, growths of all kinds in the vicinity must be reckoned with.

The general complications such as syphilis, Bright's disease, and diabetes, etc., all interpose obstacles to successful treatment. Again, when bacteria of a specially virulent type find shelter here, a favorable prognosis must be given with caution.

Almost every rhinologist meets with certain individuals who suffer from a chronic sinusitis of one sinus or another of one form or another, and in spite of surgery, topical applications, vaccines, tonics and change of climate, the sinus changes but little as time goes on.

The nasal tissues seem to have acquired a habit of secreting abnormal material and the physician seems helpless to eradicate this habit.

Whether we are dealing with an acquired habit of inherited condition of the tissues he was not able to state. Of course, there always remained the possibility of there being a hidden cause that had not been recognized.

In considering faulty surgical technic we are reminded that most of this is performed by the general surgeon, who cleans out normal structures of the nose as readily and as expeditiously as he cleans out a post-partum uterus. The poor deluded patient is destined to finish his worldly career with an incurable nasal catarrh, which is avoidable if the surgeon had been as conversant with the modern surgical procedure of the nose as the rhinologist.

It is only thirty-nine years ago that we were told that the sphenoid sinus "was beyond the range of manual and instrumental attack," but we are now able to carve its borders with much satisfaction to ourselves and still more to our suffering patient.

Then we have some patients who absolutely refuse any operation whatever, but thanks to the higher educational standards of our fraternity, this class of individuals are becoming more scarce.

The first case which Dr. Long presented was a woman who came to him May 22nd, 1920, complaining of noises in the ear, pounding and some deafness; she had had a feeling of closure in the ear for ten days. There was dried secretion in the mouth every morning. The nose was obstructed, especially in the right side.

An X-ray picture, taken May 26th, did not indicate sinusitis, or pus in the nasopharynx; there was no discharge from the nose. He removed the middle turbinal and exenterated the posterior ethmoid cells which contained small polypi. The pus from the sphenoid sinus was irrigated and the osteum was enlarged to about 4 by 6 m. m. A few days after the operation the ear symptoms subsided and have not returned since. From the middle of October to the Christmas season the patient was practically well.                                        .

The other case was that of a man who complained of frontal headaches. The eyes were refracted and the pain partially relieved. On November 23rd, 1920, he had the left middle turbinal, a spur from the right side of the septum and the uvula removed. A tonsillectomy had been performed in May, 1919.

Examination of the nose showed a high deflection to the left; the posterior ethmoid cells were discharging at the site of the recent operation on the middle turbinal, and a synechia between the remnant of the middle turbinal and the septum. On January 8th the posterior ethmoid cells were removed and the sphenoid irrigated, removing considerable pus; the ostea was enlarged and a small polypi removed. On March 3rd, the nasal and ethmoid walls of the sphenoid were removed.

Paper, "Pulsating Sphenoiditis."*<br>By Harry L. Pollock, M. D.

Dr. Frank Brawley presented the following report of a
Case of Subdural Abscess, Secondary to Sphenoid Infection

This patient gave a history of meningitis in early life. For more than ten years she suffered attacks, epileptoid in character and was very much depressed mentally, considering epilepsy to be a disgrace.

She came to Dr. Brawley for examination, at the suggestion of Dr. John R. Newcomb, of Indianapolis, December 15, 1917. At this time she was suffering from severe headache, temporal and occipital in character. Slight relief only was obtained from opiates. These headaches had followed an intranasal operation on the left side. The left eye showed great injection of the vessels of the bulbar conjunctiva and puffy red lids. The left vision was 6/12—. The visual fields showed large paracentral scotomata in both eyes.

The nose showed partially exenterated anterior ethmoid cells and a partial removal of the middle turbinal on the left side. Suction showed slight secretion in the recessus sphenoethmoidalis.

---

*See page 744.

There was rough bone in this area. The left antrum after opening and irrigation was negative. The left anterior sphenoidal wall measured 6 c. m. from the pyriform margin and this was confirmed by radiographs. The ethmoidal and sphenoidal walls were eburnated.

As suction at once relieved the severe headache, drainage of the posterior ethmoidal cells and sphenoid was decided upon. Operation on the left sphenoid and ethmoid was performed on December 21, 1917. There was moderate hypertrophy of the mucosa in the ethmoid cells and the laminae and cell walls were eburnated. The sphenoid was very shallow and when a portion of the anterior wall had been removed an opening with rough bone edges was seen in the posterior wall in the superior external region, through which the dura protruded and around the dura as it pulsated in the opening, a thin pus exuded. The distance to the floor of the subdural space was measured through this perforation and a long slot cut with the burr through the posterior sphenoidal wall near the floor for drainage. To enlarge the original opening would have made an opening impossible to close afterward. For about ten days thick greenish pus and blood drained from the lower opening. A probe was passed 10 c. m. from the pyriform margin or 3½ c. m. beyond the posterior sphenoidal wall. Progress was uneventful. The vision improved from 6/12— to 6/5+. The enlarged blind spot contracted to normal and the entire left field of vision became normal. The perforation and operative openings were closed by trichloracetic acid stimulation of granulations. The paracentral scotomata first observed proved to be excessive enlargement of the blind spot.

The patient returned to her home, but on March 8, 1918, came for examination because of epistaxis and pain about the right eye and ear following rhinitis. The left operative field was negative. The right sphenoid contained mucopurulent secretion which was removed with compressed air several times and symptoms subsided.

July 9, 1919, following an attack of influenza, the eyes were much inflamed with injected conjunctival vessels over the globe. There was vertical pain extending to the right ear. The cultures from the conjunctival sac were negative. The right posterior ethmoid showed hypertrophies and suction brought a thick, bloody mucopus followed by relief of pain. Vision had dropped to 6/12 in the right eye. Some vertigo and right-sided tinnitus were present. The ethmoid and sphenoid of the right side were opened and drained, and the headache and nasal drainage relieved. The visual field of the right eye was very irregularly contracted with paracentral scotomata. Vestibular tests were begun, showing lowering of all labyrinth reactions. These were not completed as the patient was given a complete rest following operation.

Following the operation on the right side, the patient remained in an epileptoid state for two hours, but was entirely normal mentally thereafter.

Dr. Brawley saw her one month ago and she stated that she had gained forty pounds and had never known such good health.

With each attack she experienced headache, markedly injected eyes and lids, short attacks of vertigo and tinnitus, lowered vision, marked enlargement of the blind spot, atypical epileptoid seizures. All these conditions immediately subsided with sinus drainage.

In searching the literature Dr. Brawley has been unable to find a parallel case; all similar cases ended fatally. No doubt the chronic nature of the infection and the fact that the staphylococcus aureus was the infecting organism contributed to make recovery possible.

## DISCUSSION.

Dr. Bertram C. Cushway stated that some experimental work had been started in the Roentgen Department at the Post Graduate Hospital in an effort to work out a method whereby the sphenoidal sinuses could be shown to better advantage, but the results so far had not been as gratifying as they wished and had hoped for. There were many difficulties to be overcome in this work. They have tried Dr. Law's position for showing the sphenoid, but it did not seem very successful. Dr. Bond of St. Louis had recommended throwing the head back or propping the patient back so that the rays shot from below through the chin, and the speaker believed this was a better method.

The idea of injecting the sinuses with barium is to bring out their exact position in order to be able to figure out the proper angle, so that they could always be definitely shown on an X-ray plate or film in such a manner that they would not be confused with surrounding structures.

So far very little that is satisfactory has been done, for in most instances the barium injection ran out of the sphenoids before a picture could be obtained.

It is difficult to determine the proper angle for this work, as individuals have different contours; also the sphenoids vary in size and shape and in some instances are absent. He has purchased a little instrument to use in figuring out the proper angle and is making a series of plates, hoping to be able to get a good average angle to use on all cases. At a later date he hopes to be able to give some interesting definite information for taking sphenoid sinuses.

Dr. John A. Cavanaugh said he had reported the use of barium suspended in buttermilk, but had noticed that many of the cases after injection complained of headache. Dr. Hubeny suggested the use of malted milk and Dr. Cavanaugh found that by substituting malted milk his patients had no more headache, so has used barium suspended in malted milk entirely. After injecting the solution, Dr. Cavanaugh always places a little piece of cotton at the opening, and has had no trouble with the solution running out before the picture was taken. After taking the picture, it is a simple matter to remove the cotton. Dr. Cavanaugh, with the aid of Dr. Hubeny, has been doing considerable work along this line during the past year, and plans to present a paper on the sphenoid a little later.

Dr. Charles H. Long said he had been disappointed in regard to the cure of the case and was glad to hear someone say that it would be two years before healing could be expected. In two of the cases he dried out the sphenoid with hot air introduced by means of a eustachian catheter attached to a little electric apparatus, and then applied carbolic acid, following this by alcohol. This produced considerable reaction, accompanied by a severe headache lasting for twenty-four hours. The later effects of this treatment seemed to have lessened the discharge and improved the patient's condition.

Dr. Charles M. Robertson stated that he had seen pulsating sinuses occasionally, although they were not common. He had seen one case with pulsation from the internal carotid artery, and had heard of a case that occurred in the sphenoid sinus in which the pulsation caused the patient's death, the artery having been injured. Curettage caused a break in the carotid artery wall and the patient succumbed in a few moments. He warned that one must be very careful in attempting curettage because statistics show that in 10 per cent. of the cases the carotid artery occupies a place in the sphenoid sinus itself and where a dehiscience exists it is usually on the uoter wall of the sinus. Ordinarily the carotid artery is pretty tough so it can be rubbed with the curette within bounds of safety, unless it is attacked from a lateral direction. If one keeps parallel to the lumen of the vessel there is not likely to be trouble. Cavernous sinus hemorrhage would not be as dangerous as the other. Dr. Robertson had seen the cavernous sinus torn in the Gasserian operation; the bleeding was very profuse but after a little tamponage it was easily controlled, requiring no pack. He used to think this was a very dangerous place, but after seeing some general surgeons do the Gasserian operation, he decided it was not so dangerous as he had thought. In one case he operated there was a terrific pulsation during the operation, which alarmed him greatly and he did not pursue the operation to any great extent after the pulsation began, but the case made an uneventful recovery.

As to the extradural abscess, Dr. Robertson had seen about four cases arising from sphenoid abscess. One interesting case was that of a man who had suffered with a chronic sphenoiditis for years. No history could be elicited, for the man did not seem to know much about himself; he had periodic attacks of insanity, during which he would disappear for a time and would probably be located in the gutter somewhere and would not know where he had been. He would straighten out and get along "like a good Methodist" for a while and then go away again. When he was first seen by Dr. Robertson he was in bed, the breathing was stertorous, the pupils contracted to pinpoint size and he was in the throes of death. It was impossible to examine the eyes because the pupils were so small, and when a light from an ophthalmoscope was thrown into his eyes they moved so it was impossible to see in. The temperature was 104° F., gradually ascending, the pulse was rapid and weak, and there was an appearance of profound sepsis. The only definite available symptom was the discharge running down the posterior pharyngeal wall. The discharge was not profuse but was of the yellow varnish type seen in the suppuration of the sphenoid. The patient had been seen by several men, neurologists among others, and the diagnosis was made of a luetic gumma, tumor or abscess. Dr. Robertson told the physician in charge he thought it was an extradural abscess from the sphenoid and that he would open it if they wished. The patient was removed to a hospital and the sphenoid was opened. It was not necessary to do any preliminary operating on account of an old atrophic condition in the nose, the anterior wall of the sphenoid being in view from either side. The sphenoid was opened, then the posterior wall was broken down and as he got into the sphenoid he could see a mass on the yellow wall. In curetting the posterior wall he got into the cranial cavity, when there was a sudden gush of blood and pus, which almost drowned the man. He thought he had broken into the internal carotid and expected the man to die. The patient was turned on his side with his face down, and within a few minutes the hemorrhage seemed to have spent itself and he found he could go through the sphenoid into the extradural space. The man was operated on without ether and the next morning was conscious and able to answer questions. He went on uninterruptedly for five or six days, when the physician in charge thought he should have some vaccine and give him a shot of 275,000,000 staphylococci. This was done at 10 o'clock in the morning, and at four in the afternoon the temperature was up to 103° and continued to rise one degree per hour until it reached 108° or 110° F., and the man died. There was necrosis of the posterior wall of the sphenoid and the hemorrhage came from the basilar plexus.

In another case the patient had a false epilepsy due to an abscess in the sphenoid. The nose was first operated and the anterior wall of the sphenoid was removed, at which time a large piece of bone was removed from the posterior wall. The sequestrum was at least 1 c. m. in diameter. A little pus oozed from the space, and on introducing Shafer's curette, it dropped in to 11 c. m., being 3 c. m. deeper than the sphenoidal wall. It was an extradural abscess and the case went on to uneventful recovery.

Another case was a syphilitis otitis in which the sphenoid was destroyed so that the curette could be put down to the posterior edge of the foramen magnum. Dr. Robertson thought this was not an unusual process.

He had had one case in which the lateral X-ray picture showed what appeared to be four sphenoidal sinuses, each below and posterior to each other. He believed in that case it was a syphilitic ostitis and the sinus or sinuses were small spaces hollowed out of the syphilitic osteitis. These cases improved on immense doses of antisyphilitic treatment, followed with mercury over a long period of time.

Dr. Joseph C. Beck stated that when he first tried the plan of compressing the jugular, it was purely by accident, because in that particular case he was thinking of the eye condition and the possibility of a cavernous sinus thrombosis. In the case of the man with the exophthalmos reported by Dr. Pollock, although the fundus did not show the condition he thought perhaps there was something behind the eye balls, so he compressed the jugulars and then saw the pouring out of the pus from the sphenoid. Subsequently, in cases where there was a similar condition, this had proved to be a valuable symptom. Dr. Brawley had a patient with recovery ·from a condition similar to some of Dr. Beck's cases with fatal termination. He had always kept away with any surgical intervention from the posterior wall of the sphenoid when it was found to be soft or eroded. In view of the fact that there was so much danger of setting up a hemorrhage, which could prove fatal, he believed one should leave the posterior wall alone, unless one was certain that there was an abscess in that region. He believed most of these cases were syphilitic.

Dr. John Cavanaugh said he was not prepared to report this case, but would give a brief outline. The patient, a man, was thrown from an automobile about eight months ago. His skull was fractured and he bled from both ears and the nose. Hemorrhages occurred at various intervals and three weeks ago he lost two pints of blood. The hemorrhage came like a cloudburst, all at once, then stopped, and it made little difference whether the nose was packed or not; the bleeding would last for about three minutes.

Dr. Cavanaugh first saw the patient two weeks ago. He was very anemic and a transfusion was done. On examination with the pharyngoscope, pulsation could be seen, evidently in the sphenoid area on the right side. On the left side there was nothing abnormal; the septum was pushed over, due to the pack on the right side. Dr. Beck, Dr. Iglauer of Cincinnati and Dr. Perry Goldsmith of Toronto examined the patient very carefully, and nothing definite was decided except that the packing should be continued. ·

The source of bleeding was still a question. A postnasal pack moistened in Monsel's solution was used, and changed every few days. The patient had improved somewhat since the packing was used and the headache had not ·been so severe. The coagulation time was five minutes. Partial optic atrophy of the right eye was present. The wife stated that about two months after the accident, after the patient had left the hospital, she noticed that there was a distinct bruit which she heard four inches from his head. She did not know how long the sound had been present. The Wassermann reaction was negative.

Dr. J. Holinger reported the history of a woman who had been treated during four or five months by a Christian Scientist for chronic headaches on the right side with gradual loss of vision in the right eye. The vision became so bad that she had to give up her work and the eye felt as if it was frozen. A sensation of total numbness was present. Examination showed that she could not count fingers at close range with the affected eye. The left eye was normal. Roentgen examination showed increased density over the whole right side, frontal ethmoid,

sphenoid, and maxillary sinuses.    The patient was first seen by
Dr. Holinger two weeks previously; when intranasal examination showed almost normal conditions, especially no pus could
be seen, either medial or lateral of the middle turbinal.    The
middle turbinal was not enlarged and pinkish.    The patient could
breathe through the right side most of the time and there was no
difficulty with the left.

The middle turbinal was removed, the history and the X-ray
findings made it necessary.    A large mass of granulations was
found underneath the turbinal.    When the rear end was removed there was a gush of very foul smelling pus, and in the
midst of the operation the patient suddenly brightened up and
said, "I am beginning to see!"    This first improvement in vision
was temporary.    It became permanent during the next few days
when the condition cleared up, and the foul odor disappeared
after daily washings with boric acid solution.    There was very
little secretion now and the vision had improved until it was
equal in both eyes.    The sphenoid was side open, so that one
could see into it, and the patient returned to work.

Dr. Holinger explained that the course of this history seemed
to throw some light on the question whether the loss of vision
was due to pressure against the optic nerve or to poisoning of
the surrounding tissues from the accumulation of decomposed
pus in the sphenoid and posterior ethmoid sinuses.    The sudden improvement as soon as drainage was effected, the disappearance of the improvement when a bloodclot filled the
sinuses towards the evening of the first day after the operation,
and, finally, the permanent and gradual improvement when in
the course of ten days of the after treatment, the blood-clot and
the secretions were gradually removed, all speak for pressure as
the cause of the loss of vision.    If poisoning of the tissues had
been the cause, the course would have been different.

Dr. Harry Pollock said that Dr. Beck had covered the points
about curettage in any case of sphenoidal trouble.    He agreed
with Dr. Beck that it is always dangerous to do any curetting
on the posterior lateral wall for fear of injuring the carotid or
cavernous.    Dr. Pollock had never seen a case of cavernous
bleeding by curetting the sphenoid.    He had reported a case of
suspected intracranial tumor before the Chicago Neurological
Society.    While investigating the sella there was a sudden rush
of blood which almost exsanquinated the patient.    They packed
in gauze, with stitches through the dura and scalp in order to
get the patient back to her room before death occurred, but
about twenty minutes afterward she said she felt fine and she
made an uneventful recovery.    The gauze was removed gradually
and the patient lived for at least a year, and gave birth to a
child during the year following operation.

In the second case Dr. Long had showed Dr. Pollock detected
a slight pulsation.    The patient said it hurt her nose a little to
dilate the nostril so he did not attempt to make a thorough
examination.    He believed if the jugulars were always compressed more cases would be found than were usually suspected.

In taking a spinal fluid and blood Wassermann tests a luetic infection is discovered in almost all of these cases, and in those cases Dr. Pollock thought there was always a necrosis, an osteitis of the floor of the lateral wall of the sphenoid, which went down to the body, probably to the basilar process. All these cases required a long time for recovery and all of them had received treatment with mercury and potassium iodid for at least a year, and all but two cases finally cleared up.

Dr. Alfred Lewy said he had also noticed the pulsation in the case of Dr. Long's and asked if Dr. Long had any explanation to make of the condition. To what did he attribute this pulsation of the mucous membrane.

Dr. Charles H. Long said he had not noticed the pulsation until his attention was called to it, and had no explanation to offer.

Dr. Frank Brawley stated that in his case repeated Wassermann tests were negative, there was no evidence of syphilis at any time, although the patient was examined most exhaustively, and there was no history of syphilis in the case. More than three years had passed since the drainage of the extradural abscess.

About two weeks previously he had seen a case with similar characteristics. There was very severe headache, which the patient attributed to the use of homatropin in refraction. There was some delay in gaining consent to examine the sinuses, but when this was permitted, he found pus streaming down over the anterior walls of both sphenoidal sinuses and from the posterior ethmoid region of both sides. The headache was so severe that after a few days the patient consented to operation. Both sphenoids and posterior ethmoids were opened and pus was found in large amount in all the cells. Roentgenograms taken before operation showed a very hazy area in the region of the sella and the posterior wall was nearly gone or enveloped in pus. No necrosis was present on the posterior wall of either sphenoid. The patient and his friends were hard to control and it was impossible to get the patient to remain in the hospital. They were able to get only one picture after the operation and that showed almost the same condition that had existed before. It was impossible to get the patient's consent to further operation, although Dr. Brawley thought the case might possibly be similar to the one he reported, or that it might need drainage though the posterior wall.

# CHICAGO LARYNGOLOGICAL AND OTOLOGICAL SOCIETY.

## *Meeting of April 4, 1921.*

THE PRESIDENT, DR. ALFRED LEWY, IN THE CHAIR.

### Presentation of Cases.

Dr. Charles Robertson presented a case of Vincent's angina. The patient had first noticed his disease four weeks previously, at which time there appeared a slight ulceration of the right tonsil. He became progressively worse despite the use of mouth washes containing chlorin. Dr. Robertson had first seen the patient on the day of presentation and exhibited him so that the younger members might see the condition present. The ulceration was sharply outlined, the edges undermined and irregular; it occupied the position of the right tonsil, the posterior pillar extending into the soft palate nearly to the base of the uvula, the uvula being swollen and elongated. The upper pole of the tonsil was almost destroyed, the posterior pillar was lost in the middle portion by the ulceration and the process was extending along the posterior wall of the pharynx. The only subjective sign was pain on deglutition. There was no rise in temperature, no involvement of the Eustachian tube with attendant ear pain and no involvement of the cervical glands. A smear showed a great preponderance of fusiform bacilli and spirillae, almost a pure culture.

The ulcer was very similar in appearance to a luetic ulceration, a point of interest in the diagnosis.

Dr. Robertson said the best method of treatment for Vincent's angina was the use of powdered salvarsan, salvarsan in solution swabbed on the ulcer, or salvarsan administered intravenously. He expected in this case to use a 20 per cent. solution of methylene blue, painting it onto the ulceration and getting it into the interstices as far as they went. He reviewed the epidemic of Vincent's angina during the war and stated that the use of methylene blue proved very successful in the management of these cases.

### Resonators as Possible Aid in Tuning Fork Tests—A Preliminary Report.*
#### By Robert Sonnenschein, M. D.
### DISCUSSION.

Dr. J. Gorden Wilson said that he had a clear recollection of the previous paper of Dr. Sonnenschein's to which he had referred. In that paper he propounded some puzzles in acoustics. In the paper tonight he had returned to this subject and left a few more puzzles to engage their attention. It was certainly astonishing to hear that while one could with the resonator magnify a tone, yet there were some diseases of the ear in which the hearing of that note

---

*See page 703.

from the resonator was not bettered. One would like to hear a little more about this.

In regard to the question of the relation of tinnitus to the ear lesion, Dr. Wilson had seen cases where it had been possible to localize the pitch of the tinnitus and in some of these cases the pitch of the tinnitus had a very important relation to the nerve involvement. How far further work would bear this out must be left to the future to determine.

Resonators in the study of the physics of hearing have been much used in the past, and the great work of Helmholtz was to a large extent based upon his use of resonators. In drawing deductions one, of course, must recognize that while resonators increase the intensity of the pitch to which they are attuned, they also magnify the amplitude of the corresponding overtones and the corresponding subtones.

Dr. Sonnenschein had drawn attention to a field which otologists have neglected. Dr. Wilson was confident that otologists would pay more attention to the cochlea and audition in the coming years. The cochlea offers a fertile field for investigation, much as the labyrinth did a decade or more ago. One would like to hope that from such work an increased knowledge would come to audition comparable to the knowledge which has come to us of the vestibular mechanism.

Dr. J. Holinger was not sure that it was permissible to say that the resonator increased any one particular sound, in the sense that it increases the amplitude of the vibrations. Through its size and configuration the resonator shuts out other sounds, and the one particular sound for which it is made is concentrated through reflection on the inside of the resonator and through the given volume of air which is in that special resonator. In order to increase or intensify a certain sound, that is, to increase the amplitude of the vibrations of that sound, new energy would have to be added to the sound, and a resonator does not produce energy.

Dr. George W. Boot said that we must consider the forces as well as the frequency of the vibrations. The amount of sound depends on these two factors, i.e., the amount of force is the product of the amplitude of the vibrations by their frequency. The resonator shuts out all sounds except the pitch to which it is tuned, hence that particular pitch is heard better.

The reason why the sound to which the resonator responds is not heard better in otosclerosis is probably because the sound is not really more forcible, but because other extraneous sounds are kept out by the resonator and these are the sounds that ordinarily would start the stapes to vibrating and permit the resonator's pitch to enter. If the resonator actually made the sound louder it should be better heard in otosclerosis, but if it only seems louder because other sounds are kept out, it is easily seen why it does not improve the hearing in otosclerosis.

Dr. Norval H. Pierce was surprised to learn that bone conduction was not increased by the resonator in cases of otosclerosis, and wondered whether the same experiments could not be made on bone conduction to see whether the resonator prolonged the bone conduction. It suggested a very interesting thought that by means of resonators we might be able to eliminate bone conduction in our experiments. One would think that in the use of resonators there would be a certain amount of bone conduction if the resonator was in contact with the bone of the auditory canal. but this did not seem to be the fact.

Dr. Alfred Lewy asked Dr. Sonnenschein to explain in just what manner the resonator apparently increases the sound. There appeared to be a difference in the meaning of certain terms rather than a difference in the actual facts in the case.

Dr. Sonnenschein (closing the discussion) thanked the gentlemen for their kind discussion, and said he was always glad to hear from Dr. Wilson, who had had so much experience in physiology and physical research. It is a fact that every tone has overtones. The first is the octave of the tone used, the next is five tones above that, and the next overtone is two octaves above the original tone. Often there are five overtones or more. the principal ones being the first three mentioned. He stated that resonators increase or reinforce sounds that have the same pitch as the fundamental tone or multiples thereof. It must be taken into consideration that when the tuning fork is used, the resonator increases the overtone as well as the fundamental tone itself, but the latter is most intensified. The fact that the cochlea is being subjected to very serious study at present is gratifying, especially as in the last few years the vestibular apparatus has claimed most attention.

Replying to Dr. Holinger, the speaker said he realized that one could not create energy or matter and cannot destroy it, but one can transform it. If a troop of infantry has to cross a bridge they are always commanded to break step so that the bridge will not be made to vibrate and possibly collapse. The same is true of the resonator. It picks out the tone which corresponds to its fundamental note and the repeated impulses coming at the same moment causes a reinforcement.

As Dr. Boot stated, there can be a change in the force and extent of the amplitude and thereby again changes in the intensity of the sound, making it louder.

Replying to Dr. Pierce, the two cases of otosclerosis were typical and yet the hearing was not increased at all by the resonator, which intensified the tone of the a' tuning fork.

The work had been carried out on only fifty cases, and Dr. Sonnenschein said he was not in a position to completely analyze the physical basis on which it rests. He regretted that he is not at present in contact with Professor Schaefer, in whose laboratory he had learned many important facts. Only by further study can the subject be elucidated and he is making a humble effort toward this end.

Dr. Charles Robertson read a paper on

### A Review of the Medical Aspects of Aviation.*
By Charles M. Robertson, M. D.
DISCUSSION.

Dr. George W. Mosher stated that he had the privilege of working with Dr. Robertson in the original testing and also of going through the Training Camp at Mineola, and as Flight Surgeon in

*See page 776.

Texas, where he put in about 100 hours flying. With the experience gained from these three ends he could corroborate what Dr. Robertson said. Probably 90 per cent. of commercial flying will be done under an elevation of 5000 feet and oxygen lack is not a factor until one is beyond that elevation. The rebreathing test is important, for if a man is to be a pursuit flyer at 20,000 feet, he must be able to stand that, but a little cold in the head, loss of sleep or a little indigestion will make a difference of 2,000 to 4,000 feet in a test record, and is of no great importance for commercial flying. The tests of the labyrinth are important. A functioning labyrinth must be a part of the man's equipment and without a perfect functioning labyrinth one cannot be sure what he will do, but a properly functioning labyrinth is of no great value to a man unless all other impulses come in right; muscle sense, vision and tactile sense when air currents strike on the cheek and in the face. It was Dr. Mosher's unpleasant duty while a flight surgeon to take off of flying permanently three different men who had passed "A" grade, which meant there was no limit to the man's endurance, according to the rebreathing test, and he could pass perfectly in the rotation chair. These men were all right in taking the ship off the ground and were all right in any altitude, but if they threw a ship into a side slip and came down in "nothing flat," those men—apparently through nothing that he could find except the sudden change in pressure—would lose control of themselves. Those men with a blood pressure of 130 m.m. of mercury before they flew had 90 m.m. of mercury afterward. Whether this was "nerves" or a direct result of failure of the circulatory apparatus, the fact remained. They were men who were absolutely unsafe, and yet their rotation tests and rebreathing tests showed them to be of the highest type.

Dr. Mosher thought the important thing to bear in mind was that the otologic test for fliers had been played up as the most important in Governmental work, while the fact is that the result of sudden change in atmospheric pressure, as experienced in actual flight, is more important than anything that a man will show in a rotation chair or in rebreathing tests; in his judgment, too great importance has been attached to repeated tests of labyrinth, and to rebreathing tests, and altogether too little value placed on the results of rapid changes of atmospheric pressure.

Dr. J. Gordon Wilson said he had listened with interest to Dr. Robertson's paper. Dr. Wilson's experience with the fliers had been early in the war, when our knowledge of the relation of aviation to otology was still very hazy. Looking back to that period, it is evident that otologists have journeyed far from the position they held in 1917. To mention but one example, it is recognized that some tests believed then to be of prime importance are now considered much less essential. It has been recognized that the stress laid on nystagmus and in past pointing have not the importance that one thought they had, and no one, so far as he knew, has demostrated that nystagmus and past pointing are related to flying ability.

Dr. Wilson thought Dr. Robertson was mistaken in saying that the authorities in Washington had said that the vacuum chamber was no good. Dr. Wilson believed it would be more correct to say that they believed a vacuum chamber gave accurate scientific data, but that it had been found by experience that such chambers were not suitable for routine examinations.

In regard to the question of oxygen tension, everyone who had anything to do with aviators was aware of the importance of oxygen. Dr. Robertson had spoken of men coming down exhausted and sleeping for hours. It had been found that if these men were supplied with oxygen, they quickly revived and showed less after-fatigue. What one desired was to ascertain the essentials necessary to safe flight and how, under the various conditions arising during flight, this safety mechanism could be disturbed, and how against such disturbances the flier could be safeguarded. Though recognizing fully the importance of alterations in atmospheric pressure with the resulting alteration in oxygen .tension, yet Dr. Wilson was not inclined to give as much importance to this as Dr. Robertson does. Dr. Wilson believes that of more essential importance in determining the ability of a man to fly are (1) his ability rapidly to coordinate the afferent impulses coming in from the ear, the eye and the kinesthetic senses, which are the impulses so essential to balancing, and (2) the control, largely automatic, which the aviator develops over this coordinating mechanism. It is this control, this automatic adjustment of the afferent impulses and their efferent responses, influenced undoubtedly from higher centers, which is conspicuously present in our best fliers and faulty when the flier goes stale.

Dr. Frank F. Novak, Jr., asked how the matter of nystagmus time was observed in this work. The method of looking at the eye from the side and timing it with a stop watch was unreliable and grossly inaccurate. A much better plan is the use of a reading microscope mounted on the side to observe the nystagmus movements, but even that is not as accurate as another method which had been devised at Urbana, that of using a "singing flame." This is simply a gas pipe with a small jet. The gas flame is about the thickness of a match and about one-fourth or one-half inch high. Over this flame is passed a glass tube of a definite length. The flame vibrates and produces a tone like a high pitched tone of the organ. In a dark room, looking straight ahead, one sees just one streak of flame, but if the eyes are moved from right to left it is no longer a single flame but a jagged series of lights. That is applied in measuring nystagmus time, depending upon the report of the individual whose nystagmus is being measured. While the nystagmus lasts, instead of seeing a single flame the individual sees a jagged series of flashes. When the nystagmus stops he sees only a single flame. This is one of the most accurate methods of measuring nystagmus that has been discovered to date. The work is being done by Bentley and Griffith at the University of Illinois.

Dr. Norval H. Pierce said he had not had much experience during the war other than turning something like 2,000 aviators in testing their labyrinth function. He believed the whole thing is a matter of development, and that we probably will arrive at entirely different conclusions in the future than those arrived at during the stress of war, but that the Department did the best it could in testing out aviators by the methods adopted.

Dr. Pierce asked Dr. Novak how long a nystagmus, which is considered normal, is found by the use of the singing flame, and what was the difference between the character and duration of nystagmus as measured by the ordinary methods and that measured by the singing flame.

Dr. Novak (replying to Dr. Pierce) said the test was rather characteristic. The time was greatly lengthened; he could not tell the number of seconds exactly but the reading by means of the vibrating flame is considerably longer than with the eye. If four or five observers watch the same eye and click their watches, there is a variation sometimes of three, four or six seconds, and sometimes the nystagmus ceases, but looking at it closely one sees a little left—a fine fibrillary twitching. The jagged light is very pronounced at first, then gradually gets finer, then ceases for a second, and then stops with a very fine motion.

Dr. Pierce thought this test by the singing flame seemed to depend upon the subjective sensation of the individual and believed he would rather depend upon the old method in examining recruits for aviation than to trust to a man's reported sensation. The inhibition of nystagmus is very interesting and is one of the problems being actively investigated at present. In the opinion of Dr. Pierce, there is an inhibitory mechanism which is disconnected from the will than enters into this phenomenon, and that belief is based upon the fact that when a man is turned and he vomits, the nystagmus ceases immediately the vomiting occurs. The nystagmus does not diminish but ceases instantaneously, and Dr. Pierce did not agree with Dr. Wilson that this is altogether a matter of control, but considers it a matter of automatic inhibition. He believed control could be cultivated under the will. There are two factors, a subconscious inhibitory mechanism and also a mechanism which is directly subservient to the will.

Dr. Wilson, replying to Dr. Pierce, said that control comes from the highest senses to the lower senses; call it inhibition or what one likes, it is control.

He thought Dr. Novak 'would photograph the method he described and get it under black and white, and thus do away with the things Dr. Pierce objected to. In his opinion Dr. Novak had something worth working out.

Dr. Charles M. Robertson stated that the reduction of nystagmus is not in the Army Medical Book. That was in the paper on the results of his investigation, which was published three years ago. In the Government book the statement is made that nystagmus will be lessened on repeated turning, but it does not give any figures at all. Dr. Robertson found the diminution in vertigo or in nystagmus after placing a man in a vacuum chamber for six minutes and taking him out was equal to 50 per cent. in most cases. There could not be any inhibition or control in that length of time, the man did not know what he was doing and one seance was not enough to educate him on control. The usual stop watch method was used in taking the nystagmus time and they could not be expected to have used a singing flame, as it was unknown three years ago, and he would not adopt it now as there were more desirable tests which did not rely upon the patient's response, which would not be accurate.

When they tested a man of average intelligence they had the man signify when his vertigo disappeared. They were never four seconds out of tune on the nystagmus period and the nystagmus time as experienced by the man and taken with the stop watch was almost the same, never being of appreciable variation. If one said to the man, "When your vertigo ceases say 'Now,'" he would say "Now" just as his eye motions would stop. That became to Dr. Robertson constant enough that in actual work in the field he would not look at the man's eye at all, and the same man tested over and over would not vary a second.

Regarding the reduction in vertigo by the vacuum test, one test of six minutes duration was not enough to train anybody in anything, but at the same time the vertigo was reduced. Even if there was a mistake of three seconds, as suggested by one speaker, in 30 or 40 per cent. the vertigo was less than before. A man who had a pulse of 72 and a blood pressure of 80D— 120S— there were certain types of men who, when they come out, had a diastolic of 90 and a systolic of 140 and the nystagmus was practically the same. On the other hand, a man who went in with 80 diastolic and 130 systolic would come out with a diastolic of 70 and a systolic of 120, and his nystagmus much reduced. In other words, some were stimulated with the stimulation in the labyrith with a rise in the blood pressure, some with a quickened pulse, some with lowered, but most with the quickened and the nystagmus the same, while, on the other hand, the blood pressure was depressed and the muscle tone depressed with the nystagmus shortened. Dr. Robertson recalled one big man who went in with a pressure of 80 diastolic and 135 systolic and came out with the nystagmus just about normal, but who had a syncope which lasted for several minutes and the systolic pressure 90 and the diastolic something like 50. Muscle fatigue can be tested more accurately with the accommodation or "near point", which is a very good test.

Dr. Robertson thought it looked as though there was in some an increase in the blood content of the labyrinth—a hyperemia and, therefore, an increased activity of the labyrinth—while there was an anemia in the labyrinth in the cases of reduction of the nystagmus due to a less stimulated labyrinth. That is his impression at present. The man that is stimulated when he goes into the air is the man who is going to come back. The man whose blood pressure is depressed is on the road to syncope and anemia in the entire body with the labyrinth which, if it continues, causes the man to become unconscious and that is the end of it as far as his flight is concerned.

Dr. Robertson had no intention of criticizing the Government; he thought they did their best, but believed they were barking up the wrong tree. He had had quite a lot of correspondence and conversation with the Department, which had all been friendly and not antagonistic.

Another point to be considered was the loss of carbondioxid in the blood. In a conversation with Prof. Green of the University of Missouri, it was agreed that he would take up this proposition at Mineola and see if there was anything in it, but it was never done. He had taken the vacuum test at Mineola and thought it was not good. The vacuum chamber was large and the pump was not powerful enough to produce conditions similar to flight. One man would take oxygen, some none, and some a little, and Dr. Robertson thought he was fair in saying that the test was of little scientific value therefore. He thought he was fair in stating his opinion, as the matter is a scientific question and anyone had a right to express his opinions. He was conversant with what the English thought of it, and Birkley had said that the oxygen want was not of so much importance as it was thought to be. It seemed to Dr. Robertson that the blood pressure change is the dominant factor.

# THE COLORADO CONGRESS OF OPHTHALMOLOGY AND OTOLARYNGOLOGY.

## Meeting of July 23 and 24, 1920.

ABSTRACT OF PROCEEDINGS OF THE OTO-LARYNGOLOGICAL SECTION.

### Infected Tonsils and Their Sequelae.

By Lewis Emmitt Brown, M. D.,
Akron, Ohio.

The tonsil is one of the greatest avenues of focal infection. Faucial tonsil infection may be the origin of the following conditions: Articular and periarticular rheumatism, endocarditis, myocarditis, pericarditis, neuritis, perineuritis, nephritis, pleuritis, tubercular adenitis, disease of the labyrinth, jugular or sinus thrombosis, gastrointestinal diseases as gastrititis and duodenal ulcers, various eye lesions, chorea and poliomyelitis.

Strong emphasis is made of the necessity of a thorough examination of each tonsil in all suspicious cases. Pressure should be exerted to expel the secretion from the crypts and, when indicated, smears of this excretion should be examined by a competent laboratory man. The size of the tonsil has little or no bearing on the infectivity. The smaller tonsils frequently contain blind abscesses from which absorption takes place; they may hamper the function of the eustachian tube and retard free drainage from the nose and upper pharynx.

Tonsillectomy may relieve obscure conditions such as Basedow's disease, otosclerosis, and persistent thymus.

Systemic sequelae must be appropriately treated when present.

Contraindications to tonsillectomy are: Acute inflammation or infections, advanced tuberculosis, cardiovascular changes, diabetes mellitus, luetic ulcerative processes, low coagulating power of the blood, high blood pressure, infants under one year of age and some grave mental diseases.

Complete removal of the tonsil with the capsule is emphasized. It is indicated in all cases of repeated tonsilitic where the tonsils are suspected of being foci of infection, on finding pus or the constant formation of cheesy plugs in the tonsil.

Summary.—1. The infected tonsil, more often than not, is the source and causative factor in the production of certain diseases.

2. It behooves each and every one of us to be more careful and exacting in our examination of all suspicious cases.

3. We must not be misled by the size of the tonsil, but must closely observe the condition of the tonsillar tissue, the secretion from the crypts and the general disease existing.

4. We must not forget that the systemic infection has already occurred and that the removal of the tonsil is merely removing the source of infection and is not an attempt at curing the systemic malady.

5. There are only a few contraindications against operation.

6. If the slightest doubt exists as to the source of infection, the teeth, sinuses, gall bladder and genitourinary tract having been eliminated as foci of infection, then circumstantial evidence is usually sufficient to justify complete enucleation of the tonsil.

## DISCUSSION.

Dr. W. R. Thompson, Fort Worth, Texas: I agree with Dr. Brown concerning the insignificant appearance of the tonsils in some cases with marked systemic manifestations. One of the most aggravated cases I ever saw of rheumatism resulted from tonsils which were almost indiscernable.

Dr. H. I. Lillie, Rochester, Minn.: I feel that at the present time we know very little about it. Dr. Brown has pointed out that there are two types of focal infection, referring to primary focus and a secondary focus. I think that this is well borne out in the case of arthritis where there apparently was no beneficial effect from the removal of the tonsil, which had been said to be in some cases the primary focus; until after the boy has been able to fight off the systemic infection. Glands in the neck secondary to the tonsils may act as secondary foci, so in our search for a possible focus for any given lesion we must not content ourselves with the mere examination of the teeth and tonsil, but we must have our internists go over these patients very carefully.

Dr. L. E. Brown (in closing): Mr. Chairman, I think, in closing, the only point that I want to make clear is in answer to Dr. Loeb, that I simply use the tonsil and the conditions existing in the tonsil as one of the possible sources of very systemic conditions that we encounter. That was the actual experience in every case.

## The Relation of Nasopharyngeal Malignancy to Other Diagnosis.

By G. B. New, M. D.,

Rochester, Minn.

In the author's review of forty-six cases of malignant tumors of the nasopharynx observed at the Mayo Clinic, he has been particularly impressed by the lack of nasal symptoms and the frequency with which such growths were overlooked before a correct diagnosis was made. The tumors include the sarcomas and epitheliomas but not the fibromas and myxomas. There were twenty-two cases of epithelioma, fourteen of sarcoma, and ten of other malignant tumors unnamed. In the diagnosis of lymphosarcoma it may be difficult for the pathologist to corroborate the clinical diagnosis without taking several specimens. The patients' ages varied from ten to seventy years; 50 per cent were between the ages of forty-one and sixty. Thirty-eight patients were males and eight were females.

The symptoms varied in duration from five weeks to three years. They were referable to pain in the ear and over the face and head, gradual loss of hearing, drooping of the eyelid, diplopia, nasal obstruction, enlarged glands of the neck, and so forth.

Seventeen patients complained of headache, earache and other sensations of pain which were always on the affected side, and extended in general to the frontal, temporal, mastoid, or cervical regions. In cases in which the gasserian ganglion was involved, there were symptoms such as pain, numbness, and tingling, over the distribution of the nerve.

Ten patients had eye symptoms such as ptosis of the upper lid, diplopia, pain about the eye, different forms of ocular palsies and varying degrees of blindness, due to extension of the tumor into the orbit.

Ear symptoms were present in eleven cases. These were fullness in and posterior to the ear, ringing and noises in the ear, earache and deafness. These symptoms were caused by the growth involvign the Eustachian tube.

Eleven of the thirty-two patients who had enlarged glands of the neck were operated on without discovery of the primary growth. On microscopic examination three of the growths were diagnosed endotheliomas. A clinical diagnosis of Hodgkins disease was made elsewhere in three cases. Extensive metastases sometimes occurred in the neck following a small primary growth in the nasopharynx. The upper cervical glands were always involved first and in some cases glands were involved on both sides of the neck.

A fact especially noted by the author was that in only twenty-four of the forty-six cases were the symptoms referable to the nose and nasopharynx. In nineteen of these there was a complaint of nasal obstruction, in three recurring attacks of bleeding, and in two increasing nasal discharge. Lack of these symptoms was due to the superficial character of the growth which appeared in the vault or lateral wall of the nasopharynx. In some cases the growth appeared as a small ridge or flattened ulceration, and in others it was large enough to fill the nasopharynx, bulging the soft palate and causing pharyngeal obstruction. This was particularly true of the sarcomas.

On account of the variability of the symptoms present with these tumors, some of the patients were subjected to various operations and treatments elsewhere, such as extraction of teeth, treatment of syphilis, removal of the glands of the neck, paracentesis of the ear drum, intranasal operation, tonsillectomy and operation for pituitary tumor, without the presence of the nasopharyngeal tumor being discovered.

The author particularly emphasizes the importance of making a careful examination of the nasopharynx in all cases in which any of the foregoing symptoms are present, especially when there are glands in the neck that may be malignant. Patients with neurologic symptoms referred to the eye, or ear, or patients with intracranial symptoms, should also have a nasopharyngeal examination.

## DISCUSSION.

Dr. Thompson, Canon City, Colo. (opening): I think the oculists should have credit for a good deal of this, because they are the ones that send the throat man the cases where there is something the matter with one eye for diagnosis. I know that if I send one I send fifty cases a year to the throat and nose man to see whether there is any trouble in the sinuses—either the ethmoid or sphenoid sinuses, and I am pretty sure that there will be something there because of the pecularity of the blindness and the visual field. What we are most solicitous about is that when the return is made to us of the condition, that there will be some reliance to be placed on it. Nearly every one of these cases goes through the hands of the otolaryngologist first, and then the X-ray man, and when the return comes to us we want to have it as certain as the Wassermann test.

I have seen quite a number of cases of tumors of the nasopharynx. Some of them may have been benign tumors, I do not know, but some of them have died. These things are beginning to be common now because of the solicitation on the part of the oculist.

Robert Levy, M. D., Denver, Colo.: This is a subject concerning which our knowledge is rather limited, and I feel my incompetency to discuss it, particularly after listening to this report of forty odd cases of so uncommon a condition. However, this may not, perhaps, be as uncommon as we have believed, being only apparently so because it is not recognized.

The recognition in the early period of nasopharyngeal growths is extremely difficult, most of them being diagnosed only after they have advanced to a degree sufficient to produce pronounced symptoms, symptoms having reference especially to the functions of hearing and breathing. Other more or less obscure symptoms escape our attention, and occurring as these neoplasms often do in children, physical signs are not determined easily, owing to the difficulty of carrying out a satisfactory nasopharyngeal examination. Palpation is our best method of examining children, but this is not always dependable.

. Where my attention has been definitely drawn to the nasopharynx, the condition appearing obscure, the nasopharyngoscope has been of much help in determining the location and character of the lesion, and if we are on the alert for tumors in this region we often will be able by this method to arrive at an early diagnosis.

Dr. William L. Benedict, Rochester, Minn.: I think ophthalmologists should be particularly interested in learning that twenty per cent of the cases described by Dr. New had symptoms definitely referable to the eye; in fact, some of them came for ocular imbalance or blindness, the cause of which might easily have been ascribed to constitutional disturbances or intracranial lesions.

The early diagnosis of ocular disturbance is becoming more involved as we learn more of the cause of the symptoms which so closely resemble symptoms of brain tumor. The invasion of the orbit in these cases must necessarily be by direct extension of the tumor mass into the orbit, often through the paranasal sinuses. An early symptom of nasopharyngeal tumor is paralysis of an external rectus muscle or ptosis.

Dr. Edward J. Brown, Minneapolis, Minn.: One of the gentlemen mentioned a series of twenty-seven cases that were published quite a number of years ago. I think one of those cases was mine. Many years ago—I have forgotten the details now—a man about fifty years of age came to me with no complaint except earache, having been in more or less pain for some weeks, possibly months, in both ears. I found a smooth, rounded growth perhaps three-quarters of an inch in diameter in the vault of the nasopharynx, having every appearance of being an adenoid, and in my youth and inexperience, I proceeded at once to remove it. I submitted the growth to a pathologist, who reported it as carcinoma. The man came to me but a very few times following that, and I lost track of him. His wife wrote to me some months later that he had died.

Dr. Gordon B. New, Rochester, Minn. (closing): I believe that Dr. Loeb's point is true that most of these patients are seen by the general surgeon first; many are also first examined by the medical consultant. The neurologist and ophthalmologist sometimes see them in consultation.

I think I answered Dr. Levy's question with regard to the possibility that some of these patients have malignancies of the sphenoid, in my paper. Most of these malignancies are situated laterally above the eustachian tube in Rosenmuller's fossa, are quite small growths, and are in no way connected with the sphenoid. It is impossible to determine just where some of the larger growths originate.

### The Closed Method of Dealing with Tonsillectomy Wounds.

By John O. McReynolds, M. D.,
Dallas, Texas.

The paper emphasizes the following points:

1. It is the aim of surgery in all parts of the body to secure complete primary union if practicable, reducing the granulating area to the minimum.

2. Rational modern surgery is asking the question: Is it necessary to deliberately convert a clean tonsillectomy wound into an open granulating surface?

3. Reasons are presented for an immediate and complete closure of the tonsillar wound, obliterating the fossa by bringing in proper apposition the denuded surfaces of the palatoglossus the palatopharyngeus and the superior constrictor of the pharynx, together with the overlying mucous membrane.

4. Nature never made an open tonsil fossa. Man is the originator of this condition.

5. Abundant experience has shown that immediate closure of the tonsil fossa not only contributes to our greatest security against all forms of hemorrhage, but also promotes the healing of all wounded strictures without the interference of unnecessary scar tissue which would restrict the free movement of the pharyngeal muscles.

### DISCUSSION.

Dr. F. L. Dennis (Colorado Springs, Colo.): A few years ago I adopted the practice originated, I believe, by Dr. Joe Beck of Chicago of suturing gauze in the tonsil fossa. I believe I am correct in saying that Dr. Beck has now given this up, and I am sure I have, principally on account of the discomfort to the patient for the ensuing twenty-four hours.

It seems to me that we ought to bear in mind what we are striving for as an end result from tonsillectomy. In the first place, we want to get the tonsil. That, of course, is self-evident. In the next place we want to have smooth healing, with as little scar remaining as possible; we want to preserve all the pillars, and we want to leave them just as free in their action as possible.

Thinking about the thing simply in a theoretical sort of way, it seems to me that Dr. McReynolds' procedure does not fulfill our needs. I do not see how binding the tissues together and forming one mass of the pillars and the muscles can preserve the individual action in these muscles.

Now, going back again to another reason for doing this: Dr. McReynolds spoke of the control of hemorrhage. That, I take it, was the reason that Dr. Beck adopted this plan of suturing gauze in. However, I don't believe it is necessary. I think that suturing the bleeding points at the time of operation will give us a very satisfactory and comfortable feeling about the subsequent hemorrhage.

To go back again to one of the results which we desire in tonsillectomies—that of preserving the pillars and preserving the wound in a perfectly smooth condition without contraction by scar—I think it is of the utmost importance to preserve the mucous membrane which lies at the summit of the tonsil fossa. Where this is carefully done the mucous membrane quickly spreads over and covers the raw surface, and wet get an ideal result in scar formation—I mean no distortion, because there must be scar formation.

One of the objections which, it seems to me, might be urged against this method of suturing pillars together is the fact that while we may have a clean wound at the end of the operation, I do not see how it is possible to keep it clean when we consider the infected area in which the wound lies.

Dr. W. R. Thompson, Fort Worth, Texas: With reference to Dr. McReynolds' operation of closing the tonsil wounds, I wish to say that I believe Dr. McReynolds is after end results. If bringing the pillars together will give us better end results I think it is what we want; and knowing as I do Dr. McReynolds' soundness on every point that he advocates, I am very much inclined to have the doctor at least give us further reports on his technic and results.

Dr. Edward J. Brown, Minneapolis: I would like to say just a word: A few weeks ago I removed a tonsil of a young bank clerk, and when I severed the main vessels there was a sharp hemorrhage. I forced the tonsil back into the fossa and held it there for a few moments and the bleeding ceased. Just a week after that he came into the office spitting blood with quite a sharp hemorrhage which required a considerable amount of time and manipulation to control.

Some years ago my small boy a dozen years old had bronchopneumonia. The family physician—a very skilled man—advised me to remove his tonsils. His tonsils were the smoothest, cleanest looking pair of tonsils I ever saw in a child's throat, I think. But I removed one of them as soon as he was fairly over his bronchopneumonia. The following day there was a very considerable swelling of the lateral tissues and he proceeded to get a sharp infection which left him with a damaged heart. I said to the internist: "I am not willing to treat my own children, or other people's children, without some safeguard against that kind of result." "Well," he said, "I have been telling the nose and throat men for years that they have no business to remove tonsils without preparing their patients by vaccine treatment." Ever since then I have refused to remove tonsils without giving four to six weeks of vaccine treatment. A year later I gave the boy five or six weekly injections of vaccine and then removed the other tonsil without the slightest reaction. That is my experience with cases treated since then.

Dr. W. S. Lamb, Washington, D. C.: I suppose the primary object of Dr. McReynolds' operation is to prevent hemorrhage, and I think if the coagulation time of blood were taken in more operations than is now in general practice, the end results would be better for everybody concerned; the surgeon would lose his anxiety and the patient would be absolutely protected against any very serious hemorrhage, because the only other kind of hemorrhage that you can have, and one which is very easily controlled, must be due to the cutting of the superior pharyngeal artery, which, of course, could be controlled.

The other point that struck me as I heard this paper was the question of the end result for the singer. I do not know whether Dr. McReynolds has had experience with this subject or not, but it is an important point, because by removing the tonsils you can sometimes gain two or three notes, and sometimes as many as six notes, in the register of the singer. I do not know whether that would be attained or offset. You might lose as much by the method suggested.

Dr. Harry L. Baum, Denver, Colo.: It seems to me that Dr. McReynolds' conception here (and it is new so far as I am concerned) has a fundamental and very excellent thought for its basis and a very logical reason. It is my understanding that this procedure is not primarily for the control of hemorrhage, as many seem to understand it, and if that were its only object I would be inclined to discard it without giving it a trial as I think the less radical means of controlling hemorrhage will be equally successful. It was my privilege to see Dr. McReynolds perform this operation, and it was my impression that his object was, in a word, to obtain primary union of the tonsillectomy wound without secondary infection and with less resultant scar, the control of hemorrhage being of secondary importance.

The matter of the effect on the voice of singers, of course, is one that is seriously to be considered. None of us can undertake operations on the throats of people of this type without serious consideration of the vocal consequences. It may be that alteration of the structural relationship to which they have been accustomed during years of practice might change their co-ordination sufficiently to interfere with the production of certain tones. However, as Dr. Lamb said, many cases result in an increased range, and an improvement in vocal quality, and I believe the patient must assume responsibility in these cases, whatever method is used. I question whether Dr. McReynolds' method would add to this risk in any way and I can see where it might lessen the contracture and resultant interference with function, and in that way come into favor with those of us who try it.

Dr. H. I. Lillie, Rochester, Minn.: In regard to Dr. McReynolds' technic, I will say that I am very much impressed with it. I do not believe that anyone can foretell the result in the throat after the best tonsillectomy. We have all had the experience of having done what we thought at the time a very nice tonsillectomy with very little trauma, with very well preserved pillars, to see that throat with the pillars coalesced. I think that this is more frequently observed in what I call the high-lying upper pole. Sometimes, however, in the scarring of the throat, patients do have an after-symptom which is rather uncomfortable.

In regard to the removal of tonsils in singers, I think as Dr. Pierce does, when he said that after careful tonsillectomy he has never known a patient with a real voice—of course there are people, who think they have real voices, who have not—to have had the voice injured. It has been my experience with singers that if the plica below is preserved, the resulting scar is less, the contraction at the base of the tongue is less, and the patients are less affected as far as voices are concerned. With regard to the change of register, my observation has been that usually the low register is affected favorably and not unfavorably. So I think in the choosing of any given singer for tonsillectomy, one must not only see the throat, but he must also see that patient, because in choosing that patient it would be uncomfortable for him if he chose the type of patient who would not have a beneficial result no matter how well the operation was performed.

In regard to bleeding after tonsillectomy, I believe that it is dependent upon one thing: The size of the vessels in the particular throat in which you are operating.

Dr. John O. McReynolds (closing): I wish to express my very deep appreciation of the kind reception which this somewhat radical paper has provoked. I have no desire to be dogmatic with reference to this subject.

This is not a perfectly new procedure with me. I am using it invariably in every case and have been now for about two years. In not every case have I carried out completely the idea expressed and which I feel ought to have been carried out.

In taking up in detail the discussion, my friend Dr. Dennis speaks of closing up the pillars of the tonsil fossa and placing gauze in this cavity. I have used that method but it is radically different from one I now employ and it is the very thing that we do not wish to do. It prevents your primary union, and it distends your fossa in such a way as to increase the hemorrhage.

As to the movability of the pillars, I think we have overestimated the physiologic importance of the palatoglossus. The majority of cases sooner or later will lose practically all vestige of anterior pillar. Then, if that is going to be the case, in the majority of cases, why not take advantage of the good features of this anterior pillar and let it cover the wound and diminish your area of granulating surface, which may finally, to some extent at least, be converted into the scar tissue?

Dr. Lamb spoke of the control of hemorrhage and rapid union, and the effect upon the voice of the singer. I have two objects in the operation: The control of all hemorrhage and the promotion of primary union. I have not observed any unfavorable effect on the vocal apparatus.

Dr. Andrews spoke of the bleeding from the pillars themselves. The pillars are not supposed to be disturbed by any modern successful tonsillectomy, I believe. The tonsil is supposed to be removed without interference with the pillars themselves. But if there should be bleeding from the exposed surface of the pillars it would be something that could be immediately controlled.

Dr. Brown spoke of secondary hemorrhage and vaccines. I feel that secondary hemorrhage is something that must be reckoned with wherever the wound is not closed. As to vaccines, I have not felt that there was sufficient necessity for providing against different kinds of infectious diseases to justify the routine employment of vaccines.

Dr. Baum has referred to the end results, which, of course, we all feel can not be sacrificed. We must secure final satisfactory end results.

I feel that rather a large, round Mayo needle is the most satisfactory. The large needle does not produce any more interference with the tissues than a small one. It is only the point that could pierce a blood vessel anyhow, and the tissues immediately close when the needle is passed through. The essential thing is that you use a needle that is not going to break. There is a needle holder which has been useful to me, one which I presented to the Academy of Ophthalmology and Otolaryngology in New York City several years ago. The handle is entirely out of your way and you have an unobstructed field.

Dr. Lillie speaks of tonsils in singers and the mental attitude of those singers. I thoroughly agree with him in that position.

Dr. Bannister spoke of the obliteration of the pockets. The purpose of the operation is really to obliterate the fossa. As stated in the paper, if you use a La Force instrument your dead spaces are all obliterated to begin with, and then your sutures simply complete the work which your La Force instrument had begun.

The question of complete removal is brought out by Dr. Loeb. I first inspect the tonsil that I have removed and see that I have it all, and then inspect the wounded area to see positively that no tonsil tissue remains.

Dr. Loeb also brought up the question of infection. We do not expect to have a perfectly sterile condition of the throat, but we do have just as sterile a condition as you have in your palate operations.

The end results, as brought out by Dr. Thompson, are satisfactory. I do not feel that we have reached the end, but I feel that we are struggling towards the end.

### Radium in Diseases of the Ear, Nose and Throat.

By Zdenko Von Dworzak,
Denver.

It is now generally accepted that radium holds a distinctive place in the treatment of neoplasms. In no class of cases is it of greater value than in the types treated by the otolaryngologist. Radium has a specific action on certain tissues as basal cell epithelioma, sarcoma, angioma and papilloma. The action of radium on any tissue is in proportion to the abundance of nuclei. The more closely the tissue approaches the embryonic type, the more amenable it will be to the radium treatment. Besides the destructive action on neoplasma, I have to mention the palliative properties of radium. I have in mind the relief of distressing symptoms in so-called hopeless cases. Radium relieves pain and controls obnoxious odor and secretions.

Presentation of cases:

1. Epithelial carcinoma, originating in the right side of the throat, invading the larynx, pyriform sinus and the right tonsil. 250 mg. radium, six hours' application at intervals of two days. Case practically cured in six weeks.

2. Scars in throat, the result of an unskilled tonsillectomy. Resorption of scars by application of radium placque, double strength, unscreened, in sessions of 20 minutes each for two weeks daily. .

3. Sarcoma maxillae. Opening of sinus by Denker's method. Cooking of the tumor by soldering iron, insertion of radium tube, 150 mg. for 24 hours. Six months after operation the cavity looks perfectly clear. Patient highly improved.

4. Papilloma laryngis. Tracheotomy was performed, 65 mg. radium inserted between the vocal cords for one hour and 35 minutes. In two months the larynx was perfectly normal. The papilloma of the larynx always responds favorably to radium treatment. In other tumors of the larynx, especially the hemorrhagic form, radium is contraindicated. The results obtained by my original experiments on tubercular conditions of larynx and epiglottis are very encouraging. Only in ulcerative tuberculosis I found a contraindication; lupus is positively benefited.

The neoplasms of the ear, sarcoma, mixoscarcoma and epithelioma have to be treated according to their scar.

Since my last publications on the value of radium application in cases of otosclerosis two years passed by, giving me a good deal of new material to work out my theory and put it on more solid basis. I proved on animal experiments that radium absorbs fibrous and bone tissue—both formations found in otosclerosis proper. Further, I found in about 75% of otosclerotics a considerable amount of uric acid present, and I ascribe a great number of changes in the capsule of the, inner ear to the irritating action of the uric acid.

I recommend the use of radium combined with the Roentgen ray and the knife. The number of patients cured by radium alone is probably very small relatively, but the number of inoperable cases that are markedly relieved and receive months and years of comfort is quite large. I do not, however, recommend radium treatment of any neoplasm that is surgical.

## DISCUSSION.

Dr. Thos. E. Carmody, Denver: My experience has been very similar, but I want to make one exception. The doctor mentioned the brutality in the amputation of the epiglottis. It is almost as brutal, of course, as taking out a tonsil, so that we should not consider that, because in some of these cases where an epiglottis needs to be removed we remove it because of the great amount of pain that the patient has. Now, whether we can wait for radium to take effect on that is a question. I would be glad if radium would help some of these cases, but at present we do not know that it will.

He spoke, also, of the glands of the neck, in the sarcoma of the antrum, if I understood him correctly, and that would be simply from infection, not metastasis, in that case. I have had two cases that were treated with radium some two years ago, in which there was a great deal of destruction, probably due to the fact that the cases were not screened sufficiently. In one of them the eye was destroyed and the whole of the cheek, and in the other one the eye and a part of the cheek, as well as the palate.

The point that the doctor brought out—of reducing the amount of screening in some of these tumors of the antrum—I think is a very good point, because we get a something out of the tumor and still get the effect of the rays on it. The screening of these cases—of those that I have treated—with simply a millimeter of silver and a millimeter of rubber, sometimes also a millimeter of gauze, has given best results, but as in the epiglottis cases I do not know whether they are cures or not. In some of them we have avoided recurrence.

Now, another point that the doctor brought out, which they are doing in Boston, and especially with the cases of amputation, is that immediately after the operation they are using the radium. We have been taught by many that we should wait for some time until the reaction from either the knife or from the cautery had subsided; but if we introduce the radium immediately after the operation we will get the best results. My experience with radium has been so small that I hesitate to speak of that part of it.

Dr. Gordon B. New, Rochester, Minn.: I believe that anyone who has seen the results of treatment in patients with malignant tumors of the head and neck by operative measures alone, and then has observed a similar group of patients treated by operative measures and radium, will undoubtedly be enthusiastic about the use of radium. The great problem in the treatment of these conditions is co-operation between the surgeon and radiologist. Many patients in whom radium should have been used have had surgical treatment, and many more patients have been treated by radium when surgery should have been employed. I believe that in order to achieve the best results there should be a close co-operation between the surgeon and the radiologist so that the surgeon will not operate just because the patient comes to him for examination, nor will the radiologist employ radium therapy merely because he sees the patient first. The patient should be given the treatment best suited to his particular case after a careful consultation with all those who are familiar with the pathologic condition. I believe this is well brought out by results at the Mayo Clinic in the treatment of such cases as nasopharyngeal malignancies, malignant tumors of the antrum, multiple papilloma of the larynx, and so forth.

## A Valuable Method Not Mentioned in Text Books for Treating Peritonsillitis.

By W. R. Thompson, M. D.,

Fort Worth, Texas.

Dr. Thompson, in brief, advocates early deep incision into the infected area around the tonsil, and the insertion of an especially constructed, self-retaining, drainage tube of small caliber into the wound. This tube is made of ordinary red rubber tubing with several turns of narrow adhesive tape taken around the end to form a shoulder and act as a retaining mechanism in the wound. The tube is cut in lengths of about one and one-quarter inches and is inserted small end first into the depths of the wound so that it is completely submerged, the end coming just flush with the surface of the mucous membrane. This procedure is instituted as soon as the diagnosis of peritonsillitis is made, not waiting for formation of pus, and in the experience of Dr. Thompson has given very remarkable results in almost complete relief from suffering in the comparatively large series of cases in which it has been tried.

### DISCUSSION.

Dr. Wm. C. Bane, Denver. When something new is brought to our attention that is of real value we are indebted to the physician who brings it.

Dr. Thompson has devised a surgical method for early drainage of a developing peritonsillar abscess by inserting a rubber drainage tube where depletion is most needed. His large experience and satisfactory results should stimulate us to thoroughly test out his method. Unfortunately, a large percentage of the patients with developing peritonsillar abscess do not apply for relief in the formative stage when depletion might abort the abscess. In perhaps ninety per cent of the cases, according to St. Clair Thompson, the abscess points above and anterior to the tonsil so that early insertion of the drainage tube will, in nearly all cases, bring about the desired depletion. For a good many years I have advocated and practiced the St. Clair Thompson method of opening a peritonsillar abscess. The opening is made with angular forceps like the Hartmann nasal dressing forceps. (Forceps exhibited.)

If an imaginary horizontal line be drawn through the base of the uvula, and a vertical line along the anterior pillar, they will intersect above the tonsil. The point for entrance with the forceps is one centimeter external to the meeting of these two lines. The closed end of the forceps is thrust backward and outward until the abscess is entered when the blades are spread and withdrawn, giving vent to the pus, and producing ample opening for drainage.

Dr. John Robinson, Colorado Springs: I would like explained just how Dr. Thompson makes his diagnoses between the ordinary tonsillitis and peritonsillitis so as to early determine his time of drainage.

Dr. Frank Albert Burton, San Diego, Cal.: I want to personally thank Dr. Thompson for calling our attention to this surgical intervention which has given such satisfaction in his practice. All laryngologists, from time to time, have to deal with peritonsillar abscesses which do not respond well to the usual surgical procedure. I have had a few such cases during the past year or so in which I have felt justified in following the advice of a certain laryngologist, whose name I do not recall, and removed the tonsil. This procedure does not especially appeal to me, but in each case the result was most satisfactory. I believe Dr. Thompson's method, in such cases, would be worth while. Following the operation in these cases, and in fact, as part of the postoperative treatment of all adult tonsillectomies, I have my patient use an aspirin gargle, dissolving five to ten grains of aspirin in a half glass of water as often as desired but regularly five minutes before each nourishment. This makes eating less uncomfortable, with the natural result that the patient loses less weight and strength.

Dr. Thos. E. Carmody, Denver: Dr. Bane brought out one point that I feel ought to be enlarged upon a little, and that is you practically always find your abscess in the supertonsillar fossa. You can drain those situated below by putting a forceps into them, slipping it under the anterior pillar with practically no trouble.

Another point which Dr. Thompson also mentioned—that most of these cases do not come to us until they are pretty well advanced, but the same thing applies. For a number of years I have been using forceps, but I have used a long pair of hemostatic forceps, after the method published by Pierce, of simply going into the abscess behind the pillars or under the plica and getting drainage. That is the natural point of drainage, and it is the damming of superior crypt that causes your supertonsillar abscess, which it should be called instead of peritonsillar as it practically always drains down. Dr. Thompson gets the same result because he is simply bringing it by the aid of gravity down along the posterior portion of the anterior pillar. The method brought out by Dr. Burton of simply removing the tonsil where you have an abscess I have not tried, although I have talked with a number of men who have, but it has happened that most of the cases that I have seen I have been able to drain in this other way. It had advanced so far and the abscess was so large that it really had broken through.

The method of Dr. Bane of putting forceps through the pillar is good, and unless it causes too much inconvenience to the patient, should be a little bit larger. It is a fact that the patient will not stand too large forceps. I can understand that because I have had an abscess myself.

Dr. Henry L. Baum, Denver: It occurs to me that Dr. Thompson's method certainly has a great deal to recommend it. It has been my experience in these cases that my patients have to endure from one to three days of suffering before I can give them relief, when they consult me early in the disease. In other words, relief can be given only by incision after pus has formed, opening the infiltrated tissues previous to breaking down having so far been unproductive of good results in my own experience. Incision is, of course, of immediate value in the late cases, but it is not this class of cases that Dr. Thompson is dealing with, and I feel that he has given us something which seems to me original and is certainly worth a trial. If it is as successful in my hands as it has been in his, I shall never cease to thank him for having helped me out of a very unpleasant experience in every case of this sort with which.I come in contact.

It appeals to me that drainage through this small opening is probably incomplete, because my experience with drainage tubes has been that if they are not very large they do not drain very well. Fibrin quickly forms from these secretions when in contact with a foreign substance, and would no $_d$o$_u$b$_t$ soon obstruct the tube, hence it may be that the drainage around the tube is more important than that through it.

Dr. Frank R. Spencer, Boulder: If I remember rightly, the late Dr. W. L. Ballenger advocated elevating the anterior pillar in order to get better drainage, and simply dissected the anterior pillar very much as you do in the beginning of a tonsillectomy. That method has been very painful, and evidently has not proven satisfactory. I have been an advocate of the method Dr. Bane mentioned of using a pair of forceps. I originally used either a tonsil knife or a sharp bistoury, but there are a few cases in which severe hemorrhage has followed the use of any sharp instrument. A pair of forceps will not cut, and you can spread them. Any method of opening a peritonsilar abscess is apt to be extremely painful.

Dr. John O. McReynolds, Dallas, Texas: I had the pleasure of hearing Dr. Thompson's original presentation of this subject at Houston last April, and I simply rise to say that I am convinced that the procedure has a very distinct degree of merit. I think there are two avenues through which you may reach the peritonsillar area successfully and then insert this tube as Dr. Thompson recommends. You can either introduce it through the anterior pillar, or you could introduce it in that space between the tonsil and the anterior pillar by simply opening up that channel as suggested by Dr. Bane with artery forceps and introducing it in that way into the peritonsillar abscess.

### The Three-Fold Manifestations of Fifth Nerve Disturbances.
#### By B. F. Andrews, M. D.
#### Chicago, Ill.

The trifacial nerve is important to those who limit their practice to the eye, ear, nose and throat, not only because of its distribution and function, but because of its interrelation to these organs, to the general system, and also the variety of its reactions to disturbing stimuli. It is the great sensory nerve of the head. It supplies every cavity in the head, including the cranial, and its meninges, with sense carrying fibers. Sensations in the orbit are made manifest through this nerve. The nasal mucosa and that lining the paranasal sinuses, namely, the frontal, the ethmoid, the sphenoid, and the maxillary, derive their sensory filaments from the same nerve.

After detailing the anatomy of the trifacial nerve and mentioning the connections it formed with all the motor nerves of the eye, the author states that irritations of the fifth nerve manifest themselves in disturbances of sensation, increased muscular activity and vasomotor changes.

As familiar examples of sensory disturbances, he mentions headache due to eyestrain or fatigue; earache due to irritations around the roots of teeth, or associated with tonsillectomies; tender scalp during a severe cold in the head; neuralgia and headaches of nasal origin, made worse during seasons of inclement weather, etc.

Familiar examples of motor manifestations are not so numerous as those of sensory.

After discussing the vasomotor manifestations resulting from peripheral irritations, the author refers to the retrograde changes which take place following active disturbances of the sympathetic.

There are three stages in long contined inflammatory processes: First, hyperemic, or the vessel dilatation stages. Second, hypertrophic or tissue overfeeding stage. Third, the atrophic or tissue contraction and starvation stage. Atrophies, whether in the nose, Eustachian tube, or ear, should be looked upon as end-products of fifth nerve disturbance. May there not be some causal relation between such disturbances and otosclerosis, or between them and intractable corneal ulcers?

## DISCUSSION.

Dr. Edward J. Brown, Minneapolis, Minn.: I have found that injecting the ganglion is not always an easy thing to do. I have been able to give temporary good results by injecting the peripheral branches. I think Dr. Andrews is right in his statement that if we carefully examine our cases and make a diagnosis of conditions, we will eliminate many of the cases that seem to require operation.

I remember one man of 80 years whom I relieved for some years by washing out his antrum. Later he went to Dr. Ball of St. Paul and was given further years of relief by an injection of the nerves. Still later, he returned to me with the same old trouble, and I was able to relieve him again by washing the antrum.

### Observations on the Management of Tuborrhea. ..Report of a Series of Twenty-five Cases.

By H. I. Lillie, M. D.,
Rochester, Minn.

The nose blowing habit is an important etiologic factor in all cases of suppurative otitis media. In the tuborrhea type of otitis media the nose blowing habit may be the causal factor of the continuance of the discharge. The usual manner in which a patient blows the nose is closing off the unobstructed side and forcibly clearing the obstructed side. The increased nasopharyngeal pressure causes the tube to be opened and the diseased ear, having lost the protection of an intact membranum typanum and the air pad within the ear, is filled with nasal secretions. Sneezing is the normal manner of clearing the nose, and during the process both sides are freed. When obstructions are present in the anterior nares, whether anatomic, physiologic, or, particularly, a combination of both, there is added danger of increased unilateral nasopharyngeal pressure and of blowing secretions into the tube and middle ear.

In studying twenty-six cases in the Mayo Clinic of tuborrhea in adults who complained of the discharge more than the discomfort, it was found that in fifteen, 57.69 per cent, the obstruction was combined anatomic and physiologic. Eight patients, 30.76 per cent, had no further trouble after they had learned to blow the nose with both nostrils open. No other treatment was used. No patient of this group had any demonstrable suppurative process in the nose and throat. Six patients had been advised elsewhere to undergo the radical mastoid operation. All six responded to our conservative treatment in a few days, and there was obviously no need for radical procedures. Thirteen patients had operations on the septum. In the local treatment of the ear all lavage was avoided, and the ear cleaned by means of suction or mechanically with cotton application. Two patients improved under the Yankaur tube procedure.

Conclusions from this study of cases are that: (1) Tuborrhea is frequently the result of incorrectly blowing the nose; (2) pathologic conditions other than suppurative processes, particularly anterior nasal obstructions in adult patients, are indirect causative factors of the condition, and (3) clinical classification of suppurative processes within the middle ear should be more exact.

### DISCUSSION.

Dr. William E. Callfas, Omaha, Neb. (opening): I want to relate a little experience of Dr. Jos. Beck in connection with trichloracetic acid. He conceived the idea from Dr. Harold Gifford, who uses trichloracetic acid to obliterate the tear sac. Dr. Beck thought this might be used to obliterate the Eustachian tube, but he had a facial paralysis following the use of the trichloracetic acid. The facial nerve was probably exposed. I think, however, that trichloracetic acid, can be used if care is taken not to have the applicator swab too moist.

Dr. Edward J. Brown, Minneapolis, Minn.: In a case of double tuborrhea I introduced through both tubes by means of a catheter, a wire with a tip wound with cotton and soaked with strong carbolic acid. One ear has been perfectly well during the past five years. The other was well until a few weeks ago when the man returned for a few days' treatment.

Dr. Lillie (closing): The point I wanted to make particularly in this paper was that the mere correction of the nose blowing habit in about twenty-five per cent of this type of tuborrhea will correct the tuborrhea without any management of the tube itself. This group, which I have talked about, has been the chronic type in adult patients. In cases of small perforations, attempts are made to close them by whatever means we can.

The group is interesting. We have seen a large number since the preparation of this paper, and it is greatly increasing. More careful clinical classification of suppurative diseases of the middle ear and appendages is to be desired.

### Primary Sarcoma of the Middle Ear.

By Wm. F. Callfas, M. D.,

Omaha, Neb.

Forty-one cases of sarcoma of the ear have been reported but sections were made in only thirty. In eleven more none were made. Also in the cases reported the origin was not in the middle ear in all cases, or at least was doubtful. Of the forty-one cases reported, the tumor was primarily in the tympanic cavity in twenty-four cases, as nearly as could be ascertained. In all the forty-one cases there was more or less involvement of the middle ear. Of all the cases reported, where diagnosis of sarcoma by sections were made, seventeen were probably primary in the middle ear.

Clinically, the cases seem to fall in two distinct groups. First, rapid growing, very malignant, occurring in children, and are always fatal, which run their course in from a few weeks to a year. In this group of forty-one cases, twenty-one occurred in persons below the age of twenty, eleven at the age of forty or over. In children and young adults operative interference seemed to increase the rapidity of the growth, while in the cases after the age of forty, the course seemed to be retarded by the operation. The clinical pictures were variable.

Deafness was almost universal. Pain in varying degrees in nearly all cases. Polypi or some external growth presented in the canal in twenty-six cases. Discharge from the ear in twenty cases. The irritative discharge was the only hint of etiology given in any case except a few of the juvenile cases, where symptoms dated from traumatism. Hemorrhage from the ear occurred in ten cases. Facial paralysis in seventeen.

Treatment: This was operative in nearly all cases. Radical operation was done in twelve cases. Simple removal of polypi one or more times, in ten cases. Only one case treated by X-ray was without effect in delaying the fatal outcome. There are only three cases reported where a cure can probably be claimed. Only one case recorded was treated by radium, but the pathologist diagnosed it as a malignant growth, not specifying whether sarcomatous or carcinomatous. The patient was given twelve applications of radium of from twenty to thirty minutes' duration over a period of one year. The growth had decreased in size, and the treatment was being continued at the time of this report.

Within the past four years I have had two cases of primary sarcoma of the middle ear.

Case 1. Date, October, 1916; made, age 33; occupation, farmer. Had discharging ear for two years, followed by pain and loss of hearing. A growth filled the middle ear, which bled freely. A portion of this growth, removed and sectioned, proved to be spindle-celled sarcoma. The middle ear and adjacent canal were thoroughly curetted and followed by radium treatment. Patient was given two treatments, 32 mg. of radium, time two hours, and in February of the following year 16 mg. of radium was used, time two hours. Patient has returned several times for examination, has improved in health and gained in weight. Up to the present time there is no sign of a return of the growth.

Case 2. Date, October, 1919; female, aged 32; housewife. Had right ear trouble when nine years old. Had much pain, followed by discharge which lasted only a few days. This was followed by right facial paralysis, which has existed for twenty-three years. When first seen, at the office, in October, 1919, she had severe pain in and around the right ear, was losing weight, and was able to walk only by assistance. A bluish mass filled the middle ear. An operation was performed much the same as for a radical mastoid. The middle ear was thoroughly curetted; the mass extended into the petrous portion of the temporal bone. When this was curetted and compeltely removed, the wall was perfectly smooth, and the internal carotid artery exposed at the bottom of the canal. A microscopic examination of the removed mass proved to be fibro-sarcoma. A tube of radium was inserted on September 24, 1919; 32 mg. of radium, time nine hours, September 25, 1919, 32 mg. of radium, time eight and one-half hours. Patient has returned several times for observation and was given one more treatment of radium. Following the operation and radium, she was free from pain for about one week. At about this time she suffered from a radium burn. This lasted for several weeks. She is now free from pain, has gained in weight, and is doing her housework.

While it may be too soon to say what the final outcome will be in these two cases, I think this much can at least be said, that the radium treatment has given the patients comfort and a new lease on life, if not a permanent cure.

## DISCUSSION.

Dr. Callfas (closing): In regard to Dr. Loeb's remarks, we never depend upon the clinical findings. We want to at least make sure, if we can, and we always have microscopic examinations made by a reliable man. The pathologist of the University is a man of a great deal of experience, and when he gives a report of carcinoma we can usually bank on it. Of course, we combine our clinical findings in each of these cases.

If there is some way of eliminating this pain following radium, I would like to know it. We have had a number of cases where the pain after the radium treatment was very severe, and if there is some way of avoiding that, I would be very glad to know of it.

### The Relation of the Eye to the Ear, Nose and Throat.

By Hanau W. Loeb, M. D., and Meyer Wiener, M. D.

St. Louis, Mo.

The writers announce that their experience and a careful survey of the literature force upon them the following conclusions:

1. Lesions of the eye and its adnexa occur far more frequently from pathologic processes involving the nose and paranasal sinuses than is generally accepted.

2. A study of the minor processes would result in a more fruitful yield, than that which has followed the interest in the exceptional and striking cases manifested up to the present time.

3. It is necessary to examine and to study in detail the nose and paranasal sinuses in all eye conditions for which they may be responsible, including conjunctivitis, lacrymal sac conditions, orbital cellulitis and abscess, corneal ulceration, iritis and its associates, maturing cataract, retinal hemorrhage, retinal detachment, optic neuritis, ocular and retrobulbar, optic atrophy, glaucoma, reduction of vision, diminution of the field and functional disturbances not otherwise explained.

4. It is most important to examine for and to record any change in the orbital or ocular tissues in all cases of acute or chronic suppurative processes involving the paranasal sinuses.

5. Persistent and intelligent study along these lines must bring about a solution of many of the vexing problems that have been uncovered by the casual study of the relation between the eye and the upper respiratory tract.

### DISCUSSION.

Dr. Frank R. Spencer, Bouler, Colo. (opening): Mr. Chairman and members: I have been deeply impressed by all that Dr. Loeb has said. He has covered the subject during the past few years in the very thorough manner. In the practice of ophthalmology we are anxious to know what percentage of these cases might have been attributed to sinus diseases which may have existed in childhood and maybe in adult life. At otolaryngologists we are anxious to do all we can to cure these cases. Dean's work on sinuses during the past few years, as well as that of Onodi and others, is yielding very gratifying results and shows that sinus diseases are much more prevalent in children than we had formerly thought. Doubtless we will find that more of the eye diseases in children are due to nasal disease than we had formerly thought.

Gradle's work, and also Peter's, in measuring the blind spot, as Dr. Loeb has intimated is of great value. The work can be done, of course, with a Bjerrum screen, but we prefer to use Peter's campimeter because it is easier of manipulation. We have been especially interested in watching cases of hyperplastic ethmoiditis and sphenoiditis because we see so many of these cases and the effect upon the eyes. I agree absolutely with Dr. Loeb when he says that a nasal examination is necessary in any case of eye pathology, because without such an examination you are not doing your best for the patient.

An X-ray examination of the nasal accessory sinuses in hyperplastic disease is sometimes disappointing, because there is very little or nothing which can be demonstrated in the radiogram. I am reminded in this connection of what Dr. Sweet of Philadelphia said regarding penetrating rays in searching for very small foreign bodies in the eye. He states that if the X-rays are too penetrating, the small particle of steel, copper or lead will sometimes not show on the film. That is sometimes a surprise because we do not expect a small white patch of exudate to cast a shadow, but we do expect a metallic foreign body to cast a shadow.

Now, probably in cases of hyperplastic disease of the sinuses—and this is the point I want to bring out—the rays may be too penetrating and we do not get the best results from the X-ray examination. Of course, we know there is rarefaction of bone in cases of hyperplasia, so that less penetrating rays might show the pathology.

I have also been interested in watching the cases which Sluder has designated as lower half headache, and which has its beginning in the sphenopalatine ganglion. Sometimes we see the congestion in the region of the ganglion of the sympathetic, and the eye can be relieved either by the proper nasal treatment or by surgery of the nose.

Dr. Melville Black, Denver: It seems to me the accepted position should be that when a patient is going blind from a postoptic neuritis, and no cause can be found, that the posterior ethmoid and sphenoid cells should be opened and dealt with according to the indications at the time of the operation. Other possible causes, such as focal infections from teeth, tonsils, etc., should not be neglected by any means, but they should not be followed too long to the neglect of a possible nasal sinus causation.

Dr. H. L. Lillie, Rochester, Minn.: I think that the intranasal method of drainage of well-chosen cases of dacryocystitis is a well-directed procedure. It is easily accomplished and gives good results. However, I am one of those who feels that we must not believe all dacryocystitis is due to an ethmoid involvement. The work of Shaffer is particularly comprehensive in the anatomic consideration of the sac and the ducts. I believe that the dacryocystitis may set up an involvement of the adjacent ethmoid secondarily. My experience in operating these nasal conditions has been that the involvement of the ethmoid is usually more adjacent to the sac, so it would take a great deal to prove to me that a small area of the involvement of the ethmoid immediately adjacent to the sac could secondarily involve that sac. It seems more reasonable for me to believe that the involvement comes from the dacryocystitis, in those cases not showing a frank ethmoiditis.

Dr. McReynolds, Dallas, Tex.: We had hoped that the X-ray would do something that would enable us to say, "Here we have a distinct lesion and here we have not," but as brought out here, the X-ray does not always show even definite foreign bodies within these cavities, or within the eye.

At the Atlantic City meeting of the American Medical Association I reported a number of foreign bodies within the eve so small that the X-ray positively would not show them, and yet they could be seen with the ophthalmoscope and were removed.

Dr. Edward J. Brown, Minneapolis, Minn.: I take pride in the fact that some thirty years ago I read before one of our local medical societies a paper in which I made the claim that a great deal of eye trouble came from nasal conditions. About that time a very remarkable paper was published, I think by Ziem, showing that much disease of the eye came from nasal diseases and especially from infected sinuses.

Dr. William L. Benedict, Rochester, Minn.: I think that every few years the subject of relation of the eye to the ear, nose and throat should be well reviewed. It has not been very long since in my own interneship, we made a careful search through our records and of the cases that were passing through our hands at the University of Michigan, of the eye conditions which could definitely be traced to disease about the nose and throat. We concluded from a review of our cases that there were very few eye conditions that were due to the trouble in the nose and throat.

A recent work by Schaeffer of Philadelphia, on "The Nose and the Olfactory Organ," has brought out the importance of paranasal sinus diseases in relation to dacryocystitis. The fact that we have so much purulent discharge from infected lacrymal sacs which keeps up in spite of more or less adequate drainage and treatment, has led us to believe that the ethmoids were involved more frequently that we had thought for, and since adopting the intranasal method of treating dacryocystitis we have discovered cases of ethmoiditis which had not been discovered by previous examination.

In reference to the question of whether choked disc follows disease of the sinus, personally I believe it does not, and I say that in spite of the fact that case reports do not seem to bear us out in that respect.

I think our greatest difficulty lies in choked disc. I agree perfectly with Dr. Wiener that we have borderline cases difficult to diagnose, and we must know that with choked disc we may have neuritis as a result of the choked disc. However, there are certain features accompanying inflammation which do not accompany pappilitis or edema of the nerve. If the inflammation should occur with its features strongly brought out, there would be no reason for confusing the two, but the more carefully one examines for the well-known evidences of the inflammation, the more often will he make the distinction. I feel sure that anyone who looks at the optic nerve as carefully as he looks at the sections under the microscope will be able to differentiate choked disc and optic neuritis.

# INDEX OF THE LITERATURE.

## SECTION 1.—LARYNGOLOGY AND OTOLOGY—GENERAL AND HISTORICAL.

**Biehl. C.** Vagotonia in relation to the ear.
Müenchen. med. Wchnschr., 1920—LXVII—1263.

**Crane, C. G.** Source of focal infection iritis.
N. York M. J., 1921—CXIII—442.

**Herrick, J. B.** Relation between the specialist and the practitioner.
J. Am. M. Ass., Chicago, 1921—LXXVI—975.

**Knox, H. A.** Protest against thoughtless radicalism in surgery of the nose, throat and mouth.
N. Jersey M. Soc. J., Orange, 1921—XVII—117.

**Loeb, Hanau W., and Wiener, Meyer.** The borderland of otolaryngology and ophthalmology.
Ann. Otol., Rhinol. & Laryngol., St. Louis, 1921—XXX—74.

**Watson, W. L.** General versus local anesthesia in operations on the nose and throat.
N. York M. J., 1921—CXIII—444.

**White, J. A.** History of ophthalmology and otolaryngology in Virginia.
Virginia M. Month., Richmond, 1921—XLVIII—59.

**Wurtz, W. J. M.** Malignant diseases of the nose and throat, with special reference to cancer of the nasal fossae, nasopharynx and tonsil.
N. York M. J., 1921—CXIII—434.

**Yankauer, S.** Borderline diseases.
Laryngoscope, St. Louis, 1921—XXXI—101.

## SECTION 2.—RESPIRATORY SYSTEM, EXCLUSIVE OF THE EAR, NOSE AND THROAT.

**Balvay, A.** Intratracheal treatment of asthma.
Paris Méd., 1921—XI—329.

**Caulfield, A. H. W|** Sensitization in bronchial asthma and hay fever.
J. Am. M. Ass., 1921—LXXVI—1071.

**Cecil, R. L., and Steffen. G. I.** Acute respiratory infection in man following inoculations with virulent bacillus influenzae.
J. Inf. Dis., Chicago, 1921—XXVIII—201.

**Sherman, G. H.** Vaccines in the treatment of asthma.
Laryngoscope, St. Louis, 1921—XXXI—239.

## SECTION'3.—ACUTE GENERAL INFECTIONS, INCLUDING DIPHTHERIA, SCARLET FEVER AND MEASLES. THE EAR, NOSE AND THROAT.

**Almand, C. A.** Diphtheria.
Georgia M. Ass. J., Atlanta, 1921—X.—382.

**Armand-Delille, P., and Marie Schick.** Reaction in the prophylaxis of diphtheria.
Bull. Soc. méd. d. hop., Paris, 1921—XLV—456.

**Babonneix.** Toxin versus endotoxin of diphtheria bacilli.
Bull. Soc. méd. d. hop., Paris, 1921—XLV—575.

**Bauer, E. L.** Eradication of diphtheria by means of toxin-antitoxin following Schick testing.
Penn. M. J., Harrisburg, 1921—XXIV—471.

**Bayer, K.** Specific treatment of influenza.
Münch. Med. Wchnschr., 1920—LXVII—1493.

**Cecil, R. L., and Steffen. G. I.** Acute respiratory infection in man following inoculations with virulent bacillus influenzae.
J. Inf. Dis., Chicago, 1921—XXVIII—201.

**Chown, G.** Schick test and toxin-antitoxin immunization in children's home, Winnipeg.
Canad. M. Ass. J., Toronto, 1921—XI—319.

**Dàrré, H.** Abnormal forms of diphtheria.
Bull. méd., Paris, 1921—XXXV—259.

**Davide, H. L.** Etiology of influenza.
Hygiea, Stockholm, 1921—LXXXIII—177.

**Dernby, K. G., and David, H.** Preparation of diphtheria toxin.
J. Path. & Bact., Edinburgh, 1921—XXIV—150.

**Dujariac de la Riviére, R.** Treatment of bacilli carriers.
Bull. Acad. Med., Paris, 1921—LXXXV—542.

**Durand.** Bacteriology of influenza.
Rif. méd., Napoli, 1921—XXXVII—126.

**Foster, J. H.** Intubation versus tracheotomy in laryngeal diphtheria.
South. M. J., Birmingham, 1921—XIV—352.

**Garcia del Diestro, J.** Febrile influenza in children.
Arch Espan. de ped., Madrid, 1921—V—99.

**Gaynor, H. E.** Influenza, past and present.
W. Virginia M. J., Huntington, 1921—XV—287.

**Gray, G. A., and Meyer, B. I.** Diphtheria carriers and their treatment with mercurochrome.
J. Inf. Dis., Chicago, 1921—XXVIII—323.

**Guthrie, M. F.** Sequels of influenza.
Glasgow M. J., 1921—XCV—267.

**Harris, W. L.** Diagnosis and treatment of diphtheria.
Virginia Med. Month., Richmond, 1921—XLVII—536.

**Hoyne, A. L.** Laryngeal diphtheria: review of five hundred and fifteen cases in which intubation was performed.
J. Am. M. Ass., Chicago, 1921—LXXVI—1305.

**Jordan, E. O., and Sharp, W. B.** Influenza studies: Effect of vaccination against influenza and some other respiratory infections.
J. Inf. Dis., Chicago, 1921—XXVIII—357.

**Kraus, R.** Vaccination against influenza.
Rev. del. inst. bacteriol., Buenos Aires, 1921—II—745.

**Kraus, R., and Sordelli, A.** Normal horse serum in the treatment of diphtheria.
Rev. del. inst. bacteriol., Buenos Aires, 1921—II—613.

**Lawder, T. A.** Tracheal diphtheria.
Practitioner, London, 1921—CVI—375.

**Lereboullet and Marie, P. L.** Schick reaction in the prophylaxis of diphtheria.
Bull. Soc. méd. d. hop., Paris, 1921—XLV—460.

**Loewe, L., and Zeman, F. D.** Cultivation of a filtrable organism from the nasopharyngeal washings in influenza.
J. Am. M. Ass., Chicago, 1921—LXXVI—986.

**Loiseau, G., and De la Rivière, D.** Doses of diphtheria antitoxin.
Bull. méd., Paris, 1921—XXXV—264.

**Martin, L., and Loiseau, G.** Bacteriology of diphtheria.
Bull. méd., Paris, 1921—XXXV—253.

**Martin, L., and Loiseau, G.** Prophylaxis of diphtheria.
Bull. méd., Paris, 1921—XXXV—267.

**Méry, H.** Schick reaction in the prophylaxis of diphtheria.
Bull. Soc. méd. d. hop., Paris, 1921—XLV—458.

**Mellon, R. R.** Studies in diphtheroids.
J. Med. Research, Boston, 1921—LXII—111.

**Mironesco, T.** Scarlet fever and angina.
Presse méd., 1921—XXIX—176.

**Moss, W. L., Guthrie, C. G., and Gelien, J.** Diphtheria bacillus carriers.
Johns Hopkins Hosp. Bull., Baltimore, 1921—XXXII—109.

**Neilson, J. L.** Treatment of influenza.
U. S. Nav. Med. Bul., Washington, 1921—XV—259.

**Opitz, H.** The paradoxic diphtheria reaction.
Jahrb. f. Kinderh., Berlin, 1921—XCIV—258.

**Palmer, W. H.** Diphtheria and follicular tonsillitis.
Brit. M. J., London, 1921—I—527.

**Park, W. H.** Practical value of toxin-antitoxin injections in immunization against diphtheria and of the Schick test as a means of identifying those that are susceptible.
Penn. M. J., Harrisburg, 1921—XXIV—474.

828 SOCIETY PROCEEDINGS.

**Park, W. H.** Prevention of diphtheria.
N. York State J. M., 1921—XXI—158.

**Pelfort.** Transient mumps meningitis in two children.
Rev. méd. del. Urug., Montevideo, 1921—XXIV—181.

**Richter, C. M.** Influenza pandemics depend on certain anticyclonic
weather for their development.
Arch. Int. Med., Chicago, 1921—XXVII—361.

**Rivers, T. M., and Leuschner, E. L.** Hemolytic influenza bacilli.
Johns Hopkins Hosp. Bull., Baltimore, 1921—XXXII—130.

**Rominger, E.** Diphtheria in the newborn.
Ztschr. f. Kinderh., Berlin, 1921—XXVIII—51.

**Simmons, J. S., Wearn, J. T., and Williams, O. B.** Diphtheria infections with particular reference to carriers and to wound
infections with B. diphtheriae.
J. Inf. Dis., Chicago, 1921—XXVIII—327.

**Sordelli and Wernicke.** Production of diphtheria toxin.
Rev. Asoc. Méd. Argent., Buenos Aires, 1921—XXXIII—662.

**Stine, D. G.** Comparison of influenza epidemic of 1918 with that of
1920 at the University of Missouri.
Missouri State M. Ass. J., St. Louis, 1921—XVIII—117.

**Tilley, H.** Role of tonsils in certain cases of diphtheria carriers.
J. Laryngol., etc., Edinburgh, 1921—XXXVI—235.

**Tocunaga, H.** Biology of the influenza· bacillus.
Deutsch. med. Wchnschr., Berlin, 1921—XLVI—135.

**Weaver, H.** Lessons in the management of diphtheria, especially
as suggested by the study of a series of one hundred and
forty-seven fatal cases.
J. Am. M. Ass., Chicago, 1921—LXXVI—1651.

**White, B.** Shick test and immunization with diphtheria toxin-
antitoxin.
Boston M. & S. J., 1921—CLXXXIV—246.

**Yabe, S.** Leucocytes in influenza; etiologic significance.
Kitasato Arch. Exp. Med., Toyko, 1921—IV—109.

## SECTION 4.—SYPHILIS.

**De Schweinitz, G. E.** Ocular symptoms in hypophyseal disease with
acquired syphilis.
Arch. Ophthalmol., N. York, 1921—L—203.

**Lloyd, J. H.** Syphilis of the eighth nerve.
Arch. Neurol. & Psychiat., Chicago, 1921—V—572.

## SECTION 5.—TUBERCULOSIS.

**Barajas y de Vilches, J. M.** Tuberculosis of the pharynx.
Siglo méd., Madrid, 1921—LXVIII—381.

**Janowski, W.** Thyrotuberculosis.
Ann. de Méd., Par., 1920—VIII—418.

**Laugier, A. R.** Adenoids and tonsil disease in the etiology of tuberculosis, malnutrition and infectious diseases of children.
Porto Rico M. Ass. Bull., San Juan, 1921—XV—67.

## SECTION 6.—ANATOMY, PHYSIOLOGY AND PATHOLOGY.

**Brooks, H.** Physiologic hyperthyroidism.
Endocrinol., Los Angeles, 1921—V—177.

**Rogers, L.** Observations on the developmental anatomy of the temporal bone.
Ann. Otol., Rhinol. & Laryngol., St. Louis, 1921—XXX—103.

**Ryder, C. T.** Lymph drainage of the accessory nasal sinuses.
Laryngoscope, St. Louis, 1921—XXXI—158.

## SECTION 7.— EXTERNAL NOSE,

**Behrend, M.** Rhinoplasty to replace a nose bitten off by a rat.
J. Am. M. Ass., Chicago, 1921—LXVI—1752.

**Cervera, E.** Bacteriology of rhinoscleroma.
Rev. Mex. d. biol., Mexico, 1920—I—61.

**Esser, J. F. S.** Nasoplasty from the upper lip.
Zentralbl. f. Chir., Leipzig, 1920—XLVII—1412.

**Sheehan, J. E.** Gillies' new method in giving support to the depressed nasal bridge and columella.
N. York M. J., 1921—CXIII—448.

## SECTION 8.—NASAL CAVITIES.

**Bisaillon, M., and Matson, R. W.** Anaphylaxis in asthma and hay fever.
Northwest. Med., Seattle, 1921—XX—84.

**Black, W. D.** Diagnosis of headaches of nasal origin.
South. M. J., Birmingham, 1921—XIV—241.

**Botey, R.** Treatment of obstruction of the nose.
Rev. espan. d. med. y. cir., Barcelona, 1920—III—639.

**Brandt, F. H.** Operative procedure in chronic persistent obstruction in the lacrimal sac.
Laryngoscope, St. Louis, 1921—XXXI—191.

**Cary, E. H.** Use of radium in epithelioma of the lateral wall of the nose.
Texas State J. M., Ft. Worth, 1921—XVI—536.

**Caulfield, A. H. W|** Sensitization in bronchial asthma and hay fever.
J. Am. M. Ass., 1921—LXXVI—1071.

**Cervera, E.** Bacteriology of rhinoscleroma.
Rev. Mex. d. biol., Mexico, 1920—I—61.

**Detweiler, H. K.** Present day conception of hay fever.
Canad. M. Ass. J., Montreal, 1921—IX—37.

**Donald, J.** Deflection of the nasal septum.
Practitioner, London, 1921—XVI—250.

**Faulkner, E. R.** Treatment of intranasal suppuration.
N. York State J. M., N. York, 1921—XXI—118.

**Freudenthal, W.** Telangiectasis of the face and mucous membranes of the nose and throat associated with severe epistaxis.
N. York M. J., 1921—CXIII—425.

**Graham, T. O.** Nasal catarrh.
Dublin J. M. Sc., 1921—IV—102.

**Griessmann.** Transient shifting of the nasal septum.
Münch. med. Wchnschr., 1921—LXVIII—486.

**Ingersoll, E. S.** Effect of intranasal conditions on the ocular muscles.
N. York State J. M., N. York, 1921—XXI—121.

**Jeandelize.** Retention catheter in the lacrimal apparatus.
Médicine, Paris, 1921—II—271.

**Key, Aberg H.** Rhinolithiasis.
Förh Svens Läk.-Sällsk., Sammank, 1921—XLVII—1.

**Lamb, H. D.** Disorders of lacrimal drainage.
Am. J. Ophthmol., Chicago, 1921—IV—197.

**McCready, J. H.** Intranasal operation for dacryocystitis.
Penn. M. J., Harrisburg, 1921—XXIV—483.

**Miller, J. W.** Intranasal operations with special reference to post-operative packing.
N. York M. J., 1921—CXIII—456.

**Monthus, A.** Chronic disease of the lacrimal apparatus.
Médicine, Paris, 1921—II—272.

**Mudd, S., Grant, S. B., and Goldman, A.** The etiology of acute inflammations of the nose pharynx and tonsils.
Ann. Otol., Rhinol. & Laryngol., St. Louis, 1921—XXX—1;
Also J. Lab. & Clin. Med., St. Louis, 1921—VI—322.

**Muecke, F.** Nasal obstruction and its consequences.
Practitioner, London, 1921—CVI—236.

**Ness, W.** Seasonal hay fever.
Canad. M. Ass. J., Toronto, 1921—XI—205.

**Newton, L. A.** Involvement of the maxillary sinus in acute rhinitis.
Oklahoma State M. Ass. J., Muskogee, 1921—XIV—50.

**Novak, F. J.** Basal metabolism in hyperesthetic rhinitis.
Wisconsin M. J., Milwaukee, 1921—XIX—534.

**Oertel, T. E.** Submucous replacement for external deviation.
Ann. Otol., Rhinol. & Laryngol., St. Louis, 1921—XXX—147.

**Senigaglia.** Sneezing may verify painful affection.
Policlin., Roma. 1921—XXVIII—477.

**Sheehan, J. E.** Gillies' new method in giving support to the depressed nasal bridge and columella.
N. York M. J., 1921—CXIII—448.

**Stucky, J. A.** Tonsils, teeth and nasal accessory sinuses as sources of focal infection.
Kentucky M. J., Bowling Green, 1921—XIX—205.

**Wurtz, W. J. M.** Malignant diseases of the nose and throat, with special reference to cancer of the nasal fossae, nasopharynx and tonsil.
N. York M. J., 1921—CXIII—434.

## SECTION 9.—ACCESSORY SINUSES.

**Bass, A. L.** Resume of nasal accessory sinuses and their importance.
Kentucky M. J., Bowling Green, 1921—XIX—120.

**Berruyer and Laqueviere.** Dermoid cyst in the frontal sinus.
J. d. radiol. et d'electrol., Paris, 1921—V—29.

**Black, W. D.** Diagnosis of headaches of nasal origin.
South. M. J., Birmingham, 1921—XIV—241.

**Black, W. D.** Symptoms and diagnosis of nasal accessory sinus disease with special reference to their complications.
Illinois M. J., Oak Park, 1921—XXXIX—313.

**Dabney, S. G.** Malignant disease of the superior maxillary bone.
Kentucky M. J., 1921—XIX—125.

**Denman, I. O.** Oral and sinus surgery in forward inclined sitting posture, under nitrous oxid oxygen anesthesia.
Penn. M. J., Harrisburg, 1921—XXIV—388.

**Dufourmentel.** Endonasal treatment of frontal sinusitis.
Bull. méd., Paris, 1921—XXXV—165.

**Faulkner, E. R.** Treatment of intranasal suppuration.
N. York State J. M., N. York, 1921—XXI—118.

**Gittins, T. R.** Acute infections of the nasal sinuses; treatment.
Iowa State M. J., Des Moines, 1921—XI—84.

**Harter, J. H.** Diseases of the ethmoid and sphenoid sinuses.
Canad. M. Ass. J., Toronto, 1921—XI—337.

**Hays, H.** Simple bloodless and painless operation for complete exenteration of the ethmoid labyrinth.
Laryngoscope, St. Louis, 1921—XXXI—186.

**Ingersoll, E. S.** Effect of intranasal conditions on the ocular muscles.
N. York State J. M., N. York, 1921—XXI—121.

**Lewis, F. O.** Four cases of radical frontal sinus operation with unusual pathologic findings.
Laryngoscope, St. Louis, 1921—XXXI—179.

**Monteleone, R.** Sinusitis from measles.
Policlin., Roma, 1921—XXVIII—616.

Morrin, F. T.  A case of carcinoma of the antrum of Highmore.
Dublin J. Med. Sc., 1921—IV—79.

Newton, L. A.  Involvement of the maxillary sinus in acute rhinitis.
Oklahoma State M. Ass. J., Muskogee, 1921—XIV—50.

Perdue, W. W.  Case of extradural abscess complicating an acute
left frontal sinusitis.
South. M. J., Birmingham, 1921—XIV—424.

Ridpath, R. F.  Practical points in the diagnosis of sinus disease,
from the point of view of a general practitioner.
N. York M. J., 1921—CXIII—460.

Ryder, C. T.  Lymph drainage of the accessory nasal sinuses.
Laryngoscope, St. Louis, 1921—XXXI—158.

Schaeffer, J. P.  The sphenoidal sinus and the temporal lobe.
J. Am. M. Ass., Chicago, 1921—LXXVI—1488.

Stucky, J. A.  Tonsils, teeth and nasal accessory sinuses as sources
of focal infection.
Kentucky M. J., Bowling Green, 1921—XIX—205.

Sweet, R. B.  Calculus in the maxillary sinus.
J. Am. M. Ass., Chicago, 1921—LXVII—1498.

Sweet, R. B.  Teeth, tonsils and sinuses.
Calif. State J. M., San Francisco, 1921—XIX—116.

Theobald, W. M.  A radical treatment for chronic suppuration of
the antrum with modification of the Canfield technic.
Ann. Otol., Rhinol. & Laryngol., St. Louis, 1921—XXX—131.

Watson-Williams, P.  Nasal sinus infection a causal factor in
appendicitis.
Practitioner, London, 1921—CVI—222.

White, F. W.  Pathologic nasal accessory sinuses in children.
Ann. Otol., Rhinol. & Laryngol., St. Louis, 1921—XXX—221.

White, J. W.  Infections of the paranasal sinuses.
Virginia M. Month., Richmond, 1921—XLVIII—87.

## SECTION 10.—PHARYNX, INCLUDING TONSILS AND ADENOIDS.

Azzi.  Temperature of the tonsil.
Rif. méd., Napoli, 1921—XXXVII—175.

Barajas y de Vilches, J. M.  Tuberculosis of the pharynx.
Siglo méd., Madrid, 1921—LXVIII—381.

Black, W. D.  Reducing dangers in tonsil operations in minimum.
Missouri State M. Ass. J., St. Louis, 1921—XVIII—90.

Burger, H.  Technic for tonsillectomy.
Nederl. Tijdschr. v. Geneesk., Amsterdam, 1921—I—1416.

Casanovas, R. T.  Arthritis of focal origin.
Rev. esp. d. med. y. cir., Barcelona, 1920—III—647.

**Loewe, L., and Zeman, F. D.** Cultivation of a filtrable organism from the nasopharyngeal washings in influenza.
J. Am. M. Ass., Chicago, 1921—LXXVI—986.

**Mérola, L.** Access to the tonsil through the side of the neck.  ·
Sem. méd., Buenos Aires, 1920—XXVII—165.

**Maselli, D.** Primary syphilitic chancre on the tonsil.
Policlin., Roma, 1921—XXVIII—404.

**McVey, F. J.** A new tonsil hemostat.
Boston M. & S. J.. 1921—CLXXXIV—524.

**Mironesco, T.** Scarlet fever and angina.
Presse méd., 1921—XXIX—176.

**Mollison, Wm.** The tonsil as a focus of infection.
J. Laryngol., etc., Edinburgh, 1921—XXXVI—188.

**Moss, W. L., Guthrie, C. G., and Gelien, J.** Diphtheria bacillus carriers.
Johns Hopkins Hosp. Bull., Baltimore, 1921—XXXII—109.

**Mudd, S., Grant, S. B., and Goldman, A.** The etiology of acute inflammations of the nose pharynx and tonsils.
Ann. Otol., Rhinol. & Laryngol., St. Louis, 1921—XXX—1;
Also J. Lab. & Clin. Med., St. Louis, 1921—VI—322.

**New, G. B., and Vinson, P. P.** Cicatricial laryngopharyngeal diaphragm.
J. Am. M. Ass., Chicago, 1921—LXXVI—996.

**Olitsky, P. K., and Gates, F. L.** Experimental studies of nasopharyngeal secretions from influenza patients. Studies of concurrent infections.
J. Exp. Med., Baltimore, 1921—XXXIII—373.

**Olitsky, P. K., and Gates, F. L.** Experimental studies of nasopharyngeal secretions from influenza patients. Filterability and resistance to glycerol.
J. Exp. Med., Baltimore, 1921—XXXIII—361.

**Palmer, W. H.** Diphtheria and follicular tonsillitis.
Brit. M. J., London, 1921—I—527.

**Reynolds, R.** Tonsillectomy in military service.
Mil. Surg., Washington, 1921—XLVIII—341.

**Rodman, H.** Diseased tonsils as a factor in focal infection.
N. York M. J., 1921—CXIII—466.

**Rogers, T. A.** Chronic tonsillar infecition.·
N. Y. State J. M., N. Y., 1921—XXI—124.

**Samengo, L.** Fulguration for tumors of the nasopharynx.
Sem. méd., Buenos Aires, 1920—XXVII—570.

**Scott, L. M.** Plea for the early removal of hypertrophied tonsils and adenoids in children.
Tennessee State M. Ass. J., 1921—XIII—468.

**Stucky, J. A.** Tonsils, teeth and nasal accessory sinuses as sources of focal infection.
Kentucky M. J., Bowling Green, 1921—XIX—205.

**Sweet, R. B.** Teeth, tonsils and sinuses.
Calif. State J. M., San Francisco, 1921—XIX—116.

**Thomasson, W. J.** Two cases of hemorrhage following peritonsillar abscess.
J. Am. M. Ass., Chicago, 1921—LXXVI—931.

**Tilley, H.** Role of tonsils in certain cases of diphtheria carriers.
J. Laryngol., etc., Edinburgh, 1921—XXXVI—235.

**Turner, A. L.** Two cases of traumatic adhesions of the soft palate to the posterior pharyngeal wall following removal of tonsils and adenoids; reestablishment of nasal respiration by operation.
J. Laryngol., etc., Edinburgh, 1921—XXXVI—237.

**Williams, F. G.** Treatment of hypertrophied tonsils and adenoids by radium.
Boston M. & S. J., 1921—CLXXXIV—256.

**Wishart, D. J. G.** Tumor of the hypopharynx in a child of eleven weeks.
N. York M. J., 1921—CXIII—458.

**Wurtz, W. J. M.** Malignant diseases of the nose and throat, with special reference to cancer of the nasal fossae, nasopharynx and tonsil.
N. York M. J., 1921—CXIII—434.

## SECTION 11.—LARYNX.

**Bolton, N. H.** Cigarette holder in the larynx.
Lancet, London, 1921—I—535.

**Brüggemann.** Use of metal bolts in laryngeal surgery.
Deutsch. med. Wchnschr., Berlin, 1921—XLVII—382.

**Burger, H.** Pedunculated cancer of the larynx.
Nederl. Tijdschr. v. Geneesk., Amsterdam, 1921—I—511.

**Cavazza, E.** Foreign bodies in the esophagus and air passages.
Policlin., Roma, 1921—XXVIII—293.

**Diggle, F. H.** Diagnosis and treatment of cancer of the larynx.
Practitioner, London, 1921—CVI—347.

**Ferreri, G.** Respiration after laryngostomy.
Policlin., Roma, 1921—XXVIII—81.

**Fletcher, G. W.** Thirty-three cases of foreign bodies in the esophaagus, bronchi and larynx.
Canad. M. Ass. J., Toronto, 1921—XI—332.

**Foster, J. H.** Intubation versus tracheotomy in laryngeal diphtheria.
South. M. J., Birmingham, 1921—XIV—352.

**Friedman, J., and Greenfield, S. D.** Case of foreign body in the larynx and esophagus.
N. York M. J., 1921—CXIII—818.

**Hickey, P. M.** Intralaryngeal application of radium for chronic papilloma.
  Am. J. Roentgenol., N. York, 1921—VIII—155.

**Hoyne, A. L.** Laryngeal diphtheria: review of five hundred and fifteen cases in which intubation was performed.
  J. Am. M. Ass., Chicago, 1921—LXXVI—1305.

**Iglauer, S.** Case of laryngocele.
  N. York, M. J., 1921—CXIII—464.

**Ingram, L. C.** Removal of foreign bodies from the air and the upper food passages.
  Florida M. Ass. J., St. Augustine, 1921—VII—137.

**Jackson, C.** High tracheotomy and other errors chief causes of chronic laryngeal stenosis.
  Surg., Gynecol. & Obstet., Chicago, 1921—XXXII—392.

**Judd, E. S.** Laryngeal function in thyroid cases.
  Ann. Surg., Philadelphia, 1921—CXXIII—321.

**Kelly, A. B.** Chorditis fibrinosa.
  J. Laryngol., etc., London, 1921—XXXVI—118.

**Ladeback, H.** Quartz laryngeal mirror for use with ultraviolet rays.
  München. med. Wchnschr., 1920—LXVII—1442.

**Lynah, H. L.** New instruments for use in laryngeal surgery.
  Laryngoscope, St. Louis, 1921—XXXI—116.

**Miégeville, R.** Caronic laryngitis.
  Bull. méd., Paris, 1921—XXXV—167.

**Moure, E. J.** Remote results of laryngectomy.
  Bull. Acad. Méd:, Paris, 1921—LXXXV—257.

**New, G. B., and Vinson, P. P.** Cicatricial laryngopharyngeal diaphragm.
  J. Am. M. Ass., Chicago, 1921—LXXVI—996.

**Noll, F.** Apparatus for the treatment of the larynx with ultraviolet rays.
  München. med. Wchnschr., 1920—LXVII—1441.

**Orton, H. B.** Nine cases of foreign bodies in the upper air and food passages.
  N. Jersey M. Soc. J., Orange, 1921—XVIII—118.

**Orton, H. B.** Open safety pin in the larynx for six months.
  Laryngoscope, St. Louis, 1921—XXXI—233.

**Tapia.** Laryngectomy.
  Siglo méd., Mádrid, 1921—LXVIII—148.

## SECTION 12.—TRACHEA AND BRONCHI.

**Balvay, A.** Intratracheal treatment of asthma.
  Paris Méd., 1921—XI—329.

**Cavazza, E.** Foreign bodies in the esophagus and air passages.
  Policlin., Roma, 1921—XXVIII—293.

**Cayce, E. B.** Primary carcinoma of the trachea.
South. M. J., Birmingham, 1921—XIV—422.

**D'Oelsnitz and Carcopino.** Tracheobronchial adenopathies.
Bull. Soc. méd. d. hop., Paris, 1921—XLV—297.

**Fletcher, G. W.** Thirty-three cases of foreign bodies in the esophagus, bronchi and larynx.
Canad. M. Ass. J., Toronto, 1921—XI—332.

**Fraenkel, E.** Cancer of the trachea.
Deutsch. Arch. f. Klin. Med., Leipzig, 1921—CXXXV—184.

**Hirsh, I. S.** Foreign body (coin) in the bronchus for 15 years.
Am. J. Roentgenol., N. York, 1921—VIII—191.

**Imperatori, C. J.** Six cases of foreign bodies in the esophagus and bronchi.
N. York M. J., 1921—CXIII—438.

**Ingram, L. C.** Removal of foreign bodies from the air and the upper food passages.
Florida M. Ass. J., St. Augustine, 1921—VII—137.

**Jackson, C.** High tracheotomy and other errors chief causes of chronic laryngeal stenosis.
Surg., Gynecol. & Obstet., Chicago, 1921—XXXII—392.

**Jackson, C., and Spencer, W. H.** Broncholith and pneumoconiotic material removed from a bronchiectatic cavity by peroral bronchoscopy.
N. York M. J., 1921—CXIII—461.

**Lawder, T. A.** Tracheal diphtheria.
Practitioner, London, 1921—CVI—375.

**Lynah, H. L., and Stewart, W. H.** Roentgenographic studies of bronchiectasis and lung abscess after direct infection of bismuth mixture through the bronchoscope.
Am. J. Roentgenol., N. York, 1921—VIII—49;
Also Ann. Surg., Philadelphia, 1921—LXXVI—362.

**Lynch, R. C.** Fluoroscopic bronchoscopy, esophagoscopy and gas troscopy.
N. York M. J., 1921—CXIII—437.

**Méry, H., and Girard, L.** Pathologic anatomy of the lung and tracheobronchial glands in children.
Presse méd., Paris, 1921—XXIX—313

**Orton, H. B.** Nine cases of foreign bodies in the upper air and food passages.
N. Jersey M. Soc. J., Orange, 1921—XVIII—118.

**Seelig, M. G.** Midline congenital cervical fistula of tracheal origin.
Arch. Surg., Chicago, 1921—II—338.

**Voegelin, A. W.** Foreign body in bronchi.
J. Am. M. Ass., Chicago, 1921—LXXVII—1230.

## SECTION 13.—VOICE AND SPEECH.

**Adam, J.** Infection of the middle ear and external auditory meatus from Vincent's organisms.
J. Laryngol., etc., Edinburgh, 1921—XXXVI—186.

**Ellison, E. M.** Sensory aphasia.
N. York M. J., 1921—CXIII—796.

**Head, H.** Aphasia.
Brain, London, 1921—XLIII—390.

**Morgne, R.** Aphasia and psychology of thinking.
Encéphale., Paris, 1921—XVI—78.

**Muck, O.** Laryngeal pellet in the treatment of aphonia.
München. med. Wchnschr., 1921—LXVIII—361.

**Osnato, M.** Speech, its development and integration with intelligence.
Neurol. Bull., N. York, 1921—III—47.

## SECTION 14.—ESOPHAGUS.

**Adam, J.** Infection of the middle ear and external auditory meatus from Vincent's organisms.
J. Laryngol., etc., Edinburgh, 1921—XXXVI—186.

**Arrowsmith, H.** Traction pulsion diverticulum of the esophagus.
N. York M. J., 1921—CXIII—463.

**Carmody, T. E.** Stenosis of the esophagus.
N. York M. J., 1921—CXIII—427;
Also Colo. Med., Denver, 1921—XVIII—95.

**Cavazza, E.** Foreign bodies in the esophagus and air passages.
Policlin., Roma, 1921—XXVIII—293.

**Fletcher, G. W.** Thirty-three cases of foreign bodies in the esophagus, bronchi and larynx.
Canad. M. Ass. J., Toronto, 1921—XI—332.

**Friedman, J., and Greenfield, S. D.** Case of foreign body in the larynx and esophagus.
N. York M. J., 1921—CXIII—818.

**Hirsch, I. S.** Congenital atresia of the esophagus. Report of two cases.
J. Am. M. Ass., Chicago, 1921—LXXVI—1491.

**Hubbard, T., and Galbraith, E. G.** Differential diagnosis of traumatisms and diseased conditions of the esophagus.
Ohio State M. J., Columbus, 1921—XVII—167.

**Imperatori, C. J.** Six cases of foreign bodies in the esophagus and bronchi.
N. York M. J., 1921—CXIII—438.

**Ingram, L. C.** Removal of foreign bodies from the air and the upper food passages.
Florida M. Ass. J., St. Augustine, 1921—VII—137.

**Kinoshita, M.** Mixed tumor of the esophagus.
Schweitz. med. Wchnschr., Basel, 1921—LI—156.

**Kully, B. M.** Removal of open safety pin from the esophagus of an infant.
Nebraska State M. J., Norfolk, 1921—VI—151.

**Lynah, H. L.** Borderline diseases of the esophagus.
Ann. Otol., Rhinol. & Laryngol., St. Louis, 1921—XXX—164.

**Lynch, R. C.** Fluoroscopic bronchoscopy, esophagoscopy and gastroscopy.
N. York M. J., 1921—CXIII—437.

**Maaloe, C. W.** Gastroscopy.
Uges. f. Laeger. Kjobenh., 1921—LXXXIII—525.

**Moutier.** Acute postoperative esophagitis.
Arch. de mal. l'appar. digest. (etc.), Paris, 1921—XI—126.

**Orton, H. B.** Nine cases of foreign bodies in the upper air and food passages.
N. Jersey M. Soc. J., Orange, 1921—XVIII—118.

**Paterson, D. H.** Case of esophagectasia in a child.
Brit. J. Child. Dis., London, 1921—XVIII—27.

**Patterson, E. J.** Aid to diagnosis of suspected foreign body in the esophagus.
N. York M. J., 1921—CXIII—447.

**Reynolds, R. P., and Morrison, W. W.** Congenital malformation of the esophagus.
Am. J. Dis. Child., Chicago, 1921—XXI—339.

**Ray, J. N.** Foreign body in the esophagus removed by external esophagotomy. Cure.
J. Laryngol., etc., Edinburgh, 1921—XXXVI—183.

**Roy, J. N.** A case of a foreign body in the esophagus removed by external esophagotomy. Cure.
Ann. Otol., Rhinol. & Laryngol., St. Louis, 1921—XXX—159.

**Schlemmer, F.** Foreign bodies in the esophagus.
Arch. f. Klin. Chir., Berlin, 1920—CXIV—269.

**Suter, E.** Radium treatment of cancer of the esophagus.
Deutsch. Ztschr. f. Chir., Leipzig, 1921—CLXII—50.

## SECTION 15.—ENDOSCOPY.

**Cavazza, E.** Foreign bodies in the esophagus and air passages.
Policlin., Roma, 1921—XXVIII—293.

**Fletcher, G. W.** Thirty-three cases of foreign bodies in the esophagus, bronchi and larynx.
Canad. M. Ass. J., Toronto, 1921—XI—332.

**Friedman, J., and Greenfield, S. D.** Case of foreign body in the larynx and esophagus.
N. York M. J., 1921—CXIII—818.

Hirsh, I. S.  Foreign body (coin) in the bronchus for 15 years.
  Am. J. Roentgenol., N. York, 1921—VIII—191.

Imperatori, C. J.  Six cases of foreign bodies in the esophagus and
  bronchi.
  N. York M. J., 1921—CXIII—438.

Ingram, L. C.  Removal of foreign bodies from the air and the
  upper food passages.
  Florida M. Ass. J., St. Augustine, 1921—VII—137.

Jackson, C., and Spencer, W. H.  Broncholith and pneumoconiotic
  material removed from a bronchiectatic cavity by peroral
  bronchoscopy.
  N. York M. J., 1921—CXIII—461.

Kully, B. M.  Removal of open safety pin from the esophagus of
  an infant.
  Nebraska State M. J., Norfolk, 1921—VI—151.

Lynah, H. L., and Stewart, W. H.  Roentgenographic studies of
  bronchiectasis and lung abscess after direct infection of
  bismuth mixture through the bronchoscope.
  Am. J. Roentgenol., N. York, 1921—VIII—49;
  Also Ann. Surg., Philadelphia, 1921—LXXVI—362.

Lynch, R. C.  Fluoroscopic bronchoscopy, esophagoscopy and gastroscopy.
  N. York M. J., 1921—CXIII—437.

Maaloe, C. W.  Gastroscopy.
  Uges. f. Laeger. Kjobenh., 1921—LXXXIII—525.

Murphy, J. W.  Qualifications a peroral endoscopist should possess.
  N. York M. J., 1921—CXIII—451.

Orton, H. B.  Nine cases of foreign bodies in the upper air and food
  passages.
  N. Jersey M. Soc. J., Orange, 1921—XVIII—118.

Orton, H. B.  Open safety pin in the larynx for six months.
  Laryngoscope, St. Louis, 1921—XXXI—233.

Ray, J. N.  Foreign body in the esophagus removed by external
  esophagotomy.  Cure.
  J. Laryngol., etc., Edinburgh, 1921—XXXVI—183.

Voegelin, A. W.  Foreign body in bronchi.
  J. Am. M. Ass., Chicago, 1921—LXXVII—1230.

## SECTION 16.—EXTERNAL EAR AND CANAL.

Amberg, E.  Some of the more important measurements of parts
  of the temporal bone.
  Laryngoscope. St. Louis, 1921—XXXI—147.

De Carvalho, A.  Eczema of the ear.
  Brazil med., Rio de Janeiro, 1921—XXXV—49.

Sheasby, H.  Swelling of the pinna, an early sign of deficient anti-
  scorbutic vitamin.  •
  Practitioner, London, 1921—CVI—215.

## SECTION 17.—MIDDLE EAR, INCLUDING TYMPANIC MEMBRANE AND EUSTACHIAN TUBE.

**Amberg, E.** Some of the more important measurements of parts of the temporal bone.
Laryngoscope, St. Louis, 1921—XXXI—147.

**Becco, R.** Otitis simulating mastoiditis.
Sem. méd., Buenos Aires, 1921—XXVIII—314.

**Bilancioni.** Large sarcoma in the middle ear.
Tumori, Roma, 1920—VII—200.

**Bonnet, Ray F.** Acute otitis media.
Bull. méd., Paris, 1921—XXXV—174.

**Boyd, G. A. A.** One hundred and eighty-eight cases of acute otitis media and mastoiditis in which the Schwartze operation was performed.
J. Laryngol., etc., Edinburgh, 1921—XXXVI—217.

**Diggle, F. H.** Chronic suppurative otitis media followed by left temporosphenoidal abscess·and meningitis.
Brit. M. J., London, 1921—I—600.

**Downey, J. W.** Diagnostic sign of progressive deafness.
Laryngoscope, St. Louis, 1921—XXXI—207.

**Gradenigo, G.** Ligation of the jugular vein in otitis.
Rif. méd., Napoli, 1921—XXXVII—126.

**Inglis, H. J.** Asthenic hypoacousis.
Ann. Otol., Rhinol. & Laryngol., St. Louis, 1921—XXX—237.

**Keeler, J. C.,** Study of acute infections of the ear as observed by the general physician.
N. Jersey M. Soc. J., Orange, 1921—XVIII—37.

**Leland, G. A.** Internal drainage of acute ears and abortion of acute mastoiditis by the use of Wright's solution.
Boston M. & S. J., 1921—CLXXXIV—251;
Also Laryngoscope, St. Louis, 1921—XXXI—106.

**Loeper and Forestier.** Epidemic hiccup plus acute otitis.
Prog. méd., Paris, 1921—XXXVI—82.

**Portmann, G.** Access to a projectile in the ear.
Presse méd., Paris, 1921—XXIX—274.

**Renon, L., and Blamontier, P.** Otogenous meningitis.
Ann. méd., Paris, 1921—IX—119.

**Rogers, L.** Observations on the developmental anatomy of the temporal bone.
Ann. Otol., Rhinol. & Laryngol., St. Louis, 1921—XXX—103.

**Shambaugh, G. E.** Chronic suppurative otitis media.
Wisconsin M. J., Milwaukee, 1921—XIX—462.

**Strauss, J. F.** Accidents in aural paracentesis.
Ann. Otol., Rhinol. & Laryngol., St. Louis, 1921—XXX—232.

## SECTION 18.—MASTOID PROCESS.

**Becco, R.** Otitis simulating mastoiditis.
Sem. méd., Buenos Aires, 1921—XXVIII—314.

**Boyd, G. A. A.** One hundred and eighty-eight cases of acute otitis media and mastoiditis in which the Schwartze operation was performed.
J. Laryngol., etc., Edinburgh, 1921—XXXVI—217.

**Callison, J. G.** Double mastoid operation; acute thyroadrenal exhaustion.
N. York M. J., 1921—CXIII—431.

**Campbell, A.** Conservative treatment of chronic middle ear suppuration.
J. Larngol., etc., London, 1921—XXXVI—121.

**Gill, Elbyrne.** A typical mastoiditis with report of three cases.
Ann. Otol., Rhinol. & Laryngol., St. Louis, 1921—XXX—228.

**Gradenigo, G.** Ligation of the jugular vein in otitis.
Rif. méd., Napoli, 1921—XXXVII—126.

**Joseph, L.** Pathogenesis and treatment of otosclerosis.
Deutsch. med. Wchnchr., Berlin, 1920—XLVI—1311.

**Koebbe, E. E.** Local anesthesia for simple mastoid operation.
J. Am. M. Ass., Chicago, 1921—LXXVI—1334.

**Layton, T. B.** When to open the mastoid antrum in acute ear disease.
Lancet, London, 1921—I—734.

**Leland, G. A.** Internal drainage of acute ears and abortion of acute mastoiditis by the use of Wright's solution.
Boston M. & S. J., 1921—CLXXXIV—251;
Also Laryngoscope, St. Louis, 1921—XXXI—106.

**Loeper and Forestier, J.** Otitis media with epidemic.
Bull. Soc. méd. de hop., Paris, 1921—XLV—221.

**Munyo, J. C.** Measles plus otitis.
Rev. méd. del Urug., Montevideo, 1921—XXIV—179.

**Portmann, G.** Access to a projectile in the ear.
Presse méd., Paris, 1921—XXIX—274.

**Renon, L., and Blamontier, P.** Otogenous meningitis.
Ann. méd., Paris, 1921—IX—119.

**Rogers, L.** Observations on the developmental anatomy of the temporal bone.
Ann. Otol., Rhinol. & Laryngol., St. Louis, 1921—XXX—103.

**Roy, Dunbar.** Paralysis of the external rectus in the right eye following mastoiditis in the left ear.
Ann. Otol.. Rhinol. & Laryngol., St. Louis, 1921—XXX—252.

**Saunders, T. L.** Acute mastoiditis in the aged.
N. York State J. M., 1921—XXI—177.

**Schoenbauer, L.** Tearing off of the mastoid process.
Arch. f. Klin. Chir., Berlin, 1920—CXIV—520.

**Siegelstein, M. J.** Encephalitis lethargica as a postoperative complication of acute mastoiditis with report of a case.
Ann. Otol., Rhinol. & Laryngol., St. Louis, 1921—XXX—201.

**Torrents, Castelltort J.** Scarlatinal mastoiditis.
Rev. Espan. d. med. y cir., Barcelona, 1920—III—646.

**White, J. W.** Report of cases: 1. Simple mastoidectomy on man, 81 years old. 2. Infective sigmoid sinus thrombosis. A positive blood culture with streptococcus mucosus capsulatus present.
Ann. Otol., Rhinol. & Laryngol., St. Louis, 1921—XXX—199.

## SECTION 19.—INTERNAL EAR.

**Amberg, E.** Some of the more important measurements of parts of the temporal bone.
Laryngoscope, St. Louis, 1921—XXXI—147.

**Barany, R.** Diagnosis of disease of the otolith apparatus.
J. Laryngol., etc., Edinburgh, 1921—XXXVI—229;
Also Hygiea, Stockholm, 1921—LXXXIII—81.

**Barré, J. A., and Reys, L.** Labyrinthine form of epidemic encephalitis.
Bull. méd., Paris, 1921—XXXV—356.

**Coates, G. M.** Blood clot dressing for simple mastoid operation.
Penn. M. J., Harrisburg, 1921—XXIV—477.

**Cushing, H.** Acoustic neuromas.
Laryngoscope, St. Louis, 1921—XXXI—209.

**Downey, J. W.** Diagnostic sign of progressive deafness.
Laryngoscope, St. Louis, 1921—XXXI—207.

**Fumarola, G.** Tumor of the auditory nerve.
Policlin., Roma, 1921—XXVIII—60.

**Hunt, J. R.** The static and kinetic systems of motility.
Ann. Méd., Paris, 1921—IX—123.

**Hunter, R. J.** Cultivating balance sense: prelude to cloud flying.
Laryngoscope, St. Louis, 1921—XXXI—229.

**Inglis, H. J.** Asthenic hypoacousis.
Ann. Otol., Rhinol. & Laryngol., St. Louis, 1921—XXX—237.

**Joseph, L.** Pathogenesis and treatment of otosclerosis.
Deutsch. med. Wchnchr., Berlin, 1920—XLVI—1311.

**Layton, T. B.** When to open the mastoid antrum in acute ear disease.
Lancet, London, 1921—I—734.

**Lloyd, J. H.** Syphilis of the eighth nerve.
Arch. Neurol. & Psychiat., Chicago, 1921—V—572.

**McCoy, J., and Gottlieb, W. J.** Tests of the auditory and static labyrinths and related intracranial pathways.
Laryngoscope, St. Louis, 1921—XXXI—78.

Portmann, G.   Access to a projectile in the ear.
Presse méd., Paris, 1921—XXIX—274.

Shea, J. J.   Barany tests.
Tennessee State M. Ass. J., Nashville, 1921—XIII—462.

## SECTION 20.—DEAFNESS AND DEAFMUTISM, AND TESTS FOR HEARING.

Dean, L. W., and Bunch, C. C.   Results obtained from one year's use
of the audiometer in otologic practice.
Laryngoscope, St. Louis, 1921—XXXI—137.

Levy, L.   Case of brain tumor showing value of Barany tests as
early diagnostic methods.
Tennessee State M. Ass. J., Nashville, 1921—XIII—460.

Löwenstein, O.   Objective test for the power of audition.
München. med. Wchnschr., 1920—LXVII—1402.

Ribon, V.   Musical sense of deafmutes.
Semana méd., Buenos Aires, 1921—XXVIII—83.

Shapiro, I. F.   Simple noise apparatus for testing ears separately.
Laryngoscope, St. Louis, 1921—XXXI—114.

Shea, J. J.   Barany tests.
Tennessee State M. Ass. J., Nashville, 1921—XIII—462.

## SECTION 21.—FOREIGN BODIES IN THE NOSE, THROAT AND EAR.

Bolton, N. H.   Cigarette holder in the larynx.
Lancet, London, 1921—I—535.

Cavazza, E.   Foreign bodies in the esophagus and air passages.
Policlin., Roma, 1921—XXVIII—293.

Fletcher, G. W.   Thirty-three cases of foreign bodies in the esophagus, bronchi and larynx.
Canad. M. Ass. J., Toronto, 1921—XI—332.

Friedman, J., and Greenfield, S. D.   Case of foreign body in the
larynx and esophagus.
N. York M. J., 1921—CXIII—818.

Hirsh, I. S.   Foreign body (coin) in the bronchus for 15 years.
Am. J. Roentgenol., N. York, 1921—VIII—191.

Imperatori, C. J.   Six cases of foreign bodies in the esophagus and
bronchi.
N. York M. J., 1921—CXIII—438.

Jackson, C., and Spencer, W. H.   Broncholith and pneumoconiotic
material removed from a bronchiectatic cavity by peroral
bronchoscopy.
N. York M. J., 1921—CXIII—461.

Kully, B. M.   Removal of open safety pin from the esophagus of
an infant.
Nebraska State M. J., Norfolk, 1921—VI—151.

**Lynch, R. C.** Fluoroscopic bronchoscopy, esophagoscopy and gastroscopy.
N. York M. J., 1921—CXIII—437.

**McDonald, C. A.** Salivary calculus.
Rhode Island M. J., Providence, 1921—IV—84.

**Orton, H. B.** Nine cases of foreign bodies in the uper air and food passages.
N. Jersey M. Soc. J., Orange, 1921—XVIII—118.

**Orton, H. B.** Open safety pin in the larynx for six months.
Laryngoscope, St. Louis, 1921—XXXI—233.

**Patterson, E. J.** Aid to diagnosis of suspected foreign body in the esophagus.
N. York M. J., 1921—CXIII—447.

**Ray, J. N.** Foreign body in the esophagus removed by external esophagotomy. Cure.
J. Laryngol., etc., Edinburgh, 1921—XXXVI—183.

**Roy, J. N.** A case of a foreign body in the esophagus removed by external esophagotomy. Cure.
Ann. Otol., Rhinol. & Laryngol., St. Louis, 1921—XXX—159.

**Sweet, R. B.** Calculus in the maxillary sinus.
J. Am. M. Ass., Chicago, 1921—LXVII—1498.

**Voegelin, A. W.** Foreign body in bronchi.
J. Am. M. Ass., Chicago, 1921—LXXVII—1230.

## SECTION 22.—ORAL CAVITY, INCLUDING TONGUE, PALATE AND INFERIOR MAXILLARY.

**Aloi, V.** Sarcoma of the tongue.
Riforma méd., Napoli, 1921—XXXVII—219.

**Antoninus, E., and Czepa, A.** Dental pathology and internal disease.
Wien. Arch. f. inn. Med., 1921—II—293.

**Bockenheimer, P.** Exposure of articulation of the jaw.
Zentralbl. f. Chir., Leipzig, 1920—XLVII—1560.

**Butler, H. B.** Importance of oral hygiene during childhood.
Am. J. Pub. Health, Boston, 1921—XI—297.

**Casanovas, R. T.** Arthritis of focal origin.
Rev. esp. d. med. y. cir., Barcelona, 1920—III—647.

**Dabney, S. G.** Malignant disease of the superior maxillary bone.
Kentucky M. J., 1921—XIX—125.

**De Lapersonne, F., Velter and Prélat.** Supernumerary teeth in the orbit.
Bull. Acad. Méd., Paris, 1921—LXXXV—308.

**Delbet.** Cancer of the tongue.
Prog. méd., Paris, 1921—XXXVI—192.

**Denman, I. O.** Oral and sinus surgery in forward inclined sitting posture, under nitrous oxid oxygen anesthesia.
Penn. M. J., Harrisburg, 1921—XXIV—388.

**Ecker, M.** Anesthesia in dental surgery.
Med. Rec., N. York, 1921—XCIX—870.

**Esser, J. F. S.** Nasoplasty from the upper lip.
Zentralbl. f. Chir., Leipzig, 1920—XLVII—1412.

**Fortacin, J. B.** Large sublingual dermoid cysts.
Siglo méd., Madrid, 1921—LXVIII—93.

**Gillies, H. D., and Fry, W. K.** A new principle in the surgical
treatment of congenital. cleft palate and its mechanical
counterpart.
Brit. M. J., London, 1921—I—335.

**Harvey, H. E.** Method of sterilization in dentistry.
U. S. Nov. Med. Bul., Washington, 1921—XV—302.

**Honigmann, F.** Primary acute suppurative parotitis.
Deutsch. Ztschrift. f. Chir., Leipzig, 1920—CLX—252.

**Howe, P.** Dental infections and their relation to disease. Viewpoint of the bacteriologist.
Boston M. & S. J., 1921—CLXXXVI—433.

**Huber.** Increase of mercurial stomatitis since the war.
München. med. Wchnschr., 1921—LXVIII—393.

**Hunter, J. W.** Extraction of teeth; study and protest.
Virginia Med. Month., Richmond, 1921—XLVIII—7.

**Hylin, W.** Septic osteitis of dental origin.
Hygiea, Stockholm, 1921—LXXXIII—122.

**Ingram, L. C.** Removal of foreign bodies from the air and the
upper food passages.
Florida M. Ass. J., St. Augustine, 1921—VII—137.

**Jorge, J. M.** Actinomycosis of the lower jaw.
Sem. Méd., Buenos Aires, 1921—XXVIII—185.

**Keyes, F. A.** Dental infections and their relation to disease; viewpoint of the dentist.
Boston M. & S. J., 1921—CLXXXIV—430.

**Köhl, E.** Lingual goiter.
Schweiz. med. Wchnschr., Basel, 1921—LI—361.

**Lipshutz, B.** Suppurative submaxillary adenitis.
N. York M. J., 1921—CXIII—440.

**Majour and Laquerrière.** Roentgenography of the teeth.
J. d. radiol., et d'electrol., Paris, 1921—V—27.

**McDonald, C. A.** Salivary calculus.
Rhode Island M. J., Providence, 1921—IV—84.

**Nicory, C.** Capillary angeiomatosis of the parotid gland.
Brit. J. Surg., Bristol, 1921—VIII—481.

**O'Brien, F. W.** Dental infections and their relation to disease.
Viewpoint of the roentgenologist.
Boston M. & S. J., 1921—CLXXXIV—427.

**Pelfort.** Transient mumps meningitis in two children.
Rev. méd. del. Urug., Montevideo, 1921—XXIV—181.

**Sebileau, P.** Perimandibular phlegmons of dental origin.
Presse méd., Paris, 1921—XXIX—213.

**Shearer, W. C.** Importance of surgical removal of teeth or work on minor oral surgery.
Northwest Med., Seattle, 1921—XXI—66.

**Sistrunk, W. E.** Mixed tumors of the parotid gland.
Minnesota Med., St. Paul, 1921—IV—155.

**Smith, H. D.** Oral infection.
Maine M. Ass. J., Portland, 1921—XI—273.

**Söderlund, G.** Actinomycosis of the salivary glands.
Acta Chir. Scand., Stockholm, 1921—LIII—189.

**Stucky, J. A.** Tonsils, teeth and nasal accessory sinuses as sources of focal infection.
Kentucky M. J., Bowling Green, 1921—XIX—205.

**Sweet, R. B.** Teeth, tonsils and sinuses.
Calif. State J. M., San Francisco, 1921—XIX—116.

**Tellier, J.** Septicemia of dental origin.
Prog. méd., Paris, 1921—XXXVI—168.

**Thoma, K. H.** Dental infections and their relation to disease. Viewpoint of the oral surgeon.
Boston M. & S. J., 1921—CLXXXVIII—434.

**Thompson, W. G.** Teeth and systemic disease.
Med. Rec., N. York, 1921—XCIX—946.

**Veau, V., and Ruppe, C.** Correction of unilateral harelip.
Presse méd., Paris, 1921—XXIX—321.

**Watts, R. C., and Mahamed, S. G.** Incidence of gingivitis among Indian troops.
Indian Med. Gaz., Calcutta, 1921—LVI—97.

**Webster, F. W.** Focal infections in the mouth.
Nebraska State M. J., Norfolk, 1921—VI—147.

## SECTION 23.—FACE.

**Behrend, M.** Rhinoplasty to replace a nose bitten off by a rat.
J. Am. M. Ass., Chicago, 1921—LXVI—1752.

**Esser, J. F. S.** Nasoplasty from the upper lip.
Zentralbl. f. Chir., Leipzig, 1920—XLVII—1412.

**Freudenthal, W.** Telangiectasis of the face and mucous membranes of the nose and throat associated with severe epistaxis.
N. York M. J., 1921—CXIII—425.

**Honigmann, F.** Primary acute suppurative parotitis.
Deutsch. Ztschrift. f. Chir., Leipzig, 1920—CLX—252.

**June, J.** New principles in plastic operations of the eyelids and face.
J. Am. M. Ass., Chicago, 1921—LXXVI—1293.

**Lindemann, A.** Reconstruction of the soft parts of the face.
Deutsch. Ztschrift. f. Chir., Leipzig, 1920—CLX—46.

**McDonald, C. A.** Salivary calculus.
Rhode Island M. J., Providence, 1921—IV—84.

**Nicory, C.** Capillary angeiomatosis of the parotid gland.
Brit. J. Surg., Bristol, 1921—VIII—481.

**Pelfort.** Transient mumps meningitis in two children.
Rev. méd. del. Urug., Montevideo, 1921—XXIV—181.

**Roy, J. N.** War surgery; plastic operations of the face by means of fat grafts.
Laryngoscope, St. Louis, 1921—XXXI—65.

**Sistrunk, W. E.** Mixed tumors of the parotid gland.
Minnesota Med., St. Paul, 1921—IV—155.

**Söderlund, G.** Actinomycosis of the salivary glands.
Acta Chir. Scand., Stockholm, 1921—LIII—189.

**Veau, V., and Ruppe, C.**....Correction of unilateral harelip.
Presse méd., Paris, 1921—XXIX—321.

## SECTION 24.—CERVICAL GLANDS AND DEEPER NECK STRUCTURES.

**Bruzzone, C.** Deep lymphoma in the neck.
Riforma méd., Napoli, 1921—XXXVII—364.

**Lipshutz, B.** Suppurative submaxillary adenitis.
N. York M. J., 1921—CXIII—440.

**Miller, L. I.** Bronchial fistulas; report of case.
Colorado Med., Denver, 1921—XVIII—110.

**Seelig, M. G.** Midline congenital cervical fistula of tracheal origin.
Arch. Surg., Chicago, 1921—II—338.

## SECTION 25.—THYROID AND THYMUS.

**Bergstrand, H.** Pathology of parathyroid glands.
Acta. Med. Scand., Stockholm, 1921—LIV—539.

**Berry, J.** Five hundred goiter operations; special reference to after-results.
Brit. J. Srug., Bristol, 1921—VIII—413.

**Blankinship, R. C.** Incidence of goiter in Wisconsin, with suggestions as to medical management.
Wisconsin M. J., Milwaukee, 1921—XIX—561.

**Brooks, H.** Physiologic hyperthyroidism.
Endocrinol., Los Angeles, 1921—V—177.

**Callison, J. G.** Double mastoid operation; acute thyroadrenal exhaustion.
N. York M. J., 1921—CXIII—431.

**Eberts, E. M.** Hyperthyroidism, diagnosis and treatment.
Canad. M. Ass. J., Toronto, 1921—XI—207.

**Else, J. E.** Interpretation of basal metabolic rate in toxic goiter.
Northwest. Med., Seattle, 1921—XX—118.

**Escudero.** Epinephrin test not specific for hyperthyroidism.
Rev. Asoc. méd. Argent., Buenos Aires, 1921—XXXIII—817.

**Escudero, P.** Thyroidin test for hyperthyroidism.
Rev. Asoc. méd. Argent., Buenos Aires, 1921—XXXIII—781.

**Fitz, R.** Relation of hyperthyroidism to diabetes mellitus.
Arch. Int. Med., Chicago, 1921—XXVII—305.

**Fritzche, R.** Malignant teratoma in the thyroid region.
Arch. f. Klin. Chir., Berlin, 1920—CXIV—317.

**Goodpasture, E. W.** Myocardial necrosis in hypothyroidism.
J. Am. M. Ass., Chicago, 1921—LXXVI—1545.

**Grubb, A. B.** Boiling water injections in hyperthyroidism.
Virginia M. Month., Richmond, 1921—XLVII—620.

**Harper, J.** Partial thyroidectomy.
J. Laryngol., etc., London, 1921—XXXVI—114.

**Hellwig, A.** Diffuse colloid goiter.
Deutsch. med. Wchnschr., Berlin, 1921—XLVII—324.

**Hill, J. A.** Surgical treatment of goiter.
Texas State J. M., Ft. Worth, 1921—XVI—544.

**Houssay, B. A.** Experimental goiter.
Rev. del inst. bacteriol., Buenos Aires, 1921—II—629.

**Houssey, B. A., and Hug, E.** Thyroidectomy in horses.
Rev. del. inst. bacteriol., Buenos Aires, 1921—II—637.

**Howard, W. F.** Toxic thyroid.
Northwest Med., Seattle, 1921—XX—110.

**Irwin, H. C.** The goiter problem.
Northwest Med., Seattle, 1921—XX—115.

**Janowski, W.** Thyrotuberculosis.
Ann. de Méd., Par., 1920—VIII—418.

**Jemma, G.** Thymic-lymphatic status with rachitis.
Pediat., Napoli, 1921—XXIX—126.

**Judd, E. S.** Laryngeal function in thyroid cases.
Ann. Surg., Philadelphia, 1921—CXXIII—321.

**Kear, L. V.** Hyperthyroidism and underacidity of the suprarenals
corrected by glandular therapy.
J. Am. M. Ass., Chicago, 1921—LXXVI—1349.

**Köhl, E.** Lingual goiter.
Schweiz. med. Wchnschr., Basel, 1921—LI—361.

**Lahey, F. H., and Jordon, S. M.** Basal metabolism as an index of
treatment in diseases of the thyroid.
Boston M. & S. J., 1921—CLXXXIV—348.

**Maranow, G.** Emotional factor in hyperthyroid states.
Ann. méd., Paris, 1921—IX—81.

**Mason, J. T.** Surgical aspects of goiter.
Northwest Med., Seattle, 1921—XX—112.

**Mayo, C. H.** The thyroid and its diseases.
Surg., Gynec. and Obs., Chicago, 1921—XXXII—209.

**Monge, C.** Endemic goiter.
Cron. méd., Lima, 1921—XXXVIII—3.

**Morris, M. F.** Hyperthyroidism.
Georgia M. Ass. J., Augusta, 1921—IX—325.

**Morris, W. F.** Value of the alimentary test in the diagnosis of mild
hyperthyroidism.
J. Am. M. Ass., Chicago, 1921—LXXVI—1566.

**Najera, F. C.**  Endemic goiter in Mexico.
Rev. Mex. d. Biol., Mexico, 1920—I—47.

**Pasman, F. R., and Mestre, R.**  Exophthalmic goiter in a pregnant woman.
Sem. méd., Buenos Aires, 1921—XXVIII—435.

**Pfahler, G. E.**  New roentgenographic technic for the study of the thyroid.
Am. J. Roentgenol., N. York, 1921—VIII—81.

**Rowley, A. M.**  Goiter—analysis of one hundred cases.
Boston M. & S. J., 1921—CLXXXIV—486.

**Schiff, E., and Peiper, A.**  Influence of thyroid treatment on the elimination of water and chlorids in infants.
Jahrb. f. Kinderh., Berlin, 1921—XCIV—285.

**Schlesinger, E.**  The thyroid in the young.
Ztschr. f. Kinderh., Berlin, 1920—XXVII—207.

**Sloan, E. P.**  Goiter operation technic.
Illinois M. J., Oak Park, 1921—XXXIX—130.

**Sweet, P. W.**  Goiter.
Northwest. Med., Seattle, 1921—XX—105.

**Terry, W. I.**  Radium emanations in the treatment of goiter; preliminary note.
J. Am. M. Ass., Chicago, 1921—LXVI—1821.

**Zanoni, G.**  Etiology of goiter.
Tumori, Roma, 1921—VII—277.

## SECTION 26.—PITUITARY.

**Aievoli, E.**  Surgery of the pituitary body.
Rif. méd., Napoli, 1921—XXXVII—162.

**Cushing, H.**  Disorders of the pituitary gland; retrospective and prophetic.
J. Am. M. Ass., Chicago, 1921—LXVI—1721.

**De Schweinitz, G. E.**  Ocular symptoms in hypophyseal disease with acquired syphilis.
Arch. Ophthalmol., N. York, 1921—L—203.

**Frazier, C. H.**  Control of pituitary lesions as affecting vision, by combined surgical, Roentgen ray and radium treatment.
Arch. Ophthalmol., N. York, 1921—L—217.

**Henry, A. K.**  New method of pituitary surgery.
Dublin J. M. Sc., 1921—163.

**Kay, M. B.**  Hypopituitarism, Froelich type.
Endocrinol., Los Angeles, 1921—V—325.

**Lockwood, B. C.**  Cholesteatomatous cystic tumor of the pituitary gland; report of case with discussion of diagnosis of pituitary disease.
J. Am. M. Ass., Chicago, 1921—LXXVII—1218.

**Redwood, F. H.**  Pituitary headache.
Virginia Hed. Month., Richmond, 1921—XLVIII—25.

Rucker, M. P., and Haskell, C. C. The dangers of pituitary extract; some clinical and experimental observations.
J. Am. M. Ass., Chicago, 1921—LXXVI—1390.

## SECTION 27.—ENDOCRANIAL AFFECTIONS AND LUMBAR PUNCTURE.

Barré, J. A., and Reys, L. Labyrinthine form of epidemic encephalitis.
Bull. méd., Paris, 1921—XXXV—356.

Bumke, O. Untoward symptoms of lumbar puncture.
Zentralb. f. Chir., Leipzig, 1921—XLVIII—449.

Cushing, H. Acoustic neuromas.
Laryngoscope, St. Louis, 1921—XXXI—209.

Diggle, F. H. Chronic suppurative otitis media followed by left temporosphenoidal abscess and meningitis.
Brit. M. J., London, 1921—I—600.

Eppler, L. R. Brain abscess following streptococcus sore throat.
Laryngoscope, St. Louis, 1921—XXXI—95.

Fowler, R. H. Gunshot wound of the lateral sinus.
N. York M. J., 1921—CXIII—453.

Fumarola, G. Tumor of the auditory nerve.
Policlin., Roma, 1921—XXVIII—60.

Gradenigo, G. Ligation of the jugular vein in otitis.
Rif. méd., Napoli, 1921—XXXVII—126.

Guthrie, D. Latent thrombosis of the lateral sinus.
J. Laryngol., etc., London, 1921—XXXVI—127.

Kyrle, J. Lumbar puncture.
Wien. klin. Wchnschr., 1921—XXIV—172.

Levy, L. Case of brain tumor showing value of Barany tests as early diagnostic methods.
Tennessee State M. Ass. J., Nashville, 1921—XIII—460.

McCoy, J., and Gottlieb, W. J. Tests of the auditory and static labyrinths and related intracranial pathways.
Laryngoscope, St. Louis, 1921—XXXI—78.

McEvoy, F. E. Simple incision for operations on the Gasserian ganglion.
Surg., Gynec. and Obs., Chicago, 1921—XXXII—271.

Pelfort. Transient mumps meningitis in two children.
Rev. méd. del. Urug., Mcntevideo, 1921—XXIV—181.

Perdue, W. W. Case of extradural abscess complicating an acute left frontal sinusitis.
South. M. J., Birmingham, 1921—XIV—424.

Renon, L., and Blamontier, P. Otogenous meningitis.
Ann. méd., Paris, 1921—IX—119.

Rodgers, T. D. Cavernous sinus thrombosis.
J. Laryngol., etc., Edinburgh, 1921—XXXVI—169.

Schaeffer, J. P. The sphenoidal sinus and the temporal lobe.
J. Am. M. Ass., Chicago, 1921—LXXVI—1488.

**Siegelstein, M. J.** Encephalitis lethargica as a postoperative complication of acute mastoiditis with report of a case.
Ann. Otol., Rhinol. & Laryngol., St. Louis, 1921—XXX—201.

**White, J. W.** Report of cases: 1. Simple mastoidectomy on man, 81 years old. 2. Infective sigmoid sinus thrombosis. A positive blood culture with streptococcus mucosus capsulatus present.
Ann. Otol., Rhinol. & Laryngol., St. Louis, 1921—XXX—199.

## SECTION 28.—CRANIAL NERVES.

**Cushing, H.** Acoustic neuromas.
Laryngoscope, St. Louis, 1921—XXXI—209.

**Fumarola, G.** Tumor of the auditory nerve.
Policlin., Roma, 1921—XXVIII—60·

**Lloyd, J. H.** Syphilis of the eighth nerve.
Arch. Neurol. & Psychiat., Chicago, 1921—V—572.

**McEvoy, F. E.** Simple incision for operations on the Gasserian ganglion.
Surg., Gynec. and Obs., Chicago, 1921—XXXII—271.

**Roy, Dunbar.** Paralysis of the external rectus in the right eye following mastoiditis in the left ear.
Ann. Otol.. Rhinol. & Laryngol., St. Louis, 1921—XXX—252.

**Sicard, J. A.** Prosthesis to correct facial paralysis.
Bull. Soc. méd. d. hop., Paris, 1921—XLV—612.

**Woods, H.** Retrobulbar neuritis.
Virginia M. Month., Richmond, 1921—XLVIII—69.

## SECTION 29.—PLASTIC SURGERY.

**Behrend, M.** Rhinoplasty to replace a nose bitten off by a rat.
J. Am. M. Ass., Chicago, 1921—LXVI—1752·

**Esser, J. F. S.** Nasoplasty from the upper lip.
Zentralbl. f. Chir., Leipzig, 1920—XLVII—1412.

**June, J.** New principles in plastic operations of the eyelids and face.
J. Am. M. Ass., Chicago, 1921—LXXVI—1293. ·

**Roy, J. N.** War surgery; plastic operations of the face by means of fat grafts.
Laryngoscope, St. Louis, 1921—XXXI—65. .

**Sheehan, J. E.** Gillies' new method in giving support to the depressed nasal bridge and columella.
N. York M. J., 1921—CXIII—448·

## SECTION 30.—INSTRUMENTS.

**Herr, A. H.** An improved and simplified technic for enucleating tonsils with special reference to soft and submerged tonsils and new instruments used.
Ohio State M. J., Columbus, 1921—XVII—324.

**Ladeback, H.** Quartz laryngeal mirror for use with ultraviolet rays.
München. med. Wchnschr., 1920—LXVII—1442.

**Lynah, H. L.** New instruments for use in laryngeal surgery.
Laryngoscope, St. Louis, 1921—XXXI—116.

**McVey, F. J.** A new tonsil hemostat.
Boston M. & S. J., 1921—CLXXXIV—524.

**Noll, F.** Apparatus for the treatment of the larynx with ultra-violet rays.
München. med. Wchnschr., 1920—LXVII—1441.

**Shapiro, I. F.** Simple noise apparatus for testing ears separately.
Laryngoscope, St. Louis, 1921—XXXI—114.

**Sicard, J. A.** Prosthesis to correct facial paralysis.
Bull. Soc. méd. d. hop., Paris, 1921—XLV—612.

## SECTION 31.—RADIOLOGY.

**Cary, E. H.** Use of radium in epithelioma of the lateral wall of the nose.
Texas State J. M., Ft. Worth, 1921—XVI—536.

**Hickey, P. M.** Intralaryngeal application of radium for chronic papilloma.
Am. J. Roentgenol., N. York, 1921—VIII—155.

**Lynah, H. L., and Stewart, W. H.** Roentgenographic studies of bronchiectasis and lung abscess after direct infection of bismuth mixture through the bronchoscope.
Am. J. Roentgenol., N. York, 1921—VIII—49;
Also Ann. Surg., Philadelphia, 1921—LXXVI—362.

**Majour and Laquerrière.** Roentgenography of the teeth.
J. d. radiol., et d'electrol., Paris, 1921—V—27.

**O'Brien, F. W.** Dental infections and their relation to disease. Viewpoint of the roentgenologist.
Boston M. & S. J., 1921—CLXXXIV—427.

**Pfahler, G. E.** New roentgenographic technic for the study of the thyroid.
Am. J. Roentgenol., N. York, 1921—VIII—81.

**Suter, E.** Radium treatment of cancer of the esophagus.
Deutsch. Ztschr. f. Chir., Leipzig, 1921—CLXII—50.

**Terry, W. I.** Radium emanations in the treatment of goiter: preliminary note.
J. Am. M. Ass., Chicago, 1921—LXVI—1821.

**Williams, F. G.** Treatment of hypertrophied tonsils and adenoids by radium.
Boston M. & S. J., 1921—CLXXXIV—256.

## SECTION 34.—EYE.

**Brandt, F. H.** Operative procedure in chronic persistent obstruction in the lacrimal sac.
Laryngoscope, St. Louis, 1921—XXXI—191.

**Crane, C. G.** Source of focal infection iritis.
N. York M. J., 1921—CXIII—442.

**De Lapersonne, F., Velter and Prélat.** Supernumerary teeth in the orbit.
Bull. Acad. Méd., Paris, 1921—LXXXV—308.

**De Schweinitz, G. E.** Ocular symptoms in hypophyseal disease with acquired syphilis.
Arch. Ophthalmol., N. York, 1921—L—203.

**Ingersoll, E. S.** Effect of intranasal conditions on the ocular muscles.
N. York State J. M., N. York, 1921—XXI—121.

**June, J.** New principles in plastic operations of the eyelids and face.
J. Am. M. Ass., Chicago, 1921—LXXVI—1293.

**Jeandelize.** Retention catheter in the lacrimal apparatus.
Médicine, Paris, 1921—II—271.

**Lamb, H. D.** Disorders of lacrimal drainage.
Am. J. Ophthmol., Chicago, 1921—IV—197.

**Loeb, Hanau W., and Wiener, Meyer.** The borderland of otolaryngology and ophthalmology.
Ann. Otol., Rhinol. & Laryngol., St. Louis, 1921—XXX—74.

**McCready, J. H.** Intranasal operation for dacryocystitis.
Penn. M. J., Harrisburg, 1921—XXIV—483.

**Monthus, A.** Chronic disease of the lacrimal apparatus.
Médicine, Paris, 1921—II—272.

**Pasman, F. R., and Mestre, R.** Exophthalmic goiter in a pregnant woman.
Sem. méd., Buenos Aires, 1921—XXVIII—435.

**White, J. A.** History of ophthalmology and otolaryngology in Virginia.
Virginia M. Month., Richmond, 1921—XLVIII—59.

**Woods, H.** Retrobulbar neuritis.
Virginia M. Month., Richmond, 1921—XLVIII—69.

# ANNALS

OF

# OTOLOGY, RHINOLOGY

AND

# LARYNGOLOGY

Incorporating the Index of Otolaryngology.

| Vol. XXX. | DECEMBER, 1921. | No. 4. |

## XLVII.

## NEURALGIAS OF THE TRIGEMINAL TRACT AND FACIAL NEURALGIAS OF OTHER ORIGIN. IMPRESSIONS DERIVED FROM A SURVEY OF 555 CASES.*

By Charles H. Frazier, M. D., Sc. D.,

SURGEON TO THE UNIVERSITY HOSPITAL, 

PHILADELPHIA.

One would expect a surgeon's thesis on the subject of facial neuralgia to deal exclusively with that particular type of neuralgia which responds to surgical treatment, and while I will present my operative experience with the major neuralgias, I should like on this occasion to include observations on certain other forms of painful affections of the face, that are of interest both from the standpoint of diagnosis and treatment. There has been much confusion in the terminology; the terms "facial neuralgia" and "trigeminal neuralgia" have been, un-

---

*Read before the meeting of the American Laryngological Association at Atlantic City, May 31, 1921.

fortunately, rather loosely used, sometimes to indicate merely certain painful zones in the trigeminal distribution, sometimes that specific form of neuralgia first described by J. Fothergill in 1776. Even for the latter, one finds in the literature a great variety of terms, such as "tic douloureux," "epileptiform neuralgia," "surgical neuralgia," not to speak of the terms of earlier writers, such as "trismus dolorificus," "la grande neuralgie," and so on. Major trigeminal neuralgia is the term I would propose as descriptive and distinctive and in order that there may be no misunderstanding as to what is implied I will briefly sketch its distinguishing and characteristic features.

Appearing suddenly and without any apparent exciting cause and with few exceptions after middle life, a sharp, shooting, stabbing, lancinating pain is experienced, at first in one of the three divisions of the trigeminal nerve, usually the second or third. The pain is likened by the patient to an electric shock, to a boring hot iron, to the tearing of flesh. The distribution of the pain has definite anatomic limitations, and without variation is referred to the terminal distribution of the nerve involved, to the lips, gums, tongue, teeth, nose, forehead. The pain comes as a bolt from the sky and vanishes like a shooting star. We speak of "attacks" as indicating certain periods of time during which the patient is subject to paroxysmal seizures. The attacks are of varying duration, a week or two at first and two or three in a year, but as time goes on the attacks are of longer duration and of greater frequency. I recall one unusual exception when the patient, whom I first saw at the age of 80, had experienced pain not more than a week in any one of ten years until the last attack, which had persisted for five weeks. During the attacks there are a series of paroxysms of short duration, usually a fraction of a minute, and of varying frequency. The paroxysms may be spontaneous, but they are almost invariably induced by talking, eating, swallowing, by hot or cold drinks, by draughts of cold air, by sudden noises, as the slamming of doors, by the slightest touch of skin or mucous membrane. The face cannot be washed or shaved, the teeth cleaned, the hair brushed, the nose blown; eating or drinking is out of the question. Between the paroxysms the patient is pain free, although complaining at times of a sense of soreness in the painful zones, and in the interval between attacks there is not a vestige or suggestion of the painful phenomena. Usually, but not invariably, patients enjoy comparative freedom from pain during the night; as a rule sleep is not disturbed. In intensity there is nothing comparable to the pain of trigeminal neuralgia unless it be the paroxysms of a tabetic crisis. The pain of renal and biliary colic is of great intensity, to be sure, but controlled at least in part by morphin. Not so the pain of trigeminal neuralgia. The habitual use of morphin is presumptive evidence that the patient is not a subject of the disease under discussion. There are certain motor, secretory and vasomotor phenomena which are only of incidental interest. This sketch, though very brief, suffices for our purpose, but that there may be no misinterpretation, permit me to mention certain facts that are of value in the differential diagnosis. A diagnosis of major trigeminal neuralgia is not justified when there is an associated area of anesthesia or hyperesthesia in the trigeminal zone, when the pain is continuous and not paroxysmal, when in the early stages there are not intervals of complete freedom, when the pain does not correspond to anatomic zones, when the pain is not referred to the terminal areas of nerve distribution.

The most important differential diagnosis to be made is between those cases which might be said to be of organic origin and those which are functional. The latter is a term that must be accepted as quite elastic and is used to include the psychoneuroses or the psychalgias. The differential diagnosis is important, because not only will the pain in the functional case not be relieved by operation, but the patient will complain as much, if not more, after the operation than he did before. I have seen a number of these neuroses, and I regret to say operated upon two of them.

SUMMARY.

A patient with severe boring pain in cheek, of intense degree and nine years' duration, after resection of two-thirds of the ganglion complains of as much pain as before operation; but after the operation the most intense pain is referred to a new territory.

Case 1 (File No. 63183). Aged 52, was admitted to my service at the University Hospital with a provisional diagno-sis of trigeminal neuralgia. The maxillary antrum had been drained seven years ago, although at the time there was no evidence of infection, and had been discharging off and on ever since. A number of teeth had been extracted. The pain was described as boring, with a sense of pressure, and was referred chiefly to the region of the cheek and malar bone and occasionally to the border of the mandible. To be sure, the pain was not paroxysmal, but it was so intense that the pa-tient was quite demoralized and pleaded for some radical means of relief. Rather against my better judgment, I finally decided to operate, and inasmuch as there was no pain re-ferred to the ophthalmic division I resected the maxillary and mandibular portions of the Gasserian ganglion.

The result was as should have been anticipated. The pa-tient stated after the operation that he had as much pain as he had before. But note that after the operation the pain was referred chiefly to the brow and the temple. While he admitted the pain in the cheek was better he was very posi-tive in his statement that on the whole he was just as miserable as before the operation. Perhaps it is easier to say what the patient did not have than what he did have. He did not have major trigeminal neuralgia, and the fact that he complained so bitterly of pain after the operation in regions of which he did not complain before should justify one in stamping the case as a neurosis. Perhaps this may be a convenient term with which to screen our ignorance as to the origin of some of these obscure pain phenomena.

That pain should be a conspicuous feature of herpes zoster one can readily understand. Not only is pain experienced during the initial illness before and after the appearance of herpetiform eruption, but in exceptional instances it persists for many years, not only in the zoster of trigeminal distribu-tion, but in those of the intercostal nerves. Postherpetic neu-ralgia must be, however, a very unusual sequel of herpes zoster. I have seen but two cases as affecting the intercostal nerves. and but one case of 520 trigeminal neuralgias.

SUMMARY.

A case of postherpetic neuralgia of five years' duration, characterized by constant pain of great severity and hyperesthesia in the first and second divisions.

Case 2. The patient, aged 66 years, had had, five years before I saw her, herpes zoster in the distribution of the supra- and infraorbital nerves. This was followed by an attack of erysipelas. The pain was described by the patient as dull, as a "constant ache"; it was referred to the cheek, the upper lip, the ala of the nose, and when she brought her tongue in contact with the roof of her mouth it excited pain and a sensation as "though her face was going to sleep." There was a sensation as though there was a pressure in the orbit from behind, and the skin in the region of the first and second divisions was hyperesthetic. While of greatest intensity during the initial "zoster" attack, it had been more or less constant ever since.

The hyperesthesia of the skin, so conspicuous in this case, I have observed as an equally conspicuous feature in the postherpetic intercostal neuralgias. Theoretically, one might assume that, of all forms of neuralgia, the radical operation on the sensory root would be peculiarly appropriate in those of herpetic origin, where the lesion is believed to be in the ganglion. There are reasons, which I will not here go into, questioning the soundness of this seemingly logical deduction, and on that account I recommended for my patient an alcoholic injection rather than the major operation.

The neuralgias due to tumor invasion may be confused with the major trigeminal neuralgias. The pain, should the tumor involve root or ganglion, is often paroxysmal, and in other respects the resemblance is quite striking. There are, however, points of distinction which, if not overlooked, are sufficient for purposes of differentiation, chief among which with tumors are the objective sensory disturbances, hyperesthesia or anesthesia, in some portion of the trigeminal distribution. We have seen in our clinic examples of these neuralgias from tumors involving the sensory root, from tumors originating in the ganglion or its dural sheath, tumors of the middle fossa with secondary invasion of the ganglion, and from tumors, extracranial, invading one or more of the three divisions. One of the most interesting of these was a tumor of the cerebello-pontine angle in a patient who, for six years, had undergone a number of operations on the supposition that he was suffering from tic douloureux. (This case was reviewed by T. H. Weisenburg, Journal of the A. M. A., May 14, 1910.)

We see frequent references in literature to the relief of the "major trigeminal neuralgias" by operation upon infective sinuses or by the treatment of dental infection. Is the neuralgia accompanying or following sinus infection one and the same as the major trigeminal form? Or to put the question in another way: Is sinus infection a recognized and accepted cause of the major trigeminal neuralgia? I scarcely venture to express an opinion before this distinguished group of specialists. On previous occasions, I acknowledge having stated in positive terms that peripheral infections, including sinus disease, played no part in the etiology. These convictions have been forced upon me by a critical analysis of my clinical experiences. On my records there are only three instances in which either at the time of my first observation or previous thereto had the patient been under treatment for sinus disease. I have not included cases in which sinus operations have been performed needlessly merely because no other apparent cause of the neuralgia could be found. That sinus infection gives rise to pain there is no doubt, but does it cause the "major trigeminal" variety? I suppose in rebuttal one might argue that my experience with the neuralgias caused by sinus infections has been limited, because the majority were relieved after sinus drainage at the hands of the rhinologist.

The following case I may quote, merely because the exception proves the rule:

Case 3. Aged 62 years. The patient was referred to my service at the University Hospital by Dr. J. M. Robinson, with the following history: She experienced her first pain— a fine needlelike prickling on the left side of the nose—nine years ago. A tooth was extracted but without relief. After a year of pain, in attempting to avulse the infraorbital nerve, the surgeon opened the maxillary antrum accidentally and saw pus escaping. Drainage continued for two weeks, and the sinus and wound were closed in six weeks. Two years later the infraorbital foramen was plugged and the antrum drained again, at first through the alveolar process, then through the nose. From that time on there has been no evidence of active infection in the antrum, but the pain soon spread to the third division. In the year prior to her coming under my observation she had had three severe attacks, a number of minor ones, and more or less continuous pain in the intervals. The attacks and paroxysms were in every respect characteristic of the major type of neuralgia. Her physical examination was negative except in so far as the roentgenogram showed a cloudy shadow of the left antrum. Even in this case the question might arise as to whether the infection was primary or accidental. At all events the pain was not relieved by the drainage operation.

What has been said of sinus infection might be said with equal force of dental infection. To be sure, the majority of cases upon which I have operated have had many teeth extracted, but in many instances there has been no evidence of infection. Sound teeth have been recklessly sacrificed, often upon the insistence of the patient, but frequently, I am afraid, at the suggestion of the dentist, because the pain is referred to or seems to be begin in one or two particular teeth.

Such evidence as I have presented or might present as to the etiology of the major neuralgias is, I confess, of a negative character. For a hundred years and more the etiology has been a matter of speculation, and we are as far today as ever from any clear cut conception or any convincing data as to the prevailing cause. Admitting, for the sake of argument only, focal infections as factors, why should these neuralgias be more common on the right than on the left side; why in the old rather than the young? The following is a table showing its prevalence in middle and later life.

In a series of 275 operations:
Number of cases between 20 and 30 years of age.......... 9
Number of cases between 30 and 40 years of age..........21
Number of cases between 40 and 50 years of age..........71
Number of cases between 50 and 60 years of age..........74
Number of cases between 60 and 70 years of age..........71
Number of cases over      70 years of age......................29

If, as I sometimes think, vascular changes, arteriosclerosis, fibrosis and a secondary anemia are causative agents, why is the disease so conspicuously a unilateral affection? Heredity has been said to play a part, but the facts do not substantiate this presumption. As a striking exception I may refer to a family under my care, a large family, to be sure, as there are twenty-two children, in which the mother and three children were victims. There have been only five bilateral cases in my entire series.

There are a great many instances of painful phenomena of the face, call them neuralgias if you will, that are associated sometimes with headaches, sometimes with hemicranias. While it does not clear up the etiology or pathology to classify them as migraine, this seems to be a common practice. I have been intensely interested in these migrainous cases, not so much so from the standpoint of accompanying headache as from the associated exhibition of pain in the face. The vasomotor disturbances one sees in migrainous subjects, as expressed by the sudden pallor or sudden flushing of the face, the pupillary dilation, the salivation, we must admit are expressions of some · derangement in the function of the sympathetic system. If this be true, has the sympathetic system anything to do with the pains or neuralgias of which these people complain in no uncertain terms? The following case will serve for purposes of illustration, although strictly speaking, it was a case of ophthalmoplegic migraine:

## SUMMARY.

An ophthalmoplegic migraine with intense pain in eye, temple and cheek, unrelieved by alcoholic injection, but immediately relieved by cocainization of the sphenopalatine ganglion.

Case 4. Aged 55 years. Patient was sent to my clinic at the University Hospital as a case of trigeminal neuralgia. The essential features of the case were these: Ever since girlhood she has been subject to sick headaches. These headaches usually lasted two or three days, recurred about twice a month and were usually induced by excitement or fatigue. About two years before admission she had had an acute tonsillar infection to which she attributes her subsequent pains and aches. Two months later she developed a hemicrania and a diplopia, and a month later violent pain in the right temple and eye.

The pain usually started in the temple and radiated to the eye; it was sharp and, as she said, "terrible at times," and would last for days at a time. There was no pain referred to the teeth, jaws, lips or tongue. The pain was aggravated by fatigue, worry and anxiety and relieved by morphin. I saw this patient daily for four weeks. There were times when she complained of headache and pain in eye and temple, times when she complained only of headache alone or of pain in eye and temple alone. There was nothing revealed in a most intensive study other than the unilateral oculomotor palsy, and this, unlike most cases of ophthalmoplegic migraine, was permanent and not transitory in character.

Now it is rather interesting to note in this case that at such times as her pains were unbearable, when I cocainized the posterior tip of the middle turbinate and indirectly the sphenopalatine ganglion, the pain within one or two minutes entirely disappeared. Can we draw any conclusion from this in building up a sympathetic hypothesis?

The relief of pain by cocainization of the sphenopalatine ganglion in this case brings to mind that pain picture out of which Sluder has constructed what he believes to be a clinical entity and to which he has given the name "nasal ganglion neurosis." I must confess in the five hundred odd cases of neuralgia that have come to my notice, not one conforms to the type as Sluder describes it with the dual picture of algesic and vasomotor phenomena. I might refer to the following case, which, though by no means a precise prototype, was relieved by alcoholic injection of the nasal ganglion.

SUMMARY.

A patient with neuralgia of the face of 12 years' duration complained of pain in eye, nose and cheek bone, radiating to the shoulder. Two carbol-alcoholic injections of the sphenopalatine ganglion were followed by remarkable improvement, but one mild attack in three months.

Case 5 (File No. 63411). Aged 34 years. Was sent to me by her husband, a physician, for the relief of what he thought was major trigeminal neuralgia. In fact, both he and she were prepared for and expected me to perform the major operation. She had complained for 12 years of pain in the right side of the face radiating to the shoulder and back of neck. The pain, which began deep in the cheek bone, was described as a steady, dull ache.. There were tender points above the eye on the inner side of the nose, over the malar bone and condyle of the jaw where the pain was severe. Occasionally there was a dull ache in the eye. The pain generally was constant and dull, though of sufficient severity to seem to warrant hypodermic injections of morphin. It was not lancinating or paroxysmal and was not referred to the teeth, gums, lips or ala of the nose. She was given at intervals of five days two injections of the sphenopalatine ganglion. Three months later her physician wrote me: "The patient is in better health than she has been for six years; in these three months she has had only one comparatively light attack; she has gained in weight and altogether has made a wonderful improvement."

In another case, not unlike this, upon the application of cocain to the sphenopalatine ganglion there was immediate relief of the sense of pain and tenderness in the eye. To use the patient's words, she felt as though the tension in the eye had been relieved instantaneously as by the cutting of a taut string. Two alcoholic injections of the nasal ganglion were given, but without any substantial relief, up to the time the patient passed from my observation.

If time permitted I could cite numerous other examples of neuralgia of the face of obscure origin, quite atypical if compared with the picture of "major trigeminal neuralgia." But these examples will suffice to illustrate the points of distinction. In many there are attacks, but in the attacks the pain is continuous, not paroxysmal. In the majority pain is referred to the eye, or rather the orbit, to the temple and to the region of the malar bone, not, mind you, to the terminal distribution of the trigeminus as the teeth, tongue, lips and nose. There are in some associated headaches or hemicranias; the pain is not described as shooting, darting, lancinating, but as burning and boring, sometimes throbbing and often with a sense of tension or pressure in the tissues. Many of these patients are relieved in part at least by opium derivatives: some are drug addicts. One can find no apparent cause, either local infection or systemic disorder. In a number I have found that cocainization of the sphenopalatine ganglion controls the pain almost immediately, but what the significance of this may be I am at a loss to say, unless we acknowledge the sympathetic system as a factor. Certainly treatment directed to the trigeminal tract is of no avail.

I scarcely venture to enter upon a discussion of the rôle of the sympathetic system as a factor in the etiology of neuralgias. The subject is not a new one, to be sure, but interest in it has been revived by observations during the war, particularly as to the relief of the pain of causalgias by the Leriche operation—stripping of the periarterial plexus. In discussing pain of sympathetic origin in different regions of the body, Tinel (La Medicine, February, 1921) describes a case in which among other sensory disorders there was an intense burning sensation, paroxysmal in character, referred to the head, neck and shoulder. This burning pain, so characteristic of the causalgias, is quite common in the facial neuralgias that are not of trigeminal origin.

Not long ago I denuded the carotid artery of a patient from whom previously I had removed the Gasserian ganglion. Despite the fact that there was total anesthesia in the trigeminal zone the patient continued to suffer intensely from pain in the region of the mandible.

### SUMMARY.

Following the persistence of pain after a Gasserectomy, the common and external carotid arteries were denuded of their plexus, but without any appreciable effect.

Case 6 (File No. 63906). Aged 30 years. Patient was admitted to the University Hospital November 10, 1917. Prior to admission the inferior dental nerve had been removed and an ineffectual attempt made to remove Meckel's ganglion. November 24, 1917, I excised the Gasserian ganglion. January 20, 1920, he returned complaining of as much pain as before, referred almost altogether to the region of the mandible. At the suggestion of Dr. Spiller, I excised the superficial cervical plexus, but to no avail. The patient was made the subject of an intensive study by Dr. A. H. Woods, who made the following notes: "There is a steady pain in the right lower alveolus, and paroxysms of electriclike pain, which shoot into the alveolus and angle of the mouth. These paroxysms may be started by apprehension of interference, by scraping, rubbing, pinching or sticking the face or adjacent cervical areas, as well as by pressure over the right cervical sympathetic trunk. There has been recently a ciliospinal paralysis, with angioneurotic edema of lips and eyelids. Because of the latter phenomena, because of the tenderness over the trunk of the cervical sympathetic and because of the apparent existence of afferent fibers (paroxysms of pain being excited by rubbing, pinching or sticking the face), Dr. Woods proposed a denudation of the arterial plexus of the common and external carotid arteries. This operation was practiced but with no appreciable effect upon the pain."

Before passing on to the question of treatment, let me summarize briefly this rather discursive presentation of our observations upon types of neuralgia. We recognize, first of all, a definite clinical entity in what we prefer to call "major trigeminal neuralgia," the symptoms of which are so characteristic that a diagnosis can be made that should admit of no discussion. The etiology is still a matter of speculation. We recognize other neuralgias in the distribution of the trigeminal nerve, some of them simulating the major type, such as the neuralgias due to tumors involving the sensory root, the ganglion or its several divisions, or the neuralgia following herpes zoster. We recognize a third group of neuralgias, involving chiefly the ophthalmic division, that we believe to be of toxic origin; symptomatically they have nothing in common with the major type. We recognize a fourth or miscellaneous group in which the pain, though of great intensity but not paroxysmal, is referred chiefly to the orbit, temple and cheek, sometimes to the neck, associated frequently with general headache or hemicrania; a group in which our suspicion has been aroused as to the part the sympathetic system may play in its origin. We recognize, finally, a fifth group, which we classify with the psychoneuroses or psychalgias.

I have led the reader through this maze of miscellaneous pain phenomena and cited so many cases with a definite purpose: I wanted to leave in the mind of the reader a very definite impression, in the first place, that there are many forms of neuralgia, and in the second place that the picture of major trigeminal neuralgia is so sharp and distinct that it should not be confused with other forms. The diagnosis is of vital importance when we come to consider the treatment, for what may be meat for one is poison for the other.

In discussing the treatment of major trigeminal neuralgia, I should like to restrict my remarks chiefly to my experience with the major operation. Of these there have been 204 avulsions or sections of the sensory root, 5 complete excisions of the ganglion and 5 partial excisions of the ganglion.

The major operation has long since been robbed of its terrors; the mortality, once 5 per cent, has been reduced to less than 1 per cent; there having been but one operative fatality in the last 177 cases of my series. One might say the method of its performance has been standardized. At one time or another I have introduced certain variations, to which I will refer in passing. For a while I substituted section of the root for avulsion, but to no advantage. In a few instances I have left intact the inner fasciculus of the sensory root, when the ophthalmic division was not involved, in the hope that by so doing trophic keratitis might be avoided. I am now waiting the results; should, in course of time, there be any recurrence in this series this modification will have to be abandoned. Latterly I have been able to conserve the motor root and thus prevent the atrophy of the temporal muscles which hitherto interfered with a perfect cosmetic result. This modification, furthermore, now makes it possible to operate on both sides in bilateral cases. All the technical difficulties have been mastered and the operation is now one of the most satisfactory the neurosurgeon is called upon to perform.

The vast majority of the patients, as one would anticipate, express complete satisfaction with the results. In fact, they are effusively grateful. There are, however, some exceptions to which I should like to call attention.

To a few the anesthesia is a source of annoyance. While the majority soon become accustomed to and disregard it, occasionally one sees the patient who, strangely enough, does not seem content with substitution of numbness for pain. One wonders sometimes whether in this case the pain before the operation was as violent as represented.

In a few instances the patients state that hearing is not as acute on the side of the operation. In every instance, when possible, I have insisted upon the patient consulting the otologist and, without exception, the report is received that hearing is as acute in one ear as the other. There is a subjective sensation of fullness in the auditory canal, such as we might have if the canal were tamponed with cotton. I have been at a loss to explain this "subjective" sense of deafness, nor has any explanation been offered by specialists whom I have consulted. This is a subject that is presented to you for discussion.

In a certain percentage of cases, about one in ten, there develop trophic lesions in the cornea. These usually appear on the second or third day, occasionally later, but in only three instances has the lesion not responded to treatment; and in two of these it has been necessary to keep the lids closed at their midpoint. In both instances the cornea is intact. Whether of advantage or not, we have adopted in our technic, preparatory to operation, a course of treatment for two days which includes installation of atropin and holocain. These with a boric acid wash and a protective shield are continued for a week after the operation. Any destructive lesion of the cornea may be prevented invariably if, upon the initial signs —i. e., the exfoliation of epithelium readily detected with a fluorescin stain, the lids are closed. Within 24 to 48 hours the corneal defect will be entirely repaired. We should not make light of this complication; while it is recognizably unavoidable in a certain percentage of cases, it is a gratification to know that if intelligently treated there will be immediate repair of the defect.

One of the most puzzling complications of the major operation is a transitory facial paralysis. Every surgeon who has operated upon any considerable number of cases has had his experience with this complication. My own includes altogether 7 cases; in the first 50 operations there were 3; in the second 50, 4, and in the last 121 there have been none. The paralyses are always transitory and do not appear until the second or third day after the operation. They are peripheral, not central, in type. I am still at a loss to account for them. It so happened that since I discontinued the use of a self-retaining retractor which forcibly separated the margins of the wound this complication has not occurred. Hutchinson attributed it to the detachment of the dura mater from the petrous bone, thus permitting blood to enter the small openings leading to the aqueductus Fallopii.

The surgical problems of major trigeminal neuralgia have been mastered. Granting no errors in diagnosis, satisfactory results are assured. Apart from our ignorance as to the etiology there is little left for the investigative mind, and our attention should now be directed to that miscellaneous group of atypical cases. Should a clear case be made out for a sphenopalatine ganglion type, permanent relief will come only when the ganglion is excised. Alcoholic injections, useful for diagnostic purposes, as a therapeutic measure are only of temporary expedience. My assistant, Dr. Grant, recently has elaborated a method of approach which, I believe, will render excision of the ganglion a simple, practical surgical problem. The part which the sphenopalatine ganglion plays in the etiology of these atypical forms cannot be definitely determined until the ganglion itself has been excised in a series of properly selected cases. In this problem and in the investigation of the rôle of the sympathetic system lies the most fertile field for future research.

XLVIII.

# LARYNGEAL TUBERCULOSIS FROM THE POINT OF VIEW OF THE PULMONARY SPECIALIST.*

By Charles L. Minor, M. D.,

Asheville, N. C.

While I am not a laryngologist, my specialty is one which makes constant demands on the doctor for the use of laryngoscopy, and no lung specialist who uses the laryngoscope systematically can fail to have unusual opportunities to detect and study those earliest changes in the larynx in this disease, whose diagnostic value is so great, and to form very definite impressions as regards the diagnosis, prognosis and treatment of laryngeal tuberculosis.

It is unfortunately true that few doctors command an easy use of the laryngoscope, or are familiar with laryngoscopic diagnosis, any more than they are with the use of the ophthalmoscope, and while we lung specialists should be an exception to this rule, this is only true of us to a limited degree. When, eleven years ago, I read a paper on the early diagnosis of laryngeal tuberculosis, before the National Tuberculosis Association in Washington, many good men admitted privately to me afterwards that they never examined the larynx as a part of their examination of the patient, were not familiar with the laryngoscope, and when the case developed symptoms referred it to the laryngologist for a diagnosis. Even today, while conditions have bettered considerably, laryngoscopy is not universally used by such workers, and very rarely, if at all, by general practitioners. The result of this failure to recognize that the larynx is an essential part of the respiratory system which must be studied in every complete pulmonary examination, has been to delay disastrously the early diagnosis of this disease in very many cases, so that it is too often not found in those stages when it is most curable, but

*Read before the Southern Section of the American Laryngological, Rhinological and Otological Society, at Asheville, N. C., January 29, 1921.

only discovered when pronounced symptoms, such as hoarseness, dysphagia, aphonia, etc., force it upon the doctor's attention. When these symptoms appear the case is sent to the laryngologist, who too often finds it so far advanced as to offer little prospect of successful treatment, and hence not only does the patient lose precious time, and too often all opportunity for a cure, but the laryngologist, unless he works in a pulmonary health resort, and hence has a chance to see this disease early, forms an unduly pessimistic view as to its curability, and thus fails to take an active interest in its treatment, for a man must be hopeful of his results if his therapeutics are to be successful.

Indeed, the laryngologist, unless he lives in a health resort, and thus has ample opportunity for seeing tuberculous cases, rarely I believe has a chance to see really incipient cases of laryngeal tuberculosis, owing to the fact that early trouble does not produce notable symptoms, such as would lead a layman to consult a throat specialist of his own accord, and also to the fault of the doctors who refer their throat cases to the throat specialist too late. A careful study of the treatment of laryngeal tuberculosis in the various handbooks on the subject shows that in the large majority the illustrations given and the descriptions written of the disease are not of its really early forms. The majority of the cases pictured are so hopelessly advanced that I feel indeed sorry for the man who has to treat them. There are some books which are notable exceptions to this rule, but they are distinctly in the minority, but I am glad to say that one of the best is by an American. I refer to the work by Lockard of Denver, which does credit both to its author and to our country.

If the use of the laryngoscope were more general, the early changes which are found in so large a number of pulmonary cases, and which with experience are not difficult to recognize, could be easily found. Various observers have reported different percentages of incidence of laryngeal tuberculosis in the course of pulmonary trouble, the rate varying from 13.8 as given by Wiligk up to 97 per cent according to Shaffer, Kidd in Albutt's system considering 50 per cent a fair average, Schech giving 30. I have not had time to look up my records for the past and to give you my statistics, but I

am very sure that 30 per cent is if anything rather an under-
than an overestimate.

The conscientious laryngologist does not fail to use his
stethoscope as an aid in the diagnosis of many doubtful cases,
even if the more careless worker, as we all know, too often
does not, and in this way I yearly see numbers of cases of
pulmonary tuberculosis which have been discovered by throat
men and sent to the pulmonary specialist, and I feel equally
that the lung specialist should always use the laryngoscope
to confirm his diagnosis of pulmonary trouble, and then send
the cases to the throat specialist for treatment. I have already
referred to the fact that a large percentage of cases with
beginning trouble in the larynx show no symptoms, or such
slight ones as not to draw the patient's attention, or indeed
the doctor's, so that without an inspection the involvement
of the larynx would not be suspected. If the doctor has to
send all his cases to the laryngologist for an opinion, many
throats will not be examined at all, whereas if he looks at
them himself, none will escape inspection, and moreover the
effect on a man's mind of seeing a thing with his own eyes
is much stronger than when the findings are reported to him
by another man. Some may urge that the recognition of early
lesions is beyond the power of any but the throat specialist,
but I cannot admit this, and I believe that any lung specialist,
who examines the larynx in every case, will in one or two
years get a very wide experience in early laryngeal lesions,
probably a wider one than the throat specialist can hope for,
since naturally the number of cases of really incipient laryngeal trouble that come of themselves to the latter must be
small.

Many men I believe hold off from using the laryngoscope
because they think it will be too difficult to learn or that it
will be too much trouble, but a few lessons in the technic,
followed by an honest inspection of the throat of every case,
will, I am sure, in six weeks or less, give the doctor an easy
command of this beautiful and simple diagnostic instrument,
and when that command is acquired it is only a question of
time, intelligence, opportunity and close observation before he
will become thoroughly familiar with the changes which suggest tuberculosis in the larynx.

I would now review my experience as to the early changes in the larynx in this disease, and I would first say that in the absence of a careful examination of the lungs, revealing to us tuberculous involvement, many of these changes in themselves are not absolutely diagnostic, whereas when the lungs have been studied and their condition is known, the diagnostic value of certain changes is enormously increased. Further it is well to remember that pachydermia, catarrh, syphilis and some other conditions can very closely simulate tuberculosis, and that therefore to think that the diagnosis of tuberculosis is always easy would lead one into great error. Here it might be apposite to quote that great authority on laryngeal matters, Schnitzler of Vienna, who has said very wisely: "With knowledge grows doubt." Of this view of Goethe's I am often unconsciously reminded when I compare my present doubt in the diagnosis of difficult cases with the confidence with which I thought I could unravel the most complicated findings. However, I do not believe any careful worker would allow himself to diagnose tuberculosis purely from a laryngoscopic inspection without searching carefully elsewhere in the body for corroboration by the discovery there of other tuberculous changes. Of course, some of the situations that meet us are very difficult, especially the combination of syphilis and tuberculosis in the same ulcer, and again the combination of tuberculosis and cancer, and the differentiation of some syphilitic from some tuberculous ulcers, but these difficult situations are not for me to discuss in this place, nor do they occur in cases where the question of extremely early diagnosis comes up.

Coming to the changes which we are studying, I would say that the departures from the normal which are of value to us can be classified as catarrhal, infiltrative, ulcerative and tumor-forming, edema not being in itself strictly diagnostic. Formerly much stress was laid on the value of changes in color of the mucous membrane, and a great deal of stress has been laid on the importance of the discovery of pallor of the mucous membrane, either of the soft palate or of the larynx proper. This view has been supported by so many excellent men in the past that one does not like to contradict it too strongly, but I am glad to say that in recent years many writers have combated it, and it is now generally recognized that while pallor is often found in the mucous membranes in laryngeal tuberculosis, it is not a reliable diagnostic feature, as a similar pallor can often be found in cases of marked general anemia and in prostrating and exhausting conditions. When, however, it is found in conjunction with other suspicious signs, it has, of course, some value. J. Solis Cohen of Philadelphia has, in speaking of the color changes in the larynx, stated very correctly that acute processes are generally ushered in by congestion, chronic ones by pallor.

As to catarrhal conditions, they are not in themselves diagnostic of tubercle, and unfortunately nontuberculous catarrh can imitate almost any of the conditions produced by a tuberculous catarrh, and this fact must be kept ever before us. A number of tuberculous patients show a generalized laryngeal catarrh, and such a general catarrh very frequently precedes the outbreak of definite tuberculous trouble, but no wise man would base a diagnosis on this. When, however, the catarrh is unilateral, patchy and persistent on one part of one cord, while the other side is normal (Figs. 2 and 3), it has great diagnostic significance and is not likely to be found in any condition but tuberculosis. There is one form of change which is common both to catarrh and to the development of tuberculosis which I have found to be of great value and to which I have elsewhere referred. I mean the grayish wrinkling and thickening of the mucous membrane of the posterior commissure (Fig. 1) found in a large number of tuberculous cases. While like other catarrhal manifestations, one cannot claim it to be diagnostic, it is yet suspicious, and if it is watched carefully, as it should be when found, it will be discovered in the tuberculous to be an early step in the development of more definite laryngeal manifestations.

A majority, however, of the diagnostic changes will come under the head of infiltration, and I think we will all agree that the commonest site of the infiltration is in the posterior commissure, more usually central, but also to one side or the other. The tablelike elevation of the posterior commissure centrally located (Figs. 2 and 3), I believe to be a very reliable early finding (though this, too, can be imitated by catarrhal change), and in this view I am entirely in accord with Schnitzler (Klinischer Atlas der Laryngologie, Vienna, 95). These elevations, if central, usually show a groove down their centers (Fig. 2) which can disappear if they thicken and enlarge. The mucous membrane is generally a pale, grayish pink, but at times it may be uniformly gray and wrinkled, and again at other times it may be reddened and angry. While, as I have said, this condition can be produced by catarrh, the longer I study the larynx in tuberculosis the more I am satisfied that such an elevation in this region is extremely diagnostic of the presence of laryngeal tuberculosis. The further course of such an elevation varies. Sometimes its center breaks down into a typical ulcer, which may stay localized, or may reach up on to the upper surface of the arytenoid region, or spread forward on to the insertion of the cord, on one or both sides (Figs. 7 and 8). Quite frequently this ulcer develops abundant granulations on its base (Fig. 5). At times, instead of abundant ones, it will throw out a hornlike, pointed one in the center (Fig. 6). At times the mass does not break down but enlarges somewhat, organizes slowly, and finally forms a firm, resistant, fibrous mass, which, if it had not been watched from its beginning, one would take for a tuberculoma (Figs. 10 and 12). Again, under treatment, it may gradually shrink and almost, but rarely totally, disappear, leaving a larynx that seems normal.

When the thickening is not central but eccentric, it is apt to involve the posterior insertion of the true cord, and thicken the posterior end of the cord at the same time (Fig. 3). Casselberry of Chicago, one of our best American students of laryngeal tuberculosis, considered a small grayish white, triangular ulcer or fissure at the insertion of the posterior cord, and in the center of this infiltration (Fig. 4), the best early diagnostic sign of tubercle which he knew, and it is unquestionably a very reliable sign, though I am inclined to believe that the tablelike elevation of which I have spoken is more frequently seen.

I might here quote part of a letter written to me by Dr. Casselberry on March 28, 1911, which well expresses his views as regards the earliest changes in the larynx in laryngeal tuberculosis:

"I lay the greater stress upon a lateral hyperplasia or infiltration which commences in the vicinity of the vocal process and as it progresses forms first a crease and later a fissure towards one side in the interarytenoid fold. I agree that central hyperplasia is a more common lesion, but do not consider that much reliance is to be placed upon it alone as a sign of tuberculosis, as it occurs in all sorts of inflammation of the larynx. That is, a nontuberculous central infiltration may be confusingly similar to that of tuberculous origin, whereas a lateral lesion, although less frequent, is in my experience quite characteristic of tuberculosis. This slight difference in the impressions gained by us is due, I think, to the variation in the run of patients coming before each. With you the tuberculous predominate, yielding of course a larger proportion of tuberculous central infiltration, while with myself the nontuberculous predominate, serving to exbibit in my mirror many central infiltrations which obviously are not tuberculous, but which, should the patient happen to be pale and thin, and so forth, the central infiltration would be indistinguishable from that of tuberculous origin."

It gives me great pleasure to thus give credit to my friend Dr. Casselberry, than whom there was no more careful student of these conditions, and to put on record his valuable views in this matter.

The infiltration of the posterior end of one or both cords is also of very great value (Fig. 1). The processus vocalis is enlarged, the whole posterior portion of the cord reddened and thickened, and if it is bilateral, as is frequently the case, the intervening mucous membrane is wrinkled and red, sometimes, however, gray. However, the inexperienced must be careful not to mistake the changes in pachydermia for the condition of which I speak. Here on the one side you have a prominent processus, on the other side a pit in the cord from the pressure of this prominence. Thickening, enlargement, and reddening of an arytenoid, on one side or the other, at once excites our suspicion (Figs. 11 and 6). The anteroposterior diameter of the central arytenoid region is increased, and the cartilages of Santorini and Wrisberg are one or both greatly thickened and rounded, the mucous membrane over them usually being reddened.

I have not found infiltrations or ulcerations of the aryepiglottic fold very early, but a reddened infiltration of the true cord localized (Fig. 11) and not involving the whole cord, as in the typical spindle shaped cord (Fig. 5), but of only a small portion of it (Fig. 1), is not, I believe, caused by anything but tubercle. While spindle shaped swellings of the cord are not as early as more localized thickenings, they are, of course, of great diagnostic value, though even here there are other conditions which can produce such swellings that cannot be told from tuberculous ones. Infiltrations of the false cord, of one side or the other, or of both (Figs. 12 and 6), have very great value, and where I find in an otherwise normal larynx an infiltrated and thickened cord on one side, not totally hiding the true cord, but encroaching upon its normal width in some portion of its course (Fig. 6), I am rarely disappointed later in finding the change to be of tuberculous origin. It is rarely, in early cases, that both true cords are hidden from sight, as they are by later thickenings of the false cords, but unlike many tuberculous changes in the larynx, you may find both false cords thickened at the same time, one, however, generally to a greater extent than the other (Fig. 12). In my experience, owing to pressure conditions, I believe, the mucous membrane of the upper surfaces of the infiltrated false cord tends to become yellowish pink, and it is at these sites that later serpiginous ulcers may develop (Fig. 6). At times the infiltration of the false cord may be very massive (Fig. 12), the enlargement being vertical as well as horizontal, and, like all changes of the false cord, very productive of at least hoarseness and often of aphonia.

The epiglottis is not, in my experience, quite so common a site of early changes as the regions already referred to, and I believe that small thickenings of the edge (Figs. 2 and 3) are more common and more early than the well known thickenings of the center of the posterior surface (Fig. 9). These small swellings of the edge are usually red and angry in their centers and pale towards their borders, and tend quite early to break down into ulcers which are very intractable (Fig. 8).

The early ulcerations of the larynx show themselves first either on the center of the posterior commissure (Fig. 8) or at the insertion of the posterior end of a cord (Fig. 4) or localized on a small area of the free edge of the cord (Fig.

9). The typical mouselike eating out of the edge of one cord (Fig. 6), which I believe to be always caused by tuberculosis, appears somewhat later. When we consider the pathologic condition of the tissues in tuberculosis of the larynx, it is evident that real tuberculous ulcerations follow infiltrations and are therefore not as early as are these, but they often appear very soon, and if treated with lactic acid or formaldehyde glycerin, my preference being for the former, the results are admirable. True, many good authorities claim that many of the ulcers in the larynx are not strictly tuberculous, but are simply erosions of the mucous membrane occurring in the larynx of a tuberculous subject, whereas the real tuberculous ulcer occurs from the breaking down of a tuberculous infiltration. Lenox-Browne quotes Heinze, who is pathologic examinations of forty-nine apparently tuberculous larynxes found 83 per cent tuberculous, 17 per cent nontuberculous. The demonstration of bacilli on their surface proves nothing, since they may have been deposited there from the sputum, and only by cutting out a portion of the ulcer and studying it microscopically could it be determined that it was or was not tuberculous in nature, and in America this is not a procedure we are likely to follow, but I am inclined to think it wise to regard and treat all ulcerations in a tuberculous larynx as tuberculous, even if it may give us a rather unduly favorable view of their curability. However, even when the ulcer shows the undermined ragged edges and the grayish deposits on its base of a typical tuberculous ulcer (Fig. 7), so that there can be no doubt about its tuberculous nature, it can still yield splendid results to local treatment. The earliest ulcers are those I have referred to as spoken of by Casselberry, small angular ones, tending to become fissures at the posterior insertion of the cord (Fig. 4). From the bases of tuberculous ulcers may arise either large rounded masses (Fig. 10), pointed pyramidal masses (Fig. 12), or many pointed granulations (Fig. 5), in the posterior commissure, and while these, of course, are not extremely early changes, they are yet so diagnostic and striking as to have great value to the physician. When they are present there seems to be a favorable fibroid tendency, so that while they do not disappear they tend to organize, shrinking somewhat and becoming firm and hard, and can remain for a long time with no bad effects except that when they are situated, as they are apt to be, on the posterior commissure, they can produce very persistent hoarseness. However, with patience and care I have seen them slowly shrink until they almost disappeared, leaving a result, both as to appearance and as to voice, that one could not have believed possible. However, this organization occurs chiefly in the rounded and pointed forms, and not in those with numerous pointed granulations, which are more apt to break down, undermine and spread (Fig. 9).

The ulcers which form on the upper surface of the false cord are sometimes typical, undermined, ragged and serpiginous, but are more apt to be like superficial erosions, but neither kind is very amenable to treatment (Fig. 6). Ulceration of the epiglottis is an extremely trying lesion because, while it can come early, it tends to spread rapidly, causes great dysphagia, and is very rebellious to treatment. Our presiding officer has gotten for me such admirable results in certain of these cases by epiglottidectomy that I do not think it worth while to treat them, if at all extensive, by other measures, and would advise their amputation as soon as possible. The results are often unbelievably brilliant.

Ulcerations of the free edge of the cord, if the patient preserves absolute silence, can give us very good results at times, but ulcerations spreading out onto the cord from an ulcerated posterior commissure (Fig. 7) and forming the well known horseshoe shape form of ulcer are of very bad prognostic significance.

Tumor formations, with one exception, are not early. The one I refer to is a small, long, pointed tumor, subglottic in origin, and appearing from underneath the anterior commissure, protruding like a small nipple (Fig. 9). It is usually slow in growth, and in my experience, rather favorable in its results, though at times it produces troublesome hoarseness. All the other changes with which the books are filled, the turbaned epiglottis, the edematous arytenoid, the extensive, dirty, spreading ulcerations, the perichondritis, etc., etc., have nothing to do with the subject of the early changes of the larynx in this trouble, and as doctors become more careful and thorough in their examinations of their cases, I believe that cases of tuberculosis of the larynx are going to come to you gentlemen in future so much earlier that you will see less and less of these unfavorable and ill omened conditions, which are responsible for the very bad repute which this disease has with the profession generally.

It is to be noted that the cases I have seen have almost all of them been known to me to have tuberculosis in their lungs before I have seen their throats, and therefore I can feel much more certain of my position than can the man who chances in a routine laryngeal examination to find some of these changes in persons who seem otherwise perfectly healthy, but a careful examination of the lungs is always at his disposal, and when any of the conditions that I have spoken of are found in the larynx, he would certainly be hopelessly derelict in his duty to his patient unless such an examination was made. By themselves, as I have said, they will not allow the doctor to be too positive and sure in his diagnosis, but, combined with the findings in the lungs, one can afford to make a positive statement. It is astonishing at times to see how even good men will fail to go into the history and condition of a patient thoroughly and thus not recognize the tuberculous nature of conditions in the throats which come to them.

Within the week I have seen an instructive case of this nature. A young man, before he went into the war in 1917, had a rather troublesome cough for some weeks, and while his health in the army-in this country and in Europe was good, the cough persisted most of the time. He came out of the army in 1919, feeling well, but still with some cough and hoarseness. He went to a prominent laryngologist in a great city, whose name I am sure is familiar to all of you. He examined him, said that he needed a tonsillectomy, the tonsils were removed, the cough continued, he treated the nose locally in various ways, and had the patient under observation for a year. The patient fearing tuberculosis, suggested this possibility to the doctor, who pooh-poohed it, saying that he looked too perfectly well for such a thing to be possible, and did not examine his sputum or his lungs—this, mind you, being a man of standing and prominence in the profession. Later he had the good fortune to be recommended to another equally well known man who at once suspected trouble, examined his sputum and put him on systematic laryngeal treatment and sent him to a lung specialist, who found trouble. Both lungs are considerably involved, and the larynx shows changes which in themselves are not typical, but which combined with the findings in the lungs are sufficient to diagnose the laryngeal involvement as tuberculous. When physicians can make mistakes of this sort, for this is not an isolated case, through a foolish cocksureness, and a failure to examine the sputum and the lungs in cases that are coughing, it is no wonder that we often see bad results. Yet many men seem to think that dysphagia must be found before they can think of the possibility of tuberculosis. It simply serves to remind us that in medicine nothing can be taken for granted and that no opinion is justified that is not backed up by a complete and conscientious examination.

A difficulty under which the laryngologist labors is that he cannot usually have his patients as closely under his eye and their lives as strictly supervised as can the lung specialist, and that thus the patient usually misses the favorable conditions yielded by sanatorium treatment and outdoor life. If, however, the cases are seen by him sufficiently early and he can arrange to get for them proper conditions of living, I believe that the general view as regards the very bad prognosis of laryngeal tuberculosis would undergo a great change and become much less pessimistic. It is not usually advisable for a lung specialist to undertake the treatment of such cases himself. He is not technically prepared to carry out the many valuable therapeutic instrumental procedures which may be necessary, and the laryngologist can well say to him: "Shoemaker, stick to your last." But I do believe that in uncomplicated cases of infiltrative tuberculosis of the larynx he can, by strict rest of the voice through silence and by carrying out what Bosworth has called the mild treatment of these cases, get very excellent results. Indeed, very active local treatment in the beginning is usually contraindicated. The mild treatment, as I have used it, consists first of local cleanliness through the use of simple alkalin sprays; second, where congestion is a feature of the trouble, the use of mild astringent sprays; third, where stimulation and healing are necessary, the use of oily sprays in which menthol, eucalyptus and gaultheria are usually elements. Catarrhal conditions, in my experience, whether tuberculous or simple, yield admirably to this very simple treatment. When, however, we find infiltration as in the changes I have described earlier, the addition to the former treatment of the insufflation of powdered iodoform will, I am satisfied, as a result of ample experience, cause in a very large number the gradual reabsorption of such infiltrations and the cure of the trouble, even if so good an authority as Lockard disbelieves in the practice. I have not found it difficult to teach the patients how to insufflate their own larynxes on wakening and on going to bed, although there are certain people with an idiosyncrasy to iodoform, in which it acts as an irritant, or whom it nauseates, and where it has to be given up. It sometimes causes a slight cough for a little while, but this is not troublesome. As to the patient's ability to blow the powder into the larynx, we all know that they succeed with orthoform, thus frequently checking severe pain, and where orthoform can go iodoform will go also. The mode of its action is simple and plain. Iodoform in the presence of living cells gives off nascent iodin, which is far more active than ordinary iodin, and than which there is no better tuberculocide known. This iodin is discharged into the infiltrated tissue and slowly causes its absorption and disappearance. I have used it for too many years (twenty-five) and in too many cases to doubt the causative relation of the disappearance of the infiltration and the use of the iodoform, or to justify the claim that it is merely a coincidence, and I can heartily recommend it to all of you. If one doubts the patient's ability to apply it correctly (naturally, the patient must be trained how to insufflate correctly while he inhales and how to put the point of the insufflator in the correct position), the patient should come in daily, but I personally think it very unwise to make a tuberculous patient come daily to the doctor's office for a treatment.

In ulcerated cases it is by no means so useful, and in any case, in these local applications are far better. Unless the lung specialist is especially skillful in the use of the laryngeal applicator, patients with ulcers had best be sent to the laryngologist for local treatment, and in these early ulcers the use of lactic acid glycerin or formaldehyde glycerin produces very brilliant results.

So essential to the laryngologist's success with these patients is the condition of the general vitality that it would be wise, if he cannot watch this featuer of the case, to have all his tuberculous larynx cases watched by a man skilled in the regulation of their lives, the raising of their vitality, and the bracing up of their morale, and I am sure in this way very much better results would be gotten than by local treatment, not re-inforced by constitutional and moral.

May I here be permitted a few words as to some of the results of laryngeal surgery, which I, seeing the cases after the laryngologist has gotten through with them, have a better opportunity to watch than you gentlemen. I refer to the not infrequent cases of the waking up of a hitherto entirely latent tuberculosis through a tonsillectomy or through some laryngeal operation. I have not rarely seen such interference the starting point of a desperate and fatal pharyngeal or laryngeal tuberculosis, or, much more frequently, the beginning of an active pulmonary tuberculous involvement, doubtless through the trauma of the operation disseminating tuberculous matter which had been hidden in the tonsils or other tissues. For this reason I believe that it is very important if the snare is used that the tonsil be very well freed before the wire is applied so that the pressure can by no means disseminate infective matter when the loop is tightened, and to do all such operations as cleanly and gently as possible.

Again, I see not a few cases of tuberculosis whose history shows that the beginning was due to the anesthetic used for a tonsillar or other operation. I will not here upon up the to me intensely interesting question of posttonsillectomy pulmonary abscess, a subject first referred to in this country, I believe, by Richardson of Washington in 1910 and 1912, for. though I see a number of such cases every year, it would divert discussion from the main subject of my paper.

In the years I have been treating tuberculosis I have seen so many cases where a history of an anesthesia by ether in a hitherto healthy person, followed by the development of a cough and then of tuberculosis, is plainly given, that I feel,

despite the fact that the great majority of patients who take
ether for these purposes escape with no bad results, that this
question of the possible danger of etherization as an initiator
of tuberculosis must be seriously considered before every
operation. Many operators would laugh at this, as they usually do not see these cases after the wound is healed and when
the new trouble begins, and it is the lung specialist, to whom
they come somewhat later, who has a chance to study them.
I fully realize the comfort to the operator of a deeply anesthetized patient, which makes his operative technic so much more
easy and exact, but the gain in these ways is more than counterbalanced when we realize that that sleeping tuberculous
focus which all of us carry may be and often is wakened into
activity by the irritation of the anesthetic in the lungs.

Moreover, I believe, it has been sufficiently demonstrated
that with the use of novocain and adrenalin a beautiful and
satisfactory anesthesia can be produced in the larynx, pharynx
or tonsils, and that, save in children who are so terrified that
they cannot be kept quiet, it should be the anesthetic of election in all laryngologic work.

Finally, since tuberculosis so often affects the larynx, your
specialty and mine are bound to be closely united, and it is
most desirable that the men working in both these branches
of our profession should seek to see these problems through
the eyes of the other specialty and not purely in the light of
their own. The lung specialist needs to command thoroughly
the use of the laryngoscope and have a comprehension of the
changes in early laryngeal tuberculosis. The laryngologist
needs to be a careful examiner of chests and to understand the
control of the patient's life and the building up of his general constitution. The former should be carefully on the
lookout for laryngeal changes and symptoms in his patients
and promptly call to his aid the laryngologist when he finds
those slight departures from normal which are either positively diagnostic or at least strongly suspicious. The laryngologist needs, I believe, to consider the condition of the lungs
of all his patients, especially those who cough, and examine
them thoroughly much more often than he now does, or at
least he must be able to take a good general history and to
recognize the symptoms and signs which point to possible

tuberculosis and then to refer the case to a competent man for examination, and he should give up the very prevalent custom of treating coughs as though they were purely of local laryngeal origin. When he does this he will find that in a large number of cases the real origin of the cough is in the lungs. To treat a cough locally unless you know the lungs are normal is in these days simple malpractice. When we look at cases in this light, not only will our two branches of the profession benefit, but what is far more important, our patients will get far better results from our treatment.

Let us hope then that our two specialties will yearly come closer together, work more in unison, comprehend better the problems which each has to face, and come together to help each other solve them. When this is done we will see fewer mistakes in diagnosis, less careless and planless treatment, and we will look with less pessimism than has hitherto been our custom on the results of the treatment of laryngeal tuberculosis.

61. NORTH FRENCH BROAD AVE.

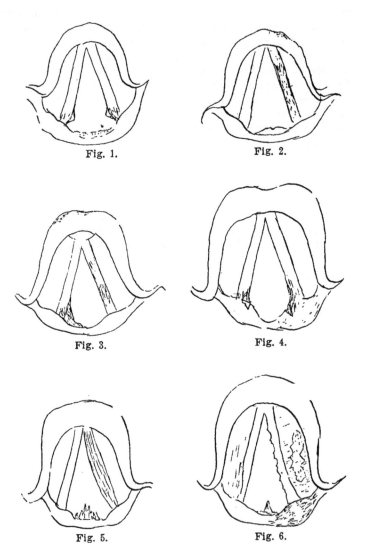

Fig. 1.

Fig. 2.

Fig. 3.

Fig. 4.

Fig. 5.

Fig. 6.

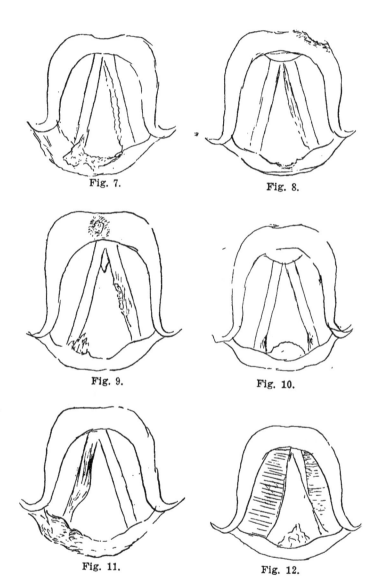

Fig. 7.

Fig. 8.

Fig. 9.

Fig. 10.

Fig. 11.

Fig. 12.

## XLIX.

## CLIMATE IN THE TREATMENT OF LARYNGEAL TUBERCULOSIS.*

By Carroll E. Edson, A. M., M. D.,
Denver.

Tuberculosis of the larynx is practically, always secondary to an active pulmonary tuberculosis. The extent and character of the primary lesion usually determine our choice of climate for the patient.

To discuss satisfactorily how the supervention of the laryngeal infection may modify this selection, we must have a clear understanding of the part climate plays in the cure of pulmonary tuberculosis. We must know just what reaction we expect to obtain when we recommend a change of climate.

The arrest of a pulmonary tuberculosis is brought about through tissue and physiologic resistance to the tubercle bacillus and its products. At present our only means of cure are those which directly or indirectly perfect, maintain or increase this resistance. The essential factors to this end are:

1. Outdoor life in pure air and sunshine,
2. Abundant nutrition,
3. Rest.

An outdoor life means living constantly in the open air. Its effectiveness is directly in proportion to the number of hours so spent out of every twenty-four. Its benefits are not secured by the patient going out occasionally for recreation, but only by passing his entire life, so far as possible, in fresh, open air; not only while at work or play but while at rest, and especially during the hours of sleep.

Abundant nutrition means, not an amount of food eaten or even of fat accumulated, but the highest maintainable balance of nutrition. It is not food ingested which counts, but food made physiologically active. To secure this maximum requires careful attention to all the patient's metabolic pro-

---

*Read by invitation before the American Laryngological Association, Atlantic City, May 30, 1921.

cesses of digestion, assimilation and especially of elimination through bowels, kidneys and skin.

Rest is economy of physiologic expenditure. Its importance in tuberculosis cannot be overestimated, but it must be carefully controlled. It is a relative term, and its meaning will vary according to the individual patient, from absolute confinement to bed over long periods, to such graded and controlled exercise as may approach full measure of work. It includes not only the limitation of muscular exercise, but control and regulation of the intellectual and emotional activity of the patient.

While all these factors are important, it does not follow that there is equal need of each for every patient. One will be most helped by rest, his nutritional balance being already well established; while another stands in urgent need of food. or may be wholly untrained to hygienic living, or the uses of fresh air. For this reason close and prolonged medical oversight is essential to secure the patient's gaining the maximum benefit from and proper distribution of the factors of rest, food and outdoor life.

What help do we gain from climate in this scheme of living?

Climate is the sum total of the meteorologic conditions prevailing in a given region over considerable periods of time. It is the average mean and range of meteorologic phenomena characterizing that place. Weather is the immediate state of those phenomena at any particular time. It is important to have this distinction always in mind. Their confusion has caused disappointment to patients and resentment against the climatologist. The weather may be very bad, wet and cold, for instance, at any one time, although the average usual conditions in that place at any time of the year are warm and sunny days. Equally a region of general cloudy or damp climate will have its pleasant days of bright sunshine.

Climate being the whole average state of meteorologic conditions prevailing in any region, every patient, wherever he dwells, lives in a climate of some kind. It is incorrect to speak of the climatic treatment of tuberculosis as one would of the quinin treatment of malaria, as if it were a specific. It is equally absurd to contrast it with medication by tuberculins or confinement in a sanatorium, as if it were a means which could be used or not, according to choice or prejudice. The climate has to be considered in every case. It cannot be avoided, for it is the environment of temperature, sunshine, humidity, rainfall, wind and barometric pressure in which the patient lives. If we keep him at home we select a climate for him as fully as if we sent him away.

The application of climate to the cure of pulmonary tuberculosis is therefore only the best utilization of these average conditions to aid in securing the fullest measure of the necessary outdoor life, in bringing some of the meteorologic components to the support or upbuilding of nutrition and tissue resistance to the disease or in maintaining physiologic rest.

A continuous outdoor life being of first importance for his cure, it follows logically that there must be an advantage to a patient with pulmonary tuberculosis in placing him promptly in a region where he can most constantly, most comfortably, with the least difficulty and fewest interruptions lead such a life.

The process of healing in a tubercular lesion is slow, and the establishment of complete arrest requires a period measured, not by days, but by months or years, during which time the patient should live out of doors. It is not the occasional pleasant day, accordingly, which counts, but the probability of such days prevailing abundantly over long periods.

Theoretically a patient can be kept out of doors in any weather, and pure air is the same everywhere; but in the actual management of a patient's life it is not the academically possible, but the easily practical, which counts the most.

The character of the weather from day to day has a great influence upon the ease and safety with which an invalid can spend his time out of doors, and the readiness with which he submits to the outdoor regime.

In one region the winter temperatuer of the air, for instance, may range so low as to require so much clothing as to be a burden to a weakened or delicate patient. It may fall so low at night as to forbid his sleeping out at all, thus depriving him of one-third of his outdoor life. In another place the summer temperature will be so high or accompanied by such humidity as to be seriously oppressive, diminishing the appetite or preventing such exercise as is desirable. A change from such a climate to a cool and breezy one will obviously be of advantage to the patient.

The degree of actual and relative humidity affects our sensation of temperature and our endurance of heat or cold. It directly influences heat loss and consequently is a factor in the metabolic balance.

The amount of sunshine, the percentage of the total possible which is actually realized in any place is of great importance to an invalid, especially if he must be inactive during the cold of winter days. In one region there may be in winter out of a hundred consecutive days an average of only twenty which are clear, while in another during the same period less than twenty will be cloudy.

Whether he be at rest or active, it is not so easy for a patient to live out of doors, even if the air be equally pure, in a place where fog or drizzly rain is frequent, as it is where week after week goes by without rain or cloud.

Similar comparative illustrations might be given of other climatic factors which are of physiologic importance to a person planning to live a long continued outdoor life; the frequency and force of high winds, influencing heat loss in cold weather or causing nervous wear if hot and dry; the regularity and extent of the diurnal range of temperature or the frequency and degree of variations from the mean.

But these examples are sufficient to indicate how the physician who is mapping the plan of life for a pulmonary invalid should consider whether he can better the conditions under which the patient is to make his fight by sending him to a more salubrious region just as he would move another patient from a dark, unventilated closet in a tenement alley to an open air ward in a municipal hospital. We improve the surroundings to the extent of our ability and the patient's means. We strive to place each patient where the climatic conditions most facilitate his leading the proper outdoor life.

If such favorable conditions are found to a greater degree or in a more constant measure in another region than the patient's home we advise him to go to that place to live; we urge him to make a change of climate. He moves into better meteorologic surroundings, as he might from a damp, poorly heated house to a dry and sunny one.

A change of climate for the purpose of facilitating an outdoor life should be prescribed, however, only when it can be made without more than counterbalancing loss in the other factors of the cure: nutrition, rest and medical control. There is no gain to a patient in placing him in the most ideal climate if to do so deprives him of the means of securing sufficient proper food or the other conditions of right living. A patient who at home might have abundance of food and care, and, even if idle, continue to have it through family assistance, may not away from home be able to command that aid in the form of money. To earn this by his own exertion may demand labor at a time when work or activity is most detrimental. Either nutrition or rest must suffer. Such a patient is better off at rest amid such conditions of outdoor life as his home climate affords.

On the other hand, one whose physical state warrants labor or whose social and financial circumstances force him to work, may often find that the gain from a more equable, milder or more bracing climate will enable him to continue at his occupatiou as he could not under the old less favorable conditions. If his only days for outdoor rest are his Sundays, he will benefit from living in a region where he can sleep out the entire year, and where forty of his weekly holidays are likely to be pleasant and sunny, instead of in a place where at most he might count on fifteen or twenty without rain or cloud.

Closely related to the question of nutrition and rest is that of proper medical supervision of the patient's life. The exceedingly elastic meaning which we must give to the term "rest" necessitates such competent medical control of the patient wherever he may live. This is especially true of cases with complications, such as laryngeal involvement, for instance, which may need local treatment. In determining upon a change of climate it is important, therefore, to know whether in the new region of better outdoor facilities the patient can have a sufficient degree of skilled medical advice. It is equally important to impress upon his mind the need for such control in the new abode. Patients too often act as if they had been told that the change to a different climate constituted the whole cure. It only affords a better opportunity to work out that cure.

Finally certain physiologic reactions to climatic factors must be borne in mind. The problem of nutrition, as we know, goes deeper than the mere question of food supply. So a change of climate may, by reason of altered conditions of temperature or sunshine, prove beneficial to one patient by stimulating appetite, digestion and assimilation. It may be unavailing to another because some factor, it may be of barometric pressure or humidity, makes demands upon his circulation or emunctories beyond their power of response. This so disturbs the physiologic balance as to offset the other advantages of easier outdoor life.

As I am now asking your attention only to the general principles controlling the selection of climate for the pulmonary invalid, it is unnecessary to go into a detailed discussion of these varied physiologic reactions. I state very briefly only those meteorologic factors of climate which experience has shown to directly influence and be most conducive to improvement in pulmonary tuberculosis.

1. Moderate or fairly high altitude. Such elevation, besides giving greater diathermance to the air and stronger sunshine, has a direct effect on hemopoiesis, promptly and decidedly increasing the formation of red corpuscles.

2. Temperature.—Cool climates are definitely conducive to nutritional improvement. Almost without exception patients make their best gain during the cold months. In southern latitudes elevation aids in securing this cooler climate.

A moderate daily range of temperature is desirable, as is a reasonably well marked annual range. Both give variety and stimulate circulatory action. Sudden, violent or long continued variations from the mean are to be avoided, as they tax the patient's physiologic response and may interrupt the routine of his outdoor life.

3. Sunshine.—The value and results obtainable from heliotherapy have been most astoundingly shown by Rollier in his clinic. The more abundant and continuous the sunshine, the better available is this valuable means of cure. The dosage must be carefully controlled, for direct sunlight, especially in high altitudes, is a powerful force not without capacity for harm. A climate of strong, continuous sunshine makes feasible an uninterrupted schedule of treatment.

4. Humidity.—The actual and especially the relative humidity of the air is perhaps the most important single factor in our comfort out of doors. It has most to do with the rate of heat loss from the body surface and with our endurance of the extremes of heat and cold. The drier the air the better each is borne, and the more enhanced the value of the direct sunlight.

5. Precipitation.—The important desiderata are a low annual rainfall and a reasonably even distribution of it through the year, so that the hot days of summer may be refreshed by short showers, and the rain or snowfall of winter be not too frequent or too long continued.

6. Wind.—A moderate regular movement of the air is most desirable for its effect on the cutaneous systems, both nervous and circulatory. It is the movement of the air upon the skin which stimulates and gives the exhilaration so associated with fresh air.

To be shunned are frequent, violent or long continued heavy winds, especially in the cold of winter or during seasons of high humidity. Equally is the close association of high wind with great dryness and dust an evil partnership for discomfort and harm.

How does climate help the patient with laryngeal tuberculosis, and what choice of meteorologic components is desirable in his case?

Tuberculosis of the larynx responds only in a general way and to a slight degree to the increased vitality induced by outdoor life and nutrition. The local laryngeal lesion is less directly affected than pulmonary tubercle by these factors. Its arrest is more dependent on the third member of the physiologic triad, rest.

Under the establishment and maintenance of complete rest the prognosis of laryngeal tuberculosis is much better than popularly believed. This complete rest, incomparably the most important part of the treatment we can bring to bear, is curiously difficult to secure.

The first, the most effective means to this end, the hardest to obtain, is silence, the absolute avoidance of all phonation. I need not enlarge upon this statement before the Laryngological Association, but I do wish to put the whole weight of my professional experience into urging you to impress upon your patients and your pupils an appreciation of its importance and value as a working therapeutic fact and not a theory only.

Next in value to silence in securing the fullest rest to the larynx is the abolition, reduction or control of cough, from whatever source it arises.

The cough of infraglottic origin, rising from the pulmonary disease, will lessen with the improvement in that lesion.

Climate, as I have shown, is a valuable aid in securing that arrest and often gives surprisingly prompt results in diminishing the cough. The local laryngeal irritation, most soothed by rest, may occasionally need local sedative applications. It is, however, to a considerable degree affected by atmospheric conditions presently to be mentioned, the control of which may greatly assuage the patient's discomfort.

The supralaryngeal cough caused by nasal, and especially pharyngeal trouble, is a factor of great importance in its wear upon the patient. From my observations it is not sufficiently appreciated or given enough detailed care. Even in purely pulmonary tuberculosis no small fraction of the most annoying cough is alleviated by proper and painstaking care of the catarrhal or obstructive congestion of the upper respiratory area. In laryngeal tuberculosis the cough from these sources is especially harmful, for it remains always a nonproductive, unnecessary cough of purely mechanical violence.

Now, it is in helping control and lessen the cough arising from the nose, the pharynx and the glottis that certain climatic factors play a definite and direct part. So important and so readily demonstrated is this role that the presence of a tubercular laryngeal lesion calls for especial consideration of them in the choice of climate. The later development of a laryngeal tuberculosis may make for the first time a change of climate advisable.

A patient with laryngeal tuberculosis does not endure well excessive heat or cold. Such patients are prone to loss of appetite and poor nutritional balance, even before any pain on swallowing has occurred. This early loss of weight and the frequent accompanying anemia is out of proportion to the added amount of tubercular disease.

I believe it is the result of anxiety, discouragement and

fear born of the knowledge and constant evidence of this complication. Consequently any added cause for poor appetite and assimilation, such as heat or humid weather, is to be avoided.

Equally do such patients suffer from great cold, especially at night, and the irritation from breathing very cold air may excite so much cough as to prevent sleeping out. Thus one of the most valuable opportunities for combining fresh air and rest will be lost. Even though the daytime cold is modified by bright sunshine, very cold nights or too wide a diurnal range in temperature are to be avoided. For these reasons it may be advisable for a patient who can afford it to make a winter sojourn in a more southern, warmer station and change to a cooler, more bracing region in the summer months.

Abrupt or marked change in the temperature of the respired air readily induces cough, as we well know. Climates characterized by such sudden or frequent changes are to be avoided.

Damp air, especially if at all cold or in motion, is an immediate excitant of cough to an inflamed larynx or sensitive rhinopharynx. Therefore the greatest benefit will accrue to the patient in a mild, equable climate, with a dry air, low relative humidity and long periods without wet weather, one, too, in which the precipitation is fairly evenly distributed in short downfalls rather than in a prolonged rainy season.

Strong winds and dusty air are sedulously to be avoided. Frequently in the same region of generally similar climatic conditions one locality will have a topography yielding shelter from the prevailing wind. It will so be entirely suitable, while a station near at hand not so protected is undesirable.

Such local details are important to consider, even after the general problem has been settled. Indeed the whole success in the cure of laryngeal tuberculosis is a matter of appreciation of, and enforcing attention to detail.

In this connection may I add a word, even if it seem a criticism? Too often we see patients sent long distances from home at a sacrificing cost to gain the advantage of a better climate for living out of doors, who, because of a laryngeal lesion, take frequent or even daily trips to the physician's office. There they sit in a crowded, often poorly ventilated room waiting their turn for local applications. This travel and waiting is undertaken frequently when the exertion involved or presence of fever should forbid should conduct. Any such patient with acute laryngeal tuberculosis which needs regular treatment should be cared for at home. If the laryngologist cannot give the time for such visits the patient will be best placed in a sanatorium where the means for local treatment are at hand, and where he does not have to pass his waiting time indoors rereading a last year's copy of Outdoor Life.

These briefly are the principles underlying the use of climate in the cure of laryngeal tuberculosis.

There is no specific climate for tuberculosis.

The disease may heal in any climate.

Some climates, however, offer the patient an incomparably better opportunity to make full use of the three requisites for cure: an outdoor life, increased nutrition, physiologic rest.

Laryngeal tuberculosis does not require a climate essentially different from that for pulmonary disease.

It does benefit, however, from attention to details. These are care in selecting a milder climate without extremes of heat or cold, especially the latter; freedom from frequent sudden changes of temperature, damp air, particularly in winter, high winds, and dust.   .             .

A careful consideration of the balance between the patient's needs, his means and the reasonable advantage to be gained from a change in surroundings is necessary to avoid disappointment or disaster. To make a correct selection the physician must understand the climatic characteristics of both the home and the contemplated resort. He must have an accurate knowledge of and an interest in meteorologic statistics and be able to interpret them properly in terms of physiologic effect upon the patient.

Future advance in the best utilization of climate will come with a greater appreciation of the fact that the physical modalities of temperature, humidity, sunlight, wind and barometric pressure are real and definite in their action. The more complete our study and knowledge of the physiologic response which they demand from a patient the better use we shall be able to make of these climatic components in the environment we select for the invalids who seek our counsel or depend upon our care.

# THE TREATMENT OF TUBERCULOUS LARYNGITIS BY SUSPENSION LARYNGOSCOPY.*

## By L. W. Dean, M. D.,

### Iowa City.

In discussing the question of the treatment of tuberculous laryngitis by suspension laryngoscopy I shall speak of this procedure only as it applies to my own work, I realize full well that while I am able to do my very best work with the larynx exposed by suspension, some others more accustomed to expose the larynx for endolaryngeal operations in a different way can do work equally well and with just as favorable results. I am fully convinced that each of us should perform endolaryngeal operations by the method with which we are most expert.

Using proper precautions, endolaryngeal operations may be performed upon the tuberculous larynx by suspension without detriment to a coexisting quiescent pulmonary condition. At least, the lung experts who keep our patients under observation cannot detect deleterious results.

During the earlier third of my laryngologic career I operated my cases of tuberculous laryngitis by indirect laryngoscopy; and during the latter third by suspension laryngoscopy and direct laryngoscopy. It is certain that during the middle third results secured were much better than those of the first, and those secured during the latter third are much better than the results of treatment during the second period. This improvement in results is not entirely due to a change in the method of doing the endolaryngeal work. However, suspension laryngoscopy helped very much.

One-half of our cases today receiving galvanopuncture, curettage, etc., have the work done by direct laryngoscopy. In my hands these patients do not get as good results as those

---

*Read before the forty-third annual congress of the American Laryngological Association, Atlantic City, N. J., May 30, 1921.

that are suspended. It is quite impossible for me to do as accurate work by direct laryngoscopy as by suspension. I have done many more endolaryngeal operations by the direct method than by suspension. I cannot place my cautery or knife as accurately by the former as by the latter method, neither can I protect the larynx so well from the cautery point. As to whether the patient is to be suspended or treated by direct laryngoscopy we will discuss later.

Unless there is some contraindication to its use, suspension laryngoscopy is to me the procedure of choice for endolaryngeal operations on the tuberculous larynx. The well illuminated larynx is thoroughly exposed. Both hands of the operator are free. He may have in one hand a spatula to expose better or to protect a certain area in the larynx, and in the other his galvanocautery point, punch or curette. He is at liberty to turn to his instrument table and select, if necessary, a different instrument without interfering with his work. He may take in his left hand a laryngeal speculum and expose the upper end of the trachea, the anterior commissure or the interarytenoid space, leaving his right hand free for operative work on the part exposed. There is no hurry. I frequently demonstrate the patient to sixteen students without the patient objecting. If there is any inconvenience from the suspension it is during the first few minutes. The patient who is suspended the first time may feel that he is suffocating. The tuberculous case is particularly favorable for suspension. The emaciated neck makes the procedure a very easy one.

Suspension laryngoscopy in laryngeal tuberculosis is indicated only in children old enough to be controlled and in adults. The use of a general anesthetic in this class of cases should not be considered. This prevents suspension laryngoscopy with young children. The work is done under local anesthesia. There is no excuse for loosening teeth. I frequently attach the tooth clips to a dental bridge, using a lead protector. There should not be the slightest danger of jaw fracture. The patient should be rapidly suspended, using every precaution for the patient's comfort. To get a good view it is not necessary to separate the jaws widely. Separating the jaws too widely may add to the patient's discomfort. It is not always necessary or advisable to bring the anterior commissure into view. It is never necessary to riase the patient's head from the table. Once suspended there is no reason for hurrying with the patient.

The anesthesia: Morphin ¼ grain, atropin 1/120 gr., is given twenty minutes preceding the operation. Ten per cent cocain is applied to the epiglottis and larynx, using a cotton swab. The swab is held in contact with the epiglottis and cords until all tendency to gagging disappears.

Immediately following the operation the patient is placed in a croup tent for six hours. We have never had a postoperative edema or hemorrhage of any consequence following the removal of the epiglottis of endolaryngeal operation on a tuberculous larynx by suspension. We have had marked edema following endolaryngeal operations by the direct method and hemorrhage following the remova lof the epiglottis without suspension. Suspension prevents these sequelæ by permitting of exact incision and cauterization when operating in the larynx and so thoroughly exposes bleeding points that they may be properly handled.

For amputating the epiglottis suspension laryngoscopy is the procedure of choice. Under local anesthesia, using the short Lynch tongue spatula, the epiglottis is distinctly exposed. It is grasped with a tenaculum forcep and, using a Lynch knife, cleanly severed at its base. I have not noted any hemorrhage of importance following this procedure. It requires but a short time.

Sometimes the shortest laryngeal spatula is too long. I then substitute the long clips used by Lynch with his tooth plate for the short clips. This brings the spatula forward on the tongue and gives a better exposure. This is more often necessary when working on the lingual tonsil by suspension.

It is not within the province of this paper to discuss the indications for endolaryngeal surgery in tuberculous laryngitis.

I will try to outline my conception of the conditions under which suspension laryngoscopy should be used and try to indicate the class of cases in which it has seemed to us to be particularly beneficial.

From July, 1919, to April 5, 1921, we had in our service 143 cases of tuberculosis of the larynx. Seventy-three received operative treatment, 37 were operated upon by direct laryngoscopy, and 36 by suspension. Dr. Scarborough, who is in charge of these cases, reports of those suspended all but a few secured improvement, most of them marked improvement, and a considerable number apparently recovered. The 37 cases are those who never were operated endolaryngoscopically except by the direct method. If we would compare the number of endolaryngeal procedures by direct laryngoscopy with those by suspension in the forty or more cases of laryngeal tuberculosis that we have under our care we would find that the number of operations by direct method would be several times greater than that by suspension. Included in the 36 cases ssuspended are all cases who had suspension perhaps only once. Most of our cases have work done on the larynges by direct laryngoscopy before the pulmonary expert considers them sufficiently quiescent for suspension laryngoscopy. After the first suspension most patients tell me that the suspension is not particularly disagreeable. Some patients seem always to have much subjective discomfort. As long as there is no pulmonary or systemic reaction we are not concerned with this. Suspension laryngoscopy, at least the first time it is used, is a decided strain on most patients, and there is greater chance of a reaction following its use than that of direct laryngoscopy. The decision as to whether the operation is to be performed by direct laryngoscopy or suspension is made by the pulmonary expert. He approves of suspension for those cases who can have the endolaryngeal work done in this way without much risk of a reaction. The suspension in our hands gives the best results, and if it can be used without detriment to the patient it is the method of choice. It is particularly desirable to suspend those cases needing cutting and curetting operations.

Early in our work several cases had reactions lasting for several days. Dr. Scarborough tells me these were of no importance and that no case has had a serious setback because of suspension. During the last year the reactions following suspension have been eliminated almost completely if not completely by a more careful supervision of the cases. A few days ago, because of rather indefinite indications that one of our cases was not doing well, the patient was not suspended.

She had a marked relapse. If she had been suspended this would have been charged to the operation.

Not only are the cases watched and studied carefully before and after suspension by the pulmonary expert, but the laryngologist gives the larynx very careful study. Three days after the operation on the larynx I go over my cases very carefully, noting just what has been the result of cautery or curettage. Then repeated careful examinations are made once a week. The frequency of suspension depends upon the needs of the larynx. Occasionally we have a case when galvanocautery is used under suspension every two weeks. These cases are usually ones that are discharged from the sanitarium whose larynges are scarred, the result of previous operations and the healing process and who have returned for cauterization of suspicious small areas in the larynx.

The patients upon whom we do suspension laryngoscopy are the favorable cases. So many of them do well that we keep them together. Those who do well help the others in carrying out their long period of treatment.

The first essential thing in treating laryngeal tuberculosis by suspension laryngoscopy is to have the patient under the supervision of a pulmonary expert who has authority to say this patient shall or shall not be suspended. Only by such a procedure can serious results be prevented. I never recommend treatment by suspension. I do advise it if the pulmonary expert thinks best. The patient must be examined and approved of by the pulmonary expert each time the patient is suspended. He must be watched carefully after each suspension. At times I find that so far as the laryngeal picture is concerned that six or eight cases should be suspended the next day. Frequently only one or two appear for the work. The pulmonary expert has not approved of the work being done at this time. Later when conditions are favorable the patient is sent for the endolaryngeal work under suspension.

Our tuberculous laryngitis cases are divided into four classes for treatment: First, those who remain in bed and receive only the simple medication; second, those who may sit up and have applied to the larynx mild astringents and antiseptics; third, those who receive rapid endolaryngeal surgical procedures by direct laryngoscopy; and lastly those who are operated upon under suspension. The pulmonary expert having before him the laryngologist's findings decides in which class the case belongs. He decides whether or not the patient is in condition to have the very careful work done in his larynx which is so beneficial and which can best be done by suspension laryngoscopy. Excepting the cases for removal of the epiglottis all cases suspended have quiescent pulmonary conditions. The endolaryngeal procedures used by direct laryngoscopy are not so extensive as those done in the quiescent cases under suspension. Excepting an occasional case whose pulmonary condition is such as to allow them to go home they are all in the sanitarium under the supervision of a pulmonary expert as long as the latter considers it advisable.

While suspension laryngoscopy seems to me to be the ideal condition for the performance of endolaryngeal operations in cases with quiescent pulmonary conditions, it is particularly adapted to the treatment of superficial tuberculous ulceration of the trachea. If these ulcerations are high up, using the laryngeal spatula these cases may be readily cauterized. If situated low down in the trachea a tracheoscope may be passed under suspension and proper treatment instituted.

# LI

# GENERAL MEASURES IN THE TREATMENT OF LARYNGEAL TUBERCULOSIS.

By Lawrason Brown, M. D.,

Saranac Lake, N. Y.

My appearance before you today must recall to your minds the opening sentences of one of Cicero's orations against Cataline. My temerity in accepting the invitation of your secretary was brought about by the fact that some laryngologists, none of whom I believe is a member of this' society, seem to consider tuberculosis of the larynx a local disease and to treat it accordingly.

While tuberculous laryngitis is rare in children and more often found at autopsy, it occurs in about 25 per cent or more of adults with pulmonary tuberculosis, slightly more in men than in women, and next to tuberculous enteritis and colitis is the most frequent complication of pulmonary tuberculosis, due most likely to direct infection of the part by the sputum. Even early cases, cases in the incipient or minimal stage, are not spared (12 per cent), but as the pulmonary disease progresses the laryngeal complication becomes more frequent (moderately advanced, 26 per cent; far advanced, 45 per cent). The importance then of a complication so frequently seen among patients with pulmonary tuberculosis cannot be exaggerated.

Laryngeal tuberculosis is rarely if ever a primary disease, a statement with which I am sure many of you will agree. I am familiar with Donellan's paper (Transactions seventh annual meeting American Laryngological, Rhinological and Otological Society, 1901, page 277); in which he attempts to prove that primary laryngeal tuberculosis is not so rare as it is usually considered. He has collected many cases which he says had the first symptoms of tuberculosis from the larynx. The lungs were normal, as experts could detect no changes.

Today since the X-rays have been widely used in pulmonary disease we know that such evidence—i. e., the usual physical examination—alone, is worthy of slight consideration. He quotes two cases with autopsies, one of which had an old diffuse tuberculous laryngitis, had "recent granulations in one apex," and the second, described by B. Frankel (D. M. W., 1886, page 490), had ulcerative tuberculous laryngitis for five years with tubercle bacilli in the sputum and normal lungs at autopsy. Birkett (Osler & McCrae's System, Vol. III, page 630) says but three cases have been described (Demme, Pogrebenski & Orth). So if it is in practically every instance secondary to tuberculosis elsewhere, usually pulmonary, as seems most probable, the problem is not the treatment of a laryngitis alone any more than the problem of typhoid fever is the treatment of a diarrhea alone. In both diseases these manifestations may thrust themselves upon our notice, demanding emphatically treatment—treatment, however, which may prove of little avail unless general treatment is enforced.

The general treatment of tuberculosis is the same, no matter what organ is involved. At the risk of repeating what is very well known to all of you, I would like to stress a few points concerned in the general treatment of laryngeal tuberculosis. Some twenty years ago we refused all patients with laryngeal tuberculosis at the Trudeau Sanatorium, for we felt the prognosis was bad, and with the treatment we used at that time it was nearly always fatal. More recently, however, we have not hesitated to admit patients with laryngeal tuberculosis, provided, of course, that it was not too extensive and that they were otherwise eligible. Our results have been very satisfactory. We are no more laryngologists today than we were then, but one vital essential in the treatment of tuberculosis has become, if I may so express it, part of us. I refer to rest. Today, to use his expression, we put the patient on silence and give the larynx absolute rest, except for such movement as occurs in breathing, swallowing and coughing. We forbid whispering, whistling and every other use of the larynx. The results from this absolute rest are just as striking as they are in the case of tuberculosis of the knee, of the hip, of the spine or indeed of any other organ that can be given nearly 100 per cent of functional rest. I have been struck by the fact that few patients who fell under my care had been kept silent. I have wondered if it were not due to a mistaken kindness on the part of some physicians who knew but who thought it almost cruel to use such drastic measures. I can assure you that while it is hard it is far from unbearable, for I myself have used a pad and pencil and uttered no sound for six weeks. Having done this myself, I have not the slightest hesitation in demanding it from my patients, and it is always a surprise to me how readily they agree to it and how conscientiously many of them carry it out. This method has changed our entire outlook upon the prognosis of laryngeal tuberculosis and, in the more slightly affected, recoveries now replace fatalities. It is true, of course, that more careful examinations of the larynx reveal earlier lesions, which are, I believe, often prevented from progressing.

Absolute rest recalls that in pulmonary tuberculosis it is at times necessary to put a lung out of commission by collapsing it, by splinting it, so to speak, with air. Absolute rest of the larynx can probably be most nearly attained by performing tracheotomy and the use of a tube. Dr. Chevalier Jackson (Trans. tenth annual meeting American Laryngological, Rhinilogical and Otological Society, 1904, page 123) has reported three cases of laryngeal tuberculosis, supposed to be primary, who wore tracheotomy tubes and got better. In the vast majority of cases such radical measures are not necessary, and in others the great amount of pulmonary secretion would certainly prove very trying and the results, I fear, would be very uncertain.

I would not imply that you do not advise rest, but I read in articles on the treatment of tuberculous laryngitis by excellent laryngologists statements such as this: "Vocal rest is a very necessary adjunct to the successful treatment of many cases of tuberculous laryngitis." "Vocal rest" may mean no singing, no shouting, no making of speeches, but as much talking as the patient desires. "The patient should not be permitted to use his voice," writes another, "except in the mildest whisper, and even this should be restricted in amount." Rest in laryngeal tuberculosis should be defined in no uncertain terms and, as I have said, should be, for a time at least, absolute. Put a card on the head of the bed stating that the patient is on silence and no conversation is permitted, as has been suggested by Robertson. How long such absolute rest should continue must depend upon how the lesion progresses. Lip whispering, than ordinary whispering, next an occasional sentence in speaking tones is the method of progression, but singing, shouting, public speaking, should be avoided for some months after recovery.

Personally I go further in the rest treatment and do not hesitate to put my patients to bed for six weeks, with wide open windows, or better still, upon a porch during the day and in a well ventilated room at night. I do this for the following reasons: Pulmonary tuberculosis is usually present, and partial rest of the lungs as much as is possible is thus effected. Cough, which may injure the larynx when excessive, is better controlled by rest in bed than by any other means, for reduction of the number of the respirations means lessened irritation of the irritable lungs, consequently lessened secretion, and in turn lessened cough, and so less sputum flowing over the larynx.

All of us believe in the conservation of natural resources. The conservation of our bodily forces in the struggle against any chronic disease like tuberculosis is far more important. Where these are conserved I like to picture to myself the increased amount of antibodies that may be formed, the increased reactions of the cells about the focus to the poison, the increased and more rapid formation of scar tissue. If this is in part hypothetical, we do know that fatigue in animals lessens resistance and decreases antibody formation.

There is still another point I would like to stress. In chronic disease, and especially in tuberculosis, almost any change under rational conditions benefits the patient. The greatest response to change of climate occurs in the first few weeks, and for this reason I urge all of my patients to take advantage of it by remaining at rest, usually in bed. I cannot help feeling that if patients with laryngeal tuberculosis were put to bed and kept silent at home at the very onset of treatment, at the time when the iron of response is hot and will yield most readily to the hammer of advice and treatment, the tendency toward recovery would be much more marked and gratifying than it is at times today, even though you cannot change his quarters and must be satisfied with open windows and no porch in his usual surroundings.

Most of you, I am sure, will agree with me that recovery from laryngeal tuberculosis depends in most instances largely upon the condition of the pulmonary tuberculosis. With advancing pulmonary disease, fever and poor nutrition, it is difficult to promote healing in a tuberculous larynx, but I have seen it done with the aid of the electrocautery. However, the lungs play such a large part in the treatment of this condition that any line of treatment that fails to consider primarily the lung disease may in the end result in the loss of the patient.

This period of rest that I have mentioned gives the patient a chance to readjust his ideas and, more important still, affords him an opportunity to become orientated and gives us a chance to educate him along the lines he must follow if he wishes to recover. As soon as I deem it advisable I put him on exercise, for a good general condition and good muscular tone, which has greatly increased under bed rest in fresh air, are conducive to a more speedy recovery.

I have dwelt upon this point, for I have thought it possible that a few laryngologists still seemed to hold to the idea that local treatment was the important thing. I do not believe less in suitable local treatment but more in local and general rest, for the usual hygienic dietetic treatment properly applied with local rest will cure about 50 per cent of all early cases.

In regard to local treatment, I feel that the laryngeal dropper, devised by Dr. Yankauer of New York, is not yet widely enough known and used, for I can now recall only one or two patients who have come to me with laryngeal tuberculosis who had ever previously employed it. One patient, I remember, an important person, had a laryngologist or his assistant pay her two visits a week (at $25.00 a visit) to drop argyrol into her larynx, which she herself learned to do in two or three days with the laryngeal dropper. The important advantage of this dropper is the fact that the patient can remain quiet and at home and apply local treatment efficaciously. I do not mean to imply that local treatment in the office can be entirely done away with, but to see a poor, weak patient dragging one foot after another, running a daily temperature of 100 to 103 degrees, coming two or three times a week to the physician's office to have his throat touched with lactic acid or formalin or some other solution, however much temporary relief it gives, is to me a sad commentary upon the art and practice of medicine, for such injurious visits should not be and are not necessary. I realize that busy men cannot treat these patients at their homes. I also realize that they demand treatment. The best solution of the problem seems to me to be for the tuberculosis specialist to acquire sufficient knowledge of local treatment to enable him to carry out the directions of the laryngologist at the patient's home.

To produce rest and to facilitate swallowing, freedom from or lessening of pain is necessary. I have tried injection of alcohol into the superior laryngeal nerve with some success, but the respites have never been long. I have not tried resection of this nerve, which has yielded some good results. (See Mayer, Ab. Br. Med. Jr., 1921, I, 35; also W. Kl. W., 1921, Jan. 6th.)

The insufflation of anesthesin or orthoform has been helpful. In these cases the laryngeal dropper has proved a godsend. Before the application of drugs I have the patient thoroughly rinse or wash out his larynx with physiologic salt solution. This removes in great part the tenacious mucus and permits the local applications to reach the surface of the ulcer. I have found that for most applications the dropper was far better than the atomizer, and just as efficacious as the intratracheal syringe in the physician's hands. Further, the patient can apply the drug before each meal and whenever the pain becomes excessive. Menthol (1 per cent) in oil is an excellent application to begin the method upon, for if the patient swallows it no harm is done. Then stronger solutions of menthol, emulsions of anesthesin, or, what I have found is best of all, Freudenthal's emulsion of orthoform and menthol, can be applied as necessary. I have by these methods been able to avoid largely cocain with its disagreeable after-results. In a few cases I have not hesitated to use morphin hypodermatically when necessary.

The apparently marked benefit produced in intestinal tuberculosis by the ultraviolet rays, or at least by some factor concerned in the treatment, have encouraged us in their use in laryngeal tuberculosis, for it can be administered in the patient's home. Some have devised special lamps for application of these rays directly to the larynx, feeling that they would act like the sun rays, which I understand have been so successfully employed in Colorado. I have used natural heliotherapy in five cases and have had excellent results in two, though two were too far advanced to hope for any benefit. On the other side, in two patients with chronic disease, general radiation was employed and excellent results obtained. I have used ultraviolet rays from a mercury vapor quartz lamp, but excellent results have been obtained (by Blegood) with the use of arc lamps, which give off much violet ray.

More recently I have been interested in the use of a thin solution of gelatin, suggested by Mr. Petroff from his studies in physical chemistry. He afterwards placed in our hands a strongly immune serum (sheep or goat). Spraying the larynx with these substances apparently afforded a few patients marked relief, but in others was of little avail.

Laryngeal tuberculosis has long been looked upon as a contraindication to pregnancy, for when this condition occurs the larynx, if at all seriously affected, often quickly grows worse. In such cases I should not hesitate to advise abortion in the first three months of pregnancy, but after this time little benefit can be hoped for from the operation. Students of tuberculosis are not yet agreed upon the causes of the bad effects in many instances of pregnancy and labor upon pulmonary and laryngeal tuberculosis.

In conclusion, I would like to state my views as follows:

About 100,000 persons die from pulmonary tuberculosis in the United States every year. At least 40 to 50 per cent of these have some laryngeal tuberculosis. If patients live on the average about three years, there must be 300,000 patients in the United States, of whom 25 to 50 per cent have laryngeal tuberculosis. In other words, about 100,000 have laryngeal tuberculosis. Many of these are people with slight or no means. Treatment of their throat condition must in large part devolve upon the medical men doing tuberculosis work. They feel their shortcomings and are eager to turn to you for help. But when they see a patient with a high fever dragged to a laryngologic dispensary, which they know is wrong, they realize that they or someone else has erred. You gentlemen can help solve this problem, for it is yours and ours. We cannot do so alone, and I venture to say that you cannot do so alone either. The tuberculosis specialist must direct the general treatment and will be, I am sure, for a long time to come the only person to give such laryngeal treatment as you advise.

# LII

# THE SURGICAL TREATMENT OF LARYNGEAL TUBERCULOSIS.*

By Robert Levy, M. D.,

Denver.

The curability of laryngeal tuberculosis is no longer a mooted question, although the means by which the cure is accomplished is still a fruitful source of difference of opinion. So many cases of spontaneous cure have been recorded that nature's method, at any rate, is accepted without objection. Man's faith in nature's wonderful achievements discourages dispute, especially when confirmed by human observation.

On the other hand, there still seems to be a large number of practitioners, general as well as special, whose belief in the virtue of active therapeutic measures is, to say the least, extremely weak, if not entirely wanting. This is particularly true of such measures as those of which this paper treats, and can be explained by the firmness with which tradition grips the profession, and the difficulty with which certain old and accepted views are uprooted.

It is within the memory of many members of this association when to attempt any active treatment for laryngeal tuberculosis was little short of criminal. No great wonder, therefore, that a radical reform should be difficult of acceptance, and especially when such reform swings the pendulum too far. The enthusiasm following Heryng's, Krause's and Goughenheim's reports, 1885 and 1887, was rather short lived, and within a very few years a reaction set in which has done much toward clarifying the treatment of this affection.

The majority of laryngologists whose practice includes many tuberculous cases have come to the conclusion that the surgical treatment in some form or other is a valuable factor in the management of this disease, and still one occasionally sees reports in which only palliative or medicinal measures are rec-

---

*Read before the meeting of the American Laryngological Association at Atlantic City, May 31, 1921.

ommended.  It is only fair to say that the most authentic of these reports are not of the most recent dates, as, for example, the one of 241 cases reported by the Rutland State Sanatorium,[1] dated 1914.  I am inclined to think that a report from such an institution made at the present time would at least mention favorably the galvanocautery.  In addition, it is the writer's personal observation that, exclusive of published opinions, there is a not inconsiderable number of men who, through lack of faith or patience in treating these cases, or who having no regular connection with a tuberculosis sanitorium, find so much to discourage them that they readily condemn all methods of treatment except the hygienic.

While the majority of writers agree that surgical treatment in some form or other is of more or less value, there is still a certain lack of definiteness as to the method, the extent of its applicability or specific indications for its use.

Under the head of surgical treatment are included:

    a. Intralaryngeal measures.

    b. Extralaryngeal measures.

The latter can be dismissed with very little discussion, for neither tracheotomy nor laryngotomy with excision of invaded parts nor laryngectomy has been used extensively enough by a sufficient number of men.  Laryngectomy is certainly making no progress in the treatment of laryngeal tuberculosis; its status seems to be about the same as stated in 1913, that "so long as success has attended simpler measures, and so long as this success is rapidly increasing the number of cures, extensive life endangering operations must be condemned."[2] Arnoldson,[3] after an elaborate compilation on external operative measures, concludes that such operations, excepting tracheotomy, can only be considered where it is possible to remove all of the disease.  This is impossible in all except early cases, and in these, other less radical measures preclude the necessity of laryngectomy or even laryngotomy.

Tracheotomy may be considered in quite a different light.  Its value as a palliative measure, whether for the relief of dyspnea or dysphagia, is well recognized in spite of the objections (Lake[4]), that it interferes with cough and expectoration, that the wound becomes seriously infected or leads to rapid extension of the disease of the lungs. These objections are more theoretical than practical.

As early as 1879 Beverly Robinson[5] recommended tracheotomy for curative as well as palliative reasons, on the same principle that Moritz Schmidt did—that is, for the purpose of putting the larynx at rest. Nevertheless, tracheotomy has received but little more encouragement than laryngectomy, and one cannot help but voice the thought that the last word as to the value of this procedure has not been said, and that some courageous, perhaps bold, operator will show us its true worth.

Intralaryngeal surgical intervention includes incision, excision, curettage and galvanocautery. Obviously, these measures should not be used indiscriminately or promiscuously. Nor are they necessarily to be exhibited only for curative purposes. The destruction or removal of diffuse tuberculous infiltration or circumscribed masses has its value for the relief of dyspnea or pain quite beyond any other method of treatment. The reason for this is based on the well known studies of Goughenheim and his pupil Dansac,[6] who showed that the pain in tuberculous laryngitis, or arytenoiditis, as they called it, was due to certain nerve lesions, producing hyperplasia of the nerve endings, "pseudoneuromata." Dansac says, "we have been struck by the relief which surgical treatment nearly always gives to the sufferings of these patients," which observation holds good today to a very large degree.

From this point of view it is easy to see that many cases which were considered unsuitable for surgical treatment may now be given the benefit of such treatment when used with discrimination.

The contraindications for surgical treatment laid down by Heryng[7] were:

"a. Advanced phthisis with hectic and wasting;

b. Diffuse miliary tubercle of the larynx and pharynx;

c. All cachectic conditions;

d. Severe stenosis of the larynx;

e. Patients exhibiting fear and nervous excitability."

Except in cases of severe stenosis prior to tracheotomy, properly selected surgical measures properly carried out, and with palliation more in mind than cure, these contraindications may be largely disregarded.   Obviously one would not indulge in extensive curettage or galvanocautery in the presence of widespread edema or intense redness with acute manifestations.   Nevertheless, the writer has seen great relief to pain following the judicious application of galvanocautery, even in diffuse miliary laryngeal and pharyngeal tuberculosis.

The ideal condition for surgical interference is one in which the tuberculous process is definitely limited or circumscribed. This occurs in socalled tuberculomata, and in the very early stage of the disease.   Unfortunately, many cases are not seen early enough, the consequence being that the area involved cannot be definitely determined—in fact, this is often impossible, even though the laryngoscope reveals a fairly well circumscribed infiltration or ulceration.

A specimen presented before the American Laryngological, Rhinological and Otological Society[8] in 1906, in which, postmortem, a section from the trachea showed tuberculosis, demonstrated how far from the site of the disease as seen with the laryngoscope the lesion may exist.   Fetterholf[9] in 1914, in a "Study of the Larynx in 100 Cases Dying of Tuberculosis," showed how extensively the disease was distributed.   Of course, this was to be expected in advanced cases, but the point is that, even though it were possible to recognize the very earliest manifestations, the fact remains that patients are not seen by a competent laryngologist until considerable involvement has taken place.

Recognizing therefore that for surgical treatment the ideal early, limited, circumscribed lesion is rarely presented, does more or less extensive involvement constitute a contraindication?   The answer is found in the many cases reported in which the patient was not only relieved of distressing symptoms but in which not infrequently the voice was restored and the disease arrested.

Saupignet[10] removed the mucosa and perichondrium over the arytenoid region by repeated operations until cicatricial tissue covered the parts, resulting in relief to dysphagia and repiration and improvement in the general condition.   This method is certainly too radical to find favor with many, but it shows what can be done in the way of healing, even in extensive diseases.   Lockard[11] showed how readily healing takes place, even though the operation does not remove all tuberculous involvement in a large number of epiglottidectomies, and his experience has been amply confirmed by others. The following is an illustrative case:

Miss A. K., 22, had pleurisy one year prior to coming to Colorado. Cough and expectoration had existed about six months. Dysphagia and slight aphonia had existed for about four weeks. There was rapid loss of weight, rapid pulse, slight fever, and physical examination showed active involvement of both lungs. The larynx was extensively affected, the epiglottis being pale with nodular tumefaction and large ragged ulcerations. The right aryepiglottic fold was pale and uniformly swollen.

The patient was highly nervous, and it was with difficulty that a satisfactory laryngoscopic examination could be made. After one month of rest and simple palliative measures, treatment by galvanocautery and excision was instituted. Now at the end of three months there is seen a moderate degree of tumefaction, which is still slightly nodular in spots, partial destruction of epiglottis, but no ulceration or other evidence of activity. The patient's general condition is greatly improved, the physical signs showing less activity and the weight increased 16 pounds.

Much has been said of the danger of wound infection and extension of the process. The effect of trauma in localizing tuberculosis or spreading a local lesion seems still to be a subject of dispute. Laboratory investigations have not been conclusive, for example: Pel Leusden[12] showed that "crushing of a kidney in rabbits, followed by the intravenous injection of tubercle bacilli, resulted in the preferred localization of the tuberculosis in the injured kidney to the exclusion of the rest of the body," while Corper[13] found that "crushing and the subcutaneous injection of chemical irritants just prior to the subcutaneous injection of virulent human tubercle bacilli in various sized doses, had no appreciable influence upon the progress of the infection as compared with that obtained in control guinea pigs."

Clinically many observers have presented instances in which trauma seems to have been a factor in etiology, as, for example, a case referred to by Walsham,[14] in which pharyngeal

ulcerations following the accidental swallowing of caustic potash became tuberculous in an individual suffering from pulmonary tuberculosis.

On the other hand, the great number of operations performed daily on tuberculous individuals is pretty good opposing evidence.

Incision.—As early as 1868 Marcet, quoted by James,[15] advocated puncture and scarification in the indurated form;
little account was taken of this until Schmidt in 1880 advised
incision, with or without lactic acid rubbings. Only a few
men besides the originators have used these procedures to
any extent. As in edema from other causes, incision is of
some value, but it cannot be considered as effective for curative purposes as other measures. In the indurative form the
contraction hoped for cannot be accomplished in any degree
as satisfactorily as by galvanocautery. Its use, therefore,
should be confined to cases of pronounced edema.

Excision.—In 1883 Schnitzler[16] removed a tuberculous
tumor endolaryngeally. Since then the excision of tuberculous
masses, whether as typical tumors, circumscribed papillomatous vegetations or localized infiltrations, has been common
practice. Even though all of the invaded structure cannot
be extirpated, as referred to above, the removal of portions
thereof is attended with satisfactory healing, relief of symptoms, and is often followed by arrest of the local lesion. This
is a much more liberal view than was taken a few years ago,
when many writers, including the author (1906), limited the
application of this operation "to those cases in which there is
a certainty or a strong probability of completely removing the
entire focus of disease."[17]

The cases best suited for excision, in addition to the well
localized ones, are those showing few acute manifestations—
in other words, the pale irregular nodular infiltrations whose
activity is manifestly sluggish. The cases presenting much red
edematous swelling, submucous gray deposits of tubercles with
general symptoms of rapidly progressing disease, such as high
fever, etc., are better adapted for other methods of local treatment. A good illustration of the value of this procedure is
found in the case recently reported by Sir Dundas Grant,[18]
in which the lesion was so extensive that the patient suffered

dyspnea and regurgitation of liquids in addition to other symptoms, and in which relief was obtained by intralaryngeal removal of tuberculous masses from the anterior and posterior commissures followed by galvanocautery to vocal and ventricular bands.

Histologic examination of masses removed from tuberculous larynges has not always shown tuberculosis except where the disease, while sluggish, was still active. Infiltration, papillomatous or smooth, often persists in the posterior commissure, constituting the principal cause of hoarseness. These masses often represent an end result, and when removed show, according to Dr. Hilkowitz, who examined them for me, "a papillary overgrowth of the surface epithelium, the corium being the seat of a round cell infiltration running between dense fibrous tissue."

The excision of the epiglottis in part or entire is not generally practiced to the extent that Lockard and a few others do, and still its value is unquestionable. Removal of small areas of infiltration, smooth or with nodular vegetations, or ulcerations involving the free margins of the epiglottis, lend themselves readily to this operation, especially if followed up with galvanocautery.

Amputation of the epiglottis is not as simple a procedure as one might infer. I have had one case of severe hemorrhage and two in which secondary cicatricial contraction caused marked stenosis. One often sees the under surface of the epiglottis covered by tuberculous ulcerations in which the temptation to remove the entire organ is very great, but judicious application of galvanocautery will usually cause satisfactory healing.

Nevertheless, epiglottidectomy is strongly advised, especially for the dysphagia when due to involvement of the epiglottis principally, and for those cases in which the tumefaction interferes with satisfactory treatment of the rest of the larynx.

Curettage.—This is less practiced than formerly, if we exclude excision by the socalled double curette. Its value is limited to surface manipulation, thus cleansing and stimulating sluggish ulcerations. It is less useful than excision for actual removal of disease areas, and less effective than galvanocautery for the relief of pain in more acute lesions.

Galvanocautery.—Of all surgical measures the galvanocautery is the most generally and favorably recommended.   Its
value seems well established, and its future as a therapeutic
agent seems assured.   Voltilini[19] in 1867 made a bold though
unsuccessful attempt to establish it.   Grünwald[20] gave us a
refinement of technic.   The names of those in whose hands
galvanocautery has given satisfaction are too numerous to mention, including Gleitzman,[21] Casselberry,[22] Iglauer,[23] Freudenthal,[24] Ruedi,[25] Killian[26] and Thomson.[27]   Casselberry warned
against its use except in skilled hands, being  fearful of untoward results.   Freudenthal speaks of Siebenmann's experience in which the reaction was so severe as to necessitate
tracheotomy.

Of course, one deprecates the performance of any intralaryngeal operation by those unskilled in laryngologic practice;
and still, if not too large an area is treated at one sitting, the
danger of serious consequences is extremely small.

Galvanocautery is applicable to a very large percentage of
cases, either for palliative or curative purposes.   Sir St. Clair
Thomson[28] found it indicated in 20.22 per cent of 178 cases.
In 100 private cases seen in the past few years, the writer used
it in 22 cases.   I am firmly convinced that its use can be extended to nearly every stage of laryngeal tuberculosis, after
the initial period of anemia or hyperemia—that is to say, in
all forms of infiltration, smooth, nodular, papillomatous; in all
varieties of ulceration, small, large, sluggish, painless or painful; even in the final stage, when necrosis is involving underlying cartilage, it may relieve suffering and help clean the
parts.   Applied superficially, its value to sluggish ulcerations
in removing necrotic tissue and in stimulating granulations is
far superior to chemical agents.

Applied by deep puncture to infiltrations its action is ideal,
for as Wood[29] puts it, "the eschar produced by burning prevents reinfection," if this were necessary, "until the tissue
has become sufficiently resistant to protect itself, sealing the
lymphatics and blood vessels."

This seems a much more reasonable explanation than that
of Ruedi,[30] who believes the thick slough acts as a protection;
at least, it is more desirable, for it does not necessitate extensive cauterization at one sitting.   Wood tells us also that

following the actual cautery "a retarding influence is exerted beyond the area actually destroyed by the heat."

Surgical treatment of laryngeal tuberculosis is not of itself the most important factor in the management of this condition. It has its limitations. There is no place here for extreme views, and its application should have a rational basis. It is only one factor in the treatment, being a valuable adjunct to other local, general, specific, hygienic and climatic measures, besides, as Dennis[31] has said, shortening the time required to bring about favorable results.

It frequently becomes necessary to institute very mild local treatment in combination with rest, fresh air, etc., before resorting to any form of surgical intervention. It may, however, be said that of all forms of local treatment, it is the most important, being the most effective. It is valuable, both as a palliative agent and as a curative measure, often being indicated for relief of symptoms when a cure is out of the question. Operation often exercises a favorable influence on the pulmonary condition, and as Ruedi has shown, galvanocautery has been of value in high altitudes which affected the lungs favorably, but which were without influence on the larynx.

In the above an attempt has been made to give surgical treatment of laryngeal tuberculosis its proper place in the management of this most serious complication and in a measure definitely to outline its special indications and applicability; but after all is said, one might paraphrase Sir St. Clair Thomson's reply to a question asked of him by Drs. Cohen and Swain at the 1919 meeting of this association. "The chief thing in determining the exact condition, local and general, for the exhibition of operative treatment is the skilled eye of the diagnostician, because it is impossible to put down in words the conditions that one sees."

### REFERENCES.

1. Lyons:  Boston Med. and Surg. Jour., July 2, 1914, p. 19.
2. Laryngeal Tuberculosis, Jour. A. M. A., May 17, 1913.
3. Archiv. f. Laryng. u. Rhin., 1913, p. 43.
4. Clinical Jour., Dec. 2, 1914, p. 678.
5. Am. Jour. Med. Sc. 1879, Vol, LXXVII. p. 407.
6. Jour. L. R. & O., June, 1894, p. 317.
7. The Jour. of Rhin. and Otol., 1894, Vol. VIII, p. 473.
8. Trans. Am. L. R. and O. Co., 1906, p. 300.

9. Trans. Am. Laryng. Assn., 1914, p. 258.
10. Rev. Hebd. de Laryng. d'Otol. et du Rhin., 1913, Vol. XXIV, p. 377.
11. Trans. Am. Laryng. Assn., 1911, p. 29.
12. Arch. f. Clin. Chir., 1911, Vol. XCV, pp. 245-91.
13. Am. Review of Tuberc., 1919, Vol. III, p. 610.
14. Channels of Infection in Tuberculosis, p. 64.
15. Brit. Med. Jour., Aug. 27, 1887, p. 457.
16. Wiener Med. Presse, 1883, Vol. XXIV, p. 446.
17. Annals of Otol., Rhin. & Laryng., Sept., 1906, p. 589.
18. Med. Press. (London), Feb. 4, 1920. p. 94.
19. Allg. Wien. Med. Zeit. No. 13, 14, 1884.
20. Die Therapie der Kehlkopf Tuberculose, etc., 1907.
21. The Laryngoscope, 1904, Vol. 14, p. 439.
22. Trans. Am. Laryng. Assn., 1911, p. 186.
23. The Laryngoscope, Oct. 1916, p. 1237.
24. Annals of Otol., Rhin. & Laryng., Sept., 1920, p. 545.
25. New York Med. Jour., July 26, 1919, p. 166.
26. Deutsche Med. Woch., March 28, 1912, p. 74.
27. Brit. Med. Jour., April 11, 1914, p. 801.
28. Ibid.
29. Trans. Am. Laryng. Assn., 1911, p. 181.
30. Brit. Med. Jour., June 21, 1919, p. 764.
31. Jour. Am. Med. Assn., Sept. 27, 1913, p. 1221.

# LIII

# CASE OF INTRANASAL ETHMOID EXENTERATION ACCOMPANIED BY UNCONTROLLABLE HEMORRHAGE; DEATH.

## By Dunbar Roy, M. D.,

### Atlanta, Ga.

Suppurative ethmoiditis occurs by no means infrequently in the practice of every rhinologist. Nasal polypi with the accompanying necrosing ethmoiditis is a familiar picture. After all the arguments have been adduced against its use, the writer is still convinced that the term necrosing ethmoiditis, attributed to Woakes, is the best general term suggestive of the real pathologic findings.

The management of these cases so as to produce a cure will tax the medical and surgical skill of the best in our profession. Whether by the use of either the external or internal operation, the fact still remains that what one would denominate as an actual cure is not always obtained. All can be benefited, but many of these will not be absolutely free from some catarrhal discharge, while in others the resulting scabby condition will be most annoying, and even the destruction of their sense of smell is by no means a remote possibility. Hence suppurative ethmoiditis must be looked upon as one of the hard problems for the rhinologist. It is not the purpose of this paper to discuss the various intranasal operative procedures which are used by different rhinologists, for the writer believes that he has obtained his fair share of success by the use of the snare, curette and punch forceps, but the object here is to present the record of one case where complications arose and where these were contributory to the final death of the patient. The more extended becomes my experience with operations on the ethmoid the more am I convinced that the exenteration of the ethmoid body is no simple procedure and should always be undertaken with the greatest precaution, and every step of the operation should be under visual inspection. The presence of suppurative ethmoiditis compels one to have great respect for the ability of nature to confine the suppurative process to these cells instead of there being a frequent extension of the same process to the cranial cavity. It is only after operative procedures that we are at all likely to have such an extension of the pathologic process, and it is for this reason that all operative work in this locality should be done with the most extreme caution. The fact that the literature will show a number of serious complications attending this operation, and even a few fatal cases, behooves us to consider it the major intranasal operation we are called upon to perform, especially if undertaken at the same time with a sphenoid involvement.

With these preliminary remarks the writer wishes to report a case of intranasal ethmoid exenteration accompanied by practically uncontrollable hemorrhage, followed by death upon the operating table where extreme measures were being instituted in our effort to save the patient.

E. J. B., age 18, a strong, robust country lad, consulted me on October 28, 1918, in reference to a very severe purulent discharge from both nasal cavities and which had been present for several years. He was also suffering with quite severe headaches. Family history was negative.

Examination of the nasal cavities revealed a suppurating ethmoiditis with numerous polypi. Transillumination showed both maxillary antrums clear, although both were punctured in order to be sure of the diagnosis, as also both frontals. X-ray plates showed practically the same thing. No blood examination was made. On the next morning an intranasal exenteration was performed on the left side. The whole ethmoid region was polypoid and soft, requiring the use of the snare, curette and cutting forceps. A good opening was also made through the nasofrontal duct and the frontal sinus thoroughly irrigated. The sphenoid was also opened, because it was very soft and a curette easily entered the antrum. No packing was used and there was no undue amount of hemorrhage. In three days the patient returned home with instructions to irrigate his nasal cavities with a saline solution.

On January 22, 1919, about four months after the first operation, the patient returned for another examination. The

left side appeared in excellent shape, with only a slight amount
of catarrhal secretion. Headache on that side had entirely
disappeared. Over the right or unoperated side there was
still present severe headaches and a profuse purulent discharge. The next morning this side was operated upon in
the same manner and with the same care and thoroughness as
the left. The frontal was irrigated and also the sphenoid.
No unusual amount of bleeding occurred and no packing was
used. The next morning the patient reported to the office
and the operated nasal cavity seemed to be in good shape.
He remained in the city for a few days so that I might irrigate the cavities myself. The operation was performed on
Thursday. On the following Monday, four days after the
operation, he came to my office late in the afternoon on account
of hemorrhage from the right side. This was checked without difficulty and without the necessity of a tampon. He remained in the office for an hour and, there being no further
bleeding, he was allowed to return to his hotel. Seen the next
morning, Tuesday, and also Wednesday, when the nasal cavity
appeared to be doing nicely. On Wednesday night, about 11
o'clock, a message from the hotel informed me that Mr. B.
seemed to be bleeding to death. I immediately told them to
rush him to the hospital in an ambulance. This was done; at
12 o'clock midnight, with the assistance of a colleague, I under-
from both sides, anteriorly and posteriorly. He had already
from both sides, anterially and posteriorly. He had already
been given a hypodermic of morphin and atropin by the house
surgeon and temporary measures had also been used. A large
sterile postnasal cotton tampon was used and both sides packed
tightly with sterile gauze from the front to the posterior opening of the nasal fossæ. He was immediately given 30 cc. of
horse serum intravenously and ⅛ gr. morphin, 1/200 gr.
atropin hypodermically every six hours. This seemed to control the hemorrhage. We left the hospital at 4 a. m.

On visiting him about 9 o'clock the next morning, only a
slight serous bloody oozing was present. Temperature, 101.2;
pulse, 110. Ice packs were kept over the nose and only liquid
diet given. It was noted that the blood coagulated readily, giving no indications of his being a hemophiliac. Horse serum
was given subcutaneously every four hours. In addition to

this, pituitrin, coagulose and other various remedies of this kind were used. At this time the patient was considerably nauseated and vomited blood. Orange albumen was administered with other liquid diets. There being considerable pain in the abdomen and evidence of gas accumulation, an enema was administered, which brought relief from these symptoms. In addition to the bloody serous discharge there was considerable flow of mucopus from both nostrils. At 6 p. m. some of the tampon was removed from the left side.

January 30th. Patient had a fairly good night. Morning temperature, 101; pulse, 102. Complains of severe headache, probably due to the damming back of the purulent discharge. Saline solution was dropped freely into both sides every hour. Small doses of calomel and soda were given to counteract the flatulency.

January 31st. Patient had a very restless night. Morning temperature, 101.2; pulse, 88. Aspirin administered for headache. No signs of bleeding. Patient feeling much more comfortable. Taking light diet. Evening temperature, 99.2; pulse, 100.

February 1st. Patient slept fairly well. Nasal cavity looked encouraging. At 6 p. m., the patient began to bleed from both nasal cavities. Ice compresses used. Morphin and atropin administered hypodermatically. Horse serum given intravenously. At 7 p. m., both sides were bleeding freely. After consultation with my colleague, Dr. Lokey, the packing in both sides was removed and the cavities irrigated with hot saline solution. The blood clotted freely. The hemorrhage was very profuse from both sides, but by exclusion and close observation the majority of the hemorrhage seemed to be coming from the left. Nothing was left to do but to repack, and this we did with iodoform gauze post-nasal and both sides of the nasal cavities. This checked the bleeding. At 9:30 p. m., horse serum was again administered. Bleeding very slight from nasal cavities and no bleeding from postnasal space.

Sunday, February 2d. Temperature, 101; pulse, 92. Patient very uncomfortable and still some blood oozing from both nasal cavities. Tampons kept saturated with adrenalin chlorid. Ice compresses continuously applied and coagulose given subcutaneously. This treatment was continued during the day.

At 8 p. m., temperature was 102, and pulse 120. He had now started bleeding profusely again from both nostrils.

We now called in consultation Dr. W. P. Nicolson, a general surgeon. As all indications pointed to the fact that most of the hemorrhage was coming from the left side, it was Dr. Nicolson's opinion that the tying of the common carotid on that side would probably stop the bleeding and that the seriousness of the case demanded radical action.

At 9 p. m., the patient was taken to the operating room, and under gas anesthesia Dr. Nicolson ligated the common carotid on the left side, Drs. Roy and Lokey assisting. While the patient was under the anesthetic both nasal cavities were cleaned and repacked with iodoform gauze and a fresh tampon placed in the nasopharynx. No bleeding could be discovered when the patient left the operating room and his general condition was very good. At 12 m. his pulse was 110; at 1:30 a. m., it was 144. Some blood oozing from both sides.

Next day, Monday, February 3d, at 6 a. m., the temperature was 100.2; pulse, 92. Patient complained of considerable pain over the right eye and both eyelids were swollen. Both eyes were kept washed with boric acid solution. Patient was quite uncomfortable, and there was considerable mucopus dripping into his throat. At 9 a. m., temperature, 100; pulse, 90. Iced applications over the nose and eyes and small doses of calomel and soda administered on account of the accumulation of gas in abdomen.

Tuesday, February 14th, 6 a. m., temperature, 98; pulse, 120. Patient very uncomfortable. Enemas given. Patient ·taking liquid diet. 6 p. m., temperature, 101.2; pulse, 110. Packing removed from left side of nose. No bleeding. Patient seems much better. Greatly troubled with mucopus in pharynx and larynx. This was removed with suction, much to the patient's comfort.

Wednesday, February 5, saline given. Soft diet readily taken. Temperature at noon, 101.2; pulse, 110. Packing removed completely from right side of nose. No bleeding. Patient much more comfortable and able to expel the mucus from his throat. Saline solution with carbolic acid used every two hours.

February 6th. Temperature, 100.3; pulse, 106. Patient had a fairly good night. Light diet being taken. 2 p. m., postnasal packing entirely removed. No bleeding. This gave the patient great relief.

Friday, February 7th. Temperature, 98.2; pulse, 100. Patient had a good night. Mouth and nose irrigated. Bowels moved normally. At 5:30 p. m., the external dressing was changed for the first time by Dr. Nicolson. One stitch abscessed. Small amount of seropus. Iodoform dressing and bandage applied.

Saturday, February 8th, 6 a. m., temperature, 99.4; pulse, 90. At 6:30 a. m., hemorrhage started from the neck incision. Dressing changed by the house surgeon and the wound tightly packed, which controlled all hemorrhage. At 10 a. m., patient had another hemorrhage from the incision. Blood clotted immediately. Dr. Nicolson again saw the patient. Given 1/6 morphin, 1/150 atropin. Wound packed again. No signs of bleeding from nose and throat. Patient had renewed hemorrhage again in afternoon.

At 8 p. m., Dr. Nicolson decided to place the patient under an anesthetic and to stop the bleeding surgically. Patient was removed to the operating room at 8:30. Gas ether anesthetic given by the same anesthetist as at the previous operation. Temperature at that time was 101.3; pulse, 100. Patient took but a few whiffs of gas when he stopped breathing. Oxygen and artificial respiration were used. The heart continued to beat for ten minutes after all breathing had ceased. Death. No autopsy was allowed, but Dr. Nicolson opened up the incision on the operating table and found a most peculiar condition. All of the neck muscles and fascia were undermined and an immense cavity found filled with clotted blood. This extended even up to the chin. The suture on the carotid was firm and there was complete ligation.

Like many others, I have operated upon a number of cases where there has been very severe hemorrhage, but this was the only case where the condition taxed my surgical ingenuity to its utmost. Knowing that the posterior ethmoid cells derived their arterial supply from the sphenopalatine, a branch of the internal maxillary, from the external carotid and from the ethmoidal branches of the ophthalmic artery, a branch from the internal carotid, we felt assured that the tying of the common carotid would take care of all the hemorrhage on the left side. This proved correct, as all bleeding ceased from the nasal cavities and all tampons were removed. But why the hemorrhage should start from the wound in the neck, and this also be so uncontrollable, is a question difficult to answer. It is of course unfortunate that no blood examination was made, but this was due to the fact that the blood clotted freely and we were expecting every moment to have the hemorrhage under control. Evidently a slow bacteremia had been progressing for some time, due to the absorption for years of pus from the ethmoid cells, and this had undermined the coats of the blood vessels as well as the integrity of other body tissues. It is undoubtedly true that the immediate cause of death was the general anesthetic, but it is equally true that the same might not have produced death had there not been such an excessive loss of blood and the whole system in such an abnormal state. So that we are not entirely in error in saying that death was due to uncontrollable hemorrhage. Such cases, while unfortunate in their termination, make us realize that these extreme cases of necrosing ethmoiditis are not without their dangers.

Arrowsmith[1] reports one case in a negro male, age 56, from whom a growth in the nose was removed by the cold snare. This was followed by severe hemorrhage and later by repeated attacks of nosebleed. On readmission to the hospital the left nostril was exposed by a lateral rhinotomy, after Moure's method, and a friable yellow mass of material which had involved and destroyed the entire left ethmoid region and inner wall of the orbit was removed. The bleeding from the field of operation was very profuse in spite of a preliminary ligation of the left external carotid. A similar tumor was removed from the supraclavicular region, where there was also considerable hemorrhage. For this reason the patient, "already greatly reduced by his previous loss of blood," died in three hours after leaving the operating room. The nasal and supraclavicular tumors were alike in gross appearance—both hypernephroma.

Felix[4] reviews many cases of fatalities following nasal operations. While he notes several deaths due to meningitis after the ethmoid operation, he makes no mention of hemorrhage as a cause of death in these cases. These cases of meningitis are included in the following notes, under the name of the author making the original report:

Dabney[3] notes three deaths following the ethmoid operation due to meningitis; none due to hemorrhage.

Hajek[5] mentions one case in which death following the ethmoid operation was due to meningitis.

In the discussion of Hajek's paper, Lack says that in over 300 ethmoid operations he had but one death. This was due to meningitis. He adds that of all other operators using his technic who reported to him, eight stated that they have had no fatalities; the other three report six deaths. All were due to meningitis. Lack says: "I have heard of no death from any other cause."

In this discussion, Ballenger states that he had but one death, also due to meningitis; he had never had any other complication "of any moment." He reported over 200 cases without his being called to check hemorrhage occurring after operation.

Halle[6] notes that he has performed 76 ethmoidal and frontal sinus operations by his intranasal technic. In one of these cases a meningitis developed that proved fatal. No mention of hemorrhage as a dangerous complication.

Hinsberg[7] reports three cases of death following intranasal exenteration of the ethmoid. All due to "infection" (meningitis). No mention of hemorrhage.

Tawse[13] reports two deaths from meningitis following the ethmoid operation.

McCullagh[8] advocates Mosher's technic for ethmoid exenteration. He states that Mosher has told him of two cases of postoperative meningitis following this operation, but not among his own cases. No fatal case of hemorrhage is noted. In regard to postoperative treatment, McCullagh says:

"The principal part of the postoperative treatment of these cases is noninterference with nature. Personally, I order no local treatment for forty-eight hours. Packing should never be used unless hemorrhage demands it or the patient is so situated as not to be within easy reach of skilled assistance if secondary hemorrhage occurs."

Pratt[10] states that he has performed between 200 and 300 operations on the ethmoid. In none of these does he record a fatal or even dangerous hemorrhage. With his technic, he says, there is little bleeding.

Shambaugh,[12] after describing the technic for the ethmoid operation, says:

"Most of the cases require no tampon if the patient remains at the hospital, where directions can be left for the introduction of a tampon in case secondary bleeding requires it. Occasionally one meets with severe bleeding at the time of operation which may require the introduction of a tampon. This should always be removed not later than the following day."

Ballenger[2] says in regard to hemorrhage following the ethmoid operation:

"Hemorrhage nearly always attends the operation, and it may either persist, or appear later as a secondary hemorrhage, though the latter is comparatively rare. By packing the nose as described, this complication may be controlled. A slight serosanguinous oozing may continue for twenty-four or forty-eight hours, in spite of the gauze packing, but it is of no serious consequence. If the patient is operated on in a hospital and remains there for three days, it will rarely be necessary to pack the nose."

Oppenheimer and Gottlieb[9] state that blood examinations should be made prior to nasal operations, and if either the coagulation time or the bleeding time vary much from the normal the operation should not be undertaken without preliminary treatment to improve the blood condition.

They report no fatal case of postoperative hemorrhage. In one case an ethmoid operation was followed by "secondary oozing for five days." The coagulation time in this case was markedly delayed.

Weinstein also notes the need for the determination of coagulation time of the blood before nasal and nasopharyngeal operations.

Pugnat[11] reports four cases of postoperative hemorrhage, not fatal, two following turbinectomy and two tonsillectomy. In all these cases there was evidence of cirrhosis of the liver or other hepatic insufficiency. Other investigators have found that hepatic insufficiency may alter the coagulability of the blood, and he believes that this factor should be considered in preparing for nasal operations.

Theisen and Fromm[14] report the use of horse serum preoperatively in nose and throat operations in any case where they expected an unusual amount of postoperative bleeding, either from a history of the patient or of the patient's family.

The ethmoid operation, they say, "is usually attended by profuse bleeding," but following the use of the serum there was very slight loss of blood in their cases.

## BIBLIOGRAPHY.

1. Arrowsmith, H.: Malignant Hypernephroma of the Ethmoidal Region. Laryngoscope, 26:909, 1916.

2. Ballenger, W. L.: Diseases of the Nose, Throat and Ear. Philadelphia, Lea & Febiger. Ed. 4, 1914.

3. Dabney, V.: Deaths Attributable to Intranasal Operations and Other Instrumentation. Surg., Gynec. & Obstet., 22:324, 1916.

4. Felix, E.: Accidents mortels a la suite d'intervention intranasales. Arch. internat. de laryngol, 37:58, 1914.

5. Hajek, L.: Lack, L. and others: Treatment of Chronic Suppurative Ethmoiditis. Brit. M. J., 1912, 2:1130.

6. Halle: Die intranasalen Operationen bei eitrigen Erkränkungen der Nebenhölen der Nase. Arch. f. Laryngol. u. Rhinol. 29:73, 1914.

7. Hinsberg: Drei Todesfälle nach intranasaler Siebbeinausräumung. Monats. f. Ohrenheil, 1255, 1913.

8. McCullagh, S.: The Treament of Ethmoiditis. New York M. J., 102:178, 1915.

9. Oppenheimer, S. and Gottlieb, M. J.: Importance of Blood Examination in the Surgery of the Nose and Throat. Am. J. Surg., 33:81, 1919; also in Laryngoscope 29:400, 1919.

10. Pratt, J. A.: Surgical Treatment of the Ethmoid. Journal-Lancet, 40:216, 1920; technic also described in Ann. Otol., Rhinol. & Laryngol., 28:1051, 1919.

11. Pugnat, A.: Les hemorragies nasales postoperatoire. Rev. de laryngol., 40—621—1919.

12. Shambaugh, G. E.: Surgery of the Ethmoid Labyrinth, J. A. M. A., 67—1901—1916.

13. Tawse, H. Bell: Some Complications and Dangers of Nasal Surgery. Lancet, 1909—2—1582.

14. Theisen, C. F., and Fromm, N. K.: Normal Horse Serum in Hemorrhage from Nose and Throat Operations. New York M. J., 100—875—1914.

15. Weinstein, J.: Nature and Control of Hemorrhage in Nasopharyngeal Operations. Laryngoscope, 27—145—1917.

# LIV

# RADIUM IN THE TREATMENT OF CARCINOMA OF THE LARYNX, WITH REVIEW OF THE LITERATURE.*

By Fielding O. Lewis, M. D.,

New York.

Laryngeal carcinoma, one of the saddest afflictions with which the laryngologist has to deal, has for many years been a vexatious problem, and indeed will no doubt remain so until the scientists and investigators have been able to determine its etiology more accurately. For this reason, no doubt, our efforts at local eradication have been much hampered.

With the advent of radium, and its effect upon cancerous growths in other regions of the body, our optimism became apparent, and during the last few years we have been striving to determine the value of radium in the treatment of cancer of the upper respiratory tract, the larynx in particular. Most of us have used it in all stages of the disease. The results are varied and confusing. Some report cures; the majority failures. Most textbooks condemn it.

Janeway, in the Memorial Hospital Report of 1917, reports twenty-seven cases of cancer of the larynx which were treated by radium. All were dead at the time of the report but one, and he was being treated for recurrence. Janeway was of the opinion that much better results should be obtained by radium in the larynx, judging from the effects on similar growths situated elsewhere. These cases were treated by means of tubes inserted into the larynx and placques applied to the neck.

Dr. Douglas C. Quick, of the same institution, exhibited before the Eastern Section of the A. L. R. & O. Society, in February of this year, two cases of carcinoma of the larynx, in which remarkable results were obtained. These cases had been treated by the insertion of radium emanations into the growth.

---

*Read before the forty-third annual congress of the American Laryngological Association, at Atlantic City, N. J., June 1, 1921.

Dr. Delavan, in the Transactions of this society for 1919, reports four cases of laryngeal carcinoma treated by radium. Two had complete laryngectomies after being thoroughly treated by radium, and two of his cases were treated by radium alone, which showed complete retrogression.

Jackson and Patterson, in his book on Peroral Endoscopy and Laryngeal Surgery, reports a laryngeal carcinoma treated by radium, which was applied directly to the growth, and the patient lived for one year following the treatment.

Dr. A. W. Watson, in the Transactions of this Society for 1917, reports one case successfully treated by external and internal applications of radium.

Dr. y de Barajas, in Medicina Ibera, Madrid, Spain, 1919, reports 58 cases treated by radium, with not one complete cure. He states that the growths undergo a process of amelioration, even to apparent cure, after the first application of radium, if dosage is adapted to the case and to the subject. All cases, however, he states, recurred in a very short time. He finds that the dosage in the larynx should not be less than 45 or 50 mg., nor more than 75 to 80 mg., with maximum duration of two hours each application, and should be made as frequently as reaction after treatment will permit. He also further states that radium merely retards the development of some varieties of cancer, hastens it in others, and completely cures none.

The writer has treated sixteen cases of carcinoma of the larynx with radium since January, 1917, with the following results:

One case in which the total laryngectomy had been performed, which had recurrence in the thyroid gland, died six months after operation. Another, in whom a complete laryngectomy was performed two weeks ago, has had large doses of radium within the larynx, and radium placques applied externally for the past year. While doing nicely, it is too early to record accurate results. Another, in which thyrotomy had been performed, with recurrence of the disease in the external wound, was treated by radium needles and died eight months after the thyrotomy. One with early involvement on the right side of the larynx was treated by radium needles inserted directly into the growth, had early retrogression, later showed signs of beginning activity, was thyrotomized, and with the assistance of Dr. William L. Clark, was treated with electric coagulation. The patient is still living and there is no evidence of recurrence after four months.

The remaining twelve cases which were considered inoperable were tracheotomized and treated vigorously by introducing needles into the growth and radium applied externally under the direction of Dr. William L. Clark. All are dead but one, who is losing ground rapidly.

In two of these remaining twelve cases there was marked retrogression of the growth, so much so that the site of the lesion was hardly perceptible, and the patient's condition remained so for several months, recurrence developed, and in spite of the use of radium they died in about a year after their first treatment.

Out of 109 cases above recorded, 10 were living at the time the reports were published, showing a mortality of about 91 per cent.

The method of applying radium in the cases which came under our observation was as follows: The first three or four cases were treated by introducing the capsule properly screened into the larynx, after the patient had been thoroughly cocainized, using a 20 per cent cocain solution within the larynx, preceded by a hypodermic of ¼ grain of morphin sulphate. The radium was held in position after the manner described by Jackson and Janeway. Later 12½ mg. needles, to which strings were securely tied, were introduced into the growth, the number depending upon the size of the growth. These were left in position, in some instances for seven to twelve hours. In addition to the needles external applications were also used.

From reports, the writer is of the opinion that more recent improved technic in the use of radium emanations, as practiced at the Memorial Hospital in New York, offers more encouraging results.

Conclusions.—From the writer's experience, and from published reports, it would seem that radium is only indicated in the socalled inoperable cases of carcinoma of the larynx, meaning those cases in which there is marked involvement of the cervical glands, epiglottis, base of the tongue, and the esophageal wall. Its analgesic effect on these cases, in moderate doses, constitutes one of the most important benefits. It is valuable for those patients who refuse operation. It perhaps exercises a beneficial effect in blocking the lymphatics before a radical operation upon the larynx. Such brilliant results have been obtained in early intrinsic malignancy of the larynx by thyrotomy that in these cases radium should not be thought of except possibly as a postoperative measure. In the more advanced type of intrinsic cancer of the larynx, laryngectomy has prolonged the lives of many by surgeons in all parts of the world. Here again radium should not be considered a means of treatment except before or after operation.

Case 1.—T. H., white, male, aged 83. Carcinoma of larynx, cervical glands and base of tongue. Admitted to Jefferson Hospital October 23, 1917. Patient died without improvement December 29, 1917.

The following is the treatment by Dr. Newcomet:

One hundred mg., 4 hrs., placed at various places on neck around tube that was inserted in throat.

Oct. 23, 1917.   100 mg., 4 hrs., on right side neck towards front.

Oct. 25, 1917.   100 mg., 3 hrs., on left side neck (front).

Oct. 27, 1917.   100 mg., 3½ hrs., under chin directly above tube.

Oct. 30, 1917.   100 mg., 4 hrs., on left side of neck, low down, below level of tube. Examined. No reaction yet. To have one more treatment on right side and one directly under tube.

Nov. 1, 1917.   100 mg., 3½ hrs., right side neck low down below level of tube.

Nov. 3, 1917.   100 mg , 3¼ hrs., on neck low down under tube. Examined. No reaction yet, but to be laid off for ten days. Return Nov. 13.

Nov. 13, 1917.   Examined. No sign of reaction yet. Patient to return in one week.

Nov. 20, 1917.   100 mg., 4 hrs., on right side of neck about level with the tube and toward side of neck.

Nov. 26, 1917.   100 mg , 4 hrs., on left side neck about level with the tube and toward side of neck.

Dec. 29, 1917.   Patient died about four days ago.

Case 2.—E. M., white, male, aged 61. Admitted to Jefferson Hospital August 9, 1920. Carcinoma of the larynx, intrinsic. Operation refused. Patient still living, but growth is beginning to involve the esophagus.

The following is the treatment by Dr. Newcomet:

Aug. 9, 1920. 50 mg., 3 hrs., on right side, median line of neck, near larynx. 50 mg., 3 hrs., on left side median line of neck. Filter 1 mm. lead, 1 in bandage.

Aug. 11, 1920. 100 mg., 3 hrs., over larynx on median line of neck. Filter 1 mm. lead, 1 in bandage.

Aug. 13-14, 1920. 100 mg., 3 hrs., on neck below level of larynx. 100 mg., 4 hrs., right side neck, high. 100 mg., 4 hrs., right side neck, low. 100 mg., 3 hrs., left side neck. 100 mg., 3 hrs., above level of larynx. Filter 1 mm. lead, 1 in bandage. (100 mg., 17 hrs., on neck.)

Case 3.—M. K., white, male, 60 years of age. Carcinoma of larynx and esophagus. Admitted to Jefferson Hospital March 13, 1920. Died April 14, 1920.

Following is the treatment by Dr. Newcomet:

Mar. 16, 1920. 50 mg., 2 hrs., in larynx. Radium in silver tube, covered with rubber, placed by Dr. Lewis.

Mar. 16, 1920. 100 mg., 3 hrs., on left side of neck above level of larynx, a little to left of median line. Radium in 2 mm. lead and 1 in bandage filter.

March 17, 1920. 100 mg., 3 hrs., on center of neck below larynx.

Mar. 17, 1920. 100 mg., 3 hrs., on right side of neck above level of larynx.

Mar. 17, 1920. 100 mg., 3½ hrs., on right side of neck below level of larynx. Patient to return April 6 for examination.

April 6, 1920. 100 mg., 3 hrs., on left side of neck under angle of jaw. 100 mg., 3 hrs., left side neck, about an inch lower than previous treatment. 100 mg., 3 hrs., left side neck, about an inch lower than previous treatment. 100 mg., 3 hrs., right side of neck under angle of jaw. 100 mg., 3 hrs., right side of neck, about 1 inch lower than in previous treatment. 100 mg., 3 hrs., right side of neck, about 1 inch lower than in previous treatment.

Patient was admitted to hospital April 2, and gastrostomy

performed. Patient had not eaten for three days. On April 6th was able to swallow water without difficulty.

Died April 14, 1920.

Case 4.—L. B. M., male, white, aged 55. Carcinoma of larynx with involvement of cervical glands. Admitted to Jefferson Hospital Aug. 26, 1919. Died Oct. 12, 1919.

The following treatment by Dr. Newcomet:

Aug. 26, 1919. 50 mg., 20 hrs.

Sept. 11, 1919. Examined. Not much reaction. Has been coughing up a great deal of mucus in the last three days. Has had several weak spells, when he almost fainted. To be treated again as before.

Sept. 11, 1919. 50 mg., 20 hrs. Radium in lead tube placed over ½ in bandage in lead collar. Radium in ten positions, moved every two hours.

Sept. 16, 1919. Examined. No change in condition. Patient still has a great deal of pain.

Oct. 2, 1919. 40 mg., 3¾ hrs., on left side of neck under ear.

Oct. 6, 1919. 50 mg., 3 hrs., on left side neck near tracheotomy tube.

Oct. 6, 1919. 40 mg., 3 hrs., on right side near tube.

Oct. 8, 1919. 40 mg., 3 hrs., on right side of neck near ear.

Oct. 8, 1919. 50 mg., 3 hrs., on left side of neck, low, near collar bone. Neck seems less swollen. Patient is feeling a little better.

Oct. 11, 1919. Patient had severe pain in right side of abdomen near border of ribs. Coughed up a great deal of very foul pus.

Oct. 12, 1919. Died. Conscious almost to time of death.

Case 5.—P. J. C., male, white, aged 64. Carcinoma of larynx, intrinsic. Laryngectomy, Aug. 21, 1919. Recurrence in the thyroid gland. Died six months after laryngectomy.

The following treatment by Dr. Newcomet:

April 19, 1920. 90 mg., 3½ hrs., left side neck; radium in 1 mm. lead 1 in bandage. 140 mg., 2½ hrs., on right side of neck, over abscess. 140 mg., 3 hrs., on right side of neck near angle of jaw. 140 mg., 3 hrs., on right side of neck on collar bone near median line. 140 mg., 3 hrs., on right side of neck about 3 inches from tracheotomy tube and level with tube. 140 mg., 3 hrs., left side of neck under angle of jaw. 140 mg., 3 hrs., on left side of neck.

Case 6.—E. R., male, white, aged 65. Carcinoma of larynx with involvement of the cervical glands. Admitted to Jefferson Hospital May 4, 1920. Died July, 1920.

The following treatment by Dr. Newcomet:

May 4, 1920. 50 mg., in larynx above cords. Radium in silver tube covered with rubber, placed by Dr. Lewis. Patient coughed up the tube after it had been in throat for less than ten minutes.

May 4, 1920. 40 mg., 3½ hrs., on median line of neck above level of larynx. 40 mg., 3 hrs., right side of neck above level of larynx, about 2 inches from median line. 40 mg., 3 hrs., right side of neck below level of larynx, 2 inches from median line. 40 mg., 3 hrs., left side of neck above level of larynx, 2 inches from median line. 40 mg., 3½ hrs., left side of neck below level of larynx, two inches from median line. 1 mm. lead, 1 in bandage filter.

May 5, 1920. 140 mg., 3½ hrs., on median line of neck at top of sternum. 140 mg., 3 hrs., left side of neck below angle of jaw near jaw bone. 140 mg., 3 hrs., left side neck below angle of jaw near collar bone. 140 mg., 3 hrs., right side neck below angle of jaw near jaw bone. 140 mg., 3⅓ hrs., on right side of neck below angle of jaw near collar bone. 1 mm. lead, 1 in bandage filter.

May 27, 1920. 100 mg., 3 hrs., on right side of larynx, a little below level of larynx.

May 28, 1920. 100 mg., 3 hrs., over larynx.

May 28, 1920. 100 mg., 3 hrs., above larynx. 100 mg., 3 hrs., left side larynx.

May 29, 1920. 100 mg., 3 hrs., right side above larynx.

June 24, 1920. Choked up. Feels poorly. To be treated 24 hrs. on neck on July 9th.

July, 1920. Patient wrote that he was unable to come for treatment. Too weak to travel. Died.

Case 7.—J. P., male, white, aged 60. Carcinoma of larynx, intrinsic. Admitted to Jefferson Hospital July 7, 1920. Operation for thyrotomy July 9, 1920. Died February, 1921.

The following treatment by Dr. Newcomet:

July 7, 1920. 100 mg., 2½ hrs., on neck at top of larynx.

100 mg., 3 hrs., on neck over larynx, a little lower than in previous treatment. 100 mg., 3 hrs., on neck at lower border of larynx. 100 mg., 3 hrs., on right side neck, about 3 inches from median line at upper edge of neck. 100 mg., 3 hrs., on right side neck at lower part of neck. 100 mg., 3 hrs., on left side neck, about 3 inches from median line, at upper edge of neck. 100 mg., 3 hrs., on left side of neck at lower border of neck. Filter 1 mm. lead, 1 in bandage.

July 24, 1920. No change.

July 27, 1920. Patient's throat, although inflamed, appeared better.

Aug. 14, 1920. Referred to dispensary.

Sept. 9, 1920. Repeat application. Treatment was considered necessary over sore spot on median line of neck.

Sept. 28, 1920. 100 mg., 3½ hrs., on median line of neck over sore area from which pus is draining. 1 mm. lead, 1 in. bandage. Examination showed that disease had not progressed but is still confined to small area around larynx. 100 mg., 3 hrs., on neck below level of pharynx. 100 mg., 3 hrs., on neck above level of pharynx. 100 mg., 3 hrs., on right side of neck (high). 100 mg., 3 hrs., on right side of neck (low). 100 mg., 3 hrs., on left side of neck (high). 100 mg., 3 hrs., on left side of neck (low). Filter 1 mm. lead, 1 in bandage. 100 mg., 23 hrs.

Sept. 29, 1920. 100 mg., 1½ hrs., on right side neck.

Oct. 25, 1920. 50 mg., 3½ hrs., over sore spot over larynx on median line of neck. 1 mm. lead, 1 in. wood filter.

Oct. 28, 1920. Examination showed extending upward from sternal notch to the caricoid cartilage midline, a scar, in the middle portion of which there was an ulceration about 1 cm. long, slitlike, surrounded by a number of small nodules. Man's voice was about the same as before operation, speaking only in a whisper.

Nov. 1, 1920. 100 mg., 24½ hrs., on neck in eight positions for about 3 hrs. each. Filter 1 mm. lead, 1 cm. wood. Four positions on right side neck, 3½, 3, 3, 3, hrs. each. Three positions on left side neck, 3 hrs. each. One position, 3 hrs., over ulcerated area on center of neck.

Nov. 9, 1920. No gross change.

Nov. 23, 1920. Patient improved. No treatment deemed necessary.

Dec. 14, 1920. Doing well.

Dec. 28, 1920. Some discomfort.

Jan. 3, 1921. 100 mg., 24 hrs., in 8 positions, 3 hrs. each on neck. 1 mm. lead, 1 cm. wood. A large quantity of pus discharging from opening in thoat. Patient feeling worse.

Feb. 1, 1921. 50 mg., 6 hrs., 4 needles around hole in neck over area of larynx, two on each side of median line, placed in skin at edge of opening.

Case 8.—H. L., male, white, aged 75. Carcinoma of larynx, with involvement of esophagus and cervical glands. Admitted to Jefferson Hospital Nov. 23, 1920. Still living, but losing ground rapidly.

The following treatment by Dr. Newcomet:

Nov. 23, 1920. 100 mg., 2½ hrs., on median line of neck above level of tracheotomy tube. 100 mg., 3 hrs., on right side of neck. 100 mg., 3 hrs., on right side of neck. 100 mg., 3 hrs., on right side of neck. 100 mg., 2 hrs., on right side of neck. 100 mg., 3 hrs., on left side of neck. 100 mg., 3 hrs., on left side of neck. 100 mg., 3 hrs., on left side of neck. 100 mg., 3 hrs., on left side of neck. Filter 2 mm. lead, 2 cm. wood (100 mg., 25½ hrs.).

Nov. 30, 1920. Felt better. Told to return in two weeks.

Dec. 14, 1920. Referred to Dr. Lewis.

Jan. 4, 1921. No over reaction.

The following cases were treated in conjunction with Dr. William L. Clark:

Case 9.—G. A., male, white, aged 55. Admitted to hospital March 8, 1919. Carcinoma of larynx and esophagus. Died about one year after the beginning of the treatment. Radium treatment began May 28, 1919. 50 mg. capsule 1 mm. brass filter covered with rubber tubing in throat 3 hrs.

July 11, 1919. 40 mg. capsule, 2½ hrs. throat.

July 25, 1919. 50 mg. capsule, 2½ hrs. throat.

Sept. 29, 1919. 50 mg. capsule, 2½ hrs. throat.

Case 10.—J. A. B., male, white, aged 43. Carcinoma of larynx with involvement of cervical glands and esophagus. Admitted to hospital May, 1919. Died in June, 1919.

May 14, 1919. 50 mg. capsule in 1 mm. brass filter covered with rubber tubing in throat 6 hrs.

June 2, 1919. Same as above.

Case 11.—J. C. S., male, white, aged 60. Carcinoma of larynx and esophagus. Admitted to hospital Aug. 30, 1920. Died Sept., 1920.

Aug. 30, 1920. 50 mg. pad 10 areas cervical region 4 hrs. each.

Sept. 8, 1920. 5-10 mg. needles, 2-5 mg. needles (60 mg.) in throat 22 hrs.

Case 12.—G. G., male, white, aged 60. Carcinoma of larynx, intrinsic. Admitted to hospital Oct. 1, 1919. Died Dec., 1919.

Oct. 1, 1919. 50 mg. capsule in throat 3 hrs.

Oct. 15, 1919. 50 mg. capsule 2¾ hrs.

Nov. 12, 1919. Five 10 mg. needles injected 12 hrs.

Dec. 8, 1919. 50 mg. pad cervical gland 3 hrs.

Case 13.—J. W. R., male, white, aged 59. Admitted to hospital June 22, 1920. Carcinoma of larynx with involvement of cervical glands, tonsil, soft palate and uvula. Died Aug., 1920.

June 22, 1920. Ten 10 mg. ½ mm. nickel and steel needles injected in throat 16 hrs. 12 areas cervical region 50 mg. pad 4 hrs. each.

Aug. 2, 1920. Ten areas cervical region 50 mg. pad 4 hrs. each.

Case 14.—K. M., male, white, aged 59. Carcinoma of epiglottis, right side of larynx and base of tongue. Admitted to hospital Dec. 16, 1919. Died July, 1920.

Dec. 16, 1919. 25 mg. capsule 1 mm. thickness brass filter in larynx 5 hrs.

March 22, 1920. Eight areas each side of neck 50 mg. radium in needles in 1 mm. thickness brass filter covered with rubber tubing with ½ in. thickness gauze pad.

May 7, 1920. 50 mg. capsule in 1 mm. thickness brass filter in opening in neck after incision of gland 20 hrs.

July 12, 1920. Five 5 mg. needles (25 mg.) in larynx 21 hours. 50 mg. pad 6 areas on neck 4 hrs. each.

Case 15.—C. M., male, white, aged 58. Carcinoma of larynx, intrinsic. Admitted to hospital June, 1920. Thyrotomy and electric coagulation. Still living and no signs of recurrence.

June 28, 1920. 5 mg. needles (20 mg.) ½ mm. thickness nickel and steel in throat 5 hrs. 6 areas cervical region 50 mg. pad 4 hrs. each.

Aug. 9, 1920. 10 areas cervical region 50 mg. pad 4 hrs. each.

Dec. 8, 1920. 21 areas cervical region 50 mg. pad 4 hrs. each.

Case 16.—S. S., male, white, aged 57. Carcinoma of larynx. Admitted to hospital May 13, 1921. Treatment with radium before operation. Laryngectomy May 14, 1921. Still living and in splendid condition.

April 27, 1921. Three 8⅓ mg. needles (25 mg.) in larynx 16 hrs. 12 areas cervical region 50 mg. pad 4 hrs. each.

# LV

# AN ANALYSIS OF OVER FIVE HUNDRED CASES OF PROGRESSIVE DEAFNESS.*

By Harold Hays, M. D.,

New York.

My intense interest in the diagnosis, treatment and general welfare of patients who have consulted me privately because of defects of hearing has led me to study very carefully the histories of those patients whom I have treated within the past five years in order to find out whether an analysis of these histories might not lead me to some more definite conclusions as to the present status of our treatment of these cases so that I might therefore be able to be more honest with myself as to the promises I could make this class of patients. It is a source of satisfaction to me to feel that otologists in general are more interested in the subject of progressive deafness and that they are getting away from the old empiric methods of treatment which often did more harm than good.

What a change has taken place during the past ten years since we have been able to make more exact interpretations of conditions because of our more accurate methods of diagnosis! I refer particularly to the more careful inspection of the nasopharynx, especially the regions of the eustachian tubes, brought about by the invention of that clever instrument, the Holmes nasopharyngoscope. One need no longer conjecture. A little time and patience is all that is necessary to give a definite concept of the picture that is present. Again the use of the electric otoscope, to which can be attached a massage apparatus, forms a valuable adjunct to our armamentarium, for by its means one is able to tell the exact condition of the membrana tympani, how much of the drum is rigid or relaxed, how much actual limitation of excursions of the drum there is, which may be accountable for a further progression of the symptoms.

For purposes of actual analysis, this paper should be statistical in nature, but statistics are dry, inaccurate and often misleading. The general conclusions at which I have arrived I feel will prove of interest. Having been able to follow many of these cases for a number of years, I feel that I am in a position to make more positive statements that if the patients had not been private ones.

Etiologic Factors.—A careful inquiry had been made in most cases as to other members of the family having had any trouble with their ears. We speak of hereditary deafness, but such a term is misapplied in any case in which deafmutism is not directly traceable through a family for generations. But that there is a hereditary predisposition to a weakness of the ear mechanism cannot be doubted, although it is not present as often as is generally supposed. In the cases under consideration, very few of the patients knew of others in the family who were hard of hearing. In a small percentage, more than one member of the family was under treatment at the same time, and in a few instances three or more members of the immediate family were deaf. It is my opinion that we should not consider the hereditary tendency of the disease as of much value in the majority of cases but that where we do find a number of members of one family suffering from this same trouble, we must advise strongly that there is great possibility that future members of the same family will have to be extremely careful of their ears.

That the diseases of childhood play a great part in altering the mechanism of the middle ear and eventually causing a progressive deafness has been forcibly brought to my mind by an analysis of these cases. There are two classes of cases which deserve particular attention—patients who have had exanthematous diseases and those who have had the recurrent colds which are so often associated with diseased tonsils and adenoids. The chief exanthematous diseases are measles and scarlet fever. If one makes careful inquiry he will find that the majority of cases of progressive deafness, which belong to what one might call the hopeless class, have had one or both of these diseases, and that frequently there was ear trouble at that time. This brings up an important point which has been emphasized by Kerr Love and others, that few of these patients have had any attention paid to their ears after the acute symptoms of the disease or the ear discharges have subsided.   Inquiry among these patients shows that, at the time of the scarlet fever, for example, the ears were well taken care of, if there had been any inflammatory reaction present or if there had been any suppuration.   But seldom were the ears examined after they went to school again, even if the family had noticed that their hearing was not as perfect as it had been before.   Oftentimes the deficiency of hearing was not sufficient to cause any apprehension, either on the part of the patient or on the part of the parents, until, perhaps, the age of puberty.   There is no doubt in my mind that an insidious process had been going on for many years and that if proper examinations had been made it would have been possible to correct the condition. From the data that we have in hand, from these cases and from the assertions that have been made by others, one is forcibly impressed with the fact that the most important treatment of progressive deafness is preventive treatment.   I am of the opinion, more than ever, that most deafness is preventable and that it is the duty of the otologist to impress this fact upon the public.

The frequent repetition of colds in childhood is intimately associated with the question of the removal of tonsils and adenoids.   Most of the cases under consideration had had their tonsils and adenoids removed at an early age.   In many cases the operation was imperfectly performed, and in a number of instances had to be done over again in adult life.   Most of these patients give a history of repeated earaches in childhood which must be seriously taken into consideration.   But I believe that it is wrong to make a definite assertion that the removal of the tonsils and adenoids alone will be sufficient to clear up any tendency to ear troubles later on in life.   An analysis of these cases shows plainly that there are many other factors, among which may be mentioned intercurrent diseases which bring about a devitalized condition of the child so that it is prone to a chronic inflammatory condition of the mucosa of the nose and throat.   Much as we feel that the proper elimination of tonsils and adenoids will bring about the results we desire, there are too many instances in which we find that their removal has not influenced the ear condition at all.   One then has to consider that the puny child who

is constantly suffering from an inflamed condition of the nose
and throat with diminished hearing, needs to be gone over
thoroughly to discover whether, for example, there is not
some trouble in the endocrine system or perhaps in the gastrointestinal tract.    It is extremely hard to get at these definite
factors.    Moreover, it has only been during the past few years
that we have had them definitely called to mind.    But I am
able to pick out isolated instances in the series, in which I
am sure that the persistent inflammatory condition in the nose,
throat and ear has been due to some defect in the general
system.    Moreover, I am so sure of this that in the more careful histories we are taking today and in the more careful
treatment we are giving children, we are paying more attention
to general treatment and its effect locally than we are to local
treatment by itself.                        •

Mention has been made of the fact that complaints of
marked defects in hearing are not made until after the age
of puberty.    In the cases under consideration, although a
definite history could be obtained of scarlet fever or some
other predisposing factor, it was seldom that the hearing was
bad enough to be noticed and to demand treatment until after
the fourteenth year.    Whatever treatment that was begun then
was given in a perfunctory manner and did little good.    It
has been my experience that children of this age cannot be
made to appreciate the seriousness of their condition and will
use every subterfuge to get out of treatment.    Most of my
adult patients have candidly admitted that they either did not
have any treatment at this time or else that they were taken
to otologists once or twice and then were told to return at
regular intervals which they never did.    This puts the blame
for future trouble on the patient himself, although it is hard
to make him see it from that point of view.

By far the majority of patients in this series have had some
nose or throat abnormality and, at an earlier date, I collected
a series of fifty of these cases to show the intimate relationship of pathologic conditions of the nose to chronic catarrhal
otitis media.    Since that time I have become more conservative and have felt that it was impossible to say, for example,
that a deviation of the septum was responsible for the ear
condition.    It is a fact that almost all these patients have some

abnormality in the nose or throat or had such an abnormality which was corrected at an earlier date. But I regret to say that the correction of the nose and throat trouble has not by any means improved the hearing. For some years I hoped that this would be so, but a proper analysis has shown me that oftentimes the damage has been done so completely before the patient came to me that no amount of operative interference could correct it. In looking over these histories I find that there is a deviation of the septum or a sinus condition or some disease of the tonsils or some adenoid tissue. And if such a condition is directly connected with some pathologic condition of the eustachian tube, which seems to me to be continued because of the nose and throat abnormality, I advise that an operation should be performed; if, on the contrary, I can see no connection, I do not hesitate to advise that no operation should be performed. It is my opinion that most of these patients have suffered from too many operations upon the nose and throat, and that they have just cause for the feeling that their condition has been made worse because of too much meddling.

Symptoms.—Naturally, the symptoms that most of these patients have complained of is deafness in one or both ears. In the majority of cases they have felt that one ear is worse than the other, but careful tests have shown that the hearing is often worse in the ear of which they complain the less. About 50 per cent of the patients have complained of tinnitus, which varies in character and degree. In the more advanced cases the complaint of the tinnitus has been more than the complaint of the deafness. It is difficult to determine when this tinnitus has first come on, but as a rule it is the forerunner of the complaint of deafness. But this does not mean that it has preceded the deafness. It is only that the deafness has not been of sufficient degree to be noticeable until after the tinnitus has made itself evident. It is my firm belief that if the majority of these patients had been properly treated at the time that they first noticed the tinnitus a great deal could have been done to prevent further trouble. Paracusis has only been present in the more advanced cases, usually in patients who have been treated by a number of physicians over a long period of years. It has been my experience that patients who have a paracusis Willisii will not respond to any treatment which we have at our command at the present time. In all probability the paracusis is due to a fixity of the ligament of the oval window which it is difficult if not impossible to overcome. Dizziness and nystagmus have seldom been noted except in those cases which demonstrate some trouble more deeply located beyond the middle ear.

There is a certain class of cases which demand our attention and which have not been differentially classified. 1 refer to patients who suffer from what I have termed "intermittent deafness." Such patients will state that their hearing is better at one time or another, is better in one climate or another. Any change in the weather seems to make a great difference in their hearing acuity. Any change in their physical condition seems to make a great difference in their hearing acuity. Over half the patients in this series, under thirty years of age, have what I call intermittent deafness. One should pay careful attention to this fact, because it indicates that the ear condition is not so bad but what it can be arrested or improved, provided one is able to get the factor which makes the change in the hearing acuity. A careful examination of these cases shows that in almost all cases the reason for the change in hearing is because the mucosa of the eustachian tube becomes inflamed at times, while at other times this inflammation subsides and the tube again becomes patent. In other words, the cause of the trouble must be found in the nasopharynx. Many of these patients have diseased tonsils which set up an irritation in the nasopharynx, as explained by Emerson. Others have adhesions in the fossa of Rosenmüller which are continually interfering with proper muscular action of the eustachian tubes. Others have definite abnormalities in the nose, particularly hyperplastic or suppurative conditions of the nasal sinuses. But by far the majority of them have a polypoid condition of the posterior tips of the inferior turbinates which act directly on the tubal orifice. Some of these polyps are small but hang directly into the tube itself, while others are so large that they block off the nasopharynx completely. Since the examination with the nasopharyngoscope has become a routine procedure in our office we have been surprised to find that polypoid tips of the inferior turbinate are present in nearly

75 per cent of the adults who come to us complaining of deafness, particularly of the intermittent type. I cannnot too strongly emphasize this point. Moreover, as will be shown later on, it is surprising in how many cases the hearing has been improved after these tips have been properly attended to.

After trying numerous classifications of cases, we have decided that a clinicopathologic classification is the best. By this I mean that the clinical evidence of the condition, as evidenced by tuning fork tests and symptoms, is joined to the pathologic evidence as shown in the middle ear and nasopharynx. In former years, the general term O. M. C. C., was used, which meant nothing. Today it is necessary to differentiate the various types of progressive deafness with which we commonly come in contact. We have found it satisfactory to place our patients in one of the groups about to be mentioned.

1. Retracted drum with stenosed tube.

2. Retracted drum with open tube.

3. Slightly retracted drum with a tube which intermittently opens and closes.

4. Slightly retracted drum which, on vibratory massage, shows only slight loss in motion.

5. The relaxed ear drum, associated or unassociated with a retracted drum.

6. Rare cases, such as otosclerosis and nerve deafness.

1. Retracted Drum With Stenosed Tube.—A large percentage of cases come in the first class. At no time is the tube open unless it is forced open by the passage of applicators or bougies. These cases cannot be Politzerized and seldom can be benefited by catheterization.

2. Retracted Drum With Open Tube.—A small percentage of cases belong to this class. The deafness is associated with an atrophic condition of the mucosa of the nose and throat, which extends up through the eustachian tubes into the ears. The retraction, in parts, may be associated with a relaxation of the drum. In other cases the drum is held rigid, due to the marked infiltration with connective tissue and the ankylosis between the articular joints.

3. Slightly Retracted Drum With a Tube Which Intermittently Opens and Closes.—By far the majority of patients

under thirty years of age belong to this class and can be benefited by proper treatment. The amount of retraction is due to
the negative air pressure in the middle ear and is most often
secondary to some condition in the nasopharynx. When this
is overcome and the tube dilated, the drum can be readily
massaged and the excursions are about normal. One has to
watch these cases carefully, because any acute inflammatory
condition of the nose and throat immediately shows its effects
on the hearing acuity.

4. Slightly Retracted Drum, Which, on Vibratory Massage,
Shows Only Slight Loss in Motion.—In a goodly percentage
of cases, examination with the otoscope, attached to a vibratory massage apparatus, will show almost normal excursions
of the drum. There may be a few adhesions which hold the
drum down in places, or there may be a slight thickening of
the drum in certain parts. The ossicular joints seem to be
freely movable. It is important to recognize this class of
cases, for it is in them that vibratory massage, if done with
intelligence, will do so much good. Almost always there is
an associated condition of the eustachian tube which needs
attention.

5. The Relaxed Ear Drum, Associated or Unassociated
With a Retracted Drum.—In numerous papers in the past I
have spoken of the relaxed ear drum, which gives rise to what
I have popularly called pocket handkerchief deafness. This
class of cases has a definite syndrome. With every act of
blowing the nose the patient has been in the habit of inflating
his ears. He has made himself deaf by overinflating his
ears, and his ears are peculiarly sensitive to all vibrations,
whether they be sound or not. A very large percentage of
cases that were originally called O. M. C. C. belong in this
class. They must be recognized, because they are the cases
which should·be left severely alone unless one feels that it
is worth while to attempt to tighten up the ear drums. Sometimes the relaxation is in certain parts of the drum only and
is accompanied by a retraction in other parts due to adhesions
between the drum and the internal wall of the middle ear or
between the ossicular joints. A definite diagnosis of this
clinicopathologic entity can readily be made by means of the
nasopharyngoscope and the otoscope.

6. Rare Cases, Such as Otosclerosis and Nerve Deafness. —No better evidence of the rarity of true nerve deafness can be given than by an analysis of these cases, which shows that there were only three cases of nerve deafness out of five hundred patients examined. All three were syphilitic in origin, or at least in all three cases there was a history of a previous syphilis. I do not wish to assert that all cases of nerve deafness are due to syphilis. There are other factors, such as meningitis and systemic infections. Yet, having heard so much about nerve deafness, I am rather surprised to find that there were only three cases in this series. And what is equally as surprising to you perhaps, I have not seen one case of otosclerosis that I could diagnose clinically. It is about time that we restricted the term otosclerosis. It is used too loosely and has become a byword in the mouths of the deaf with the result that a great many patients who are told that they have this condition give up in despair and become hopeless despondents. Not having seen a case of otosclerosis in over five hundred cases of deafness makes me feel that the condition is very rare, and this is further corroborated by the statements of investigators who declare that a very minimum percentage of cases of deafness examined pathologically after death show the lesions of otosclerosis.

Improved Methods of Examination.—Our conception of the pathologies of progressive deafness has expanded considerably since the introduction of more precise methods of examination. The cursory examination of the ear drum with an ordinary speculum and the examination of the nasopharynx with the small rhinoscopic mirror will not suffice. There are three new essential instruments with which the otologist cannot get along without—the Holmes nasopharyngoscope (a great improvement on my original instrument, the pharyngoscope), the electric otoscope with attachments for pneumomassage of the drum, and the various applicators, sounds and bougies, the best of which are patterned after Yankauer's instruments. In the earlier cases of this series we did not have these valuable instruments to aid us in diagnosis, but now that we use them as a routine procedure it is hard to believe that we ever got along without them. Direct inspection of the eustachian orifice is of most importance, and we are amazed at the amount of information we derive from this examination. The otoscope allows us to ascertain the exact excursions of the ear drum, which is of equal importance. The determination of the character of the mucosa of the eustachian tube can only be properly determined by the passage of applicators, sounds and bougies through it. The information that can be derived from such a procedure I described in a paper read last year before our State society.

Value of Tuning Fork Tests.—Tests of hearing acuity by means of tuning forks as well as by the watch, whisper and spoken voice are a part of our usual procedure. But the more I have recourse to such examination, the less value I place upon it. Not for one moment would I give up these tests in order to differentiate the kind of deafness that is present or in order to make comparative observations, but the personal equation enters into the tests to a great extent. But what is of most importance, the amount of improvement which the patient derives from treatment cannot be measured by instruments but only by his own interpretation of the amount of improvement that has taken place. I am not as anxious to know whether my tuning forks show any improvement in my patient's hearing as I am in knowing whether he feels that he is hearing better in the practical everyday life that he leads. In analyzing this series I find that in many cases the patient thinks that he hears better, although my technical examination shows no improvement. A considerable number of these patients have stood by me for years, and they are content that I can keep them from getting worse. From my own personal point of view, I am not satisfied, but the patient is and that is what counts in the end. There is no instrument that I know which is an accurate test of hearing at the present time, unless we accept the audiometer, which Dean has written of in a recent issue of the Laryngoscope.

Prognosis.—The cases in this series divide themselves into two classes: patients who are moderately deaf and in whom there is some hope of improvement, and cases that are hopelessly deaf from the medical point of view. More of the latter class are consulting me year by year, perhaps because the otologists of the country are using me as a court of last resort. Mental reconstruction of the deafened is becoming more and more the duty of the otologist, and this latter class can be handled only in that way. The prognosis, therefore, depends upon the type of case one is treating. I believe that the results I am beginning to attain in the mildly progressive type of case means a great deal for the future. I know that I am getting better results than I did as short a time as three years ago. I cannot help but feel that the future is full of promise if the otologists of the country will delve into this problem with the same thoroughness with which they have handled all other problems in their field. First of all, the prognostications of the future will depend on how much educational propaganda can be spread about so that the proper preventive measures in early childhood will be used. Secondly, otologists must be impressed with the fact that a proper clinicopathologic picture must be revealed before any attempt is made at treatment. Thirdly, we must get away from the time worn idea that inflation of the ears is the only treatment. The prognosis of the socalled hopeless cases will depend upon our ability to make these patients take up lip reading at the earliest opportunity. That is the salvation of these patients.

Treatment.—It will not be my purpose to outline any definite treatment as the result of my careful perusal of these cases. The most important thing to my mind is that I have become more and more convinced that the only hope of relief lies in the proper attention to pathologic conditions of the nasopharynx which exercises any influence on the eustachian tube. Tubal patency is of the utmost importance and must be permanently, not temporarily, established. Having assumed that everything of an ameliorative nature, be it operative or otherwise, has been attempted, there is often still a degree of inflammation at the orifice of the eustachian tube or in the tube itself which must be overcome. After having tried every kind of medicament we have come to the conclusion that the high frequency current, properly applied, does the most good. The ultraviolet ray may be applied by direct vacuum tubes, or one may use the modified nasopharyngoscope which I have recently had made, into which can be fitted a fine electrode for fulguration. The vacuum tubes are made on the same lines as a eustachian catheter, and are wound with silk ribbon which is coated with shellac so that if they break in the nose no harm will be done. They are inserted into the orifice of the eustachian tube and the current is applied directly for from five to ten minutes. The results are very gratifying. After one to two treatments the tube remains open and stays open for a considerable length of time. We have treated about fifty patients in this way during the past six months, and in many instances the hearing has been markedly improved without making use of dilators in the tube of any kind. The fulguration treatment is of particular value in those cases in which polypoid tips of the inferior turbinates are overhanging the eustachian orifices and where there are evidences of glandular excrescences on the promontory of the tube, in the fossa of Rosenmuller or in the mouth of the tube itself. The current is applied in the same manner as when one desires to get rid of a growth in the bladder. As the fulguration is performed under direct inspection no harm can be done.

What conclusions can be arrived at as a result of an analysis of this large number of cases? Surely we must feel that the results are not very gratifying, as far as cures are concerned. But the future is full of promise. First and foremost, we must classify our cases in a different manner than we have in the past. A clinicopathologic classification must be established, as it seems almost hopeless to get at a pathologic classification by itself. Secondly, we must pay more attention to the etiologic factors in childhood and recognize the fact that most of the harm is done before it is discovered, and therefore be able to instruct parents and family physicians more carefully. Thirdly, we must separate those cases for whom something can be done medically from those for whom nothing can be done medically, and give these patients the benefit of our honest advice. It is a sad commentary on our treatment in the past that we have so many hopelessly deaf patients who have to resort to lip reading to overcome their handicap. Lastly, the newer and precise methods of diagnosis and direct treatment which we feared to use until a few years ago have become common knowledge and encourage us to feel that in the course of time we shall be able to treat these patients with intelligence and be able to give them honest encouragement.

2178 BROADWAY.

# LVI

# CERTAIN OBSERVATIONS IN RELATION TO THE SURGERY OF THE SPHENOID SINUS.

By B. N. Colver, M. D.,

Battle Creek.

Introduction.—About ten years ago opportunity was afforded to observe a very puzzling case in the clinic of a well known internist. This patient was seen by a number of consultants, but the diagnosis was established only at autopsy. It was abscess of a sphenoid sinus with meningitis. At this time I was also fortunate to be able to study with Skillern. He was then working on the material for the first edition of his excellent book, "The Accessory Sinus." Ever since, the lure of the sphenoid sinus has been persistent and insistent. This interest has been stimulated by the writings of Skillern, Sluder, Loeb, and others. In our own clinic we have been struck with the more than occasional case in which the sphenoid sinus seemed to be the site of persistent pathology. In many cases of multiple sinusitis it is inevitable that the sphenoid should participate. Shambaugh[1] reports a case of acute abscess of one sphenoid sinus in which the posterior ethmoid cells were also involved. He remarks that infection restricted to the sphenoid sinus in which other nasal accessory sinuses are not involved is rather the exception. In this he evidently refers to the acute cases. But in not a few chronic cases, where either in our own clinic or in other clinics the pathology of septum, middle turbinates, and other sinuses had been either corrected or excluded, the patient continued to suffer with obscure symptoms apparently of nasal origin. Persistent nasopharyngitis, lateral pharyngitis, recurrent rhinitis and indefinite aches and pains in the head without evident cause led us more and more frequently to suspect the sphenoid sinus. The recognition of the more severe cases by the obvious clinical picture invited us to seek the milder and less clearcut ones. Further, the conclusion was reached that it is just as logical to expect a residual infection of low grade in one or both sphenoid

sinuses after an intense rhinitis, as it is to look for the same
in a maxillary or frontal sinus. Each spring brings its after-
math of chronic cases, secondary to the neglected acute rhinitis cases of the winter.[2] In many of these the ethmoid labyrinth may have recovered completely from the acute infection
and the general nasal mucosa look normal. Remaining, however, there may be a frontal, a maxillary, or a sphenoidal relic
with the more or less indefinite mild chronic course. It is to
the surgical care of such sphenoid cases that there observations
are directed.

### THE SUBMUCOUS SPHENOID SINUS OPERATION.

Surgical Procedure.—The surgical procedure that has been
followed in the later of these cases consists in a submucous
resection of the nasal septum, with the removal of considerable of the anterior wall of the sinuses down to the lower angle,
and when possible even a bit of the floor of the sinus. The
septum between the sinuses may be partially or completely removed as indicated by the pathologic condition present.

When the septal operation is carried far back the vertical
plate leads to the sphenoidal crest. This is covered below by
the anterior portion of the base of the vomer, under which it
runs into the rostrum of the sphenoid. The alæ of the vomer,
anteriorly, spread laterally to cover the inner borders of the
sphenoturbinals. After the crest is reached the mucous membrane over the anterior surface of the sphenoid is elevated,
thus giving wide exposure of the field. Slits are next made
in the thin bony wall of the sinuses between the crest and the
sphenoturbinals. These slits may be continued downward into
the thinner borders of the alæ of the base of the vomer. Occasionally this may be done and the anterior bony wall of the
sinuses removed without lacerating the sinus mucosa. The
only difficulty arises from the varying anatomy and relations
of the sinuses to each other.

After the slits are made forceps may be slipped astride the
upper portion of the crest, which is removed as far as the base
of the vomer. Considerable difficulty is experienced if an
attempt is made to remove the crest without first delimiting
and partially freeing it as mentioned. The removal may be
continued downward to insure good exposure of the anterior

wall of the sinuses and of the floor as well. This includes the biting away of the anterior portion of the vomer back to the rostrum. The especial advantage of this is to obviate the leaving of a lip or retaining wall at the floor of the sinus. This clean removal permits the chimney action during inspiration, described by Canfield, in relation to the maxillary sinus. In his operation he urges the removal of the deepest portion of the median wall for this purpose. The anterior inferior angle of the sphenoid sinus, while not acutely angulated, often presents a sort of reservoir or cupping. This lays it open to suspicion as an area of persistent pathology, as pointed out by Denker, in relation to the anterior superior angle of the maxillary sinus.

In the course of the operation we have found occasion to correct middle turbinate pathology also by such procedures as infraction and proper placement of turbinates in relation to the straightened septum and correction of the socalled cystic middle turbinates. The first step with such a cellular turbinate is to plunge the angle knife into the center of its anterior end. The contained cell is thus punctured. The blade of the scissors is now introduced and the incision continued inferiorly and posteriorly, and superiorly and posteriorly to the extent of the cell. A snare is slipped over the lateral half of the split turbinate and that half thus removed slightly back of the posterior end of the cell. This reduces the lateral diameter of the turbinate from 60 to 75 per cent without diminishing the area of mucous membrane and with a minimum area of surgical wound. The remaining median shell may be squeezed or compressed by a flat forceps and infracted, and thus straightened, moulded, and placed to best advantage in relation to the new septal plane. This also facilitates the inspection and work upon the anterior sphenoidal wall.

, After the bone work is complete and the turbinates are infracted, the mucous membrane of the anterior walls of the sphenoid sinuses may be removed by knife, forceps and scissors. This is done through a long nasal speculum that gently presses aside the septum and the posterior end of the opposing turbinate.

The after-care is the after-care of the submucous resection. A light gauze packing is used for the septal flaps, but not carried far back in the nose. We have not packed any sinus. In some of our cases the Lynch septal splints have been used.

In two or three cases the thickness of the lower portion of the bony sinus wall has made a bone biting forceps inadequate to remove as low as desired. A chisel has been held with the edge vertical or at right angles to the floor of the sinus, and two or three nicks cut into the heavier bone. After this, gentle rocking of the demarked fragments easily removes them. In one case considerable bleeding was encountered but it was not serious. The sinus mucous membrane is pushed aside rather than lacerated. Only at the conclusion of the bony operation is the nasal mucous membrane removed overlying the sinus, and finally the sinus mucous membrane itself correspondingly trimmed away.

No irrigation or antiseptics have been used in the sinuses. The rhinorrhea cerebrospinalis noted by Skillern has not been observed.

In opening these sinuses we have found mucus varying from nearly clear to decidedly purulent. We have found the mucosa apparently normal after being wiped out and have found it congested, swollen and thickened in local areas.

Cavanaugh reports one of his cases in which the opening of a dry sinus was followed by the immediate relief of a long continued pressure. He believes this to have been a vacuum sphenoidal sinus.

Classification.—In diagnosis and decision, the classification given by Skillern[3] has been followed.

1. Acute Inflammation.—These cases are incidental to acute nasal infections and are not surgical. Under proper care practically all of them should resolve.

2. Chronic Catarrhal Inflammation.—This is the mildest, most common and least recognized form of sinusitis. Its history and symptoms are persistent pharyngitis sicca, pharyngitis lateralis, postnasal discharge, fullness and dryness in the nasopharynx and hawking and rasping of the throat in the morning. It rarely becomes frankly purulent or shows marked exacerbations, but continues about the same indefinitely.

3. Chronic Purulent Inflammation.—In this form the mucosa is infected in local areas, some portions being more or

less healthy. ᵔ The characteristics of this type are remittent. There are exacerbations with pronounced symptoms, such as profuse discharge and typical headaches. During the quiescent stage the symptoms abate, but there is always some postnasal discharge, dull headache, and an extreme tendency to "catch cold."

In both of these chronic forms Skillern advocates his conservative operation. In this operation the normal nasal structures are almost undisturbed. It would appear that these cases are also quite suitable for the procedure outlined herein, especially when the anatomic conformation of the septum and turbinates calls for correction. The microscopic examination made of tissue taken at autopsy from the sphenoid sinus by J. D. Cowie and J. S. Fraser (quoted by Cavanaugh) shows that slight catarrhal changes in the mucous membrane were often found, but genuine suppuration was rare.

4.—Chronic Purulent Inflammation with Permanent Pathologic Changes in the Mucosa and Underlying Bone.—These cases are more severe or advanced cases and more rare than the other two. They are the typical sphenoidal empyema of the textbooks. All the classical symptoms appear and are marked. There are headache, mental symptoms, cacosmia, marked postnasal secretion, sore throat, hoarseness, disturbances of bronchi and stomach and ocular symptoms. From such cases we believe the sphenopalatine ganglion syndrome may often arise.. These are the cases of hyperplastic sphenoiditis described by Sluder. They probably result from long continued irritation of the cavity. If diagnosed in the early stage and properly handled they would never develop into this type, and many cases of ganglion symptoms could be avoided.[4] It was for such chronic cases that sphenoid surgery was first utilized and the radical intranasal operation devised, as described by Hajek. Inasmuch as the posterior ethmoid cells are usually involved, it would seem that the radical operation is the one of choice.

5. Mucocele.—Such pent up collections of mucoid material are more or less rare. Skillern advises the radical operation, but it would seem that the submucous sphenoid operation would be justifiable, at least as the first attempt, in any case with deviated septum.

6. Pyocele.—This collection of pent up pus resulting from a sudden closure of ostium or an acute infection of a mucocele, is indeed a rare incident. It is, on the other hand, a very grave condition and is probably the class to which belongs the case noted above. A prompt and radical operation is indicated. It is likely that the packing, congestion and edema incidental to the submucous operation would negative even the trial of the same for such cases. In such a case presenting marked septal deviation the operation might be carried to the removal of the sphenoid crest and then completed outside the septal flaps. This would mean the removal of the mucosa overlying the anterior surface of the sinus before the bone wall was attacked. Further, the more virulent nature of the pus would lead to the possibility of a complication of healing of the septal flaps. In none of the cases performed for sinuses of suitable type has there been any complicating infection or trouble with septal healing.

Examination.—Cavanaugh[4] suggests that "Compared with the general interest in the other sinuses, the attention given to the sphenoid sinus is slight, due, maybe, to the fact that it is harder to reach and examine. It is of greater importance, due to closer association to vital structures, and when affected is more liable to complications."

Loeb[5] says "that we do not know why the sinus should escape infection when every necessary condition is present so far as our knowledge goes; at any rate the opportunity is abundant, the attack is rare." It is a question whether the attack is really as rare as this would indicate. Surely the incidence of the chronic cases does not coincide with infrequency of acute infection. The violent or obstructed cases fortunately enough are rare, but the mild and moderate cases are common.

The history of these cases, together with the negative findings in the anterior two-thirds of the nose, has been of greatest value in the diagnosis. The tentative diagnosis may be made by a careful study of the clinical course and by elimination of the sinuses of the anterior series.

Cavanaugh states his indications for a careful sphenoid research to be postnasal dripping, obscure cases of tinnitus aurium, headaches, obscure eustachian tube infections, postauricular pains without special local findings, pressure back of the eyes and tenderness of the eyeball. He also suggests that, "It is possible that many disorders of the pituitary body are secondary to the primary disturbance of the sphenoid sinus. Dr. Cushing in his book on "The Pituitary Body and Its Disorders," states that it is not unusual for patients to mention an occasional unexpected and intermittent discharge of mucus in the pharynx. Dr. Cushing would lead one to infer that this is the result of the diseased gland, but it is a question whether the sinus pathology may not precede."

Anterior rhinoscopy is usually of no conclusive value. Especially is this true if the septum is deviated to any extent and the middle turbinates more or less crowded. Occasionally the mucosa in the region of the anterior sphenoidal wall may be seen and redness, swelling or discharge noted. In the wide open nose such inspection is relatively easy, though the incidence of sphenoid disease is correspondingly less frequent.

Posterior rhinoscopy, with particular attention to the lateral folds of the pharynx and vault of the nasopharynx, gives more evidence of value, especially after the sinuses of the anterior series have been excluded. In particular, the nasopharyngoscope (Holmes) is of greatest value. By cocainizing the inferior meatus only, the nasopharyngoscope can be freely used and yet the suspected field not altered by the medication. By this means pathologic hyperemia, edema, mucus, mucopus, pus or polypoid degeneration can be detected, especially if several observations are made at different times of the day and at intervals during the same visit. One very marked and frequent finding is the irritative thickening of the septal mucosa opposite and extending down from the sphenoethmoidal angle. If only one method of examination were permitted the nasopharyngoscope would be the one of first choice. We have not tried the hand burr, as suggested by Grayson,[6] as the repeated use of the nasopharyngoscope has given the equivalent diagnostic information.

The X-ray examination has not been of great dependability in these cases. This is due partly to the difficulty of separating the sphenoid sinuses from the posterior ethmoid cells in roentgenologic study. A greater factor, however, is the likelihood of no alteration in the density of the tissues to the X-ray.

Loeb[5] states that "roentgenography has so far been of little value in the diagnosis of sphenoid empyema."

Iglauer[7] has found that "the roentgenogram is a great aid to diagnosis and should be combined with careful clinical study." In this he agrees with Law,[8] who says, "It is necessary to know the history, symptoms and the clinical findings before attempting a diagnosis."

Jervey[9] also agrees that "as a matter of preference, I would not be without its aid, for it often adds weight to the positiveness of the diagnosis." In a case of primary tuberculosis of the sphenoid Kernan[10] reports marked clouding.

Shambaugh[11] reports that "transillumination and the X-ray were of no particular value in the diagnosis of sphenoid sinus trouble in an acute case, "but in an abscess of one sphenoid sinus "the evidence was of definite value."

Cavanaugh probes the ostium, dilates with bougies and then uses a small transilluminator. The most he expects from transillumination, apparently, is anatomic information.

The examination of the fundus is always to be made, though only of corroborative value. There is nothing pathognomonic or constant. After studying a considerable number of proven cases, Dr. L. V. Stegman epitomizes the fundus findings as follows: "Sometimes the picture is that of a mild optic neuritis. The disc is usually slightly blurred, the margins of the papilla and retina 'fusing.' The vessels show only slight change, if any, the veins being slightly darker and broader, and maybe a trifle tortuous. There is also contraction of the color fields, especially for red and green, and the blind spot may be a trifle enlarged."

Other Treatment.—Most of these cases being essentially chronic, have had previous treatment, and many of them have had nasal operations. For a long time we have tried various methods, such as vacuum treatments, corrective surgery to the septum and turbinates, vaccines, general therapeutics, as regulation of the diet and of the gastrointestinal tract, and other measures looking toward the improvement of constitutional vigor. Cases which do not show marked improvement within a few weeks are unlikely to yield short of sphenoid surgery. Some cases have been advised climatic change, and in the milder ones, where the other nasal pathology has already been corrected this has been very satisfactory. In some cases, however, the return to the northern climate, with the changeable seasons, has been followed within a relatively short time by a recurrence of the annoying symptoms. In some of the catarrhal cases where a definite diagnosis of sphenoid disease could not be made, the surgery has been confined to the correction of septal and turbinal pathology. Turbinates that have been in contact with or in close proximity to marked septal deviation have been thus relieved from such a relation. The vicious circle of turbinate hyperemia and edema, irritating pressure against the irregular septum and retained secretions has thus been broken. In the course of a few months the condition of the turbinates has been wonderfully improved. With this the irritation in the sphenoethmoidal angle has subsided. Whether or not these were true cases of sinus catarrh is not easy to say.

### SUMMARY.

During the past year fifteen cases have been found where the sphenoid pathology and the irregularities of septum and turbinates have seemed to indicate this operation.

In these cases, where septal irregularity intervenes, this can be corrected, and the further work on the sphenoid sinus adds but little to the operation. If a radical operation should be done later the septal work of the first operation would be a help or step toward the second.

. The pathology of the middle turbinates is corrected, and yet the turbinate preserved. No functionally necessary tissues are destroyed.

The technic permits of free inspection of the depths and angles of the sphenoid sinus.

The anterior wall, and especially the lower angle, may be removed freely and recovery thus insured.

In the nose with straight septum and a free view, either the conservative operation of Skillern or possibly an exploratory opening as suggested by Grayson is indicated. Skillern points out, however, that some cases otherwise suitable for the conservative operation may not be done when the anatomy of the septum and superior turbinate results in a mere slit. Such cases would not contraindicate the submucous sphenoid operation but rather would be entirely suitable for the same.

## BIBLIOGRAPHY.

1. Shambaugh: Acute Sphenoid Sinusitis. Surg. Clin. of Chicago, p. 1193, Dec., 1920.

2. Thomson: Treatment of Acute Nasal Sinusitis. The Practitioner, CVL. No. 1, p. 1, Jan., 1921.

3. Skillern: Sphenoid Sinus: Present Day Value of Surgical Procedure. J. A. M. A., LXVII, No. 27, Dec. 23, 1916, p. 1896.

4. Cavanaugh: The Sphenoid Sinus. Ill. Med. Jour., XXVII, No. 5, May, 1920 p. 331.

5. Loeb: The Sphenoid Sinus. J. A. M. A., LXVII, No. 27, Dec. 30. 1916, p. 1991.

6. Grayson: The Exploratory Opening of the Sphenoid Sinus. The Laryngoscope, XXV, No. 2, Feb., 1915, p. 65.

7. Iglauer: The Oblique Method of Roentogenography of the Ethmoid and Sphenoid Cells. J. A. M. A., LXVII, No. 26, Dec. 23, 1916, p. 1905.

8. Law: Am. J. of Roentgenology, Aug., 1917. (Quoted by Jervey.)

9. Jervey: X-ray Aid in the Diagnosis of Nasal Accessory Sinus Disease. Southern Med. Jour., XIII. No. 4, April, 1920, p. 291.

10. Kernan: A Case of Tuberculosis of the Sphenoid Sinus. The Laryngoscope, XXIX. No. 5, May, 1919, p. 276.

11. Shambaugh: Abscess of the Sphenoid Sinus. Surg. Clinics of Chicago, II, No. 3, June, 1918, p. 675.

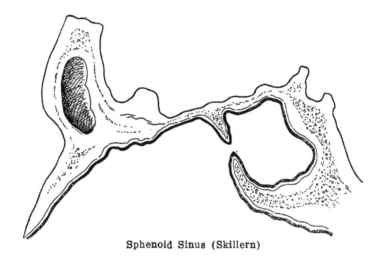

Sphenoid Sinus (Skillern)

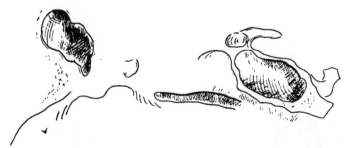

Varied Conformations of Anterior-
Inferior angle of the Sphenoid Sinus.

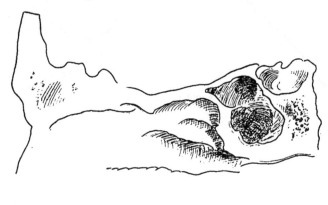

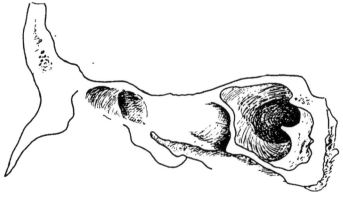

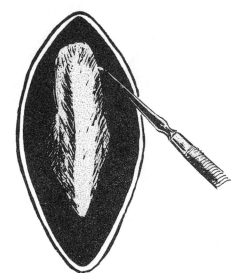

Separating the Sphenoidal Crest

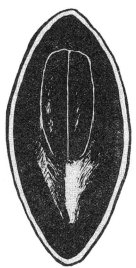

The Sinus Exposed

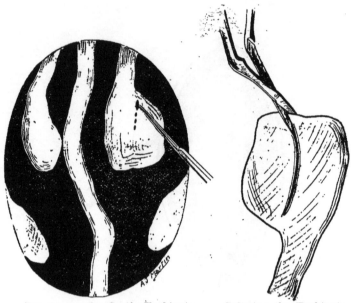

Puncturing the Cystic Turbinate      Splitting the Turbinate
with Scissors

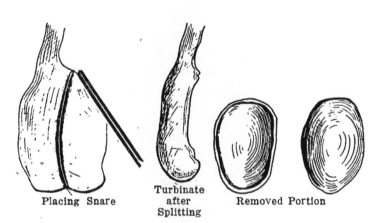

Placing Snare     Turbinate     Removed Portion
after
Splitting

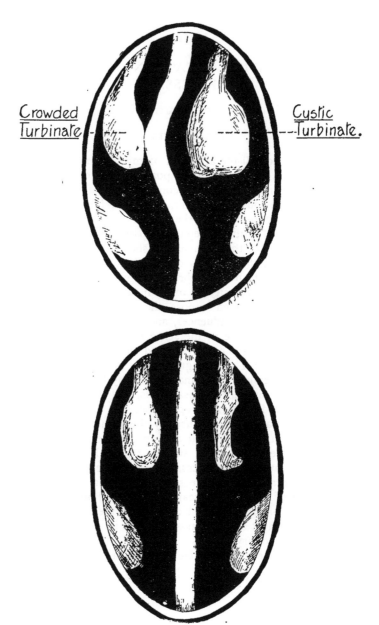

Crowded
Turbinate

Cystic
Turbinate.

Septal and Turbinal Relation Corrected

## LVII.

## POSTOPERATIVE TREATMENT OF BRAIN ABSCESS.*

### By S. MacCuen Smith, M. D.,

Philadelphia.

I should like to call the attention of my hearers to the fact that I have been restricted to the postoperative care of brain abscess and am not expected to consider any other phase of the subject. Obviously, however, some brief statements of fact are necessary to elucidate the text.

In all cases of otitic encephalic abscess formations, the route of selection for their evacuation should be through mastoid exenteration; this enables one to follow the avenue of infection and explore both cerebrum and cerebellum; furthermore, it avoids the necessity, in most instances, of various trephining operations, which expose the dura and underlying structures to infectious influences, and actually do not always provide efficient drainage in the sense of a gravity outlet.

A cerebellar abscess is best evacuated via the posterointernal wall of the antrum. This triangular space is bounded in front by the posterior semicircular canal, behind by the lateral sinus, and above by the superior petrosal sinus, and this area is well exposed by the radical mastoid operation.

As superficial abscesses are usually the result of disease in the posterior mastoid cells and are directly beneath the tentorium and close to the outer surface of the lateral lobe, in hunting for a superficial abscess, therefore, we explore from behind the lateral sinus, whereas we may begin our explorations in front of the sinus to search the cerebellum for deeply seated abscess formations, which are usually the result of labyrinthine involvement and are mostly found in close proximity to the internal auditory meatus.

Should it be deemed advisable to make a counter opening

---

*Read at the annual meeting of the American Otological Society, at Atlantic City, N. J., June 1, 1921.

through the squama, the location for the same can be readily determined after the abscess cavity has been located through the tegmen. In such instances it is conceivable that irrigation might be employed to advantage.

In cases of unencapsulated abscess, the brain forceps is to be preferred. Personally I have not had any difficulty in entering an encapsulated abscess with this instrument. The opening can be enlarged very readily with a minimum of disturbance by gently separating the blades.

At the time of the first packing, great care must be exercised to manipulate the brain substance gently and just as little as possiible. When a drainage tube is used and allowed to protrude, considerable damage may be caused by placing over it flat dressings. Indeed, I have seen several cases where this has been done progress well for a time, but finally develop some complication, which I attributed to this undue and unwise pressure. It is much better to place a quantity of loose gauze packing at the outer end of the drain.

Some operators get good results by the use of one or preferably two tubes. The cigarette, rolled rubber or gauze drain is used with equal efficiency by other men. Whatever drain is selected (I personally prefer the cigarette), care must be taken that it is inserted to the full depth of the abscess cavity. If for any reason this must be changed, everything should be ready to introduce a fresh drain to the full depth of the cavity immediately on withdrawing the original one. In the case of a child in which I evacuated an abscess from three different parts of the brain, I used for each operation—they were about two weeks apart—a double cigarette drain. In this particular instance the drainage was ample, the patient making a complete recovery, having been employed in a responsible position since her recovery, about seven years ago.

In case iodoform gauze is used—and this is advisàble in almost all primary packings—we should bear in mind that a continuation of its use over an extended period may cause symptoms of iodoform absorption. If iodoform packing has been used at the time of operation, and the cavity is large and the pus foul, it is sometimes advisable to replace the same by one or preferably two drainage tubes at the first dressing, and under these circumstances irrigation is indicated.

Personally I have found it necessary to use lavage or irrigation in but a few cases of brain abscess. However, if it is deemed advisable to wash out the cavity, either at the time of operation or subsequently, two tubes must always be used. The tube provided for the return flow must be of larger caliber than that used to introduce the fluid. I wish again to state that I think it unwise to use irrigation at the primary operation, for fear of disseminating the infection. I also believe it unwise to use irrigation at any time as a routine procedure, although it is not only advisable but necessary in some instances, notably in chronic cases. When, in the judgment of the operator, irrigation is called for, the more useful solutions are those ranging from the simple normal salt or boric acid solution to one of carbolic acid, bichlorid of mercury, or the Carrel-Dakin solution, the selection being governed by the virulence of the infection.

If the opening into the abscess is sufficiently large, intracranial pressure, under the stimulus of gauze packing, can be depended upon to empty the cavity of its secretion and necrotic tissue. If irrigation is used, the fluid should be under low pressure and, as above stated, ample provision is to be made for the return flow.

The Whiting encephaloscope is useful for exploring the cavity after the abscess has been opened, and also for the repeated introduction of gauze into the cavity in suitable cases, as it reduces to a minimum trauma or disturbance to the brain substance. Another efficient means of promoting drainage, and one which causes but little disturbance in selected cases, is the introduction of the finger into the abscess cavity at each dressing, until the discharge materially decreases. Finger explorations are especially indicated if symptoms of imperfect drainage become manifest.

I have not had any personal experience with Mosher's copper wire gauze drain nor the British Army drain, but the principle is sound. It is claimed that they provide efficient drainage when combined with the use of glycerin, which softens the necrotic brain tissue and facilitates its escape with other débris.

It would seem that the character of the permanent drain must be decided almost wholly by the operator according to the findings in individual cases. There are objections to the prolonged use of rubber tubing because the beating of the intracranial vessels against the same tends to destroy the parenchyma, and yet practically all of our early cases were treated in this manner, with a creditable percentage of success. If we felt quite secure in following Macewen's custom of removing the drain in twenty-four to forty-eight hours, then the above objection would be overcome and the rubber tubing drain would be ideal. However, most of us would exhibit the vacillation of a doubting Thomas anent the abscess cavity having been rendered thoroughly sterile—a requisite unconditionally essential for the fulfillment of Macewen's ideal.

It has been my custom to change the dressings every day or two, or even twice daily if necessary to keep them clean. The patient is more comfortable by following this procedure, and I am a believer in keeping the wound free from accumulated débris. Furthermore, I think it aids in promoting free drainage by perhaps stimulating capillary attraction, which cannot possibly obtain with a dressing that has become dried and "dead."

The encapsulated form of abscess requires a longer period for healing through the development of granulations, and therefore must be drained for a longer time than the unencapsulated type. The drain here, of whatever selection, must be withdrawn very gradually. Only the operator's personal experience and the conditions of individual cases can determine when to abandon the effort to keep the drainage tract patulous. It is better to continue this somewhat too long than to run the chance of not having thoroughly evacuated the infectious material from the abscess cavity, as well as the tract leading to the same.

It is not my habit to make especially large dural openings, hence it has not been necessary to make an attempt to suture the dura after the draining process has ceased. Indeed, I consider this an unwise procedure in most instances, as experience has shown that there will be some escape of fluid even after the methods to promote drainage have been abandoned. Suturing the dura, under such circumstances, would be harmful. The usual methods of protecting the dura from infection before and following the operation, such as walling off with iodoform gauze, etc., should be scrupulously carried out afterwards until the abscess has entirely healed and the wound closed.

If the healing of the bone opening is retarded by a hernia cerebri, an attempt should be made to correct the same by exerting pressure by means of gauze pads made in cone shape and held in position by the usual bandage. In case this does not succeed, the mass, which is mostly granulation tissue, should be excised, provided the hernia does not include the cerebellum or motor cortical region. The exposed surface is then dusted with iodoform or other antiseptic powder, and the gauze pads above mentioned continued. One of my cases presenting an obstinate hernia through the tegmen was treated in this way, with the result that the depression is barely noticeable.

I believe that on account of the seemingly necessary haste in operating, the average case of brain abscess is not properly prepared for such a grave procedure. However necessary it is to promote elimination, I deem it most unwise to resort to violent purgation, on account of its depleting effect. It has been my custom before operation, at intervals of eight hours when such time is available, to give high enemas of normal salt solution, and this is continued at intervals of four or five hours subsequent to the operation, as indicated. In the case of the child to whom I referred above, the condition was so grave that we resorted to the administration of normal salt solution intravenously. The beneficial effect of normal salt solution in such cases is truly surprising and is well worthy of your consideration. It is most important that the patient should be kept quiet and free from all annoyances, even after the serious symptoms have subsided.

As all otitic brain abscess formations are subject to recurrence, the patient should be cautioned not to engage in any activities that increase intracranial congestion for at least one year. This restriction embraces everything that enters into a well regulated life, including food, drink, recreation, amusement, mental activity and sleep, and of these an abundance of sleep is most essential.

The patient's improvement following evacuation of pus from the brain is truly astounding in some instances. This is especially shown in the way the pulse and temperature will return to normal or above, from their subnormal state, and even more noticeable is the improved mental condition, the patient emerging from a state of dulness or even perhaps a comatose state, and resuming the alertness of the normal mind and again taking interest in his surroundings, and recognizing his friends and objects, and even asking for food. The transition is amazing, and I know of no other condition where the changes are so marked, and relatively so immediate, as in those cases where the functional impairment is due to inflammatory pressure and not to necrotic destruction. The latter cases are always critical and in event of ultimate cure recovery is prolonged even to several years.

# LVIII.

# MONOCULAR RETROBULBAR OPTIC NEURITIS CAUSED BY PURULENT MAXILLARY SINUSITIS.*

By J. W. Jervey, M. D.,

Greenville, S. C.

In discussing a paper by L. A. Coffin of New York, read at the annual meeting of the American Laryngological, Rhinological and Otological Society in 1917, on the subject of the relationship of the nasal accessory sinuses to diseases of the eye, E. S. Thomson of New York remarked that it was hardly necessary to take the maxillary antrum into consideration. Whereupon J. A. White of Richmond related a case of a middle aged lady who had a retrobulbar neuritis which was blinding her and which promptly cleared up on washing out the antrum.

At the 1920 meeting of the Midwestern Section of the Laryngological, Rhinological and Otological Society, H. B. Lemere of Omaha recounted a case of optic neuritis which responded to treatment of the maxillary antra.

These are the only two cases I can recall or find after a hasty review of the past few years' literature which directly connect pathology of the antrum of Highmore with optic nerve pathology.

In the past fifteen or twenty years much has been said and written about ocular and orbital disease secondary to disease of the paranasal sinuses, and a few years ago the late Christian Holmes of Cincinnati even went so far as to say that he believed 40 per cent of all eye diseases had their origin in the nasal accessory sinuses. Owing, however, to the close juxtaposition, amounting almost to contiguity of the optic nerve with the posterior ethmoid cell and the sphenoid sinus, it seems to have been more or less commonly accepted that optic

*Read at the annual meeting of the Southern Section of the American Laryngological, Rhinological and Otological Society, at Asheville, N. C., January 29, 1921.

neuritis, when due to sinus infection, is the result of pathologic changes in these posterior sinuses.

L. E. White of Boston, in a very interesting and valuable contribution read at the annual meeting of the Laryngological, Rhinological and Otological Society in 1919, reported some seventeen cases of retrobulbar neuritis, occurring as a result of infection of the posterior ethmoid and sphenoid sinuses. He gave an enlightening resume of the literature, but in no case was there any reference to the maxillary antrum in this connection. But inasmuch as a large part of the orbital floor is constituted of the roof of the maxillary antrum, it would seem to require no great endowment of genius or credulity to conceive and believe that antral infection could and does at times involve the first nerve and its environs in the orbital apex.

I am glad to be able to supplement the two cases referred to at the beginning of this paper with one of my own, seen in the fall of 1920.

Case.—Miss B. J., a country girl of 16 years, of good health and strong physique, consulted Dr. C. E. Crosby of Greenwood, S. C., in September, 1920, complaining of styes on the lids of both eyes. He found she had a high compound hyperopic astigmatism, which, upon correction, gave a best vision in the right eye of 20/40, and in the left eye, counting fingers at eight feet. (Note: It was the left eye in which vision was the worse, and this fact supplied an interesting feature of the case.) One week later the patient said she "felt something pop in the upper part of her left eye," and on returning to Dr. Crosby, he found V. R. with correction equaled 20/20, V. L. equaled light perception only. At this time blanching of the left papilla was noted and some enlargement of retinal vessels. Diseased tonsils were discovered and their removal advised.

About one week later the vision in the right eye began to fail, and various X-ray and laboratory examinations failed to reveal the cause of the trouble. In other words, a thorough preliminary study of the case had been made, when at this point I was called into consultation.

October 18. Examination discloses V. R. equals 20/200, with correction equals 20/100. V. L. equals light perception only. The field of vision of the right eye (campimeter) proved to be severely narrowed, having central vision and only five degrees in upper and nasal fields, with about twenty degrees in lower field and ten degrees on the temporal side. The vision of the left eye was too bad to chart the field. The ophthalmoscope showed normal eyegrounds, all media clear. There was noticeable tenderness on pressure over whole of right maxillary antrum, and radiographs showed a faint cloudiness of this sinus. Transillumination by palatoorbital route also revealed definite though not marked cloudiness in this area. Right middle turbinate cystic. No discharge in nares. Large chronic inflamed tonsils and a large adenoid were noted. The history of the case seemed to indicate that the left eye was amblyopic as a result of the high refractive error, and the probable diagnosis of right retrobulbar neuritis, previously made by Dr. Crosby, was concurred in.

October 19. The right middle turbinate was resected and the whole ethmoid line was opened. No pus or granulations were found. There appeared to be no sphenoid opening in the anterior wall, and entrance was made with a Grayson burr. The sphenoid was seen to be absolutely sound and normal. The nasoantral wall was then opened and the antrum irrigated, a large quantity of pus being evacuated.

October 21. V. R. (with correction) equaled 20/70.

October 22. Irrigated antrum.

October 28. V. R. (with correction) equaled 20/50.

On October 29 the tonsils and adenoid were removed. Antrum irrigations were continued every two or three days.

November 2. V. R. (with correction) equaled 20/40, very little pus remaining in antrum.

November 4. V. R. (with correction) equaled 20/20, pus gradually disappearing from antrum.

December 7. V. R. (with correction) equaled 20/15; antrum seems to be clean. The left eye remained amblyopic.

It is true the tonsils and adenoid were removed during the course of treatment, but inasmuch as the ocular condition had shown immediate and continuing marked improvement following the evacuation of the antral pus, steadily progressing during and after tonsil operation, it seems fair to conclude that the maxillary sinus was the real atrium of infection.

# LIX.

## MUST IT ALWAYS BE A TONSILLECTOMY?*

### By Henry L. Swain, M. D.,

#### New Haven.

In every community there is a large number of persons who stand in need of something done to their tonsils. In these days a conscientious operator, stressed a bit, perhaps by popular opinion, lay and professional, feels that he is negligent in his duty to his patients and colleagues if he does not always do a tonsillectomy when the tonsils are the objects of suspicion. If he is in "the swim," so much work in that line stares him in the face that he feels that he must

> "Count that day lost
> Whose low descending sun
> Views from his hand
> No tonsillectomy done."

If he is obsessed with the idea that there is no other way to meet the requirement of an honest opinion of "the tonsil menace" except to enucleate, then the above couplet is not merely slightly satirical, but really a confession of faith, his form of fanaticism.

Every once in a while one nowadays hears an echo of remonstrance, gradually swelling into a real murmur of protest, as was recently expressed to me by a wealthy lady, whose erudite medical consultant wished to give her the benefit of every doubt, and so four years ago they started to put her through a variety of "stunts" to find out the cause of her rapid heart action. The empirical surgery of the day was called into requisition—rank empiricism, she chose to term it—a perfectly just criticism of the spirit of the times. If somebody gets relief from having his tonsils out, then why not try it on everybody who has the same symptoms?

If an appendix made one person have certain troubles, why may it not do so to the next? Teeth, appendix and tonsils can

---

*Read before the Forty-third Congress of the American Laryngological Association, Atlantic City, June 1st, 1921.

and do make a lot of trouble.  Let's eliminate them, and so we often do without much evidence of a positive nature.  This removal of "organa non grata" occurs so frequently and safely in these days, thanks to the skill and wonderful technic of the surgeon and operating room personnel, that we become a bit callous and forget some sad facts.  For instance, in one year of my own small sphere of activity, I know of several cases of lung abscess and all that they sometimes mean, and one death, just to settle the question of a possible connection of the tonsils with focal disease.  And one in which an innocent and valued life was shortened when he consulted a stomach specialist, who advised that the teeth be removed. The dentist did some, the undertaker the rest.  And this happens now and then everywhere.  Is it right?

But to return to the lady.  First she had her teeth out, because so many seemed to possibly be the source of trouble. Failing here, they eliminated her tonsils, a most uncomfortable, distressing and weakening experience for a woman of sixty years plus.  As she somewhat naively put it, "and I am now consulting you for the sore throats which were surely to be relieved by this mild (?) procedure."

Failing again, they attacked a rectal condition as surely the cause of the trouble.  Incidentally they did some local good there, although the heart still went on its merry, rapid, tantalizing way.  Then they did something else—I seem to have forgotten that; failing there, she went to Johns Hopkins, where elaborate X-ray, laboratory tests and other things were done to her.  She was threatened with another flight of surgery, but went home to consult her family.  While seated in the train she fell into conversation with a very well known medical man, who himself had been the victim of much empiricism, and who was advised—equally empirically—to see if milk and milk products were not the cause of his trouble.  They were, and he advised her to try it, and in her case they also were. If she avoids milk and milk products, except a sparing amount of well made butter, she has no trouble, and this was three years ago.  Previously she had been for a long time on a purin free diet.  When she contemplates, with a degree of charity which is as rare as it is exalted, what a well meaning surgery has done to and for her, she sighs, and merely says she wishes she had her teeth back. I was only with the greatest struggle prevented from reciting to her what a wag friend of mine delights in flaunting before me from time to time,

"The lives of rich men oft remind us
Of the operations that are done
Not always because sore needed,
But because they have got the 'mon.' "

In what precedes in the history of the lady in question we see what always arouses the most violent protest in my soul—a lot of guesswork, with surgery as the potent factor. In her case, she still lives, but ought we not to labor without ceasing to arrive at more exact methods?

Are we forever to go on trying with knife and guillotine to undo the mischief done instead of ever pausing to consider the mischiefmaker? Shall we never have time when trying to put out the fire to consider ways and means to prevent its origin and spread? How much time do we, who are thus assembled to listen to discursive remarks like these, ever give to the question whence came these germs whose unwilling hosts we are? Do we sufficiently encourage by even the briefest review the patient work of the laboratory man who, if we would listen to him, could tell us much about the life history of many a germ? And might he not do more if we all went to him and helped him in his studies by giving them the human touch, so to speak? He knows now that you can take the most virulent germ and by passing it through certain cultures entirely change its characteristics. Acid-fast may become non-acid-fast and vice versa, pathogenic may become non-pathogenic and vice versa. Properly encouraged and stimulated by your broad minded personal interest, might we not learn the earlier sources of these germs and prevent them from becoming pathogenic? And would not that be the greater miracle? However, we must so far, as the result of our mental habits, ever devote our earnest endeavor to put out the fires already started, but in doing so should we not when the question, for instance, of focal disease in an adult is concerned, ask ourselves, Is there not some other way, sane and sure, to prove the tonsil either as guilty or of making it guiltless, or both, without putting all patients always through an ordeal of tonsillectomy?

For years in cases not seeming to require very radical measures I have been working with a method which has turned out to do exactly what is suggested in the last sentence. While debating whether my conclusions were worth chronicling before this distinguished body, I have learned that others, by other processes, have accomplished very brilliant results and proved to be true the very conclusions which I have drawn. The three methods which give class and distinction to this work are, first, that of Irvin Moore, in the use of caustic paste in the shrinking and actual removal of undesired and undesirable tonsil tissue, and very lately the splendid idea of using the potent X-ray, as has been done now by numerous operators, but which was first called to my attention by the articles of Wetherby, and by Murphy and his collaborators, who are working at the Rockefeller Institute in New York. And lastly, and by no means least, we are to hear from our beloved and distinguished fellow member, Dr. Delavan, of the use of radium for this same purpose. The action of the two last is similar, but in the case of the latter so simple in its application, as is evidenced by F. H. Williams,* when compared to the extensive apparatus necessary for properly controlled dosage by X-ray.

The object of all is to eliminate the tonsil as the troublemaker, and at this point might it not be profitable to consider the question, If a faucial tonsil is projecting more morbid matter into the system than any other part of the ring of Waldeyer, what part of the tonsil does it? What constitutes the difference between the tonsil which does and the one which does not? If any one not accustomed to giving the subject much consideration will take the pains to pass a probe with a right right angled curve into any of the usual crypts of the tonsils he will be wonderfully surprised at the ease and frequency with which the probe can be made to slip under and come out through another cryptal opening. This tract leading from one to the others is usually at the bottom of the crypt, often right up against the capsule, and communicates with the bottom of another crypt or crypts.

---

*Treatment of Hypertrophied Tonsils and Adenoids by Radium. A Preliminary Statement. Boston Medical and Surgical Journal, March 10, 1921.

Such fistulous tracts probably come because the deepest parts of such crypts have been dilated when evacuation was interfered with by the swelling at the outlet, and the simple pressure on the intervening walls caused absorption, or when particularly virulent matter may have caused active erosion to penetrate the wall and thus make a single cavity in the depth with two or more outlets. These caves or cisterns are full of fluid matter at all times and never sterile.

It is the crypts with recesses and tunnels beneath the surface which cannot cleanse or evacuate themselves which usually constitute the threat or menace of an evil tonsil, suspected of causing focal disease. At times the more fluid parts run out, leaving the cell detritus behind, and we have a. cheesy substance which, when large enough, comes out as a separate mass, quite odorous and often complained of by the patient. These masses, to my mind, are never as momentous as is the menace of the fluid stuff which preceded them. Unless actually diseased, as in tuberculosis, syphilis, cancer, which are not being considered at this point, the usual tissue intervening between the crypts of the tonsils, absorbs perhaps, but practically never in itself constitutes any threat. If it does, then every tonsil does, and there are many square inches of such threatening tissue all over the base of the tongue, tonsillar lingual folds (French), lateral columns, and posterior walls of the pharynx, and, worst of all, in the region of the vault of the pharynx, where the pharynx, tonsil, adenoid is or was. So I think it logical to say that the lymphoid tissue in itself, even when thickened and hypertrophied, constitutes no actual menace. It is only when it harbors exudate in pockets which cannot be easily cleansed and flushed out by overflowing secretions of the racemose glands, which always empty numerously and copiously, into the apex of the crypts, that it will make trouble.

Said retention areas unquestionably exist wherever the crypts or pockets communicate under the surface. Speaking as we are of faucial tonsils, we should bear in mind that they are completely delimited by a definite, firm capsule, which a wise and beneficent Providence created so that those of us who almost always operate with a snare tonsillectome, can do a neat, clean job and remove the mass in toto. This limiting membrane is so constituted as not of itself to absorb, and during operations is penetrated, when not too much traumatized, only by the lymphatics and blood vessels.

When these pockets constitute real abscess cavities, as they appear sometimes to do, then this very squeezing to which we subject them when the tonsil is removed entirely and solely by the cold snare, must force the fluids of these submerged pockets into the lymphatics and general circulation, and once in a while it produces a severe constitutional reaction immediately following the operation. Otherwise we see this matter ooze onto the surface of every tonsil as the snare cleaves it from its bed.

This very foul secretion gets down into the blood and secretions in the throat at the time of operating under general anesthetic, and so gets into the lungs, sometimes making the much dreaded lung abscess. This possibility of forcing poisonous matter into the system constitutes my reason for invariably adhering to the plan, never, if possible to avoid it, to operate while acute inflammation renders the germ activity of all the fluids in the tonsillar crypts more potent for evil. That others have operated in the midst of a quinsy or other acute seizures with impunity by no means leads me to go against my reason, and some very unhappy results have occurred.

On account of the above mentioned facts, even when intending later to do a tonsillectomy, I like to proceed just the other way. I like to slit up all the pockets, to get rid of all known and accessible retention areas, subdue all active inflammation and then see what happens. If favorable results occur, all well and good. If not, then the tonsil is freed from any adhesion it may have with the pillars of the palate, or plica, no pockets of matter are ready to burst into the lymphatics, as well as towards the surface, and the whole tonsillectomy takes place with ease. Particularly does this line of treatment commend itself in tonsillectomy on the adult when one expects to do the operation under local anesthesia, or better still, nerve blocking.

Since I have worked in this way, a number of interesting things have come to light. First, one can frequently establish by the simple slitting beyond all peradventure, that certain focal symptoms are due to the tonsil. Secondly, one can so successfully conduct the work as to free the tonsils of a definite menace, for example, the streptococcus viridans.

Three years ago I had a patient who for over a year had a bursitis in the shoulder, and later, after I saw her, a tender joint in the foot. She had been advised to have her tonsils removed, and the date was set. Her dentist steered her to me because she had definite pus pockets in the gums around two teeth. This pus and the crypts of her tonsils contained streptococcus viridans. She being nothing loth, even if the dentist was a bit doubtful, we went to work, he to cure the Rigg's disease, and I to eliminate the retention pockets in the tonsils. The gums and tonsils ultimately became free from streptococcus, the shoulder and the foot well, and the patient has remained well ever since. A vaccine was also used to eliminate all question.

The first treatment of the right tonsil gave immediate relief to her shoulder, and as that was before anything else was done and was greater than anything else that had previously been accomplished, there could be no question as to the relation of cause and effect. Also, vaccines alone have notoriously failed to cure these cases. I think here that the gums were first infected, and later the germs infected the whole mouth and tonsils. While I agree with you that "It takes more than one swallow to make a summer," a swallow is a swallow, "for a' that." And were this the only instance, it would be worth the chronicling, but I have observed this almost magical relief from thus simlpy cleaning up the crypts too many times to have any doubt in the matter, any more than when it has occurred afetr that exceedingly impressive and spectacular encounter known as tonsillectomy. That is—please observe—we have both established the connection between the tonsil and the distant disease, and cured the patient at the same time.

The recent article already referred to in the Journal of the American Medical Association for January 22, 1921, by Murphy and others working in the Rockefeller Institute, demonstrates that not only can tonsils be shrunk in size by X-ray treatment but the crypts become free from streptococci while being thus treated. My own observations are thus corroborated. Their explanation is the same as mine. The shrinking in size lessens the retention in the crypts and the germs die.

They deny any special or specific action of the X-ray on the germs themselves.

This is, however, no more, you will remember, than Dr. French has told us he can do by curettement, or, on another occasion, we were told by Dr. Delavan that he accomplished when he positively demonstrated that he could eliminate carriers of disease by his complete disinfection of the nose and throat by his method of using dichloramin-T.

As these cases of my own have multiplied and have been observed, some for perhaps ten years, I felt so sure of the matter that I was almost ready to say that I could in the above way always deetrmine when a tonsil is or is not a menace.

A young man, directly following a sore throat, had multiple joint symptoms and was permanently invalided. I was asked if I thought his tonsils caused the trouble. Matter could sometimes be squeezed out of them when adroitly and firmly compressed. I said I could not rule them out, but I would treat them so they would constitute no further menace. This I did, so thoroughly that I felt justified in saying that I thought I had them all right. Then he went away to a sanatorium noted the country over for its insistence that the tonsils be removed as a sine qua non.

They took cultures from the remnants of the tonsils, they introduced hyperdermic needles into the tissue of the tonsils and sucked the matter from the deepest accessible area, and in the end they told him "they guessed they would look elsewhere for the trouble." "Perhaps a gallstone operation or a diet would restore the youth," and they improved him by the latter.

Another instance where the tonsils must be removed. Nothing doing, unless patient complied. Slitting and clipping reduced the tonsils to a sterile mass, and the doctor was told that a-complete removal had been accomplished. He was more than pleased with the "beautiful tonsillectomy," and then, at my request, as an obstinate iritis was now coming on, with further search a pus tube was diagnosed and removed. Patient is in blooming health. (I forgot to add that previous to my efforts she had many of her teeth out, and with no effect.)

Case after case seems to prove that if there is no glandular —lymph node—swelling in the neck, which always means unquestionable absorption, and the crypts are cleansed and sterilized of any suspicious streptococci, one is justified in claiming such a tonsil is not producing evil of itself, the reason being that these treatments can be so thorough that nothing need be left which will harbor pathogenic germs.

Every once in a while one will score a failure, just as he often does when he does a major tonsillectomy, a very good argument, it seems to me, in favor of giving the weak and timid a chance to get by without the harder, dangerous work.

I have particularly in mind as I write these words, meeting on one occasion, socially, a very blooming specimen of comely womanhood. The young matron greeted me by name, and as I presume my face did not show the response she expected, she laughingly accused me of not recognizing her. Then suddenly I exclaimed, "Yes I do; but what has happened to you?" 'Nothing but your own handiwork.'" She had some two years previously been compelled by family happenings to discontinue work which I had been doing on the tonsils, and I remember at the time that I regretted very much indeed not being able to finish up. She had been very strongly urged to have the tonsils out (as you will see, most excellent advice), but dreaded it because she was so weak and miserable. She had a lot of various things the matter with her, and there was enough glandular infiltration in the neck to make one suspicious of the connection with the tonsils. I proceeded as usual to slit up the crypts, and punch out all undermined areas, finding in one tonsil a real abscess. Although her course of treatment was only about half done, she was compelled to stop, but had already begun to improve. In spite of ceasing all treatment, she gained twenty pounds, lost her pallor, recovered her initiative, and was the transformed individual ·I discovered. Some weary wag will say, "Think what might have happened if the whole of her tonsils had been taken out?" That you will have to conjecture. I was perfectly satisfied with what my efforts had accomplished. Certainly no perfect tonsillectomy, by whomsoever performed, had ever done more. Some tonsil tissue remains, but the pockets are removed.

I can surely and safely affirm that this has happened so often that I know I am not taking too grave chances, that I am never trifling with anybody's lease of life, or happiness, by suggesting it as an alternative to tonsillectomy. Please let me again state it is only an alternative, a substitute for tonsillectomy, when from choice or necessity you cannot do the more radical procedure.

The question of daring to do surely enters into a situation such as the one which follows. A lady of some forty-six summers had a most uncomfortable joint affection flitting around from one to the other, and apparently finally settled in the hands and feet, she being some of the time unable to use either, a predicament hard to beat. In addition the heart action was irregular. She lived out of town, and was brought to me a number of times to see if the simple slitting would settle the question whether the tonsils were the cause of the trouble. She was certainly the kind of a case where if one could avoid a serious operation it ought to be carefully shunned. The tonsils were small and yet what we would term suspicious, as indicated by French's transilluminator, a much too little used instrument. Nothing very serious in the way of accumulation of matter in the tonsils was found, but with no other difference in the daily routine from that of the previous months, she began to improve, and no one could possibly convince either her or me that the tonsil work did not cure her. Certainly she went through the two hardest winters of her life, the first, while undergoing treatment, where, owing to the circumstance of her husband being in Washington and her help all taken away by war activities, she did her own work at home and no end of Red Cross work, thus as you perceive having the use of her hands, feet, head and heart; and the previous winter she had been waited on hand and foot. The relief began after four treatments.

I cannot think of anything I have overlooked in making up my mind that these treatments have been the cause of the improvement noted, but in several instances, when, as a tonsillectomy itself often does, it seemed not to have relieved successive attacks of sore throat, a little more thorough treatment applied in the same way to the tonsils themselves did the trick.

Often when the work done to the tonsils seems to have failed a bit of attention to the nose and the much neglected nasopharynx will turn the tide from failure to success. Also we have been recently shown by Dr. French of Brooklyn that accessory tonsil tissue, with well developed, massive crypts, capsule—all the elements of a middle tonsil—often exists in the region between the faucial tonsil and the lingual tonsil. This tissue he was bold enough to attack with a Sluder tonsillectome, having by his transilluminator proved it guilty of criminal possibilities if not intent.

Such conspicuous masses have been removed, so well ensapculated, so cleanly and smoothly enucleated, that one could readily pass them off as enucleated tonsils. That these can make trouble by absorption and can be made innocuous by milder measures I have successfully demonstrated this last year, and am sure this explains why, when both faucial and lingual tonsils have had their fair meed of attention, I may have failed by having overlooked this region just mentioned. This region is often forgotten, when a real hard tonsillectomy has been done, and this brings us to a final suggestion before describing the simple methods I have used in the actual work.

It is not a terrible crime, in my judgment, to have omitted a bit of lymphoid tissue. I do not believe it can be helped. In any case, the best operators in the country (which means the world), do and always will occasionally leave tissue behind if for no other reason that it is too small to see, and it later grows to take the place of the removed tonsil. Small bits are, apparently, frequently overlooked, and especially when working with local anesthesia or nerve blocking, not merely because of the pain but because the gagging, bleeding, fainting or other bad actions on the patient's part make us desist from further trial to the patient. I repeat, I consider it no crime to have thus omitted some tissue. By simple slitting and punching out, and the galvanocautery shrinking, one can later care for this tissue with accuracy and safety, and thus oftentimes avoid an injury to the palate, base of the tongue and the deep tissues of the neck, which can all too easily ensue when rapidly, at the end of a bloody operation, attempting to gather into the snare whatever small fragments it will grasp. The clean cases which do not bleed are the very ones which seldom need any extra work.

Please understand that in most of what I have said in this paper I have in mind the adult who, having had symptoms of focal disease, is having the tonsils eliminated, but it may be adapted to tonsils of any age. To young children, and the young timorous adult the best work to my mind is always done under a general anesthetic, and naturally when one operates radically he always removes all adenoids from the nasopharynx.

And now a few words as to the method. After a thorough cocainization of the crypts, inside and out, with a finder one discovers all adhesions with the plica and pillars of the palate and the intercommunicating crypts of the tonsil, and generously and freely opens them up, the bulk of the work being done with Leland's or similarly constructed probe pointed knives. Then with simple punch forceps bite out or off any tissue which would seem to be liable to grow together again, which will often occur when left to drop together with nothing more than a simple slitting. The tissue between the crypts often has to be snipped out so as to make the cavities cup shaped or grooved, in which condition when healed over they offer no place for retention of matter deleterious to the system. The rule of the work is to do what is convenient and easy of accomplishment on one side and a week later the other, alternating back and forth until all pockets are abolished. If the tonsil is large and the crypts and the pockets deep, one has the choice of snipping and removing the superfluous hypertrophied tissue, or one can use the electric cautery or both. In my own case both are very frequently used. When the tonsils have been thus handled they are not very sore following the treatments, and one can accomplish just as much in the way of shrinking as he chooses, so much so that one can be greeted, as I stated in one of my cases, with the remark, "What a beautiful tonsillectomy." And it was; at least there was less tonsil visible than after many a socalled tonsillectomy. Furthermore, one rarely gets serious bleeding, accomplishes his purpose without upsetting the even tenor of a patient's life, even by a hair, does not distort or amputate any portion of the palate, and if his work—as we all so carefully do nowadays—is done cleanly, almost no infection can take place. One has rarely to work more than three times on the same tonsil—five weeks of little or no discomfort at all, as contrasted to a patient I have recently seen for the second time, who was two months getting over the effects of his tonsillectomy, forever has a distorted palate and troublesome adhesions at the base of the tongue, nearly died from hemorrhage, having to be transfused, all to prove that the tonsil did not cause his sore throats and colds. I have treated him several times since the operation, which I distinctly advised against as probably unnecessary. I say when one contrasts and, as I sincerely believe, can by the former way rule out the tonsil absolutely as the cause of the trouble, why not do it in that way, where appropriate occasion presents itself, especially when if, as before stated, the tonsil should continue to rebel, a later tonsillectomy has usually only been facilitated.

The genesis of an idea or plan of procedure sometimes is interesting, often revealing. Years ago when removing adenoids my custom was not always to rip out the tonsils, as is now done as the invariable routine. Then we did it only when the tonsils were large. When I did not remove the tonsils I formed the habit of always, with finger or instrument, liberating the tonsils from the plica and perhaps anterior pillar of the palate, and was much impressed at the shrinking in size which this produced. Later I started to do this to the tonsils in cases where I was about to shrink them by ignipuncture.

Probably I have shrunk more tonsils in this way (ignipuncture) than almost any other extant operator. Naturally, some of my cases have since been tonsillectomized, and heads wagged at the failure of the method, but no oftener than enucleation itself has failed. Since I have done the preliminary slitting, fewer case have relapsed, and by my present method I can more often completely get rid of all bad tissue than by any but the slickest kind of tonsillectomy. I have done all of this for so many years, with careful checking up, that I am venturing to offer this as a substitute in suitable cases for the much more serious, and in adults, painful enucleation. In presenting these thoughts for your attention there is nothing new or startling in them. It is only that they represent something definite and positive, and, after all, I beg of you, do not

for one moment think that I do not deem it wise to tonsillecto-
mize my own clientele, nor do I desire to cast any slightest
reflection on the splendid work of my fellow conspirators.
Quite on the contrary. I merely reaffirm that if one does not
care to do a tonsillectomy for any reason, I have in this manner accomplished just as spectacular, just as wonderful, just
as enduring results as I or any one else has by the major operation, and all that I have said is really in the way of emphasizing, not minimizing, the importance of tonsil work.

May I not, in closing, quote from the eminent English observer, Dr. Irvin Moore, who, as before mentioned, in the
British Journal of Laryngology, October, 1919, writes along
similar lines and suggests when, for any reason, it is deemed
unwise or contraindicated to perform tonsillectomy, the application of caustic paste to the tonsils? He shows some very
ingenious cup to hold the paste against the tonsil. The paste
is composed of equal parts of caustic soda and hydrated lime
mixed with a little alcohol. "This escharotic not only destroys
in successive layers a portion of the tissue by a process of dis-
integration, but also devitalizes a subjacent layer, causing it to
become soft and friable. During the devitalizing process the
tonsil undergoes general shrinkage. The largest tonsils have
been reduced to normal size, whilst in the case of diseased tonsils there has been no blocking up or sealing up of septic crypts
as may occur with the galvanocautery.

Though this treatment by this escharotic paste can never be
expected to take the place in suitable cases of complete removal of the tonsils by operative methods, yet experience has
undoubtedly shown that it is a highly effective and valuable
alternative in cases so frequently met where risks of excision
have to be seriously considered or where the radical operation
is refused."

Now that it has been so definitely proven what can be
accomplished by these various methods, and especially by
the X-ray and radium, the pendulum may be expected to swing
well over to the other side of the arc, but for myself, when
advising patients I shall continue to do as I have already done
in numerous instances. First get rid of the main pockets and
adhesions as outlined here. Then have them have their X-ray
or radium treatment. This should prove to be adequate to

produce all needed elimination when it is elected as the method of choice—but, as suggested by Stewart, New York Medical Journal, January 4, 1919—it can never be expected to exceed in efficiency a clean, perfect tonsillectomy, except as the effect of the rays shrinks other parts of the Waldeyer's ring of lymphoid tissue, as well as faucial tonsils. Also it will be reasonable to expect that certain shriveled up, sclerosed and atrophied tonsils, even when presenting some considerable mass, will not shrink or be altered by the radiant activity, by whatever means administered, as will others even smaller when composed of the usual type of tonsil tissue.

195 Church St.

## LX.

## PERCEPTION DEAFNESS.*

By Francis P. Emerson, M. D.,

Surgeon Massachusetts Charitable Eye and Ear Infirmary,
Boston.

Etiology.—In considering the etiology of nonsuppurative
deafness there have been two theories that have divided otologists into camps. First, those who have believed in the theory
of negative pressure, and second, those who have believed in
infection as the primary cause. Of late years the advocates
of infection have been the more numerous. Judging from
the treatment generally accepted by otologists, it is fair to
assume that the second class have believed that deafness was
the result of an acute infection that damaged the conduction
apparatus and then ceased to be a factor in the further progress of the disease. The deafness was then progressive by
further attacks of tubotympanic catarrh that was the result of
a fresh infection. The writer wishes to take issue with this
position and to claim that all deafness is the result of a deep
infection in the lymphoid tissue; that the infection then exists
as a chronic focus subject to acute exacerbations; that the
resulting deafness does not occur from the extension by continuity of the infected tissue through the tubes and middle ear
so much as it is the result of a toxin acting on the perception
apparatus. That is, we have perception deafness from the
beginning that can be demonstrated throughout its course until
the end result, which is either nerve degeneration or perception
deafness, without regard to the tissue reaction in the middle
ear.

If we carefully analyze our histories of chronic deafness
we find in one class that there was otalgia in childhood, and
in these cases we all attribute the middle ear involvement to
a blocked tube secondary to infection of the lymphoid tissue.

---

*Read before the meeting of the American Otological Society at
Atlantic City, N. J., June 1, 1921.

Until adolescence, lymphoid tissue predominates, and beyond this period it is replaced by fibrous and mucoid elements (Jonathan Wright). With the change in structure the lymphoid tissue undergoes retrograde changes, becomes less functionally active, and is therefore more susceptible to infection. The next class of cases follow the infectious diseases and are characterized by a more virulent infection which, in many instances, results in chronic foci subject to acute exacerbations throughout life. For a long time the foci may remain as a walled off local process. If the resistance of the host is lowered, the virulence of the organism increased or necrotic tissue changes destroy the leukocytic barrier, then we have systemic complications with remote tissue reactions. Why this takes place in a particular joint, endocardium or middle ear, we do not know, but once having occurred the tissue reactions go on in the same organs indefinitely. The history clearly shows that the patient was never deaf until a certain time when he had influenza, measles, diphtheria, etc. Following this infection the deafness was progressive, and especially noticeable after acute exacerbations. Cultures of the throat show some form of virulent bacteria present in the lymphoid tissue. The vessels of the anterior pillars are injected, the tonsillar crypts contains pus, mucopus or débris. The secretions of the pharynx are changed—i. e., there is a low grade pharyngitis, and the deep cervical glands under the angle of the jaw are enlarged. With acute exacerbations of the focal process these glands are sensitive on palpation. While there is a tendency for the infection to extend to the lining of the eustachian tube with gradual extension to the middle ear, the gross tissue changes are of only secondary importance to the accompanying infection in the problem of deafness. The conduction apparatus, when considered as a mechanism for the protection of the nicely adjusted perception apparatus, is wonderfully arranged. With the tissue reactions following a focal infection due to a particular strain of bacteria in all forms of deafness, there seem to be changes in the conduction apparatus analogous to those taking place in other organs which are damaged as the result of a similar focal infection. In all cases there is a functional disturbance of the perception apparatus, and in the organ of hearing, as in other organs, the restoration of function is dependent on whether its special nerve mechanism is irreparably damaged or only functionally disturbed.

Many otologists since the days of William Meyer have recognized the importance of removing infected adenoids and tonsils. Many now recognize that adults carry infection throughout life in the lymphoid tissue with an accompanying low grade pharyngitis. It is not only necessary to remove these foci in cases of deafness, but all contributory infective areas in the teeth, sinuses or chronic mastoids, that drain through the lymphatics. In a given individual the balance between the infective agent and the natural immunity of the patient due to the bactericidal and antitoxic powers of the tissues, blood plasma and cells, varies markedly. When this balance is once disturbed by any cause that lowers the resistance of the host and systemic infection results, the remotely involved tissue becomes sensitized, and less toxin than would affect a normal individual suffices to continue the morbid process. This makes the presence of innumerable saprophytes in the mouth and pharynx and such pathogenic bacteria as the streptococcus mucosus, viridans and hemolysins, the micrococcus catarrhalis, pneumococcus, bacillus mucosus capsulatus, grippe bacillus, diphtheria and pseudodiphtheria bacilli, which may be found in infected lymphoid tissue and the sinuses, particularly dangerous to the carrier. Furthermore, such infectious foci of the head may be associated with secondary infection of the lymph nodes of the neck and mediastinum. These patients have low resistance, and overwork is as potent in activating the focal process as is exposure. With these conditions present, and judging from the analogy of similar tissue reactions in other organs and from clinical experience, it is the conviction of the writer that deafness is the manifestation of a systemic infection resulting from a special strain of bacteria, the toxin acting on the perception apparatus from the beginning and continuing so to act until the terminal stage of marked perception deafness or nerve degeneration, the accompanying gross tissue changes in the conduction apparatus playing but a minor rôle in deafness.

Deafness may be defined as an impairment or loss of tone perception. Corti's cells are supposed to constitute the clearing house where sound waves are differentiated and conveyed through the auditory nerve to the cortical centers. It is at the acoustic centers that wave impulses are interpreted as sound. We say then that anything that obstructs or interferes with these wave impulses reaching the perception apparatus results in deafness. Is this the true explanation? Let us assume that deafness has its beginning in infection. Now, not all infections are followed by impairment of hearing. In some cases of infection in which tone perception is impaired there is a complete restoration of hearing with the clearing up of the infection. These are the few cases in which inflation and the usual methods of treatment of the eustachian tube are indicated. There are deep infections, however, that do not clear up with the subsidence of the acute symptoms, either from the virulence of the infection, the lowered resistance of the host or poor drainage, and these infections cause most of our cases of deafness. These chronic foci may, with acute exacerbations, for a long time give only local symptoms. When the local barrier is once broken down we have systemic manifestations and but mild local symptoms. When this occurs the remote tissue reactions seem to remain constant and are further damaged with recurring exacerbations of the focal process. If the systemic infection was followed by myalgia, infectious arthritis, endocarditis or nephritis, it continues to do damage to the tissues originally involved. A joint may be involved as the result of local chemical, circulatory or traumatic causes or, as Rosenow says, because of the selective action of a special strain of bacteria. If we consider for a moment the resulting pathology in a large joint it may help us to understand the changes in the organ of hearing which are accompanied by deafness. First, there are circulatory changes followed by the pouring out of leukocytes from the blood stream and increased secretion. This is followed by the formation of new connective tissue, pressure symptoms, the absorption of cartilage, etc., depending on how far the process may go. The nerve supply shows at once functional disturbance of its sensory fibers by pain, and of the motor nerves by changes in its terminal filaments. We may cause the inflammatory products about the joint to disappear, but restoration of function depends on the integrity of its special nerve supply. Now, in the organ of special sense we see somewhat similar phenomena. With a primary infection that was accompanied by deafness each recurring exacerbation adds to the damage of the tissues originally involved. That is, if the tissue reaction was in the mucous membrane, the fibrous tissue or bone, it continues as such, and we have a progressive chronic catarrhal, catarrhal adhesive otitis media or possibly otosclerosis as long as the chronic focus is active or secondary foci continue the same type of infection. We have the same circulatory changes, the same pouring out of leukocytes from the blood stream and increased secretion with the formation of fibrous bands or the deposition of new bone. The analogy goes further, for we have at once functional disturbance of the end organ—that is, the acoustic centers and tinnitus. This occurs at once in every form of deafness. We may cause absorption of the inflammatory products in the tube or middle ear, but the restoration of hearing depends on whether the perception apparatus can be functionally restored.

For these reasons the writer has been forced to the conclusion that deafness is from the first concerned with the perception and that the conduction apparatus plays but a minor rôle. We have studied minutely the obvious gross tissue changes but have lost sight of the fact that the perception apparatus is impaired from the first and continues to lose in function throughout the course of the disease. With the loss of tone perception there is tinnitus. Hearing tests show a loss in perception for the whispered voice and also a raising of the low limits. As the blocked tube becomes open the low limits become normal, but if the process is progressive the perception for the whispered voice diminishes. The low limits are not again raised until the function of the perception apparatus is markedly impaired. With the raising of the low limits we begin to have a negative Rinné, marked perception impairment of the upper limits, and, in some cases, involvement of the cochlear nerve. The impairment of the perception for the 2048C[4] fork is often noticed and frequently tone gaps. In fulminating cases where in a short time the membrana propria, malleus and incus are destroyed and yet the hearing remains good and may be nearly normal for years, the functional impairment of the hearing may be so pronounced that tone perception is wholly lost for the spoken voice. If this comes on suddenly as the result of the toxic action of a virulent infection that quickly clears up, the hearing returns because the perception apparatus is not permanently damaged. Metallic instruments are of no practical value in indicating the beginning of nerve deafness. When bone conduction is lowered for the $256C^1$ or $512C^2$ forks nerve deafness has been present for a long time. Deafness results from the action of a toxin on its special end organ in constitutional diseases and also in those chronic focal infections which so many patients have throughout life. The writer does not believe that alcohol and tobacco ever cause deafness with patients who have a normal throat. Both, however, cause a pharyngeal congestion and activate the focal process in the lymphoid tissue, increasing the absorption of the virus originally responsible for their impairment of tone perception. In the same way pyogenic foci in the teeth and sinuses are contributory causes of deafness because they drain into the lymphatics of the throat. Gross changes from hypertrophic processes in the conduction apparatus resulting in increased connective tissue, fibrous bands or bony ankylosis, are of minor importance in deafness compared with the perception impairment which started with the original infection and had progressed with the more obvious tissue changes. Skilled otologists have difficulty in interpreting certain hearing tests because they try to analyze them to conform to certain types of deafness. Diminished tone perception is indicated in the same way at the beginning of all middle ear diseases, whatever the tissue reaction from a given infection. After perception impairment is far advanced in those cases involving the cochlear we make a diagnosis of nerve deafness. It is obvious that this must have been going on for a long time before nerve deafness can be detected by a metallic instrument. Tinnitus, which is the only way that the acoustic apparatus can react to stimulation or irritation, is present with the first impairment of tone perception. As we know, clinically these subjective sounds are intermittent at first, but with the progress of the disease they become continuous and change in character.

While the gross changes in the eustachian tube and middle ear interfere with the transmission of sonorous vibrations these do not come within the range of ordinary conversation.

Furthermore, the low limits clear up with the unblocking of the tube in acute conditions, even though perception for the whispered voice may be further lost. What is of more importance in the loss of tone perception resulting from a blocked tube is pressure on the stapes. While this seems to effect only sonorous vibrations and therefore is of secondary importance in the treatment of deafness, it undoubtedly is important in causing tinnitus. Now, tinnitus is another term for labyrinthine stimulation or irritation, so that pressure and toxemia seem to be important factors in the gradual loss of tone perception.

We have, then, in every deep chronic infection of the lymphoid tissue which has been followed by deafness, two ways in which its progress is manifest. First, by gross changes affecting the conduction apparatus but playing but a minor rôle in the loss of tone perception. Second, by the action of a toxin on the end organ impairing the function of the acoustic centers or, in a less number of cases, manifestly involving the cochlear nerve.

It would seem that the profound loss of tone perception in nerve deafness was due to changes in the terminal filaments of the auditory nerve rather than to changes in the cortical centers themselves. Cases of advanced progressive deafness often show a bilateral hearing test that does not vary throughout the scale. This could be explained on the ground that it is probable that the auditory fibers from each ear end partly on the same side and partly or mainly on the opposite side of the cerebrum (Howell).

Treatment.—While the writer has treated deafness on the above outline of its etiology for ten years, emphasizing the importance of infection, and failing to get results from inflation except in recent cases, the interpretation of the way in which deafness resulted has only been reached in the last few years. Obviously we remove the primary focus and all contributory foci tending to reinfect the lymphoid tissue. This makes it necessary to do radical surgery and not merely convert a chronic antrum into a latent one, or improve a pharyngitis without removing the cause above or below. Many latent antra with atrophic changes and without a pyogenic focus will still reinfect the lymphoid tissue and eustachian tube. Gross changes in the nares have not been considered as affecting deafness unless infection was present. Submerged tonsils have been removed in adults in all ages up to seventy years whenever there was a change in the secretions of the pharynx or enlarged cervical glands under the angle of the jaw. Enlarged cervical glands following an acute infection that do not subside within a few weeks presuppose that the focal infection has not cleared up. Metabolic changes have not been considered as coming primarily from the intestinal tract but as having originated from the upper respiratory tract, as pointed out by Billings. With the removal of infection general measures are instituted to overcome the effects of a long continued toxic process. While the iodids, pilocarpin, strychnin, electricity, auditory reeducation, etc., are indicated, it is also necessary to improve the general condition. The loss of tone perception through depressed nerve states seem best treated on broad general lines. Many cases of deafness that have existed over a long term of years will improve markedly. In others the duration may be short and yet the treatment is hopeless. At present there seems to be no way of determining how far the perception apparatus is damaged or, in case of nerve involvement, whether degeneration is far advanced. Progressive or perception deafness has a most hopeful outlook if treated early and energetically when the cochlear is not involved. All patients who have had a deep infection as a result of measles, scarlet fever, diphtheria or flu should have an interval tonsil and adenoid operation as a routine procedure without regard to age. Every patient who has a blocked tube and tinnitus accompanying a socalled acute infection should be carefully examined for a definite focus which should be treated surgically before secondary foci result. After this the follow up treatment should be local and general. All cases of long standing focal infections are about 20 per cent anemic and many have cardiac and renal conditions needing general medical care. The usual methods of treatment are all indicated under special conditions. In chronic progressive deafness, until the low limits are raised, however, the two important indications are the prevention of tubotympanic catarrh by the removal of chronic streptococcal foci and the recognition that impairment of tone perception is constantly going on.

### INFECTED ADENOIDS.

Case 1.—S. S., 8 years, blocked tubes, pressure on stapes; Dec. 27, 1919. Past history: T. and A. operation three years ago. Two months ago following measles commenced to be deaf. Tinnitus marked in both ears. Examination: Epipharynx blocked by infected lymphoid tissue. Sinuses: Ethmoids transilluminate poorly. Antra clear. A. D.: M. T., ground glass appearance; indrawn. L. R. broken. A. S.: Same. Hearing test:

| R | | L |
|---|---|---|
| 2/25 | W.V. | 2/25 |
| 14 | R ac | 16 |
| 6 | 256C¹bc | 6 |
| | Weber | |
| 64 | L.L. | 64 |

Diagnosis: Blocked tubes. Pressure on stapes.

Dec. 31, 1919. Adenoid removed under gas.

Oct. 28, 1920:

| R | | L |
|---|---|---|
| 25/25 | W.V. | 25/25 |
| 32 | L.L. | 64 |

P. S.—Tinnitus persisted several months and gradually disappeared as the infection cleared up.

Treat.: No inflation. Epipharynx treated after adenectomy until infection cleared up.

Key to hearing test: W. V., whispered voice; Cons., conversation; R., Rinné ac—bc; W., Weber; U. L., upper limit (Galton whistle) ; L. L., lower limit (Dench fork).

Case 2.—I. B., 12½ years, B. O. M. C. C., May 24, 1919. Past history: Measles, 9 years. Chickenpox, 9 years. Whooping cough, 7 years. Has been growing slightly deaf, especially following colds. Several attacks of tonsillitis. Throat does not feel right in the a. m. Examination: B. cryptic tonsillar disease. Septum, high deviation to left. Turbinates, posterior ends of inferior turbinates markedly enlarged, especially on the left side. Hearing test—

| R | | L |
|---|---|---|
| 20/25 | W.V. | 25/25 |
| 37 | R ac | 45 |
| 8 | 256C¹ bc | 10 |
| | + < Weber | |
| 32 | L.L. | 32 |

July 1, 1919. Tonsillectomy; ether.

| R | | | L |
|---|---|---|---|
| 15/25 | | W.V. | 20/25 |
| 20 | R | ac | 19 |
| — | | — | — |
| 10 | 256C¹ | bc | 9 |
| | | . + < Weber | |
| 32 | | L.L. | 64 |

March 1, 1920. Attack of mumps. Following this attack hearing less acute.

July 1, 1920. Went to New Hampshire camp for the summer.

Sept. 10, 1920. Epipharyngitis. Marked swelling of posterior ends of inferior turbinates.

| R | | | L |
|---|---|---|---|
| 15/25 | | W.V. | 20/25 |
| 18 | R | ac | 18 |
| — | | — | — |
| 8 | 256C¹ | bc | 8 |
| — | | + < Weber | — |
| 32 | | L.L. | 32 |

Treatment: No inflation. Treatment of infection. Sprays, normal salt solution and 20 per cent argyrol.

October 26, 1920—

| R | | L |
|---|---|---|
| 23/25 | W.V. | 23/25 |
| 32 | L.L. | 32 |

November 16, 1920—

| R | | L |
|---|---|---|
| 25/25 | W.V. | 25/25 |
| 32 | L.L. | 32 |

Note.—Although this patient was out of doors all summer her ears did not clear up, owing to a persistent epipharyngitis with blocking of the left posterior naris. As soon as the infection was removed the hearing returned to normal.

Case 3.—H. L., 51 years, January 11, 1916, single, American. Past history: Measles, chickenpox, scarlet fever (mild). History of abscesses in childhood. Last three or four years history of swelling in one ear and then the other. No loss of hearing patient thinks. Head colds frequent. Occipital headaches with tenderness of the scalp at times. Rheumatism since April in knees and fingers. Is being treated for rheumatic iritis. Tinnitus continues since August in both ears. General health always poor. History of abscess in intestine and of mucous colitis. Examination: Septum to left with a large posterior basal spur. Turbinates, hypertrophic changes. Do not shrink under cocain. Sinuses, negative. Teeth, negative. Tonsils, R. shows cheesy débris.. Hearing test:

| R | | | L |
|---|---|---|---|
| 6/25 | | W.V. | 12/25 |
| 19 | R | ac | 19 |
| — | | — | |
| 8 | 256C¹ | bc | 8 |
| | | + < Weber | |
| 32 | | L.L. | 32 |
| N | | U.L. | N |

Treatment: Tonsillectomy. Submucous resection. Treatment of infection. Teeth looked after.

April 5, 1917. Gall bladder operation.
Dec. 29, 1919. Otalgia dentalis.
Mar. 28, 1921. No rheumatism or iritis since tonsillectomy.

| R | | | | | L |
|---|---|---|---|---|---|
| 25/25 | | R | ac | | 25/25 |
| Not taken | { | | — | } | Not taken |
| | | | bc | | |
| — | | | Weber | | — |
| 32 | | | L.L. | | 32 |

Note.—See history. Infection in teeth and throat followed by headache. Rheumatism, rheumatic iritis, infection of gall bladder. Deafness, cured by removing the chronic foci without inflation.

Case 4.—E. G., 8 years, Nov. 16, 1920, only child, mother and father living, L. antrum, deafness. Past history: Measles at 3 years with aural discharge. T. and A. operation one year ago. Oct. 8, second T. and A. operation. Deafness worse than before. No discharge, but ear feels sore to touch. Otalgia 3 days ago. Head cold. Pus in left naris. X-ray shows left antrum. Wassermann negative. A. D.: Drum dull and retracted with thickening and healed perforation, anteriorly and below. Ear dry. A. S.: Same as A. D. except for more retraction. Hearing test—

| R | | | L |
|---|---|---|---|
| 2/25 | | W.V. | 2/25 |
| 20 | R | ac | 30 |
| — | | — | — |
| 28 | 256C¹ | bc | 24 |
| | | Weber $>$ $+$ | |
| 64 | | L.L. | 32 |

Dec. 2, 1920. Left radical antrum operation.

May 27, 1921. Light reflex in right ear slightly broken. Drum retracted. Old scar anteriorly. Left ear, drum retracted. Fairly good light reflex. Slight thickening.

May 20, 1921—

| R | | | L |
|---|---|---|---|
| 3/25 | | W.V. | 20/25 |
| 17 | R | ac | 30 |
| — | | — | — |
| 28 | 256C¹ | bc | 24 |
| | | Weber $>$ $+$ | |
| N | | U.L. | N |
| 64 | | L.L. | 32 |

Note.—No inflation. Infection cleared up and best ear improved from two to twenty feet for whispered voice.

Case 5.—R. Eff, O. M. S. L. O. M. S. Ch. Cum. Grans. J. C., 25 years, barber, married. May 25, 1921. Past history: History of discharge from left ear as a child, then for short and infrequent periods until two years ago. While at Camp Devens in 1919 had double pneumonia and the discharge has been at shorter intervals. No pain, no vertigo or headaches. Colds frequent. Chronic catarrh. History of diseases of childhood uncertain. Examination: B. cryptic tonsillar disease. Large central adenoid. Transillumination not so clear on the left side. M. M. of nares injected. Large gland under angle of left jaw.

Aural examination: Right ear. Healed horseshoe perforation involving greater part of membrana propria. Short process visible. Long process foreshortened and apparently tied down to the promontory. Large calcarious deposits in the scar tissue anterior to the long process over the region of the tube and in the posterior superior quadrant. Malleus does not move under otoscope. L. ear. Posterior superior half of drum grayish in color and thickened. Short process indistinct. Anterior and inferior half of drum filled with pale granulation tissue. Discharge moderate. Almost entire anterior half of drum replaced by granulation tissue. Hearing test:

| R | | | L |
|---|---|---|---|
| 25/25 | | W.V. | 25/25 |
| 16 | R | ac | 16 |
| — | | | — |
| 8 | 256C¹ | bc | 9 |
| — | | Weber | — |
| N | | U.L. | N |
| 32 | | L.L. | 32 |

Note.—Here was a history dating back to childhood of intermittent discharge, in which the conduction apparatus was seriously involved and yet there is normal hearing.

### CONCLUSIONS.

1. Every case of loss of tone perception seems to result from the action of the toxin of a chronic pyogenic focus on the end organ.

2. The toxin is probably due to a special strain of bacteria with a selective action on the organ of hearing.

3. The gross tissue changes seem analogous to those taking place in other organs, as the result of a focal infection, the return of function in each case depending on the integrity of its special nerve mechanism—either the acoustic centers or cochlear nerve.

4. Diminished tone perception seems to start with the onset of the deafness and is more important than the changes in the conduction apparatus. The early raising of the low limits due to the blocked tube clears up as the tube opens. Following this the tube is more open on the side of the deaf ear as atrophy succeeds the hypertrophic salpingitis.

5. When the 256C¹ or 512C² fork shows lowered bone conduction nerve deafness is already far advanced.

6. The end result in chronic progressive deafness is marked perception impairment or nerve degeneration.

7. No hearing test is characteristic of any particular form of middle ear disease.

8. Gross tissue changes in the middle ear follow the original type of infection and do not change.

9. Alcohol and tobacco seem to cause eighth nerve deafness by causing a pharyngeal congestion with increased absorption of the toxin from the chronic focus.

10. Patients treated early have every right to expect recovery if the primary focus is removed and the deafness is confined to a functional disturbance of the acoustic centers.

# LXI.

## THE PROGNOSIS OF THE TUBERCULOUS LARYNX.*

By John B. Gregg, A. B., M. S., M. D.,

Sioux Falls, S. D.

The subject of tuberculosis of the larynx is of vital importance to the laryngologist, due to its common occurrence, to the great desire to alleviate the conditions imposed by the disease, and to its influence on the prognosis of pulmonary tuberculosis, which is always rendered more grave by the presence of a laryngeal involvement. The relative frequency of the laryngeal complication of pulmonary tuberculosis necessitates very careful study and well directed effort, in order that the system may be relieved of this additional lesion and thereby enabled to better carry on its battles with the main source of infection in the lungs or elsewhere.

In all cases of pulmonary tuberculosis early and frequently repeated laryngeal examinations should be made by a skilled laryngologist. This results in the discovery of many cases of incipient laryngeal involvement at a time when proper treatment will be most beneficial to the larynx. Not infrequently we have patients come to us because of the laryngeal condition who have had no symptoms indicating a pulmonary lesion. In but a few cases the diagnosis of tuberculosis of the larynx is made before any demonstrable lesion elsewhere can be found. One such patient had a definite tuberculous larynx, demonstrated by microscopic examination of a section, two years before the internist could find involvement elsewhere.

Although laryngeal tuberculosis is most frequently coexistent with or complicates pulmonary tuberculosis, yet Orth, Demme, Frankel, Progebinisky, Manasse and Steiner have each reported one case of primary tuberculosis where postmortem findings have substantiated the clinical diagnosis. Per-

---

*Candidate's thesis for the American Laryngological, Rhinological and Otological Society.

sonally I have never seen a case of verified primary tuberculosis of the larynx.

The purpose of this article will be to give the results of the observations of the writer in his work at the Iowa State Sanatorium for the Treatment of Tuberculosis. The endeavor will be made to show how many different factors enter into the prognosis of the tuberculous larynx. At the outset I wish to state that all these cases were in Doctor Dean's service, with whom the writer was so fortunate as to be associated.

The report consists of 122 cases of laryngeal tuberculosis found in 610 cases of pulmonary tuberculosis at the sanatorium during the year 1919-1920. Criticism may be offered that the length of observation has been too short, but the writer's problem has been more to determine what factors enter into the consideration of the laryngeal prognosis. These cases were examined by the writer at regular weekly intervals, and an accurate record made of the condition found at each examination. At every examination the internist in charge of the case was present, in order to correlate the findings of the internist and laryngologist to the best interests of the patient. We have always felt that the decision as to whether any operation shall or shall not be done should be left to the internist, who is thoroughly conversant with every phase of the patient's condition, and that there should be the closest cooperation at all times. The larynx of every case which enters the sanatorium is examined, and even if found negative is reexamined at frequent intervals, for often a patient with a negative larynx on entrance will develop tuberculous laryngitis within six weeks.

Frequency of Laryngeal Tuberculosis.—Laryngeal involvement exists in a varying percentage of the cases of pulmonary tuberculosis, the exact percentage being in a measure determined by the accuracy and persistency of examinations. Osler[1] gives 18 to 30 per cent, while Willigk estimates the percentage at 13. Schroeder[2] estimates that 20 per cent of all cases of chronic pulmonary tuberculosis have laryngeal complications. Sir St. Clair Thomson in a report[3] based on the study of 693 sanatorium cases found 25.6 per cent with laryngeal complication, while Fetterolf[10] in a clinical postmortem study of 100 cases dying of pulmonary tuberculosis found the larynx grossly involved in 83 per cent.

From the statistics of the Iowa Sanatorium we find that in 1737 cases of pulmonary tuberculosis there were 474 cases of laryngeal involvement, or in 27 per cent of the total number of cases. The 1737 pulmonary cases may be divided into 322 incipient cases, 722 moderately advanced cases and 693 far advanced cases. In the 322 incipient cases laryngeal tuberculosis was found in 31, or in 10 per cent. In the 722 moderately advanced cases laryngeal tuberculosis was found in 151, or in 21 per cent of the cases. In 693 far advanced pulmonary cases laryngeal involvement was found in 292, or in 42 per cent of cases.

Among 379 deaths at the sanatorium in the last five years, laryngeal tuberculosis was present in 165, or in 43 per cent of cases. The series of cases especially studied consists of 122 cases of laryngeal tuberculosis, or 20 per cent found in 610 pulmonary cases.

Sex.—Among the 122 cases of laryngeal tuberculosis females were affected in 57 per cent and males in 43 per cent of the cases. These figures show a discrepancy inasmuch as women preponderate at the institution. Taking the larger number of cases of laryngeal tuberculosis, the sex ratio is about equal.

Age.—Among the 122 cases studied 9 per cent, or 11 cases, were between the ages of 10 and 20. Thirty-eight per cent, or 46 cases, were between 21 and 30; 33 per cent, or 46 cases between 31 and 40; 15 per cent, or 18 cases between 41 and 50, and 5 per cent, or 6 cases, were between the ages of 51 and 60 years.

The above figures show the greatest number of cases (71 per cent) between the ages of 20 and 40; next come the cases between 40 and 50 years (15 per cent), then the cases occurring in youth (9 per cent), and lastly (5 per cent) the cases occurring between the age of 50 and 60 years. Wide extremes in the age may occasionally be encountered, varying from 12 months to 76 years. The percentage for young adults and children in this report may be small, due to the fact that there is but limited accommodation for children at this institution.

Among the eleven cases between the ages of 10 to 20 years,

the larynx remained unimproved in 6 (55 per cent) and improved in 5 (45 per cent).

In the 46 cases between 21 and 30 years of age, the larynx
remained unimproved in 25 (54 per cent), improved in 11
(24 per cent), and arrested in 10 (22 per cent).

Of the 41 cases between 31 and 40 years of age the larynx
remained unimproved in 21 (31 per cent), improved in 12
(29 per cent) and arrested in 8 (20 per cent).

Considering the 18 cases between the ages of 41 and 50
years of age, the larynx was unimproved in 13 (72 per cent),
improved in 1 (6 per cent) and arrested in 4 (22 per cent.).

Among the six cases between 51 and 60 years of age the
larynx remained unimproved in three (50 per cent), improved
in one (17 per cent), and arrested in two (33 per cent).

Of interest from the above data is the information that the
percentage of unimproved larynges is higher between the ages
of 41 and 50 years (72 per cent) than it is for all other ages
(50 to 55 per cent).

Tubercle Bacilli.—Tubercle bacilli were found in the sputum
in 87 per cent of the 122 cases.

Pulmonary hemorrhage occurred in 44 cases or in 36 per
cent of all laryngeal cases. It has not been uncommon for
the patient to date his laryngeal trouble from the time of the
hemorrhage.

Definitions.—Before taking up the subject further it will
be necessary to define terms to be employed.

Incipient: The incipient case is one in which there are slight
or no constitutional symptoms (including especially gastric
or intestinal disturbance or rapid loss of weight), slight or
no elevation of temperature or acceleration of pulse; slight
infiltration limited to the apex of one or both lungs or a small
part of one lobe; no tuberculous complications.

Moderately advanced cases (M. A.), shows no marked impairment of function, either local or constitutional; marked
infiltration more extensive than under incipient, with little or
no evidence of cavity formation, no serious tuberculous complications.

The far advanced cases (F. A.) show marked impairment
of function, local and constitutional; extensive localized infiltration or consolidation in one or more lobes, or disseminated

areas of cavity formation, or serious tuberculous complications.

Pulmonary classification on discharge:

Arrested (a.), all constitutional symptoms and expectoration with bacilli absent for a period of six months, the physical signs those of a healed lesion.

Apparently arrested (aa.), all constitutional symptoms and expectoration with bacilli absent for a period of three months, the physical signs to be those of a healed lesion.

Quiescent (Quies.) Absence of all constitutional symptoms; expectoration and bacilli may or may not be present; physical signs stationary or retrogressive; the foregoing conditions existing for at least three months.

Improved (Imp.) : Constitutional symptoms lessened or entirely absent; physical signs improved or unchanged; cough and expectoration with bacilli usually present.

Unimproved (Unimp.) : All essential symptoms and signs unabated or increased.

Laryngeal condition on discharge:

Arrested (a.) : Laryngeal condition healed for six months or more.

Improved (Imp.) : Laryngeal condition lessened markedly or a healed larynx of less than six months' duration.

Unimproved (Unimp.) : Laryngeal condition unabated or increased in severity.

Pulmonary Condition on Admission.—In 122 cases of laryngeal tuberculosis the pulmonary involvement was incipient in 3, moderately advanced in 31, and far advanced in 88 cases.

A tabulated report of the pulmonary and laryngeal results is here given.

| Incipient Cases: | Cases | Per Cent |
|---|---|---|
| Lungs improved with larynx improved | 1 | 33.3 |
| Lungs improved with larynx arrested | 1 | 33.3 |
| Lungs arrested with larynx arrested | 1 | 33.3 |
| Moderately advanced cases: | | |
| Death with larynx unimproved | 3 | 10 |
| Lungs unimproved with larynx unimproved | 3 | 10 |
| Lungs unimproved with larynx improved | 7 | 22 |
| Lungs improved with larynx unimproved | 4 | 13 |
| Lungs improved with larynx improved | 6 | 20 |
| Lungs quiescent with larynx unimproved | 0 | 0 |

|                                              | Cases | Per Copy |
|----------------------------------------------|-------|----------|
| Lungs quiescent with larynx improved         | 2     | 6        |
| Lungs quiescent with larynx arrested         | 5     | 16       |
| Total                                        | 31    |          |

Thus in the moderately advanced cases the larynx process was arrested in 16 per cent, improved in 48 per cent and un-improved in 33 per cent of cases. It is of interest to note that the larynx improved while the lungs remained unimproved in seven (22 per cent) of the cases, also that the larynx re-mained unimproved while the lungs improved in four (13 per cent) of cases.

In the moderately advanced cases the pulmonary condition became quiescent in 7 (22 per cent), improved in 10 (32 per cent), unimproved in 10 (32 per cent), and death occurred in 3 (10 per cent).

| Far advanced cases:                               | Cases | Per Cent |
|---------------------------------------------------|-------|----------|
| Death with larynx unimproved                      | 31    | 35       |
| Death with larynx improved                        | 1     | 1        |
| Lungs unimproved with larynx unimproved           | 24    | 27       |
| Lungs unimproved with larynx improved             | 5     | 6        |
| Lungs improved with larynx unimproved             | 2     | 2        |
| Lungs improved with larynx improved               | 8     | 9        |
| Lungs improved with larynx arrested               | 5     | 6        |
| Lungs quiescent with larynx improved              | 2     | 2        |
| Lungs quiescent with larynx arrested              | 6     | 7        |
| Lungs apparently arrested with larynx arrested    | 2     | 2        |
| Lungs arrested with larynx arrested               | 2     | 2        |
| Total                                             | 88    |          |

In the far advanced cases the larynx process was arrested in 18 per cent, improved in 17 per cent and unimproved in 64 per cent of cases. The larynx improved while the lungs remained unimproved in five cases (6 per cent) and the larynx remained unimproved while the lungs improved in two cases (2 per cent).

The pulmonary condition in the far advanced cases was arrested in 2 (2 per cent), apparently arrested in 2 (2 per cent), became quiescent in 8 (9 per cent), improved in 15

(17 per cent), unimproved in 29 (33 per cent), and death occurrde in 32 cases (36 per cent).

Our number of incipient cases is too small to be of any value, but we learn from comparison of the laryngeal results in the moderately advanced and far advanced cases that our prospects of improving the larynx are twice as good in the moderately advanced cases (64 per cent) as in the far advanced cases (35 per cent). In other words, the laryngeal prognosis varies directly with the extent of pulmonary involvement.

Consulting the records of 1737 cases of pulmonary tuberculosis whose histories can be traced at the sanatorium, we find laryngeal involvement in 474 cases, or in 27 per cent of the total number. In 322 incipient cases lrayngeal tuberculosis was found in 31, or in 10 per cent of cases. Considering these 31 incipient pulmonary cases with laryngeal involvement, 8, or 25 per cent, died; 2, or 6 per cent, were discharged unimproved, 2 or 6 per cent as improved, 12 or 38 per cent as quiescent, 7 or 22 per cent as apparently arrested, and 1 or 3 per cent as arrested; this rating being from the pulmonary and general condition.

In the 291 cases of incipient pulmonary tuberculosis without laryngeal involvement, 23 or 8 per cent died, 29 or 10 per cent were discharged with lungs unimproved, 71 or 24 per cent as improved, 63 or 22 per cent as quiescent, 85 or 29 per cent as apparently arrested, and 20 or 7 per cent as arrested.

In 722 moderately advanced cases laryngeal tuberculosis occurred in 151 or 21 per cent of cases. Of these 151 cases of moderately advanced tuberculosis with laryngeal involvement 25 or 17 per cent died, 55 or 36 per cent were discharged with lungs unimproved, 28 or 18 per cent as improved, 27 or 18 per cent as quiescent, 13 or 9 per cent as apparently arrested and 3 or 2 per cent as arrested.

In the 571 cases of moderately advanced pulmonary tuberculosis without laryngeal involvement, 57 or 10 per cent died, 116 or 20 per cent were discharged with lungs unimproved, 143 or 25 per cent as improved, 146 or 25 per cent as quiescent, 89 or 16 per cent as apparently arrested and 20 or 4 per cent as arrested.

In 693 far advanced pulmonary cases, laryngeal tuberculosis was found in 292 or in 42 per cent of cases. Of these 292 cases, 132 or 45 per cent died, 82 or 28 per cent were discharged with lungs improved, 62 or 21 per cent as improved, 13 or 5 per cent as quiescent, 1 or 3 per cent as apparently arrested, and 2 or 6 per cent as arrested. Of the 401 cases of far advanced pulmonary tuberculosis without laryngeal involvement 132 or 33 per cent died, 111 or 28 per cent were discharged with lungs unimproved, 54 or 13 per cent as improved, 77 or 19 per cent as quiescent, 24 or 6 per cent as apparently arrested and 3 or 1 per cent as arrested.

Of paramount interest in the above tabulations is the fact that the percentage of deaths in incipient tuberculosis with laryngeal involvement is three times as great (25 per cent) as is found in the pulmonary involvement alone (8 per cent). In moderately advanced tuberculosis with laryngeal involvement the mortality was 17 per cent, while in cases without the laryngeal complication the mortality was but 10 per cent.

In far advanced pulmonary tuberculosis with the laryngeal complication the mortality was 45 per cent, while in the same class of cases without the complication the mortality was 33 per cent.

General Condition.—By the general condition, we mean the evident ability or lack of ability of the individual to fight against the infection; with or without the tendency toward tissue repair as shown by the previous history. The patient's general condition is classified as favorable, guardedly favorable or unfavorable by the internist at the time of his admission to the sanatorium.

In our series of cases the general condition was favorable in 8, guardedly favorable in 15, and unfavorable in 99 cases. The laryngeal condition was arrested in 75 per cent of the favorable cases, and improved in the remaining 25 per cent. The laryngeal condition was arrested in 27 per cent, improved in 27 per cent and unimproved in 47 per cent of the guardedly favorable cases.

Among the 99 unfavorable cases, the laryngeal condition was arrested in 13 per cent, improved in 25 per cent and unimproved in 62 per cent of the cases.

Thus we realize that our laryngeal prognosis varies directly with a favorable or unfavorable general condition.

Digestion.—Whether of not digestion is impaired is to be considered, inasmuch as impaired digestion makes its results manifest on the system as a whole, with the laryngeal improvement or lack of improvement directly affected.

In our series of cases digestion was impaired in 34 and unimpaired in 88 cases. Of those in which digestion was impaired, the larynx process was arrested in 3 per cent, improved in 24 per cent and unimproved in 73 per cent of cases. Among those where digestion was unimpaired the larynx was arrested in 25 per cent, improved in 28 per cent and unimproved in 47 per cent of cases.

To show the pulmonary results: among those with impaired digestion 3 per cent were discharged as arrested, 3 per cent as quiescent, 15 per cent as improved, 26 per cent as unimproved, and 53 per cent died.

Among those with unimpaired digestion 4 per cent were discharged as arrested, 16 per cent as quiescent, 28 per cent as improved, 34 per cent as unimproved and 18 per cent died.

The presence of a tuberculosis enteritis or colitis is of marked importance when occurring in a case of pulmonary tuberculosis with laryngeal involvement. In this series of 122 cases there were 19 such cases, of which 14 died and 4 remained unimproved as regards general condition. The larynx was arrested in 1 case, improved in 2 cases and remained unimproved in 16 cases, or 84 per cent.

In a study of the general prognostic significance of laryngeal and intestinal tuberculosis occurring together with a pulmonary affair, our records for the last few years have been used. In a series of 239 cases of pulmonary and laryngeal tuberculosis without intestinal involvement there has been death in 72 or in 30 per cent of cases. In a series of 95 cases of pulmonary and intestinal tuberculosis without laryngeal involvement there was death in 36 or 38 per cent of cases. In a series of 49 cases of combined pulmonary laryngeal and intestinal tuberculosis death occurred in 30 or in 61 per cent of cases.

In brief, the more extensive the infection, the higher the

mortality and the poorer the prospect for improvement in the laryngeal condition.

Pregnancy.—Pregnancy has long been considered a dangerous complication of tuberculosis. Godskesen of Copenhagen has laid special emphasis on this condition as a complication of laryngeal tuberculosis. He reports 55 cases, 24 from literature, 31 from his own experience. Of his 31 cases, 26 developed the condition of the larynx during pregnancy. The larynx in only five of the cases was materially improved by active treatment.

In this series of cases pregnancy was present in two cases. The larynx rapidly became worse and death resulted in each case. In our six other cases of pregnancy complicating laryngeal tuberculosis, two died and four are alive. Thus in the total of eight cases, death resulted in 50 per cent of cases. The larynx was improved in only two cases after delivery.

Symptoms.—Laryngologists seem to be well agreed that there are no distinctly pathognomonic symptoms of tuberculosis of the larynx. The more extensive his experience, the fewer positive signs does he consider. The early symptoms are usually those of simple chronic laryngitis, tickling in the throat, feeling of dryness (rare in our experience) and slight huskiness. As the process extends, there is a cough of a "husky, ineffectual type." This huskiness develops into hoarseness and may go on to complete aphonia. It is well to remember that the hoarseness may be due to a paresis of the recurrent laryngeal nerve, caused by pressure of tuberculous glands, the larynx itself being uninvolved. With the development of tuberculomata in the larynx, dyspnea may supervene, although this is rare. The writer has been compelled to do a tracheotomy in but one case where there was extensive involvement with edema of the whole larynx.

Reverting to the question of hoarseness in laryngeal tuberculosis: the writer while assigned to the British Royal Army Medical Corps, picked up at least a score of cases of laryngeal tuberculosis, the laryngeal disease evidently having developed subsequent to the severe laryngitis produced by mustard gas.

In our series of cases, hoarseness at some time or other was the most common symptom, being present in 99, or 81 per cent of cases. This condition varied, of course, from a slight huskiness to complete aphonia, and in duration from a month to several years. The hoarseness in 30 per cent of cases began soon after the onset of marked coughing. Dysphagia was present in 23 cases, of which number 17 had marked involvement of the epigiottis. Ten cases with involvement of the epiglottis gave no history of dysphagia. As a factor in the production of dysphagia, marked infiltration with ulceration of the arytenoids and aryepiglottidean folds has been found by us to be of importance.

In twenty (16 per cent) cases of laryngeal tuberculosis there were no laryngeal symptoms whatsoever.

Laryngeal Involvement.—Examination of the larynx shows early a condition resembling chronic simple laryngitis—that is, a hyperemia of the mucosa of the cords and interarytenoid space. Slight infiltration may be added to the above picture early. The site of the early infiltration is usually the interarytenoid space, seen as a circumscribed swelling forming a convex projection during deep inspiration. It is usually located in the midline, but may be found on one or both sides, in the latter case giving the central portion a sunken or punched out appearance. The swelling may be a broad based, flat affair or a definite tumorlike mass, in nearly all cases presenting on its surface a grayish roughened appearance due to the breaking down of the surface epithelium. In rare cases it may take on a papillomatous aspect.

In the vocal cords, the infiltrate may take on the form of a diffuse or circumscribed redness with moderate swelling strongly suggestive of a simple chronic laryngitis. The tuberculous process usually involves one side, or one side to a greater extent than the other. There may be circumscribed infiltration, most common on the vocal processes and generally found in connection with hyperplasia of the interarytenoidal mucosa. In such cases the posterior ends of the cords are of a deep pink or red color, somewhat uneven or notched along the free edge and rounded in form with an apparent increase in both width and thickness.[10] There may be simply alteration in color, either as a redness or loss of pearly luster, and even this slight change limited to one cord is highly suggestive. There may be slight infiltration of the anterior commissure affecting either the angle of the cords or the region above or below it and resulting markedly in interference with ad-duction and phonation. As the infiltration persists, reaching the central portion of the cords, they assume their character-istic cylindrical form. This swelling may assume large pro-portions, the cords becoming several times their normal size, and as in other portions of the larynx, the surface epithelium of the cord may be quickly eroded, leaving shallow ragged ulcers.

The arytenoid cartilages may also be affected, unilaterally most frequently, and bilaterally in many cases as the disease progresses. The process here consists of infiltration showing as a swelling of deep red or purplish color, the extremities of which extend upward and outward until lost in the aryepi-glottic folds. If the infiltration is of long standing, the mucosa becomes pale and translucent, movement of the cords is me-chanically hindered by the enlarged cartilage as well as by ankylosis of the cricoarytenoid joint. There is usually more or less edema present about the cartilage and along the usually infiltrated aryepiglottidean folds, which tend in some cases, where the swelling is marked, to close off the entrance to the larynx resulting in a marked dyspnea and dysphagia.

The epiglottis is usually affected later, and in the milder cases presents an appearance of being thickened, with the edges slightly rolled on themselves, bright red or pale in color. In more advanced cases it may be greatly swollen, assuming the characteristic turban shape, with either slight or extensive ulceration and destruction. Severe pain is usually associated with involvement of the epiglottis, and slight infiltration de-stroys its mobility. In some cases the epiglottis may be almost entirely eroded.

The tuberculoma is of comparatively frequent appearance. They may be found in all portions of the larynx, being the most common in the ventricles, in the interarytenoid space and under the angle of the glottis.

Any and all of the above lesions may go on to ulceration which may be superficial or deep and destructive. The most frequent sites of ulceration include the vocal cords, interary-tenoid sulcus, arytenoid cartilages and epiglottis. Ulceration may occur, however, on all segments of the larynx.

In our series of 122 cases, the epiglottis was involved in 27, or in 22 per cent of cases. There was infiltration alone in 8 cases and infiltration with ulceration in 19 cases. Of the 27 cases showing involvement of the epiglottis death occurred in 12 cases (44 per cent) within one year, 6 cases (22 per cent) were discharged as unimproved, 7 (26 per cent) as improved, 1 (4 per cent) as quiescent, and 1 (4 per cent) apparently arrested from the pulmonary standpoint. The laryngeal condition remained unimproved in 20 cases (74 per cent), was improved in 4 cases (15 per cent) and became arrested in 3 cases (11 per cent).

The writer remembers distinctly two cases in which the laryngeal involvement was limited entirely to the epiglottis. The epiglottis was amputated, proven tuberculous on section, and the larynx and pulmonary condition, which had remained stationary previous to the amputation, went on to recovery.

The arytenoids were involved in 36 or in 29 per cent of the laryngeal cases. They showed infiltration in 27 and infiltration with ulceration in 9 cases.

The interarytenoid space was infiltrated in 57, and infiltrated with ulceration in 16, giving the total involvement as 73 cases, or 59 per cent.

The vocal cords were infiltrated in 25 and ulcerated in 35, giving a total involvement of 60, or 49 per cent of the total number of cases.

The false cords were infiltrated in eleven and showed infiltration with ulceration in 5 cases. With a total of 16 cases this would give an involvement of 13 per cent.

The whole larynx was involved in 13 cases or in 12 per cent of the total number. Of these 13 cases, 9 or 69 per cent died within one year, two (15 per cent) were discharged unimproved, and 2 (15 per cent) as improved. The larynx remained unimproved in 11 cases (85 per cent) and improved in 2 cases (15 per cent).

It is very evident, therefore, that involvement of the epiglottis or extensive involvement throughout the larynx, indicates a poor prognosis both as regards life and as regards probability of improving the laryngeal condition.

Treatment.—In the treatment of laryngeal tuberculosis there are certain general features on which all are agreed. The first of these is the influence of careful supervision of the daily life of the patient, his rest, diet, hygiene, exercise, and so on. One should insist that the patient be under sanatorium or hospital treatment, for those who will not place themselves under such care are hampering their progress, and in many instances turning the balance from recovery to a fatal termination. All of our cases were patients at the State Sanatorium, with which we have the closest cooperation, and it has been largely due to this cooperation that good results have been obtained. Much depends on the patient's determination to do his part, and this unquestionably is made easier by the carefully regulated sanatorium life.

Absolute rest of voice is insisted upon for all, regardless of what their other treatment may be. Some cases of laryngeal tuberculosis are cured wholly by silence.

Steam inhalations, using compound tincture of benzoin twice daily, are given at the sanatorium.

Lactic acid in 50 per cent solution is applied daily to the larynx, the exact lesion being brushed carefully with it. Formalin is used in some cases, beginning with a very weak solution and gradually increasing the strength as rapidly and as far as the patient seems to do well on it. We have applied it in 2 per cent solution with no discomfort to the patient. Some larynges will do best under one form of treatment; others will demand different treatment. It is only by keeping close watch of the larynx that one gains the best results.

For relief of dysphagia we use orthoform, anesthesia, injection of the superior laryngeal nerves, and where the epiglottis is involved, amputation of this structure. It is well to state here that aside from the relief of pain, the laryngeal lesion is in some cases favorably affected by removal of the epiglottis. This is due more indirectly than directly, deglutition is made easier and the increased alimentation results in improvement in the general condition.

In cases whose general condition is very poor, or where there is a continued pronounced breaking down in the lungs, the above treatment only is used. This is also true of those cases in which practically the entire larynx is involved.

Given cases who have a fair chance of recovery from the general standpoint, this method is combined with surgical treatment. The object in this, as in any form of treatment of laryngeal tuberculosis, may be summed up in the one word, fibrosis.

As a rule, when the diagnosis of laryngeal tuberculosis is made, local applications are first tried; lactic acid, 50 per cent, applied to the larynx daily. If there develops a small infiltration of the vocal angle or interarytenoid space, the cautery is tried, repeating every fortnight. The local applications are continued as before. If the infiltration does not yield to this treatment, the infiltrated area is curetted. If the infiltration now subsides, the cautery is resumed; if not, the curette is again used in two weeks.

If there is a tuberculoma in the interarytenoid space or a well circumscribed tuberculoma of the false cords, or a small tuberculoma or ulcer on the true cord, this is removed by the laryngeal forceps. If there is an interarytenoid tuberculoma in addition to the excision the base is curetted. Following this the cautery is used, or the curette, the choice being dependent upon the return of infiltration or tumor. Tuberculomas may require several excisions, but as a rule two or three excisions bring them down to the point where they can be controlled by other methods.

If the local application of lactic acid does not seem to be causing the lesion to fibrose, a change is made to formalin, usually 1 per cent. It must be emphasized that the success of treatment is based upon constant observation and a prompt change of treatment when change is indicated.

The results obtained in the treatment of laryngeal tuberculosis have, on the whole, been gratifying. The fact that many cases of tuberculosis have a better result in the larynx than they do in the pulmonary lesion shows very markedly the efficacy of the treatment. When one recalls that less than 25 years ago the presence of a laryngeal tuberculosis was considered a death warrant, one may be pardoned for showing considerable optimism.

All of our cases received the regular routine treatment: sanatorium care, rest of voice, steam inhalations and the local application of lactic acid or formalin as indicated. Forty-one cases received this routine treatment only, while 81 cases received combined routine and surgical treatment. Amputation of the epiglottis was done in 17 cases with good results. Injection of the superior laryngeal nerve was done in 13 cases. It was usually found necessary to reinject about once a week, although some cases were relieved of pain by a single injection. Curettement alone was used in six, cautery alone in twenty, and combined curettment and cautery in thirty-five cases. In these cases 111 curettments were done and 213 cauteries. All the amputations of the epiglottis and curettments were done by the suspension method; also a majority of the cauteries. Using this method we feel that the treatment is more accurate and thorough.

Results.—Considering the total number, or 122 cases, the laryngeal condition remained unimproved in 68, or in 56 per cent; it was improved in 30, or in 25 per cent, and arrested in 24, or 19 per cent. Combining the improved and arrested cases, we have a total improvement, considering all cases, of 44 per cent.

Among the 41 cases not treated surgically the larynx in 37, or 90 per cent, remained unimproved, while 4, or 10 per cent, were improved. These cases were considered by the internist as unfit for surgical treatment, due to marked, progressive involvement of lungs. Of the 81 cases treated surgically, 31 or 38 per cent remained unimproved, 26 or 32 per cent improved, and 24 or 20 per cent were arrested. Combining the improved and arrested cases, we have a total laryngeal improvement of 62 per cent in those cases treated by the combined routine and surgical method.

If the pulmonary and general condition of the patient on discharge is considered and compared with the laryngeal condition on discharge, it is found that in 35 cases who died the laryngeal condition was unimproved in 34 or 97 per cent and was arrested in 1 case or 3 per cent.

The laryngeal condition in 42 cases who were discharged with lungs unimproved, was unimproved in 28 or 67 per cent, improved in 13 or 31 per cent, and became arrested in 1 case or 2 per cent.

In 25 cases discharged with the lungs improved the laryngeal condition was unimproved in 6 or 24 per cent, improved in 13 or 52 per cent, and became arrested in 6 or 24 per cent. Combining improved and arrested larynges we find a total improvement of 76 per cent in cases where the pulmonary and general condition was definitely improved.

Among 15 cases discharged with lungs quiescent, the laryngeal condition was unimproved in 1 case or 7 per cent. The laryngeal condition was improved in 3 or 20 per cent and arrested in 11 or 53 per cent, giving a total improvement of 73 per cent.

Five cases were discharged as apparently arrested from the pulmonary and general standpoint, and in each case or 100 per cent the larynx was arrested.

The development of tuberculosis of the larynx without any question renders the final outcome of the disease process less hopeful. This is true, not only because of the added lesion which the body must resist, but it is an added evidence, in early cases, of either a lack of resistance or of a very virulent type of infection. In the average case it is an evidence that the disease is progressing, that the bodily defenses are being broken down; in other words, the disease has reached an advanced stage.

Not so many years ago the development of laryngeal tuberculosis was considered as a notice to the physician and the patient that further attempts at resistance were useless. With the advances made in the past 20 years in the treatment of this complication this gloomy outlook no longer obtains, although it must not be forgotten that it is serious.

Considering the laryngeal lesion, the most that physicians could hope to do 20 years ago was to relieve pain and hope for euthanasia. Contrasted with this, we now find a very different attitude among laryngologists and tuberculosis specialists. All admit that the situation demands careful, conservative judgment and united action on the part of physician and patient; but the records show that a gradually growing and gratifying percentage of cases do recover, and well authenticated cases of permanent cures are many.

A definite laryngeal prognosis is, however, very difficult. An early diagnosis, of course, is essential to a favorable prognosis. Other factors must be weighed: age, stage of the pulmonary condition, general condition, digestion, other complications, extent of laryngeal involvement, progress of pulmonary condition, cooperation of the patient, general supervisory control, and the skill and experience of the laryngologist. The laryngeal prognosis depends on the sum total of the above factors.

### CONCLUSIONS.

1. Laryngeal tuberculosis is found in 10 per cent of incipient cases, in 21 per cent of moderately advanced cases, and in 42 per cent of far advanced cases of pulmonary tuberculosis.

2. The percentage of unimproved larynges is higher between the ages of 40 to 50 (72 per cent) than it is for all other decades (50 to 55 per cent).

3. The percentage of improved larynges was twice as high in the moderately advanced (64 per cent) as it was in the far advanced cases of pulmonary tuberculosis, 35 per cent. In other words, the laryngeal prognosis varies directly with the extent of the pulmonary involvement.

4. The mortality within one year in incipient pulmonary tuberculosis with laryngeal involvement is three times as great (25 per cent) as is found in the same type of pulmonary cases without the laryngeal complication.

The mortality within one year, in moderately advanced pulmonary tuberculosis with laryngeal involvement, is twice as great (17 per cent) as is found in the same type of cases without the laryngeal complication (10 per cent).

In far advanced pulmonary tuberculosis with the laryngeal complication, the mortality was 45 per cent or but 12 per cent higher than in the same class of cases without the laryngeal involvement (33 per cent).

5. The laryngeal prognosis varies directly with a favorable or unfavorable general condition.

6. In cases with unimpaired digestion, the percentage of unimproved larynges was 47, while in those with impaired digestion 73 per cent of the larynges were unimproved.

7. Intestinal tuberculosis occurring in cases of pulmonary and laryngeal tuberculosis gave a mortality of 74 per cent within one year and unimprovement in the larynx in 84 per cent of cases.

8. Involvement of the epiglottis, or extensive involvement throughout the larynx, indicates a poor prognosis both as regards life and as regards probability of improving the laryngeal condition.

9. The improvement or lack of improvement in the larynx, if treated carefully, parallels closely (with exceptions) the improvement or lack of improvement in the lungs and general condition.

## CASE REPORTS.

Case 1.—Sex, female; pulmonary condition on admission, FAC.; involvement, TIII; side involved, R. III., L. III; duration of lesion, pulmonary, 5 years; general condition, unfavorable; digestion, impaired; tubercle bacilli, +; hemorrhage, +; other complications, tuberpleuritis; laryngeal symptoms, hoarseness; laryngeal involvement, ulceration L. false cord and each true cord; much interarytenoid infiltration.

Case 2.—Sex, male; pulmonary condition on admission, Maa.; involvement, TII.; side involved, RI., LII.; duration of lesion, pulmonary, 8 years; general condition, guardedly favorable; digestion, impaired; tubercle bacilli, +; hemorrhage, —; laryngeal symptoms, none; laryngeal involvement, tuberculoma posterior end T. cord and interarytenoid; each cord ulcerated.

Case 3.—Sex, male: pulmonary condition on admission, FAC.; involvement, T. III.; side involved, R. III., L. III.; duration of lesion, pulmonary, 2 years; general condition, unfavorable; digestion, unimpaired; tubercle bacilli, +; hemorrhage, —; laryngeal symptoms, hoarseness, 15 mo.; laryngeal involvement, interarytenoid tuberculoma.

Case 4.—Sex, female; pulmonary condition on admission, FAC.; involvement, T. III.; side involved, R. III., L. III.; duration of lesion, pulmonary, 7 years; general condition, unfavorable; digestion, impaired; tubercle bacilli, +; hemorrhage, —; other complications, T. B. of left kidney, enteritis colitis; laryngeal symptoms, hoarseness and dysphagia; laryngeal involvement, infiltration and ulceration epiglottis, much arytenoid and interarytenoid infiltration.

Case 5.—Sex, male; pulmonary condition on admission, FAC.; involvement, T. III.; side involved, R. III., L. II.; duration of lesion, pulmonary, 5 years; general condition, unfavorable; digestion, unimproved; tubercle bacilli, +; hemorrhage, —; other complications, myocarditis; laryngeal symptoms, hoarseness; laryngeal involvement, arytenoid and interarytenoid space infiltrated.

Case 6.—Sex, female; pulmonary condition on admission, FAB.; involvement, T. III.; side involved, R. II., L. III.; duration of lesion, pulmonary, 3 years; general condition, unfavorable; digestion, unimpaired; tubercle bacilli, +; hemorrhage, +; other complications, pleurisy; laryngeal symptoms, hoarseness 4 years; laryngeal involvement, cords thickened, reddened.

Case 7.—Sex, male; pulmonary condition on admission, MAB.; involvement, T. II.; side involved, R. I., L. II.; duration of lesion, pulmonary, 4 years; general condition, unfavorable; digestion, unimpaired; tubercle bacilli, +; hemorrhage, —.

Case 8.—Sex, female; age, 23; pulmonary condition on admission, FAC.; involvement T. III.; side involved, R. III., L. III.; duration of lesion, pulmonary, 8 mo.; general condition, unfavorable; digestion, impaired; tubercle bacilli, +; hemorrhage, —; laryngeal symptoms, hoarseness, 1 mo.; laryngeal involvement, left cord infiltrated, arytenoids infiltrated, interarytenoid space ulcerated.

Case 9.—Sex, male; age, 23; pulmonary condition on admission, FAA.; involvement, T. III.; side involved, R. I., L. I.; duration of lesion, pulmonary, 13 mo.; general condition, unfavorable; digestion, unimpaired; tubercle bacilli, +; hemorrhage, —; other complications, fibroplastic endocarditis; laryngeal symptoms, hoarseness, 1 year; laryngeal involvement, epiglottis thickened, infiltration each arytenoid and interarytenoid space.

Case 10.—Sex, male; age, 31; pulmonary condition on admission, MAC.; involvement, T. II.; side involved, R. I., L. I.; duration of lesion, pulmonary, 2 years; general condition, unfavorable; digestion, unimproved; tubercle bacilli, +; hemorrhage, —; laryngeal symptoms, hoarseness, 1 year; laryngeal involvement, epiglottis enormous thickened and ulcerated, infiltrated throughout while larynx.

Case 11.—Sex, female; age, 10; pulmonary condition on admission, MAB.; involvement, T. II.; side involved, R. I., R. I.; duration of lesion, pulmonary, 8 mo.; general condition, guardedly unfavorable; digestion, unimpaired; tubercle bacilla, +; hemorrhage, —; laryngeal symptoms, hoarseness 2 years and dysphagia 4 mo.; laryngeal involvement, infiltration of interarytenoid space with slight thickening each true cord.

Case 12.—Sex, female; age, 20; pulmonary condition on admission, FAC.; involvement, T. III.; side involved, R. I., R. III.; duration of lesion, pulmonary, 2 years; general condition, unfavorable; digestion, unimpaired; tubercle bacilli, +; hemorrhage, +; laryngeal symptoms, cough and hoarseness, 5 mo.; laryngeal involvement, interarytenoid tuberculoma.

Case 1.—Laryngeal treatment, routine; larynx when discharged, unimproved; lung condition on discharge, unimproved.

Case 2.—Laryngeal treatment, curette and cautery; larynx when discharged, improved; lung condition on discharge, quiescent.

Case 3.—Laryngeal treatment, routine; larynx when discharged, unimproved; lung condition on discharge, unimproved.

Case 4.—Laryngeal treatment, routine; larynx when discharged, unimproved; lung condition on discharge, unimproved.

Case 5.—Laryngeal treatment, amputation epiglottis; larynx when discharged, unimproved; lung condition on discharge, died.

Case 6.—Laryngeal treatment, routine; larynx when discharged, unimproved; lung condition on discharge, died.

Case 7.—Laryngeal treatment, cautery; larynx when discharged, A.; lung condition on discharge, quiescent.

Case 8.—Laryngeal treatment, curette and cautery; larynx when discharged, improved; lung condition on discharge, improved.

Case 9.—Laryngeal treatment, routine; larynx when discharged, unimproved; lung condition on discharge, unimproved.

Case 10.—Laryngeal treatment, amputation epiglottis, curette and cautery; larynx when discharged, improved; lung condition on discharge, unimproved.

Case 11.—Laryngeal treatment, cautery; larynx when discharged, improved; lung condition on discharge, unimproved.

Case 12.—Laryngeal treatment, curette, cautery; larynx when discharged, improved; lung condition on discharge, improved.

Case 13.—Sex, female; age, 28; pulmonary condition on admission, FAB.; involvement, T. III.; side involved, R. II., L. III.; duration of pulmonary lesion, 2 years; general condi-

tion, unfavorable; digestion, impaired; tubercle bacilli, +;
hemorrhage, +; laryngeal symptoms, hoarseness, 1 mo.; laryngeal involvement, interarytenoid tuberculoma; laryngeal treatment, routine; larynx when discharged, unimproved; lung
condition on discharge, unimproved.

Case 14.—Sex, female; age, 36; pulmonary condition on admission, FAC.; involvement, T. III.; side involved, R. III.,
L. II.; duration of pulmonary lesion, 6 years; general condition, unfavorable; digestion, unimpaired; tubercle bacilli, +;
hemorrhage, —; laryngeal symptoms, hoarseness, 4 mo.; laryngeal involvement, ulceration posterior end L. true cord, infiltration of interarytenoid space; laryngeal treatment, routine;
larynx when discharged, unimpaired; lung condition on discharge, unimproved.

Case 15.—Sex, female; age, 33; pulmonary condition on admission, FAB.; involvement, T. III.; side involved, R. II., L.
III.; duration of pulmonary lesion, 21 years; general condition,
unfavorable; digestion, unimproved; tubercle bacilli, +; hemorrhage, —; laryngeal symptoms, hoarseness, 6 mo.; laryngeal
involvement, interarytenoid infiltration with superficial ulceration; laryngeal treatment, injection superior laryngeal; larynx
when discharged, improved; lung condition on discharge, unimproved.

Case 16.—Sex, female; age, 20; pulmonary condition on
admission, FAB.; involvement T. III.; side involved, R. III.,
L. III.; duration of pulmonary lesion, 2 years; general condition, unfavorable; digestion, unimpaired; tubercle bacilli,
—; hemorrhage, —; laryngeal symptoms, hoarseness, dysphagia; laryngeal involvement, tuberculoma interarytenoid
space, infiltration R. false cord; laryngeal treatment, curette,
cautery; larynx when discharged, unimproved; lung condition
on discharge, unimproved.

Case 17.—Sex, male; age, 26; pulmonary condition on admission, FAB.; involvement, T. III.; side involved, R. III., L.
III.; duration of pulmonary lesion, 1 year; general condition,
unfavorable; digestion, unimpaired; tubercle bacilli, +; hemorrhage, —; laryngeal symptoms, hoarseness, cough; laryngeal
involvement, larynx waxy appearance throughout, cords infiltrated; larynx when discharged, improved; lung condition on
discharge, improved.

Case 18.—Sex, male; age, 33; pulmonary condition on admission, FAB.: involvement, T. III.; side involved, R. III.; L.
III.; duration of pulmonary lesion, 1 year; general condition,
unfavorable; digestion, impaired; tubercle bacilli, +; hemorrhage, —; other complications, T. B., pleuritis, T. B. tongue;
laryngeal symptoms, hoarseness; laryngeal involvement, ulceration each vocal cord, interarytenoid ulceration; laryngeal
treatment, routine; larynx when discharged, unimproved; lung
condition on discharge, died.

Case 19.—Sex, female; age, 20; pulmonary condition on admission, FAB.; involvement, T. III; side involved, R. III., L.
III.; duration of pulmonary lesion, 2 years; general condition,
unfavorable; digestion, impaired; tubercle bacilli, +; hemorrhage, +; other complications, T. B., pleuritis; laryngeal
symptoms, hoarseness, dysphagia; laryngeal involvement, infiltration left cord and left arytenoid; laryngeal treatment,
routine; larynx when discharged; unimproved; lung condition on discharge, died.

Case 20.—Sex, female; age, 26; pulmonary condition on admission, FAB.; involvement, T. III.; side involved, R. I., L.
III.; duration of pulmonary lesion, 9 years; general condition,
unfavorable; digestion, unimpaired; tubercle bacilli, +; hemorrhage, —; laryngeal symptoms, hoarseness, dryness; laryngeal involvement, infiltration arytenoid and interarytenoid
space; laryngeal treatment, curette; larynx when discharged,
unimproved; lung condition on discharge, unimproved.

Case 21.—Sex, female; age, 23; pulmonary condition on
admission, FAC.; involvement, T. III.; side involved, R. II.,
L. III.; duration of pulmonary lesion, 4 years; general condition, unfavorable; digestion, unimproved; tubercle bacilli, +;
hemorrhage, +; laryngeal symptoms, hoarseness; laryngeal
involvement, interarytenoid infiltration and ulceration; laryngeal treatment, curette; larynx when discharged, unimproved;
lung condition on discharge, died.

Case 22.—Sex, female; age, 21; pulmonary condition on admission, MAC.; involvement, T. II.; side involved, R. II.; L.
II.; duration of pulmonary lesion, 5 years; general condition,
unfavorable; digestion, unimpaired; tubercle bacilli, +; hemorrhage, —; laryngeal symptoms, hoarseness; laryngeal involvement, much ulceration each vocal cord; laryngeal treat-

ment, routine; larynx when discharged, unimproved; lung
condition on discharge, improved.

Case 23.—Sex, male; age, 33; pulmonary condition on admission, FAB.; involvement, T. II.; duration of pulmonary
lesion, 2 years; side involved, R. III., L. III.; general condition, favorable; digestion, unimpaired; tubercle bacilli, —;
hemorrhage, —; laryngeal symptoms, hoarseness 1 year; laryngeal involvement, interarytenoid infiltration with ulceration, R.
cord; laryngeal treatment, curette, cautery; larynx when discharged, A.; lung condition on discharge, AA.

Case 24.—Sex, female; age, 24; pulmonary condition on
admission, MAB.; involvement, T. II.; duration of pulmonary
lesion, 1 year; side involved, R. I., L. II.; general condition,
favorable; digestion, unimpaired; tubercle bacilli, +; hemorrhage, —; laryngeal symptoms, none; laryngeal involvement,
interarytenoid infiltration; laryngeal treatment, curette and
cautery; larynx when discharged, A.; lung condition on discharge, quiescent.

Case 25.—Sex, female; age, 37; pulmonary condition on
admission, MAC.; involvement, T. II.; duration of pulmonary
lesion, 4 years; side involved, R. III., L. I.; general condition,
unfavorable; digestion, impaired; tubercle bacilli, +; hemorrhage, +; laryngeal symptoms, hoarseness; laryngeal involvement, ulcerated cord; laryngeal treatment, cautery; larynx
when discharged, improved; lung condition on discharge, unimproved.

Case 26.—Sex, female; age, 37; pulmonary condition on admission, FAC.; involvement, T. III.; duration of pulmonary
lesion, 5 years; side involved, R. III., L. II.; general condition,
unfavorable; digestion, impaired; tubercle bacilli, +; hemorrhage, —; laryngeal symptoms, hoarseness; laryngeal involvement, extensive involvement, perichrondritis, epiglottis eroded.
amputation epiglottis, injections; larynx when discharged, unimproved; lung condition on discharge, died.

Case 27.—Sex, male; age, 42; pulmonary condition on admission, MAB.; involvement, T. II.; duration of pulmonary
lesion, 9 mo.; side involved, R. II., L. II.; general condition,
G. favorable; digestion, unimpaired; tubercle bacilli, +; hemorrhage, —; laryngeal symptoms, hoarseness; laryngeal involvement, left cord infiltrated, both false cords infiltrated:

laryngeal treatment, routine; larynx when discharged, unimproved; lung condition on discharge, unimproved.

Case 28.—Sex, male; age, 23; pulmonary condition on admission, MAA.; involvement, T. III.; duration of pulmonary lesion, 16 mo.; side involved, R. III., L. I.; general condition, unfavorable; digestion, unimpaired; tubercle bacilli, +; hemorrhage, —; laryngeal involvement, R. cord ulcerated, interarytenoid infiltration; laryngeal treatment, routine; larynx when discharged, improved; lung condition on discharge, unimproved.

Case 29.—Sex, male; age, 49; pulmonary condition on admission, FAB.; involvement, T. III.; side involved, R. III., L. III.; duration of pulmonary lesion, 15 years; general condition, unfavorable; digestion, unimpaired; tubercle bacilli, +; hemorrhage, +; laryngeal symptoms, hoarseness; laryngeal involvement, R. cord ulcerated, interarytenoid infiltrated; laryngeal treatment, refused treatment; larynx on discharge, unimproved; lung condition on discharge, quiescent.

Case 30.—Sex, male; age, 31; pulmonary condition on admission, FAC.; involvement, T. III.; side involved, R. III., L. III.; duration of pulmonary lesion, 10 years; general condition, unfavorable; digestion, impaired; tubercle bacilli, +; hemorrhage, —; laryngeal symptoms, sore throat, dysphagia, hoarseness; laryngeal involvement, whole larynx involved, infiltrated; laryngeal treatment, nerve injections; larynx on discharge, unimproved; lung condition on discharge, died.

Case 31.—Sex, male; age, 35; pulmonary condition on admission, MAB.; involvement, T. III.; side involved, R. III., L. I.; duration of pulmonary lesion, 5 years; general condition, favorable; digestion, unimpaired; tubercle bacilli, +; hemorrhage, —; laryngeal symptoms, hoarseness; laryngeal involvement, infiltration L. false cord, also R. cord; laryngeal treatment, routine; larynx on discharge, improved; lung condition on discharge, quiescent.

Case 32.—Sex, female; age, 25; pulmonary condition on admission, FAC.; involvement, T. III.; side involved, R. III., L. II.; duration of pulmonary lesion, 1 year; general condition, unfavorable; digestion, unimpaired; tubercle bacilli, +; hemorrhage, —; laryngeal symptoms, hoarseness; laryngeal involvement, interarytenoid infiltration, also R. cord; laryngeal treatment, routine; larynx on discharge, unimproved; lung condition on discharge, unimproved.

Case 33:—Sex, male; age, 59; pulmonary condition on admission, FAC.; involvement, T. III.; side involved, R. III., L. II.; duration of pulmonary lesion, 18 mo.; general condition, unfavorable; digestion, impaired; tubercle bacilli, +; hemorrhage, —; other complications, toxic myocarditis; laryngeal symptoms, hoarseness, dysphagia, 6 mo.; laryngeal involvement, infiltration with superficial ulceration throughout larynx, epiglottis ulcerated; laryngeal treatment, amputation epiglottis, routine; larynx on discharge, unimproved; lung condition on discharge, died.

Case 34.—Sex, male; age, 26; pulmonary condition on admission, MAB.; involvement, R. III., L. I.; side involved, T. II.; duration of pulmonary lesion, 5 years; general condition, unfavorable; digestion, unimpaired; tubercle bacilli, +; hemorrhage, —; laryngeal symptoms, hoarseness, 3 mo.; laryngeal involvement, true cords and left arytenoid infiltrated; laryngeal treatment, cautery; laryngeal condition on discharge, A.; lung condition on discharge, unimproved.

Case 35.—Sex, female; age, 34; pulmonary condition on admission, FAB.; involvement, R. III., L. III.; side involved, T. III.; duration of pulmonary lesion, 10 mo.; general condition, unfavorable; digestion, unimpaired; tubercle bacilli, +; hemorrhage, —; laryngeal symptoms, none; laryngeal involvement, interarytenoid infiltration; laryngeal treatment, cautery; laryngeal condition on discharge, unimproved; lung condition on discharge, unimproved.

Case 36.—Sex, female; age, 29; pulmonary condition on admission, FAC.; involvement, R. II., L. II.; side involved, T. III.; duration of pulmonary lesion, 3 years; general condition, unfavorable; digestion, unimpaired; tubercle bacilli, +; hemorrhage, —; other complications, enteritis, colitis, hoarseness. dryness, dysphagia, interarytenoid ulceration, each cord ulcerated, upper border epiglottis ulcerated; laryngeal treatment, amputation; laryngeal condition on discharge. unimproved; lung condition on discharge, died.

Case 37.—Sex, male; age, 25; pulmonary condition on admission, AC.; involvement, R. III., L. III.; side involved, T. III.; duration of pulmonary involvement, 8 years; general con-

dition, unfavorable; digestion, unimpaired; tubercle bacilli,
+; hemorrhage, —; other complications, enteritis, colitis,
hoarseness following gassing, dysphagia, whole larynx infiltrated and ulcerated, including epiglottis; laryngeal treatment,
amputation; laryngeal condition on discharge, unimproved;
lung condition on discharge, unimproved.

Case 38.—Sex, female; age, 26; pulmonary condition on admission, FAC.; involvement, R. II., L. III.; side involved, T.
III.; duration of pulmonary lesion, 6 years; general condition, unfavorable; digestion, impaired; tubercle bacilli, +;
hemorrhage, +; other complications, enteritis colitis; laryngeal symptoms, hoarseness; laryngeal involvement, whole larynx infiltrated, ulceration of cords; laryngeal treatment; routine; laryngeal condition on discharge, unimproved; lung condition on discharge, died.

Case 39.—Sex, female; age, 24; pulmonary condition on admission, FAC.; involvement, T. III.; side involved, R. III., L.
III.; duration of pulmonary lesion, 4 years; general condition,
unfavorable; digestion, unimpaired; tubercle bacilli, +.; hemorrhage, —; other complications, myocarditis; laryngeal symptoms, hoarseness, 3 mo.; laryngeal involvement, infiltration of
interarytenoid space, both arytenoid and R. true cord; laryngeal treatment, routine; larynx on discharge, unimproved;
lung condition on discharge, died.

Case 40.—Sex, female; age, 23; pulmonary condition on
admission, FAB.; involvement, T. III.; side involved, R. III.,
L. III.; duration of pulmonary lesion, 10 mo.; general condition, unfavorable; digestion, unimpaired; tubercle bacilli, +;
hemorrhage, +; other complications, enteritis colitis; laryngeal symptoms, hoarseness; laryngeal involvement, infiltration
L. arytenoid and inter.; laryngeal treatment, cautery; larynx
on discharge, unimproved; lung condition on discharge, died.

Case 41.—Sex, male; age, 30; pulmonary condition on admission, MAA.; involvement, T. I.; side involved, R. II., L. I.;
duration of pulmonary lesion, 4 years; general condition, favorable; digestion, unimpaired; tubercle bacilla, +.; hemorrhage, +; laryngeal symptoms, none; laryngeal involvement,
ulceration T. cord, infiltration S. arytenoid; laryngeal treatment, curette, cautery; larynx on discharge, unimproved; lung
condition on discharge, died.

Case 42.—Sex, female; age, 34; pulmonary condition on admission, FAA.; involvement, T. II.; side involved, R. I., L. II.; general condition, unfavorable; digestion, unimpaired; tubercle bacilli, +; hemorrhage, —; laryngeal symptoms, none; laryngeal involvement, epiglottis infiltration, interarytenoid infiltration; laryngeal treatment, curette, cautery; larynx on discharge, A.; lung condition on discharge, quiescent.

Case 43.—Sex, female; age, 34; pulmonary condition on admission, FAB.; involvement, T. II.; side involved, R. III., L. I.; duration of pulmonary lesion, 12 years; general condition, unfavorable; digestion, unimpaired; tubercle bacilli, +; hemorrhage, +; laryngeal symptoms, slight hoarseness; laryngeal involvement, interarytenoid tuberculoma; laryngeal treatment, amputation; larynx on discharge, improved; lung condition on discharge, improved.

Case 44.—Sex, female; age, 34; pulmonary condition on admission, FAC.; involvement, T. III.; side involved, R. III., L. III.; duration of pulmonary lesion, 16 years; general condition, unfavorable; digestion, impaired; tubercle bacilli, +; hemorrhage, +; laryngeal symptoms, huskiness, dysphagia; laryngeal involvement, epiglottis infiltration and ulceration whole of left side, larynx invo.; laryngeal treatment, amputation; larynx on discharge, A.; lung condition on discharge, quiescent.

Case 45.—Sex, female; age, 34; pulmonary condition on admission, FAB.; involvement, T. III.; side involved, R. III., L. III.; duration of pulmonary lesion, 2 years; general condition, unfavorable; digestion, unimpaired; tubercle bacilli, +; hemorrhage, +; other complications, enteritis colitis; laryngeal symptoms, hoarseness, dysphagia; laryngeal involvement, marked infiltration of arytenoid; laryngeal treatment, cautery; larynx on discharge, unimproved; lungs on discharge, died.

Case 46.—Sex, female; age, 30; pulmonary condition on admission, MAB.; involvement, T. II.; side involved, R. I., L. III.; duration of pulmonary lesion, 2 years; general condition, unfavorable; digestion, unimpaired; tubercle bacilli, +; hemorrhage, +; other complications, T. B. append pluer; laryngeal symptoms, effusion, hoarseness; laryngeal involvement, interarytenoid space and L. arytenoid; laryngeal treatment, cautery; larynx on discharge, unimproved; lungs on discharge, died.

Case 47.—Sex, female; age, 28; pulmonary condition on admission, FAC.; involvement, T. III.; side involved, R. III., L. II.; duration of pulmonary lesion, 1 year; general condition, unfavorable; digestion, impaired; tubercle bacilli, —; hemorrhage, —; laryngeal treatment, routine; larynx on discharge, unimproved; lungs on discharge, died.

Case 48.—Sex, female; age, 31; pulmonary condition on admission, MAB.; involvement, T. II.; side involved, R. II.. L. II.; duration of pulmonary lesion, 2 years; general condition, unfavorable; digestion, unimpaired; tubercle bacilli, +: hemorrhage, —; other complications, pregnancy; laryngeal symptoms, hoarseness; laryngeal involvement, infiltration and ulceration epiglottis, edema; laryngeal treatment, none; larynx on discharge, unimproved; lungs on discharge, died.

Case 49.—Sex, male; age, 51; pulmonary condition on admission, FAB.; involvement, T. III.; side involved, R. II., L. I.; duration of pulmonary lesion, 12 years; general condition, unfavorable; digestion, unimpaired; tubercle bacilli, +; hemorrhage, —; laryngeal symptoms, dysphagia; laryngeal involvement, ulceration each vocal cord; laryngeal treatment. cautery; larynx on discharge, A.; lungs on discharge, improved.

Case 50.—Sex, male; age, 49: pulmonary condition on admission, FAB.; involvement, T. III.; side involved R. III., L. III.; duration of pulmonary lesion, 10 mo.; general condition, unfavorable; digestion, unimpaired; tubercle bacilli, +; hemorrhage, —; laryngeal symptoms, hoarseness: laryngeal involvement, false cords; laryngeal treatment, routine: larynx on discharge, unimproved; lungs on discharge, unimproved.

Case 51.—Sex, female; age, 28; pulmonary condition on admission, FAC.; involvement, T. III.; side involved, R. II., L. III.; duration of pulmonary lesion, 2 years; general condition, unfavorable; digestion, unimpaired; tubercle bacilli, +; hemorrhage, —; laryngeal treatment, routine; larynx on discharge, unimproved; lungs on discharge, died.

Case 52.—Sex, female, age, 35; pulmonary condition on admission, MAA.; involvement, T. III.; side involved, R. II., L. II.; duration of pulmonary lesion, 1 year; general condition, unfavorable; digestion, impaired; tubercle bacilli, +;

hemorrhage, —; laryngeal symptoms, hoarse, 6 mo.; laryngeal treatment, cautery; laryngeal involvement, ulcer false cord, lf arytenoid swollen; larynx on discharge, improved; lung condition on discharge, unimproved.

Case 53.—Sex, female; age, 28; pulmonary condition on admission, FAB.; involvement, T. III.; side involved, R. III., L. I.; duration of pulmonary lesion, 18 mo.; general condition, unfavorable; digestion, unimpaired; tubercle bacilli, +; hemorrhage, —; laryngeal symptoms, hoarseness; laryngeal treatment, cautery; laryngeal involvement, interarytenoid infiltration; larynx on discharge, unimproved; lung condition on discharge, unimproved.

Case 54.—Sex, male; age, 59; pulmonary condition on admission, FAA.; involvement, T. II.; side involved, R. II., L. II.; duration of pulmonary lesion, 3 years; general condition, unfavorable; digestion, unimpaired; tubercle bacilli, +; hemorrhage, —; laryngeal symptoms, hoarseness; laryngeal treatment, routine; laryngeal involvement, ulceration each cord; larynx on discharge, unimproved; lung condition on discharge, unimproved.

Case 55.—Sex, female; age, 19; pulmonary condition on admission, MAB.; involvement, T. III.; side involved, R. III., L. I.; duration of pulmonary lesion, 5 years; general condition, unfavorable; digestion, impaired; tubercle bacilli, +; hemorrhage, +; laryngeal symptoms, none; laryngeal treatment, cautery; laryngeal involvement, false cords; larynx on discharge, improved; lung condition on discharge, unimproved.

Case 56.—Sex, female; age, 34; pulmonary condition on admission, FAC.; involvement, T. III.; side involved, R. III., L. II.; duration of pulmonary lesion, 19 years; general condition, unfavorable; digestion, impaired; tubercle bacilli, +; hemorrhage, —; other complications, pregnancy; laryngeal symptoms, none; laryngeal treatment, amputation; larynx on discharge, unimproved; lung condition on discharge, died.

Case 57.—Sex, male; age, 17; pulmonary condition on admission, FAB.; involvement, T. III.; side involved, R. III., L. II.; duration of pulmonary lesion, 10 years; general condition, unfavorable; digestion, unimpaired; tubercle bacilli, +; hemorrhage, +; laryngeal treatment, cautery; laryngeal involvement, interarytenoid; larynx on discharge, unimproved; lung condition on discharge, improved.

Case 58.—Sex, male; age, 24; pulmonary condition on admission, FAB.; involvement, T. III.; side involved, R. II., L. II.; duration of pulmonary lesion, 5 mo.; general condition, unfavorable; digestion, impaired; tubercle bacilli, +; hemorrhage, —; other complications, enteritis; laryngeal treatment, cautery; laryngeal involvement, ulceration; larynx on discharge, unimproved; lung condition on discharge, died.

Case 59.—Sex, female; age, 25; pulmonary condition on admission, MAB.; involvement, T. II.; side involved, R. II., L. II.; duration of pulmonary lesion, 1 year; general condition, unfavorable; digestion, unimpaired; tubercle bacilli, +; hemorrhage +; other complications, arthritis; laryngeal symptoms, none; laryngeal involvement, interarytenoid infiltration; laryngeal treatment, cautery; larynx on discharge, improved; lung condition on discharge, unimproved.

Case 60.—Sex, female; age, 28; pulmonary condition on admission, FAC.; involvement, T. II.; side involved, R. III., L. III.; duration of pulmonary lesion, 9 mo.; general condition, unfavorable; digestion, impaired; tubercle bacilli, +; hemorrhage, —; other complications, none; laryngeal symptoms, hoarseness; laryngeal involvement, erosion epiglottis; laryngeal treatment, routine; larynx on discharge, unimproved; lung condition on discharge, died.

Case 61.—Sex, male; age, 36; pulmonary condition on admission, FAB.; involvement, T. III.; side involved, R. III., L. III.; duration of pulmonary lesion, 1 year; general condition, unfavorable; digestion, unimpaired; tubercle bacilli, +; hemorrhage, —; other complications, arthritis; laryngeal symptoms, hoarseness; laryngeal involvement, L. cord ulceration; laryngeal treatment, routine; larynx on discharge, improved; lung condition on discharge, unimproved.

Case 62.—Sex, female; age, 40; pulmonary condition on admission, FAB.; involvement, T. III.; side involved, R. I., L. III.; duration of pulmonary lesion, 20 years; general condition, unfavorable; digestion, unimpaired; tubercle bacilli, +; hemorrhage, +; other complications, arthritis; laryngeal symptoms, hoarseness; laryngeal involvement, L. cord ulceration;

laryngeal treatment, cautery; larynx on discharge, unimproved; lung condition on discharge, unimproved.

Case 63.—Sex, male; age, 35;.pulmonary condition on admission, FAC.; involvement, T. III.; side involved, R. III., L. III.; duration of pulmonary lesion, 8 mo.; general condition, unfavorable; digestion, impaired; tubercle bacilli, +; hemorrhage, —; laryngeal symptoms, hoarseness; laryngeal involvement, epiglottis infiltration; laryngeal treatment, routine; larynx on discharge, unimproved; lung condition on discharge, died.

Case 64.—Sex, male; age, 17; pulmonary condition on admission, FAC.; involvement, T. III.; side involved, R. II., L. III.; duration of pulmonary lesion, 1 year; general condition, unfavorable; digestion, impaired; tubercle bacilli, +; hemorrhage, +; other complications, T. B. hip, epiglottis; laryngeal symptoms, hoarseness; laryngeal involvement, whole larynx infiltrated; laryngeal treatment, nerve injection; larynx on discharge, unimproved; lung condition on discharge, died.

Case 65.—Sex, female; age, 22; pulmonary condition on admission, FAB.; involvement, T. II.; side involved, R. II., L. I.; duration of pulmonary lesion, 8 mo.; general condition, unfavorable; digestion, unimpaired; tubercle bacilli, —; hemorrhage, +; other complications, arthritis colitis; laryngeal symptoms, pain in throat and hoarseness; laryngeal involvement, epiglottis thickened; laryngeal treatment, amputation; larynx on discharge, unimproved; lung condition on discharge, died.

Case 66.—Sex, female; age, 31; pulmonary condition on admission, FAC.; involvement, T. III.; side involved, R. III., L. III.; duration of pulmonary lesion, 5 years; general condition, unfavorable; digestion, impaired; tubercle bacilli, +; hemorrhage, —; laryngeal symptoms, hoarseness; laryngeal involvement, ulcer R. vocal cord, R. false cord, R. arytenoid; laryngeal treatment, routine; larynx on discharge, unimproved; lung condition on discharge, died.

Case 67.—Sex, male; age, 43; pulmonary condition on admission, FAC.; involvement, T. III.; side involved, R. III., L. III.; duration of pulmonary lesion, 1 year; general condition, unfavorable; digestion, impaired; tubercle bacilli, +; hemorrhage, —; laryngeal symptoms, hoarseness; laryngeal involvement, ulceration R. cord, infiltration R. arytenoid; laryngeal treatment, routine; larynx on discharge, unimproved; lung condition on discharge, died.

Case 68.—Sex, male; age, 35; pulmonary condition on admission, FAC.; involvement, T. III.; side involved, R. III., L. II.; duration of lesion, 2 years; general condition, unfavorable; digestion, impaired; tubercle bacilli, +; hemorrhage, —; laryngeal symptoms, hoarseness; laryngeal involvement, R. arytenoid; laryngeal treatment, tracheotomy; larynx on discharge, unimproved; lung condition on discharge, died.

Case 69.—Sex, female; age, 36; pulmonary condition on admission, MAB.; involvement, T. III.; side involved, R. II., L. III.; duration of pulmonary lesion, 7 mo.; general condition, favorable; digestion, unimpaired; tubercle bacilli, +; hemorrhage, —; other complications, arthritis colitis; laryngeal symptoms, none; laryngeal involvement, arytenoid and cords infiltrated and edematous; laryngeal treatment, routine; larynx on discharge, unimproved; lung condition on discharge, died.

Case 70.—Sex, male; age, 23; pulmonary condition on admission, FAB.; involvement, T. III.; side involved, R. III., L. II.; duration of pulmonary lesion, 3 years; general condition, unfavorable; digestion, unimpaired; tubercle bacilli, +; hemorrhage, —; laryngeal symptoms, none; laryngeal treatment, cautery; larynx on discharge, unimproved; lung condition on discharge, unimproved.

Case 71.—Sex, male; age, 50; pulmonary condition on admission, MAB.; involvement, T. II.; side involved, R. II., L. II.; duration of pulmonary lesion, 1 year; general condition, favorable; digestion, unimpaired; tubercle bacilli, +; hemorrhage, —; laryngeal symptoms, none; laryngeal involvement, interarytenoid infiltration and each arytenoid; laryngeal treatment, cautery; larynx on discharge, A.; lung condition on discharge, quiescent.

Case 72.—Sex, male; age, 50; pulmonary condition on admission, FAB.; involvement, T. III.; side involved, R. III., L. II.; duration of pulmonary lesion, 4 mo.; general condition, unfavorable; digestion, unimpaired; tubercle bacilli, +; hemorrhage, —; laryngeal symptoms, none; laryngeal involvement, infiltration arytenoid, infilt. and dach. arytenoid; laryngeal treatment, curette; larynx on discharge, unimproved; lung condition on discharge, improved.

Case 73.—Sex, male; age, 20; pulmonary condition on admission, MAB.; involvement, T. II.; side involved, R. II., L. I.; duration of pulmonary lesion, 6 mo.; general condition, favorable; digestion, unimpaired; tubercle bacilli, +; hemorrhage, +; laryngeal symptoms, none; laryngeal involvement, tuberculoma interarytenoid; laryngeal treatment, curette; larynx on discharge improved; lung condition on discharge, unimproved.

Case 74.—Sex, male; age, 27; pulmonary condition on admission, MAA.; involvement, T. III.; side involved, R. I., L. I.; duration of pulmonary lesion, 18 mo.; general condition, favorable; digestion, unimpaired; tubercle bacilli, +; hemorrhage, +; other complications, arytenoid false cords and both walls of larynx infiltrated, ulceration interarytenoid; laryngeal symptoms, hoarseness; laryngeal involvement, arytenoid false cords; laryngeal treatment, cautery; larynx on discharge, improved; lungs on discharge, improved.

Case 75.—Sex, male; age, 18; pulmonary condition on admission, MAB.; involvement, T. III.; side involved, R. II., L. II.; duration of lesion, 3 years; general condition, unfavorable; digestion, impaired; tubercle bacilli, —; hemorrhage, +; laryngeal symptoms, none; larynx on discharge, improved; lungs on discharge, improved.

Case 76.—Sex, female; age, 37; pulmonary condition on admission, FAA.; involvement, T. III.; side involved, R. III., L. II.; duration of lesion, 9 years; general condition, unfavorable; digestion, unimpaired; tubercle bacilli, +; hemorrhage, —; other complications, infiltration interarytenoid space; laryngeal symptoms, hoarseness; laryngeal involvement, infiltration interarytenoid of t. cords; laryngeal treatment, cautery; larynx on discharge, A.; lungs on discharge, died.

Case 77.—Sex, female; age, 37; pulmonary condition on admission, FAB.; involvement, T. III.; side involved, R. III., L. III.; duration of lesion, 8 mo.; general condition, unfavorable; digestion, unimpaired; tubercle bacilli, +; hemorrhage, —; other complications, cords rough, ulcerated, infiltrated; laryngeal symptoms, huskiness; laryngeal involvement, cords rough, ulcerated; laryngeal treatment, cautery; larynx on discharge, unimproved; lungs on discharge, died.

Case 78.—Sex, female; age, 34; pulmonary condition on admission, FAC.; involvement, T. III.; side involved, R. III., L. II.; duration of lesion, 16 years; general condition, unfavorable; digestion, unimpaired; tubercle bacilli, +; hemorrhage, —; other complications, ulcerated epiglottis; laryngeal symptoms, hoarseness; laryngeal involvement, ulcerated epiglottis; laryngeal treatment, cautery; larynx on discharge, unimproved; lungs on discharge, died.

Case 79.—Sex, male; age, 37; pulmonary condition on admission, FAB.; involvement, T. III.; side involved, R. III., L. II.; duration of lesion, 12 years; general condition, unfavorable; digestion, unimpaired; tubercle bacilli, +; hemorrhage, —; other complications, R. arytenoid and R. false cord ulcerated; laryngeal symptoms, hoarseness; laryngeal involvement, R. false cord; laryngeal treatment, amputation epiglottis; larynx on discharge, unimproved; lungs on discharge, died.

Case 80.—Sex, male; age, 44; pulmonary condition on admission, FAC.; involvement, T. III.; side involved, R. III., L. III.; duration of lesion, 1 year; general condition, unfavorable; digestion; unimpaired; tubercle bacilli, +; hemorrhage, +; other complications, infiltration true cords and interarytenoid space; laryngeal symptoms, none; laryngeal involvement, infiltrated interarytenoid; laryngeal treatment, cautery; larynx on discharge, unimproved; lungs on discharge, died.

Case 81.—Sex, male; age, 38; pulmonary condition on admission, FAB.; involvement, T. III.; side involved, R. II., L. III.; duration of lesion, 8 mo.; general condition, unfavorable; digestion, unimpaired; tubercle bacilli, —; hemorrhage, +; laryngeal involvement, tuberculoma base of epiglottis; laryngeal treatment, cautery; larynx on discharge, improved; lungs on discharge, quiescent.

Case 82.—Sex, male; age, 38; pulmonary condition on admission, FAA.; involvement, T. II.; side involved, R. II., L. I.; duration of lesion, 1 year; general condition, unfavorable; tubercle bacilli, +; hemorrhage, —; laryngeal involvement, left half infiltrated; laryngeal treatment, amputation; larynx on discharge, improved; lungs on discharge, improved.

Case 83.—Sex, male; age, 40; pulmonary condition on admission, MA.; involvement, T. III.; side involved, R. III., L. I.; duration of lesion 2½ years; general condition, favorable; digestion, unimpaired; tubercle bacilli, —; hemorrhage, —; laryngeal involvement, L. cord thickened and red; laryngeal treatment, cautery; larynx on discharge, A.; lungs on discharge, quiescent.

Case 84.—Sex, male; age, 32; pulmonary condition on admission, FAB.; involvement, T. III.; side involved, R. III., L. II.; duration of lesion, 3 years; general condition, unfavorable; digestion, unimpaired; tubercle bacilli, +; hemorrhage, —; laryngeal symptoms, hoarseness; laryngeal involvement, interarytenoid infiltration; laryngeal treatment, cautery; larynx on discharge, unimproved; lungs on discharge, unimproved.

Case 85.—Sex, female; age, 34; pulmonary condition on admission, FAC.; involvement, T. III.; side involved, R. II., L. III.; duration of lesion, 1 year; general condition, unfavorable; digestion, unimpaired; tubercle bacilli, +; hemorrhage, —; laryngeal symptoms, hoarseness; laryngeal involvement, interarytenoid infiltration; laryngeal treatment, nerve injection; larynx on discharge, unimproved; lungs on discharge, died.

Case 86.—Sex, female; age, 28; pulmonary condition on discharge, FAC.; involvement, T. III.; side involved, R. III., L. III.; duration of lesion, 15 years; general condition, unfavorable; digestion, impaired; tubercle bacilli, +; hemorrhage, +; laryngeal symptoms, hoarseness; laryngeal involvement, infiltration interarytenoid; laryngeal treatment, routine; larynx on discharge, unimproved; lungs on discharge, died.

Case 87.—Sex, female; age, 36; pulmonary condition on admission, FAA.; involvement, T. II.; side involved, R. I., L. I.; duration of lesion, 5 mo.; general condition, unfavorable; digestion, unimpaired; tubercle bacilli, +; hemorrhage, +; laryngeal symptoms, hoarseness; laryngeal involvement, false cords; laryngeal treatment, cautery; larynx on discharge, unimproved; lungs on discharge, unimproved.

Case 89.—Sex, female; age, 45; pulmonary condition on admission, FAC.; involvement, T. III.; side involved, R.

III., L. II.; duration of lesion, 4 mo.; general condition, unfavorable; digestion, unimpaired; tubercle bacilli, +; hemorrhage, —; laryngeal symptoms, aphonia 2 mo., cough 5 mo.; laryngeal involvement, small tuberculoma interarytenoid space, infiltration both false cords; laryngeal treatment, routine; larynx on discharge, unimproved; lungs on discharge, unimproved.

Case 90.—Sex, female; age, 28; pulmonary condition on admission, FAA.; involvement, T. III.; side involved, R. II., L. II.; duration of lesion, 7 mo.; general condition, favorable; digestion unimpaired; tubercle bacilli, +; hemorrhage, —; laryngeal symptoms, huskiness; laryngeal involvement. posterior end Rt. cord ulcerated, slight interarytenoid infiltration; laryngeal treatment, curette; larynx on discharge, A.; lungs on discharge, improved.

Case 91.—Sex, female; age, 22; pulmonary condition on admission, MAC.; involvement, T. II.; side involved, R. II., L. I.; duration of lesion, 5 mo.; general condition, unfavorable; digestion, unimpaired; tubercle bacilli, +; hemorrhage, —; laryngeal symptoms, hoarseness 4 mo., dysphagia 5 mo.; laryngeal involvement, infiltration with ulceration throughout larynx, epiglottis thickened and ulcerated; laryngeal treatment, amputation epiglottis, injection sup. laryngeal nerves; larynx on discharge, unimproved; lungs on discharge, unimproved.

Case 92.—Sex, male; age, 29; pulmonary condition on admission, FAC.; involvement, T. III.; side involved, R. III., L. I.; duration of lesion, 18 mo.; general condition, unfavorable; digestion, unimpaired; tubercle bacilli, +; hemorrhage, +; laryngeal symptoms, hoarseness 7 mo., cough; laryngeal involvement, infiltration each border in cord, infiltration with superficial ulceration space; laryngeal treatment, curette and cautery; larynx on discharge, improved; lungs on discharge, improved.

Case 93.—Sex, male; age, 32; pulmonary condition on admission, FAB.; involvement, T. III.; side involved, R. III., L. II.; duration of lesion, 3 years; general condition, G. favorable; digestion, unimpaired; tubercle bacilli, +; hemorrhage, +; laryngeal symptoms, none: laryngeal involvement, posterior end each cord infiltrated with ulceration left cord, interarytenoid space; laryngeal treatment, curette and cautery; larynx on discharge, unimproved; lungs on discharge, unimproved.

Case 94.—Sex, male; age, 24; pulmonary condition on admission, FAC.; involvement, T. II.; side involved, R. III., L. II.; duration, 9 mo.; general condition, unfavorable; digestion, impaired; tubercle bacilli, +; hemorrhage, +; laryngeal symptoms, hoarseness; laryngeal involvement, ulceration interarytenoid space, true cord infiltrated; laryngeal treatment, routine; larynx on discharge, improved; lungs on discharge, improved.

Case 95.—Sex, male; age, 29; pulmonary condition on admission, FAC.; involvement, T. III.; side involved, R. II., L. III.; duration of lesion, 4 years; general condition, G. favorable; digestion, unimpaired; tubercle bacilli, +; hemorrhage, +; other complications, induced phenorrhax; laryngeal symptoms, none; laryngeal involvement, infiltration each arytenoid and interarytenoid space; laryngeal treatment, cautery; larynx on discharge, A.; lungs on discharge, quiescent.

Case 96.—Sex, male; age, 37; pulmonary condition on admission, MAB.; involvement, T. II.; side involved, R. II., L. II.; duration, 2 years; general condition, G. favorable; digestion, unimpaired; tubercle bacilli, +; hemorrhage, +; laryngeal symptoms, hoarseness 1 year, followed by hemoptysis, cough; laryngeal involvement, cough, larynx infiltrated throughout, slight thickening superior border of epiglottis, infiltration of true and false cords, interarytenoid space; laryngeal treatment, routine; larynx on discharge, unimproved; lungs on discharge, improved.

Case 97.—Sex, female; age, 46; pulmonary condition on admission, FAB.; involvement, T. III.; side involved, R. II., L. III.; duration of lesion, 15 years; general condition, unfavorable; digestion, unimpaired; tubercle bacilli, +; hemorrhage, +; laryngeal symptoms, hoarseness, dysphagia; laryngeal involvement, epiglottis infiltrated, also right false cord; laryngeal treatment, amputation; larynx on discharge, unimproved; lungs on discharge, unimproved.

Case 98.—Sex, female; age, 29; pulmonary condition on admission, FAC.; involvement, T. III.; side involved, R. III., L. III.; duration of lesion, 6 mo.; general condition, unfavorable; digestion, unimpaired; tubercle bacilli, +; hemorrhage, —; other complications, tuberculous vulgaris, T. B. salpingitis right; laryngeal symptoms, T. B. tonsil, hoarseness, dysphagia; laryngeal involvement, true cords infiltrated, infiltration and ulceration of interarytenoid space; laryngeal treatment, routine; larynx on discharge, unimproved; lungs on discharge, improved.

Case 99.—Sex, female; age, 15; pulmonary condition on admission, FAB.; involvement, T. III.; side involved, R. II., L. I.; duration of lesion, 10 mo.; general condition, unfavorable; digestion, unimproved; tubercle bacilli, +; hemorrhage, —; laryngeal symptoms, hard palate, hoarseness and cough; laryngeal involvement, epiglottis right infiltrated, tuberculoma interarytenoid space; laryngeal treatment, cautery; larynx on discharge, unimproved; lungs on discharge, improved.

Case 100.—Sex, female; age, 35; pulmonary condition on admission, FAB.; involvement, T. III.; side involved, R. III., L. III.; duration of lesion, 7 mo.; general condition, unfavorable; digestion, unimpaired; tubercle bacilli, +; hemorrhage, —; laryngeal symptoms, hoarseness; laryngeal involvement, tuberculoma interarytenoid space, ulceration right true cord: laryngeal treatment, routine; larynx on discharge, improved; lungs on discharge, unimproved.

Case 101.—Sex, female; age, 21; pulmonary condition on admission, FAC.; involvement, T. III.; side involved, R. II., L. III.; duration of lesion, 5 years; general condition, impaired; digestion, impaired; tubercle bacilli, +; hemorrhage, +; laryngeal symptoms, hoarseness 2 years; laryngeal involvement, ulceration superior border of epiglottis, slight interarytenoid infiltration; laryngeal treatment, amputation; larynx on discharge, A.; lungs on discharge, improved.

Case 102.—Sex, male; age, 29; pulmonary condition on admission, FAB.; involvement, T. III.; side involved, R. III., L. II.; duration of lesion, 1 year; general condition, unimproved; digestion, unimpaired; tubercle bacilli, +; hemorrhage, +; laryngeal symptoms, hoarseness, 4 mo.; laryngeal involvement, thickening of superior border epiglottis, infiltration false cords, interarytenoid space, ulceration posterior end each true cord; laryngeal treatment, patient refused; larynx on discharge, unimproved; lungs on discharge, unimproved.

Case 103.—Sex, female; age, 50; pulmonary condition on admission, FAC.; involvement, T. III.; side involved, R. III., L. III.; duration of lesion, 15 years; general condition, unimproved; digestion, unimpaired; tubercle bacilli, —; hemorrhage, +; laryngeal symptoms, dysphagia, hoarseness; laryngeal involvement, epiglottis infiltrated, true cords ulcerated; laryngeal treatment, amputation; larynx on discharge, unimproved; lungs on discharge, unimproved.

Case 104.—Sex, male; age, 41; pulmonary condition on admission, FAA.; involvement, T. II.; side involved, R. II.; L. III.; duration of lesion, 4 mo.; general condition, unfavorable; digestion, unimpaired; tubercle bacilli, —; hemorrhage, —; laryngeal symptoms, hoarseness 2 mo., much cough; laryngeal involvement, rt. false cord infiltrated, reddened, rt. arytenoid infiltrated; laryngeal treatment, curette; larynx on discharge, A.; lungs on discharge, improved.

Case 105.—Sex, male; age, 32; pulmonary condition on admission, MAA.; involvement, T. III.; side involved, R. III., L. III.; duration of lesion, 3 years; general condition, unfavorable; digestion, unimpaired; tubercle bacilli, +; hemorrhage, +; laryngeal symptoms, hoarseness, 2 years; laryngeal involvement, interarytenoid space infiltrated and ulcerated cord; laryngeal treatment, curette; larynx on discharge, improved; lungs on discharge, improved.

Case 106.—Sex, male; age, 28; pulmonary condition on admission, incip. A.; involvement, T. I.; side involved, R. II., L. I.; duration of lesion, 2 years; general condition, unfavorable; digestion, unimproved; tubercle bacilli, —; hemorrhage, —; laryngeal symptoms, hoarseness; laryngeal involvement, posterior end left cord ulcerated in post., slight infiltration interarytenoid space; laryngeal treatment, curette; larynx on discharge, A.; lungs on discharge, improved.

Case 107.—Sex, female; age, 41; pulmonary condition on admission, FAA.; involvement, T. II.; side involved, R. II., L. III.; duration of lesion, 4 mo.; general condition, unfavorable; digestion, unimpaired; tubercle bacilli, —; hemorrhage, +; other complications, media spinal lymph gland; laryngeal symptoms, hoarseness; laryngeal involvement, right cord infiltrated and ulcerated, in post. one third slight infiltration;

laryngeal treatment, cautery; larynx on discharge, A.; lungs on discharge, A.

Case 108.—Sex, female; age, 32; pulmonary condition on admission, MAA.; involvement, T. III.; side involved, R. III., L. III.; duration of lesion, 3 years; general condition, unfavorable; digestion, unimpaired; tubercle bacilli, —; hemorrhage, —; laryngeal symptoms, none; laryngeal involvement, interarytenoid, ulceration each true cord; laryngeal treatment, curette; larynx on discharge, A.; lungs on discharge, A.

Case 109.—Sex, male; age, 28; pulmonary condition on admission, incip. A.; involvement, T. I.; side involved, R. II., L., 0.; duration of lesion, 2 years; general condition, favorable; digestion, unimpaired; tubercle bacilli, +; hemorrhage, —; laryngeal symptoms, hoarseness and dysphagia; laryngeal involvement, true cords infiltrated, left cord stationary, interv. space infiltrated; laryngeal treatment, curette; larynx on discharge, improved; lungs on discharge, improved.

Case 110.—Sex, female; age, 30; pulmonary condition on admission, incip.; involvement, T. I.; side involved, R. 0., L. II.; duration of lesion, 9 years; general condition, favorable; digestion, unimpaired; tubercle bacilli, + hemorrhage, +; laryngeal symptoms, hoarseness, 3 mo.; laryngeal involvement, inter. space infiltration and ulceration; laryngeal treatment, routine; larynx on discharge, improved; lungs on discharge, slight improvement.

Case 111.—Sex, female; age, 34; pulmonary condition on admission, FAB.; involvement, T. II.; side involved, T. II., L. I.; duration of lesion, 15 years; general condition, unfavorable; digestion, unimpaired; tubercle bacilli, +; hemorrhage, —; laryngeal symptoms, hoarseness, 4 mo.; laryngeal involvement, infiltration with ulceration of intery. space; laryngeal treatment, curette; larynx on discharge, improved; lungs on discharge, quiescent.

Case 112.—Sex, male; age, 45; pulmonary condition on admission, MA.; involvement, T. II.; side involved, R. III., L. I.; duration of lesion, 3 mo.; general condition, unfavorable; digestion, unimpaired; tubercle bacilli, —; hemorrhage, —; laryngeal symptoms, hoarseness, dysphagia; laryngeal involvement, interarytenoid tuberculoma, infiltration and ulceration true cords and ulceration epiglottis; laryngeal treatment, amputation; larynx on discharge, A.; lungs on discharge, quiescent.

Case 113.—Sex, female; age, 29; pulmonary condition on admission, MAB.; involvement, T. II.; side involved, R. II., L. II.; duration of lesion, 8 years; general condition, unfavorable; digestion, unimpaired; tubercle bacilli, +; hemorrhage, +; laryngeal symptoms, hoarseness; laryngeal involvement, interarytenoid space infiltration; laryngeal treatment, curette and cautery; larynx on discharge, improved; lungs on discharge, unimproved.

Case 114.—Sex, female; age, 35; pulmonary condition on admission, MAB.; involvement, T. III.; side involved, R. III., L. II.; duration of lesion, 17 years; general condition, G. favorable; digestion, impaired; tubercle bacilli, +; hemorrhage, +; laryngeal symptoms, hoarseness; laryngeal involvement, infiltration of interarytenoid space and each arytenoid, ulceration true cords; laryngeal treatment, routine; larynx on discharge, unimproved; lungs on discharge, improved.

Case 115.—Sex, female; age, 25; pulmonary condition on admission, incip. A.; involvement, T. I.; side involved, R. I., L. 0.; duration of lesion, 4 mo.; general condition, favorable; digestion, unimpaired; tubercle bacilli, —; hemorrhage, —; laryngeal symptoms, slight hoarseness, dryness of throat; laryngeal involvement, arytenoids infiltrated; laryngeal treatment, routine; larynx on discharge, improved; lungs on discharge, improved.

Case 116.—Sex, female; age, 32; pulmonary condition on admission, FAB.; involvement, T. II.; side involved, R. II., L. I.; duration of lesion, 7 mo.; general condition, unfavorable; digestion, unimpaired; tubercle bacilli, +; hemorrhage, —; laryngeal symptoms, hoarseness, 4 mo.; laryngeal involvement, each false cord infiltrated, right more marked, interarytenoid space infiltrated; laryngeal treatment, curette; larynx on discharge, A.; lungs on discharge, quiescent.

Case 117.—Sex, female; age, 22; pulmonary condition on admission, FA.; involvement, T. III.; side involved, R. IIII., L. II.; duration of lesion, 18 mo.; general condition, unfavorable; digestion, unimpaired; tubercle bacilli, +; hemorrhage, —; laryngeal symptoms, hoarseness, 2 years; laryngeal involvement, interarytenoid infiltration; laryngeal treatment, curette; larynx on discharge, A.; lungs on discharge, quiescent.

Case 118.—Sex, female; age, 28; pulmonary condition on admission, FAB.; involvement, T. II.; side involved, R. IIII., L. IIII.; duration of lesion, 2 years; general condition, unfavorable; digestion, impaired; tubercle bacilli, +; hemorrhage, +; other complications, tuberculous enteritis; laryngeal symptoms, hoarseness, 8 mo.; laryngeal involvement, interarytenoid infiltration, left cord; laryngeal treatment, curette; larynx on discharge, improved; lungs on discharge, unimproved.

Case 119.—Sex, male; age, 34; pulmonary condition on admission, FAB.; involvement, T. III.; side involved, R. III., L. II.; duration of lesion, 4 years; general condition, G. favorable; digestion, unimpaired; tubercle bacilli, +; hemorrhage, —; laryngeal symptoms, hoarseness; laryngeal involvement, epiglottis infiltration, ulcerated interarytenoid, infiltration left cord; laryngeal treatment, epiglottis removed, arytenoid curettement; larynx on discharge, A.; lungs on discharge, AA.

Case 120.—Sex, female; age, 52; pulmonary condition on admission, FAV.; involvement, T. III.; side involved, R. II., L. III.; duration of lesion, 7 mo.; general condition, unfavorable; digestion, impaired; tubercle bacilli, —; hemorrhage, —: laryngeal symptoms, hoarseness, 8 mo.; larynx involvement, infiltration of each arytenoid, each true cord; laryngeal treatment, curette and cautery; larynx on discharge, A.; lungs on discharge, A.

Case 121.—Sex, male; age, 44; pulmonary condition on admission, MAB.; involvement, T. II.; side involved, R. III., L. I.; duration of lesion, 2½ years; general condition, unfavorable; digestion, unimpaired; tubercle bacilli, +; hemorrhage, +; laryngeal symptoms, pain right tonsil region; laryngeal involvement, arytenoid infiltrated, ulceration each true cord; laryngeal treatment, routine; larynx on discharge, unimproved; lungs on discharge, improved.

Case 122.—Sex, female; age, 20; pulmonary condition on admission, FAB.; involvement, T. III.; side involved, R. II., L. III.; duration of lesion, 1 year; general condition, unfavorable; digestion, impaired; tubercle bacilli, +; hemorrhage. —; laryngeal symptoms, hoarseness 1 year, dysphagia 1 mo.: larynx involvement, epiglottis infiltrated with deep ulceration, interarytenoid space infiltrated, cords ulcerated; laryngeal treatment, amputation of epiglottis; larynx on discharge, unimproved; lungs on discharge, unimproved.

### BIBLIOGRAPHY.

1. Osler:   Practice of Medicine, Ed. VIII.
2. Schroeder:   Deutsche Med. Wochenschrift, Vol. 36, p. 45.
3. St. Clair Thomson:   Practitioner, London.
4. Lockhard:   "Tuberculosis of the Nose and Throat."
5. Steiner:   Archives fur Laryngologic, 26 424, 1912.
6. Turban:   Pulmonary Tuberculosis.
7. Heryng:   Ann. Otol. Rhinol. and Laryngol., 1908, p. 1003.
8. Ruedi:   Zeilschr. fur Ohrenheilknnde, Bd., 73 Hft., 3, 1915, p. 174.
9. St. Clair Thomson:   Lancet, Oct. 18, 1919.
10. Fetterolf:   Laryngoscope, Vol. 26, 1916.

# LXII.

## NAUSEA AS A NASAL REFLEX.

By Greenfield Sluder, M. D.,

St. Louis.

Nausea is a symptom of innumerable clinical conditions. It has been mentioned frequently as a symptom of nasal disorders of one kind or another, descriptions of which may be found on perusal of the literature of the past thirty years. It has, however, always been one of a dozen or more symptoms, all of which might have accompanied any acute inflammatory disease with pain.

Nausea, as an isolated specific reflex from the nose, as far as I know, has not hitherto been observed.

My interest in this phenomenon began ten years ago when I injected the nasal (sphenopalatine-Meckel's) ganglion with plain 95 per cent alcohol. It was not uncommon then to produce nausea by that injection. I have seen such a case in which the patient was nauseated instantly by the injection, vomit for six days, intermittently. I have seen this phenomenon also follow the postethmoidsphenoid operation. Since I have added carbolic acid to the alcohol injection, nausea has been much less frequent, but still sometimes follows. Frequently, in the throes of severe pain produced by any cause, nausea and vomiting occur, a fact which has been well known probably throughout all time. Anything which will stop the pain under these conditions will stop the nausea. So it has happened that on many occasions a severe nasal ganglion neuralgia has been accompanied by nausea, which ceased with the cessation of the pain by anesthetizing the ganglion. Such cases have been quite frequent in my experience; but within the past year I have had a number where there was not any pain, although the nausea was severe. In one severe nasal neuralgia, on many occasions pain was absent, although a purposeless vomiting had continued for twelve hours, and was stopped in five minutes by the application of one drop of 90

per cent cocain to the nasal ganglion district. This has been
repeated many times in this patient.

In another case, one of hyperplastic nonsuppurative sphenoidal headache, marked nausea without headache is sometimes manifest. Applications of one drop of 90 per cent cocain solution to the floor of the sphenoidal cell stops it in about
ten minutes. In this cell the Vidian canal may be felt elevated from the floor about one-half centimeter.

These are two anatomic subdivisions of cases which are to
be thought of as one type, namely, that of sympathetic nervous
system irritations; or at least I should think so. I say this
because of the intrasphenoidal cocainization of the Vidian
nerve in the Vidian canal. Beyond this, I am unable to specu-
late as to the mechanism of this apparently well defined reflex.

These observations indicate that the power of making nausea reflex from the nasal ganglion or the Vidian trunk is independent of any pain complement. They suggest, however,
that in whatever way the reflex is made it is probably not unrelated to that which makes the pain, inasmuch as it is relieved by cocain locally applied, just as the pain reflex is so
stopped. Overdosing with cocain makes nausea return in
these cases.

In this association of speculative thought please see "Asthma
as a Nasal Reflex," by Greenfield Sluder, M. D., Trans. Am.
Med. Assn., Sect. Laryngol., Rhinol. and Otol., 1919.

# LXIII.

## A CASE OF NODULAR HEADACHE OF NASAL (SPHENOPALATINE-MECKEL'S) GANGLIONIC ORIGIN.

By Greenfield Sluder, M. D.,

St. Louis.

Nodular or rheumatic headache, as it is sometimes called, is not frequent compared to other headaches. It is characterized by the presence of nodules from the size of a pea to that of a hazelnut, in some part of the scalp or the nape of the neck, which are supposed to be the cause of the headache. Sometimes they are spoken of as being found lower down in the shoulders.

The theories of their origin and their relation to the headache and the literature concerning the problem are profuse. Those interested will find much in the monographs on migráin.

The case I report is striking.

A lady, 40 years old, gives a clear history of a "lower-half headache" of great severity from her childhood, stating that when it was very bad "knots" came in her neck and over her scalp. She has been my patient for fifteen years, but I never succeeded in seeing her when the "knots" were present until one month ago. At this time she had an unusually severe attack of nasal ganglion neuralgia, for which she consulted me. She spoke of the severity of the attack and called attention to some "knots" in her neck. At the lowermost part of the occiput were two nodules near the middle line, each side, one centimeter wide, and two centimeters long, tender to touch. Full cocainization of the nasal ganglion relieved the pain, and an hour later the node of the right had disappeared. That of the left side was present 24 hours later, but smaller and less sensitive. It disappeared in ten days more.

These are the cases that are spoken of by massage advocates. Auerbach describes them as constant chronic headaches with nodules. Patrick described them as acute or chronic.

Auerbach cut a specimen of one of them out for microscopic examination but could prove nothing. I cannot help thinking that these nodes are manifestations on the part of the sympathetic not unrelated to some of the skin lesions of neurotic sensory or trophic origin. One case, however, must be remembered merely as one case.

I have seen some cases latterly where the nodules were at the locations of lymphatic glands. In these cases the question arose as to whether they were not in reality lymph glands and that the enlargement was brought about through the sympathetic nervous system.

## LXIV.

## RESULT OF THE USE OF THE HEAT HYPEREMIA IN THE ESOPHAGEAL STRICTURE.*

### By L. W. Dean, M. D.,

### Iowa City, Iowa.

The genitourinary specialists have for many years used heat hyperemia to soften the strictures of the urethra before dilating them. Heat has been applied to the strictured part by the use of bags containing hot water and by using electrically heated bougies.

Since last summer we have been using electrically heated flexible esophageal bougies for dilating fibrous esophageal strictures. This procedure has hastened very much the dilating process. In using these bougies for dilating fibrous strictures we have not confined the action of the heat to the production only of heat hyperemia but have used the heat until an edema was produced. In dilating urethral strictures the edema must be avoided because of the blocking of the urethra by the swollen membrane. In esophageal work a slight edema is of advantage; too much edema will close the esophagus, a condition to be avoided.

These elastic electrical bougies are used as follows: A bougie is selected that will fit tightly in the stricture, using a mouth gag to prevent the patient biting the bougie. It is inserted tightly into the stricture. Before insertion the bougie is warmed to 40 degrees centigrade and is left in place for thirty minutes, the bougie remaining at a constant temperature during this time. When the bougie is removed the strictured area is hyperemic; the fibrous tissue appears moist; it is edematous and softened. The dilation is continued immediately after the removal of the heated bougie with nonheated flexible bougies.

These esophageal bougies are made by V. Mueller & Co.

*Read before the Fourth Annual Meeting of the Association of American Peroral Endoscopists, Atlantic City, June, 1921.

Within the bougie and in contact with its wall is a radiator. The temperature of the radiator is controlled by a light socket controller of the Wappler type. A thermometer is inserted into the current to indicate the temperature of the bougie.

· We have secured our best results in old fibrous strictures of adults.

# LXV.

## DOUBLE MASTOIDITIS; PERISINUS ABSCESS; PRO-LONGED POSTOPERATIVE TEMPERATURE; UNUSUAL BLOOD COUNT; RECOVERY WITHOUT FURTHER OPERATION.

By J. L. Maybaum, M. D.,

New York.

Sophie A., age 13 years, was admitted to the Manhattan Eye, Ear and Throat Hospital, April 24, 1920, service of Dr. T. P. Berens, with an acute mastoiditis involving the left ear. Past history as to general and aural disease, negative. There was a history of influenza two months previously, followed by pain in the right ear; ear drum ruptured spontaneously; moderate purulent discharge. She had had considerable pain in the region of the left mastoid for a period of one week before entering the hospital.

Examination on admission: Fairly well nourished, anemic individual. She appeared to be quite ill; temperature, 102; pulse, 84; respirations, 18.

Left ear: Profuse discharge from the middle ear, under tension; small insufficient perforation in left inferior quadrant. Posterior superior wall decidedly sagging. Hearing markedly impaired. Periosteal thickening, extreme tenderness, left mastoid.

Right ear: Slight mucopurulent discharge, perforation in posterior inferior quadrant; drum injected and thickened; landmarks absent excepting short process of the malleus. Hearing function, whisper 10 feet. Resolving right middle ear.

I did a simple mastoidectomy (left) the same evening and found extensively involved mastoid. Free pus under pressure and pale gelatinous granulation throughout. Sigmoid sinus covered with pus and granulations—perisinus abscess.

*Read at the Section on Otology, November 12, 1920.

On the ninth day following the operation on the left mastoid patient began to complain of a recurrence of pain in the right ear. Temperature rose in a few hours from 100 to 104, pulse 90, respirations 22. Right drum bulging and showing small amount of pulsating pus from the perforation in the posterior inferior quadrant.

Although the temperature dropped gradually after the paracentesis and the aural discharge was quite profuse, the pain in the right ear continued during the next twenty-four hours. Slight mastoid tenderness and periosteal thickening. X-ray examination May 2nd, disclosed pus and granulations with beginning bone absorption. The operative findings on the right side differed little from that found at the operation on the left mastoid, except that the perisinus abscess here was smaller in extent and the sinus in the region one-half inch posterior to the knee was covered with granulations. The patient's convalescence from then on was uneventful, and on the 25th of May she left the hospital, returning to the clinic for her dressings. The subsequent course was rather interesting.

On May 29th, she was readmitted to the hospital. She had been feeling well until the evening before, when she became feverish and complained of severe frontal headache. Temperature, 105; pulse, 140; respirations, 24. Dr. Stowell reported general examination, as to heart, lungs and abdomen, negative. Reflexes normal. Both mastoid wounds very satisfactory, showing healthy granulations and slight amount of mucopurulent discharge. During the next two days the temperature fluctuated between 102 and 104 degrees; pulse, 124 to 138; respirations, 24. Two general examinations during this period reported negative. Laboratory reports will be detailed later. On the 7th, 8th, 11th and 24th of June the patient had a distinct sharp rise of temperature, from 99 to 104, 105 and 106 degrees, respectively, followed in each instance by a rapid decline to normal, the third time to subnormal, within twelve hours. A chill of five minutes' duration, the only one throughout her illness, preceded the second rise of temperature.

There was an interval of twenty-four hours between the first and second rises of temperature. Three days between the second and third elevations of temperature, followed during the next two weeks by practically normal temperature, during which the patient's general condition was excellent. There occurred another rise of temperature within a few hours from 100 to 106 degrees and again a rapid decline to normal. From then on the temperature remained within normal limits. The patient left the hospital July 5th, refusing to remain for further observation. At the height of each temperature rise the pulse relative to the temperature was slow, ranging between 100 and 108. Except for general malaise during each elevation of temperature, the patient continued to show a steady improvement in health. The patient returned to the clinic during the next two weeks for her mastoid dressings, at the end of which time she was discharged fully restored to health.

As to laboratory findings: Three blood cultures were taken, showing no growth after fifty-six hours' incubation.

Seven blood counts were made with the following results: May 1, 1919—Leucocytes, 18,600; large mononuclear lymphocytes, 10 per cent; small mononuclear lymphocytes, 2 per cent; polynuclears, 88 per cent. May 2—Leucocytes, 18,200; L. M. L., 10 per cent; S. M. L., 28 per cent; polys., 62 per cent. May 21—Leucocytes, 10,200; L. M. L., 7 per cent; S. M. L., 25 per cent; polys., 68 per cent. June 1, 1919—Leucocytes, 5,600; L. M. L., 40 per cent; S. M. L., 43 per cent; polys., 17 per cent. June 5—Leucocytes, 5,000; L. M. L., 42 per cent; S. M. L., 29 per cent; polys., 28 per cent. June 11—Leucocytes, 7,200; L. M. L., 34 per cent; S. M. L., 8 per cent; polys., 58 per cent. July 3—Leucocytes, 8,400; L. M. L., 28 per cent; S. M. L., 4 per cent; polys., 68 per cent.

The first three blood counts were taken at various times before the first sharp rise of temperature. The second three were taken during the period of temperature rises. The final count was taken ten days after the last temperature elevation. Wassermann, negative. Urine examination, negative. Culture from each mastoid showed streptococcus pyogenes.

A presumptive diagnosis may be made in this case of a sinus thrombosis, the symptoms, considering the various facts in the case, being accounted for by the presence of an aseptic clot in either lateral sinus. The exclusion of any other possible factor responsible for the rises of temperature, together with the general well being of the patient, and three negative blood culture findings would tend to substantiate this diagnosis.

A possible tubercular process was constantly kept in mind because of the repeated findings of lymphocytosis, but physical examinations failed to disclose anything abnormal.

In children a lymphocytosis not infrequently takes the place of a polynucleosis during infectious processes.

Among the factors influencing me in adopting a conservative attitude in this case as to further·surgical interference were:

1. The continued general well being of the patient throughout in spite of her rises of temperature. She could be kept in bed only with the greatest difficulty.

2. The long interval between the third and fourth rises of temperature and the absence of any further rise.

3. Three negative blood cultures.

4. Absence of leucocytosis and polynucleosis, following double mastoidectomy, although typical "sinus thrombosis" temperature rises occurred.

17 EAST 38TH ST.

# LXVI.

## CAVERNOUS SINUS THROMBOSIS OF OTITIC ORIGIN.*

### By J. L. Maybaum, M. D.,

#### New York.

Frank L., 12 years of age, was seen by me at the Manhattan Eye, Ear and Throat Hospital, August 15, 1918, service of Dr. T. P. Berens. The history which he gave was as follows: Previous aural history negative. The patient's parents did not recall that the boy had any of the infectious diseases of childhood; was always in good health until two years ago. At that time he was struck by a brick just above the left ear. He was immediately taken to the Presbyterian Hospital, where he was operated upon for fracture of the skull. After remaining at the hospital for three weeks, he returned home practically restored to health. From then until four weeks ago he had been in excellent health. While bathing at the seashore he developed severe pain in the left ear, frontal headache, followed two days later by a profuse aural discharge. He was treated by his physician for a few days and then referred to a general hospital. His ear symptoms subsided somewhat, but he began to have attacks of continued nausea and vomiting; was treated for a few days for a gastrointestinal condition. At the end of five days he was brought to the Manhattan Hospital, complaining on admission of considerable pain in the left ear and mastoid headache. Two chilly attacks during the last thirty-six hours; fever, nausea and vomiting.

On admission the afternoon of August 15th, the patient appeared extremely ill. His temperature was 103, pulse 96, respirations 20. The temperature rose from 100 to 105 degrees in a few hours; pulse, 110; respirations, 24.

Examination of left ear: A large perforation in postero-superior quadrant, from which foul smelling discharge was

---

*Read at the Section on Otology, November 12, 1921.

escaping.   Marked sagging of the superior bony canal wall.
There was some edema over the right mastoid and exquisite
tenderness, especially over the emissary.   Hearing of the right
ear very much impaired.   No spontaneous nystagmus.   Both
labyrinths reacted within a minute to caloric stimulation.   Pupils react sluggishly.   Some rigidity of the neck present.
Kernig absent.   Knee and abdominal reflexes normal.

Blood count August 15th showed: Leucocytes, 18,500;
polynuclears, 84 per cent.

Nothing abnormal was found on thorough physical examination of the heart, lungs and abdomen.

I did a lumbar puncture before operating and withdrew
10 cc. of cloudy spinal fluid under increased pressure.

On operating that evening, I found an extensively involved
mastoid.   Large perisinus abscess.   The sigmoid sinus from
the knee down had a dirty yellow grayish appearance, and pus
could be seen oozing from an area of the sinus about one-
fourth of an inch in diameter near the knee.   The sinus exposure was carried back for a distance of more than half way
toward the torcular end before normal appearing sinus wall
was reached.   This part of the sinus was covered with granulations.   The usual degree of exposure of the sigmoid sinus at
the lower limit was carried out.   There were no granulations
covering this part of the sinus from the perforated sloughed
area to the lower end of the exposure.   The sinus wall, however, had a grayish, thickened, lusterless appearance.   An
extradural abscess was found in the region of the posterior
fossa near the knee.   Exposure of dura of middle fossa over
tegmen antri disclosed nothing abnormal.

A jugular resection was done.   The vein was collapsed
almost to the clavicular end.

On opening the sinus a partly disintegrated clot was found
in the sigmoid sinus—no bleeding from the jugular end.   There
was a firmer clot in horizontal part of the sinus, upon removal
of which free bleeding occurred.

The patient reacted fairly well following the operation.   On
visiting him the next morning I noticed considerable edema of
the left eyelid.   Other evidences of a cavernous sinus throm-

bosis soon followed. Exophthalmos became marked. The ocular conjunctiva showed a pronounced chemosis; pupil of left eye dilated and fixed. Because of the dulled sensorium of the patient and rapidly increasing edema of the eyelid, the question of ocular mobility could not be determined. The symptoms which were present previous to operation—evidences of meningeal involvement—continued unabated. Daily fluctuations of temperature between 100 and 104 degrees. The last three days the temperature continued high, remissions being less marked. On the third day following the operation the right eye became similarly involved. The condition grew progressively worse, the patient lapsing into coma, dying the seventh day after his admission to the hospital. No autopsy was permitted.

Laboratory findings: Culture from the mastoid, streptococcus mucosus. Blood culture negative. Cerebrospinal fluid at the time of operation, turbid; sugar absent; trace of albumen, marked degree of lactic acid, contained abundant mononuclear and polynuclear leucocytes. Bacteriologic examination negative.

The findings in the cerebrospinal fluid together with the symptoms on admission would indicate that the patient had on entering the hospital, in addition to a jugular thrombophlebitis, at least a circumscribed purulent meningitis.

The above case of cavernous sinus thrombosis is reported not only because of the comparative rarity of that form of otitic sinus disease, but because of the lesion since then derived from this experience. The prognosis of these cases is recognized to be quite hopeless, because of the inaccessibility of the cavernous sinus to such surgical procedures as are applicable to the lateral sinus.

Wherever in a case of lateral sinus thrombosis the bleeding from the jugular end is absent or where, after the lateral sinus has been opened, clinical evidence of septic absorption continues from a clot on the bulb, the jugular bulb should be opened and drained, provided, however, the general condition of the patient permits of such a procedure. During the past few years Dr. Whiting has repeatedly demonstrated this to be

feasible.   I believe he has not as yet published his work along
these lines.   Dr. Friesner time and again, during the last year,
has demonstrated upon the cadaver the comparative ease with
which the jugular bulb can be thoroughly opened and drained
without endangering the facial nerve.   He further enlarges
the approach to the bulb by removing the jugular process of
the occiput.   I have followed this procedure upon the cadaver
a considerable number of times during the past year and have
myself noted the facility and safety with which this operation
can be performed.

17 EAST 38TH ST.

# SOCIETY PROCEEDINGS.

## THE FORTY-THIRD ANNUAL CONGRESS OF THE AMERICAN LARYNGOLOGICAL ASSOCIATION, HELD AT ATLANTIC CITY, MAY 30 TO JUNE 1, 1921.

Reported by

Emil Mayer, M. D., Abstract Editor, and

C. J. Imperatori, M. D., Assistant Abstract Editor.

### President's Address.

After expressing his gratification at the honor bestowed upon him by his election to the presidency of this Association, and introducing the distinguished guests, Dr. Mosher presented the following as part of his presidential address:

### The Liver Tunnel and Cardiospasm.

By Harris P. Mosher, M. D.,

Boston, Mass.

Last year I reported the cadaver findings in thirty cases of the injected esophagus and stomach of adults and sixty injected and dissected babies. I have recently supplemented these by clinical observations. One set of findings has proved to supplement the other. The result of my observations can be summed up as follows: First, a free passage through the subdiaphragmatic esophagus depends upon the potency of the liver tunnel; second, in ten cases of cardiospasms of which I have sufficient data to draw conclusions, there was either a partical crescentic stricture, or a full annular stricture at the beginning of the liver tunnel and opposite the upper edge of the left lobe of the liver. So far as my cases go, stricture and not spasm was found to be the chief causative factor. More cases are necessary in order to determine whether or not the high percentage of stricture in cases of cardio spasm which I found is constant.

The basic fact of my paper of last year was that the liver is chiefly responsible for the shape of the lower end of the esophagus. The subdiaphragmatic portion of the esophagus runs in a tunnel of liver, and according to the closeness of the investing liver, is either flaring and trumpet shaped, or narrow and cone shaped. Plates of the lower end of the esophagus often show it ending in a nipple like point. Between this and the fundus of the stomach there is a gap. This gap is the closed liver tunnel. I demonstrated in my last paper that the upper edge of the liver often makes a crease in the front wall of the espohagus, and that this crease is present at birth. The left crus makes a crease in the posterior wall of the esophagus and a marked notch in its left edge. Experiments on the cadaver show that the crescentic mound which is often seen through the esophagus in the right half of the field as the liver is approached, is made by the upper rim of the liver. I asked Dr. Gordon of the X-Ray Department of the Massachusetts General Hospital to prove, if possible, that the upper border of the liver exerted appreciable pressure on the front surface of the esophagus in the living. The result of our combined observations is that in a majority of normal cases there is an appreciable delay of the bismuth milk at the upper border of the liver when a patient swallows. Dr. Gordon made the further observation that when the diaphragm is lowered the bismuth milk, which is held back momentarily by the liver edge, shoots at once into the stomach. Putting the patient in a position which causes the liver to fall away from the esophagus and so relieving the esophagus of liver pressure, also to make the fluid pass into the stomach more easily.

I have found in the cadaver four specimens of annular stricture of the lower part of the esophagus. Each one caps a circumscribed dilatation of the esophagus, which is bounded below by the constriction caused by the left crus. Each stricture is on a level with the upper edge of the left lobe of the liver.

In three cases of cardiospasm of which I have good records, the diaphragm was moderately lowered in one and markedly lowered in the other two.

In grouping my cases of cardiospasm I find that there is an element of stricture in the majority of them, and this stricture is by preference at the beginning of the liver tunnel at the upper edge of the liver.

The stricture element found in my cases varied from a slight crescentic fold in the right quadrant of the esophagoscope in the region of the hiatus to a full annular stricture with a central opening. In the cases which showed the crescentic fold, steady pressure with the end of the esophagus usually resulted in the tube slipping by into the normal esophagus below and through this into the stomach. The withdrawal of the tube disclosed a vertical slit in the mucous membrane of the esophagus. I have held these cases to be analagous to partial webs at the mouth of the esophagus. I have records of three cases in which there was a full stricture with a central opening. This stricture was at the hiatus, or rather at the upper edge of the liver. On divulsing the stricture with the mechanical dilator a crescentic mounding was seen in the right field. Steady pressure with the tube caused the tube to pass this and enter the subdiaphragmatic esophagus and then continue on into the stomach. This mound I now believe to be the upper edge of the liver.

I have one case which showed a narrowing of the whole length of the liver tunnel. We have, then, as my cases show, strictures at the upper or lower edge of the liver tunnel, or anywhere in its course, or we can have a narrowed liver tunnel or a stiffened tunnel through which the food runs slowly. My observations would seem to show that spasm is a minor element in these cases, that some form of stricture is generally present. I believe that the strictures are due to some inflammatory process either within the liver tunnel or in the vicinity of the cone of the diaphragm.

What causes these partial and full strictures to form at the upper edge of the liver tunnel? I found one case in which there was healed tubercular process of the lumbar vertebra opposite the upper edge of the liver and opposite the stricture. The fact that in the majority of normal cases the upper edge of the liver causes a momentary delay in swallowing and that the knifelike edge of the liver often markedly indents the front face of the esophagus makes this part of the esophagus vulnerable and subject to trauma. I feel that narrowing of the liver tunnel due to an inflammatory involvement of the lesser omentum will be found in the future to play a large part, if not the greatest part, in producing these strictures connected with cases of cardiospasm. Where does the inflammation originate? It can originate in any part of the peritoneal cavity. Below the diaphragm the peritoneum runs from the lesser curvature of the stomach to the liver, making the lesser omentum and bounding the foramen of Winslow. The subdiaphragmatic esophagus is bathed in this peritoneal tissue. This shares in the inflammations, acute and chronic, of the rest of the peritoneal tissue of the abdominal cavity. When the lesser omentum becomes involved, the liver tunnel becomes less flexible, the liver and diaphragm less mobile, and we have the familiar result which has been styled temporary cardiospasm, that is, there is difficulty in swallowing. It is well known that disease of the gall bladder, cancer of the lesser curvature of the stomach, and if cancer can cause it, ulcer can do the same, and disease of the appendix are associated with cardiospasm. In one of my cases of full stricture the patient, when an infant, swallowed a two-cent piece. In another case, the patient gave a history of general peritonitis twenty years ago.

I have proved to my satisfaction that many of these so-called cases of cardiospasm are mainly cases of stricture of the upper end of the liver tunnel.

### Tonsillectomies in Adults for Rheumatism With Critical Review of Results.

By Hill Hastings, M. D.,

Los Angeles, Cal.

Much that has been written of the tonsil operation deals with the surgical technic. Comparatively little has appeared in laryngological literature dealing with clinical problems or the results from the patient's standpoint.

The limitations are:

First. All adult cases in which tonsillectomies were done solely for ear, nose and throat diseased conditions are excluded.

Second. Cases that date back over six years are excluded.

Third. All cases are excluded that are of shorter duration of observation than four months.

Tables are presented showing ages, duration of rheumatism, parts affected, character of rheumatism with results of tonsillectomy, throat history, and subsequent history of 130 cases.

The subsequent results are based on personal examination of the patients by the writer, by the internists or by the orthopedist, and checked up by questionnaires received from all of the 130 cases, except 26 who could not be located. 39.5% were improved. Some of them gradually growing worse, some of the remaining stationary. In this whole series of tonsillectomies there were no hopelessly chronic cases operated, and it would seem that the percentage of "not improved," i.e., 21% should not have been so high; nevertheless, one feels that many of the cases that were marked "improved" might have become hopelessly chronic but for the tonsil surgery. A review of the cases of rheumatism marked "cured" is worth while. Of the 40 cases in which apparent cure resulted, 22 were diagnosed "chronic arthritis mild"; 11 were acute arthritis cases, and 5 were diagnosed "myalgia". A general survey of these cases showed that most of these patients had suffered for years, but not continuously, with pain and stiffness in one or several joints, at times acute and temporarily crippling. A few were crippled for months before operation. Orthopedic measures of various kinds had been tried. A few of them gave a history of symptoms of tonsil trouble; some no history of throat trouble. In 7 cases the history showed an acute tonsillitis as a forerunner of the rheumatism. In other cases an accumulation in a tonsil crypt caused rheumatic symptoms.

It has been the writer's experience to find that adult patients suffering from toxic symptoms are referred to the laryngologist for his decision as to whether or not the tonsil is the seat of a chronic infection. Other patients come with the statements that their tonsils have been pronounced infected or that a culture that has been made from the crypts showed chronic infection. The writer has taken some pains to inform all such patients that every adult's tonsil is a chronic infected tonsil, from which a positive culture can be made. The same is probably true of most tonsils in children. Therefore, the necessity for a tonsillectomy depends not solely upon the examination by a laryngologist, but upon a complete study of the patient to determine all possible factors responsible for the invalidism, rheumatism, heart trouble, etc.

### Results of the Treatment by X-Ray and Radium of Diseased Tonsils and Adenoids.

By D. Bryson Delavan, M. D.,
New York City.

Suggestions have recently been made that lymphoid hypertrophies can be radically cured by radiation, both from the X-Ray and from radium. Investigations have been carried on under exceptionally favorable conditions and several interesting results have been obtained.

Whether the presence of pathogenic organisms in the tonsillar crypts is the result of hypertrophy or whether the hypertrophy arises from another set of conditions, there is no question that enlarged tonsils with resultant poorly drained crypts have a pathologic significance. The other lymphoid deposits which occur in various parts of the pharynx, usually at the vault, lateral walls and base of the tongue, commonly show alterations similar to those found in the tonsil. It has been proved in general that lymph cells are powerfully influenced by radiation, doses very much smaller than those required to affect other tissues being sufficient to destroy them.

To summarize: Very small amounts of X-Ray are sufficient for the reduction of lymphoid tissue, doses so small than no injury, it is claimed, results to other parts from its application. The current used is too weak to affect even the external integument, but sufficiently strong, nevertheless, to destroy the lymphoid tissue, and no scar tissue is left behind. The rays themselves do not destroy bacteria, hence they do not affect concealed abscesses of the tissue. They act by so modifying the crypts that free drainage from them is secured, and thus the crypts continue to empty themselves of all offending contents. As the tonsil atrophies, the infection will disappear from the opening up and drainage of the crypts. The principle of this procedure, long recognized, has been carried out surgically for many years, in many cases with excellent results. Dr. Murphy maintains that little atrophy will result in the case of fibrous tonsils, since the rays have no effect upon fibrous tissue. This being true, such cases must continue to be treated surgically, as heretofore.

Moreover, since radiation does not affect bacteria, its application in cases of concealed chronic abscesses of the tonsil will be ineffective, an unfortunate circumstance, in view of the prevalence of this condition.

That the method of treatment by radiation will quickly come into general use is improbable. The region of the neck is one containing numerous important anatomical structures which must be carefully guarded against injury. All agree that knowledge of the safe and effective use of both X-ray and radium is acquired only through highly intelligent study and much experience. Far better that experiments be carried on by those qualified for the work than that the success of a method of such good promise should be compromised and perhaps discredited through errors due to incomplete understanding of the medium, or to faulty technic in its application. Knowledge of the subject is in its infancy, and far more study and observation are needed to prove the value of the few theories already suggested; but what has already been done has dveloped questions of greatest interest, not to be settled by theoretical discussion but by painstaking experimentation and accurate scientific observation.

## Must It Always Be Tonsillectomy?

By Henry L. Swain, M. D.

New Haven, Conn.

Dr. Swain, having in mind the frequency with which in late years the tonsil was looked upon as the cause of an astonishingly large number of diseases and symptoms affecting the comfort and menacing the lives of patients, and while recognizing the perfectly laudable desire on the part of the operator to get rid of the tonsil—root and branch—felt that we as a profession ought not to leave out of our consideration the fact that there are other methods than tonsillectomy, which are safe, sane, sure, and enduring in their results, whenever we wished to employ them. These methods did not endanger life, did not subject the patient to the often very distressing effects of serious hemorrhage, avoided the chance of lung abscess, brought the patient out of the affray with undistorted and nonadherent palates, and without even the disturbance of their daily routine of life. From his own experience with a simple method of slitting up intercommunicating crypts and other retention pockets, punching out undesirable tissue areas and, if necessary, shrinking the tonsils by galvanocautery procedures, he was able, very often, by the same process, to prove tonsils guilty, and to make them cease from troubling, achieving frequently as spectacular and permanent results thereby as he or anybody else ever attained by perfect tonsillectomies. While preparing this paper he not only discovered that he was not, as he thought, alone, but many others had had similar results by other means, and had only lately been made acquainted with the brilliant results of work by X-ray exposures.

With all these observations well carried out and thoroughly followed up in his own case for years, he felt that the original question was answered, that it was not always necessary to do a complete tonsillectomy, to remove the threat and menace of the faucial tonsil.

## DISCUSSION.

Dr. Joseph L. Goodale, Boston, Mass.: I think that the Society is extremely fortunate in having listened to these three papers, which show that there is still something to be said in regard to the subject of the tonsil. I want to ask Dr. Hastings to tell us whether in these cases it is possible for him to ascertain absolutely whether there has been an unusually large proportion of what we might call anaphylactic types among the twenty per cent of arthritic cases that failed to show improvement? I ask this, because he suggested the hypothesis that certain arthritic cases may conceivably be explained on the ground of previous sensitization of the joints, which, in subsequent infection, were again brought into prominence—not through direct penetration of bacteria, but through toxins generated in the tonsils finding response in the joints. I have myself seen a case of what I have called ingestion anaphylaxis giving rise to arthritis. At the suggestion of the orthopedic surgeon. I tested the patient with various proteids and got a definite reaction to meat and potato. These two articles were then omitted from his dietary; and within ten days the joint symptoms disappeared. He then gave these foods up, and again the joint symptoms disappeared; and he has been well ever since. I have not seen him for a year; but when I last saw him, he was entirely well.

In regard to Dr. Delavan's paper, the cases that we can influence are chiefly the juvenile. In the senile ones, with evident symptoms resulting from absorption, I question whether we can accomplish so much.

Dr. Joseph H. Bryan, Washington, D. C.: My experience is confined to five or six cases. I will report three of these. The others are still under observation. In case 1, the patient, a gentleman, came down last September with influenza, and then suddenly developed localized pneumonia with endocarditis and nephritis. He was critically ill for a few days, and finally overcame the invasion of bacteria; but he had a marked prostration, which continued for several months. He was unable even to walk to my office. a distance of only three blocks, and had to take a cab. The nephritis continued long after the other complications had cleared up, and while I knew that he had had bad tonsils, it did not appear to me that they might be the cause of the continued nephritic condition. The tonsils were buried in fibrous tissue and examinations of them showed the presence of two kinds of streptococcus, viridans and hemolyticus. The patient received six applications of the X-rays. and the nephritis cleared up completely, although the bacterial contents of the tonsils remained the same. The organisms were not destroyed. The man was a bad surgical risk and could not have had a tonsillectomy performed under local anesthesia on account of the condition of his throat; and he could not have taken a general anesthetic. I do not know whether the good results in this case was due to opening the crypts and increasing the drainage, or to shutting off the lymphatics and preventing invasion of the system by the bacteria from the tonsils; but the case was successful.. In the second case, there was marked fibrosis of the tonsils on both sides, with arthritis of the knee. The patient was a woman of sixty-five years, who had refused to have the tonsils taken out, and I was glad that she had come to that decision. I had the X-rays applied. She had marked streptococcus hemolyticus infection. There has been no reduction in the amount of tonsil tissue, so far as we can. tell. There may be in the amount of the lymphoid tissue, but the mass as a whole is the same as before; and the organisms are as numerous as formerly. I do not believe that any improvement at all occurred. In the third case. the patient was a lady of seventy-three years who had glaucoma and infected tonsils. The tonsils were small and soft and contained streptococcus hemolyticus and viridans. The X-ray was applied, and the tonsils have been completely absorbed. They were twice the size of a marrowfat pea. The organism has been changed from viridans to hemolyticus. There has been great improvement in her general health and in her eye. We have had remarkable results in this case. I believe that her general health benefit will continue, and the ophthalmologist feels that there is a possibility of further improvement to the eye. Of the other cases, I have had one case in a child of twelve years. who had tonsils and adenoids combined. I am not able to report on that condition yet. I believe that this is a valuable adjunct to our treatment. particularly in selected cases, but I do not believe that it will supplant surgery.

Dr. Cornelius G. Coakley, New York City: About ten days ago, I reported before the New York Academy of Medicine the results of our survey of tonsils that we had operated on during the past twelve years (about one hundred and forty-six) for rheumatism; and our results were above eighty-five per cent of very marked improvement or cure. It is very disappointing, especially in a case of acute polyarthritis, to find that some patients will have acute polyarthritis in spite of complete enucleation of the tonsil and as much of the lymphoid tissue as possible. With reference to the use of the X-ray on the tonsil, if there are fifty-five thousand people in New York who need treatment of the tonsil, apparently the X-ray is not going to be of much benefit in reducing this number. The actual time of using the ray is three to five minutes, but it has to be repeated from five to seven times. Therefore, the total time consumed is certainly more per individual patient than that when surgery is employed. There is no question that the X-ray will reduce the size of the lymphoid tissue. It has been used for years for that purpose in the case of severe lymph nodes in the neck. thymus gland cases and some cases of sarcoma, producing a reduction in the size of the tissue. The question, however, comes up, "What effect will simply reducing the size of the tissue have on the infective material?" The first statement made was that the tonsil was sterilized as the result of this procedure. The Rockefeller Institute cultured the tonsils before and after it, and found various organisms before and also afterwards, and all the tonsils were sterile afterwards. It just happens that three persons so treated, complaining of various socalled rheumatisms, have come under my care. One of these patients I had seen before being X-rayed, but I had not cultured the tonsil. I cultured it afterwards and found streptococci. The symptoms of none of these patients were in any way ameliorated as the result of the treatment, and they were very bad operative risks. One, a man sixty-five years of age, with more than two per cent of sugar and diacetic acid, did not have his symptoms a bit relieved. We have had two cases besides these three in which we advocated the use of the X-ray in the hope that it would do something for them in the way of reducing the size of the lymphoid tissue and reducing the severity of the symptoms. I am afraid that it will be found eventually that the X-ray or radium will unquestionably reduce the size of the tonsils; but whether it will put the tonsils in such a shape as to free them from infection, especially in the case of small sized tonsils, I have great doubt.

Dr. Lewis A. Coffin, New York City: The trouble seems to be altogether with those tonsils that do not free themselves of pus or crypt secretion and accumulation. The retained matter acting as an irritant or infecting agent causes local inflammatory or distant infectious conditions. The size of the tonsil per se has nothing to do with it. We all know that the large Irish potato-looking tonsil, filling out half of the pharynx, is the most innocent of tonsils except for its physical in-the-wayness.

The problem of the tonsil is solved if the crypts are thoroughly drained or rendered aseptic. If radium or the X-ray when safely used will do this (which I doubt) then hands up for radium or the X-ray.

Dr. Swain accomplished the desired ends by splitting up the crypts and the application of some of the various antiseptics. Probably every man present has accomplished the same end by the same means.

Interesting questions are why some tonsils develop and interfere with their own drainage, and again. can one do anything to prevent such development.

Dr. J. Payson Clark, Boston, Mass.: I should like to report briefly a case which I think worth recording, both on account of the age of the patient and on account of the happy result of tonsillectomy. She was sixty-nine years old and had had rheumatism in the chief joints with considerable pain. She had had tonsillitis three years in succession. followed by a stiffness in the finger joints. There were buried tonsils, full of cheesy material, especially in the crypts of the tonsils. In this case, the history and the appearance of the tonsil seemed to point pretty conclusively to this being the source of the trouble, yet in a patient of that age, I hesitated to advise tonsillectomy. I referred her to an orthopedist, who gave her a thorough examination, and said the arthritis was of combined origin. He thought the tonsillar ailment important, but advised simple measures first. She went under treatment for several months without improvement. Finally she said that she had decided to have the tonsil out. I removed the tonsils on the 17th of May, 1918. She had remarkably little trouble afterwards. She was able to eat by the next day. I was apprehensive that she might have a great deal of pain and discomfort. The right tonsil was very adherent. She went to the country on the 19th, and I got a letter on the 24th saying that she had had no more pain in the joints. but that they were still stiff. This chronic process had been going on for so many years that there were changes in the joints that could not be relieved by operation. Two years afterwards she said that she was free from pain and could walk with more ease, and that she was much pleased with the result of the operation. Slitting the tonsils, of course, is a procedure which has been successful in the hands of many. of us. Suction in the crypts, I think a valuable treatment in suitable cases.

Dr. George L. Richards, Fall River, Mass.. I should like Dr. Delavan to tell us about the tendency to dryness of the mouth and throat. Even with ordinary tonsillectomies, there is a certain amount of dryness resulting in a certain percentage of cases. All forms of new treatment pass through a stage of enthusiasms, a stage of criticism, and a stage of hostility. Is that going to ensue with this type of work, roentgen and radium? There is no doubt that the X-ray and radium will destroy lymphatic tissue, but is it not possible that in this destruction we shall have ill results, not in a year, but in some later period?

Dr. Harmon Smith, New York City: I will omit answering Dr. Swain and Dr. Hastings. and confine myself what I have to say to the X-ray and radium. We all know that in the application of both X-ray and radium they benefit a malignant tumor by the production of endarteritis. The application does not destroy the tumor; it shuts off the blood supply, and shrinks down the mass. The first blood supply is very primitive. When we cut it off, the diseased tissue shrinks in due course of time; but nature establishes a new blood supply of more lasting character; and the tumor begins to grow again. When, in the application of raying, it does not destroy the lymphatic tissue but shuts off the blood supply to the lymphatic channels. the tissue shrinks; and when the blood supply begins to reestablish itself, as it will, if the patient live long enough, you will have an increased growth of the mass.

. Dr. John R. Winslow, Baltimore, Md.: The X-ray and radium will destroy tissue, lymphoid tissue included. Radium has been used for that purpose; what proof have we that it will not destroy more important structures in the neck? If it will destroy these tissues, why will it not destroy important endocrine structures—the parathyroids, for instance? In applying the X-ray to the naso-pharynx, I think that there is a certain possibility of the production of a meningitis. In fact. this has occurred in the treatment of tumors in this region with radium. These are points that I should like to present to you. In the treatment of comparatively simple hypertrophy, such as that of tonsils and adenoids, I do not think that the time element is much reduced or that the safety is much greater, as compared with surgery.

Dr. Hastings, Los Angeles, Cal. (closing): We should study our cases thoroughly before deciding for or against operation. It would be interesting to study those cases in which we did not operate to see if secondary focal symptoms developed. It would also be interesting to study a group of cardiovascular cases in the same way I have attempted to study this group of rheumatic cases.

Dr. Goodale asked whether there had been anaphylactic reactions noticed in the uncured cases. My attention was not brought to such reactions. Such may have been the factor in the case reported where the patient starved himself for twenty-six days on account of rheumatism with marked improvement, symptoms recurring on beginning to eat.

Dr. Delavan, New York City (closing): The thesis just presented was prepared at the request of the president of the Association, who desired that the subject of the treatment of diseased tonsils by X-ray and radium be brought before the Association for explanation and discussion. My object has been to record the latest facts and theories pertaining to it, not yet venturing positive opinions of my own. In the present stage of the investigation. it would seem that our attitude should be one of receptivity. This seems to have been submerged in a wave of rather premature objection. By no means all of the propositions regarding the use of radium in this connection have been scientifically established. Much more must be learned and proved before the method can be accepted as effective and safe. One fact, however, seems to have been definitely demonstrated, namely, that radium exerts a powerful influence upon lymphoid tissue. even when applied in very small doses. It has also been proved that there are certain other things which it will not do. One of these is to reduce fibrous tissue. Another is to destroy the activity of septic germs. By so much at least its value in the treatment of the tonsils is negative. In certain other conditions referred to in the paper the success of its application seems fully to warrant more extended investigation. The worth of the method is being scientifically tested in the best hands. When the tests have been carried on for a sufficient length of time, we shall know more about the subject. At present the situation is tentative.

Dr. Swain, New Haven, Conn. (closing): I have worked a good

deal on what I have presented to you. It has been conscientiously done. so.that I am able to assure you that the details have been carefully gone over, and I think that there are several safe methods to eliminate the tonsil, as the cause of trouble. You can do it in one of these ways, and not do a tonsillectomy. I agree with Dr. Hastings' experience in one of his cases in considering these focal infection cases, that we must remember that we have twenty-six feet of intestines of which the tonsil is only the beginning.

### Ventriculocordectomy—A New Operation for the Cure of Goitrous Paralytic Laryngeal Stenosis.

By Chevalier Jackson, M. D.,
Philadelphia.

The literature of laryngeal stenosis is so burdened by the premature reports of cases that the author has waited for the lapse of time to prove the permanency of what he believes to be an ideal operation for the cure of that form of stenosis associated with bilateral recurrent paralysis when the stenosis is due solely to the paralysis. In these cases, tracheotomy has usually been already done for urgent dyspnea, and the patient comes to the laryngologist for decannulation.

Technic: No anesthetic, general or local. was used in children. In adults, cocaine was painted on with a swab and a sedative of morphine gr. ¼, was given hypodermatically an hour before operation. The larynx was exposed with the direct laryngoscope and through it the punch forceps were inserted. The ventricular band was elevated and the forceps applied. Thus the floor of the ventricle and part of the mucosa of its outer wall was removed at one clip. A clear cut is necessary. The tissues must not be hacked. In some cases the ventricular bands were in tight apposition, so that the forceps were insinuated between them before expanding the jaws. Great care should be taken to avoid getting too far outward between the thyroid and cricoid cartilages lest the cricoarytenoideus lateralis be injured. With the forceps used, this accident is easily avoided. Great care should also be taken not to excise any part of the arytenoid cartilage. The clipping off of the extreme tip of the vocal process of the arytenoid was necessary in some of the cases because of the shortness of the cord; but the excision of more than this is unnecessary and should be avoided. It may not be amiss here to state that, judging from experience in postgraduate teaching at the Bronchoscopic Clinic, few laryngologists seem to realize how far the vocal process of the arytenoid projects forward toward the anterior commissure. To perform the operation, however, requires education of the eye and the fingers in endoscopic technic. Of course, the excision of cord and ventricular floor can be done by laryngofissure, but here we have, though not a serious operation, yet one that will appear much more formidable to the patient. No after treatment is necessary. The surface of the wound is covered with an exudate under which healing by granulation progresses. In one case, a granuloma appeared at the site of the wound, and excision was done lest it later lessen the lumen of the airway. In two cases a slight degree of perichondritis was present, after the excision of the second cord and ventricular floor; but it subsided spontaneously in about a month. In one case the lumen of the airway was not quite sufficient, and prolonged treatment with the McKee divulsor was necessary to increase it. Bouginage can be used for this purpose after ventriculocordectomy, though it or any other form of dilation is useless before removal of the obstructive cord and its supporting tissues. The duration of the operation done endoscopically on one side only, was never over one minute in any case, not counting the time required to paint on the cocaine solution. The healing has not required more than three weeks in any case and in some cases healing was completed in 10 days.

Conclusions: 1. In ventriculocordectomy I believe we have a simple endoscopic operation that can be done under local anesthesia and that will cure almost every case of laryngeal stenosis due solely to abductor paralysis if the case is not complicated by a faulty tracheotomy.

2. Ventriculocordectomy is indicated in cases of stenosis resulting from a hopelessly paralyzed larynx.

3. This or any other form of operative clearing of the airway is contraindicated in the first six months of abductor laryngeal paralysis. In most cases it is wise to wait a year.

4. The best means of affording relief of dyspnea and safety of the patient during this waiting period is by prompt low tracheotomy. High tracheotomy is the cause of more cases of cicatrical laryngeal stenosis than any other one thing. With a low tracheotomy, a pair of proper cannulae and a daily toilet of the fistula there is nothing lost by waiting.

5. Out of 18 cases ventriculocordectomized the 7 that were uncomplicated by cicatricial stenosis were afforded by this procedure alone satisfactory relief of dyspnea. One required divulsion in addition.

6. The chief functions of the larynx are phonetic, protective and expectorative. Considered in the light of the degree of preservation of these functions, ventriculocordectomy, I venture to think, not only surpasses any previously devised operation, but is simply ideal for those cases in which neural and muscular atrophy has rendered resumption of normal cordal motility hopeless by either spontaneous recovery or neuroplastic surgery.

## DISCUSSION.

Dr. D. Bryson Delavan. New York City: We know that methods similar to this have been employed, not only in the surgery of the human being, but in veterinary surgery; and any betterment in the process and what might be called standardization of the treatment is welcome.

Dr. Robert Clyde Lynch, New Orleans, La.: I have seen but two or three cases of this type of paralysis, but it struck me, during his description of the reason for the regeneration of the vocal cord. that in these cases of infralaryngeal carcinoma which I have operated on by suspension, and in which I have evidently removed a good portion of the vocal process of arytenoid cartilege and muscle, there has been no effort on the part of nature to reform any portion of the cord whatever. I was at a loss to know why this has occurred; since in cases of thyrotomy, the cords do reform, or something reforms which takes the place of the vocal cords. That has been noticed in the cases that I have operated on by intralaryngeal resection. None of the cases have shown any disposition to renew the cord. The space remained wide open, and as if this were rubbed out entirely. Possibly this may add something to the theory of regeneration of the cord.

Dr. Cornelius G. Coakley, New York City: We have seen, in this connection, in our service at the Bellevue Hospital, two or three cases a year. The only treatment that we have been using has been that of tracheotomy. Most of our cases are those which come as the result of central lesions or bulbar paralyses. I should like to ask Dr. Jackson, first, whether he considers that it is necessary, in long standing, slowly developing cases of bulbar paralysis. to do the tracheotomy; and second, how much hemorrhage he gets during the operation on small children?

Dr. Joseph B. Greene, Ashville, N. C.: I have several patients under observation at the present time who should have some treatment, and I shall refer them to Dr. Jackson.

Dr. Henry L. Swain, New Haven, Conn.: I should like to know what proportion of cases have to have the double ventriculocordectomy, and what vocal results Dr. Jackson gets—what proportion of patients can speak audibly enough to be understood in a noisy place.

Dr. Emil Mayer, New York City: I should like to ask Dr. Jackson to let us know what local anesthetic he uses; what is the manner of application; and the strength of that particular local anesthetic.

Dr. Swain, New Haven, Conn.: Is that forceps big enough for a grown man? Will it give space enough?

Dr. Chevalier Jackson, Philadelphia, Pa. (closing): In these cases of tabes, disseminated sclerosis and other conditions that are eventually fatal, although not for a long period of years, it is a question for the patient to decide as to whether or not he will get along with tracheotomy palliation. or whether he wants this operation done. In many of these patients the paralysis becomes total. That is, the cord assumes a cadaveric position in the first cord before the other becomes paralyzed. In that case, where one cord becomes cadaveric before the other one, the patient has a chink large enough to get along with. When the second cord becomes paralyzed, he does not asphyxiate because the other cord is in the cadaveric position.

In regard to the matter of the voice, the patients must be told that the voice will be reduced to a whisper for quite a number of months. Then it will be a stage whisper, and later they will phonate; and in a year or so, they will have a voice that can be heard across the room. It is a deep, rough voice, without modulation; but abundantly loud for all ordinary purposes. It is particularly to the goitrous cases that the operation is adapted. Their expectation of life is longer than in other cases. In tabes and disseminated sclerosis, it is not so long; although many survive for years.

With regard to Dr. Swain's question about the necessity of doing a double operation, after making a section on one side, usually about a month elapses before I do the second cord. If the patient should feel that he has plenty of air to get along with, the second cord may not need operation; but I should not feel justified in abandoning the tracheotomy canula in that case.

Regarding the name of the operation, the floor of the ventricle is excised; and that is why I use the term ventroculocordectomy, faulty though it may seem.

With regard to Dr. Mayer's question about the anesthetic, twenty percent cocaine was sufficient in most cases. Most of the patients were adults; but one was a child, in whom no anesthetic, local or general, was needed.

Dr. Coakley. My questions were not answered. Is preliminary tracheotomy necessary? Has there been much hemorrhage?

Dr. Jackson: With regard to preliminary tracheotomy, in the cases of bilateral paralysis in which one cord had become cadaveric, the patients will get along without tracheotomy; but I always feel that it is better to tracheotomize both, rather than to wait a year to see if movement will be recovered. If no motility appears within a year, abduction will never come back. Ventriculocordectomy is indicated. Regarding the hemorrhage, it is extremely insignificant, or very slight in amount. Probably the pinching of the forceps pinches off the blood vessels and prevents the hemorrhage.

### Papilloma of the Larynx in Children, With the Report of an Unusual Case.

By O. A. M. McKimmie, M. D.,
Washington. D. C.

In carrying out the review of the literature on this subject, I have been impressed with the following facts: That our knowledge of the causation of papilloma has not increased; that nearly all writers during this period state their conviction that removal by use of the direct laryngoscope is the preferable method if removal, seems best.

The youngest children operated by the direct method were one 17 months old and one of 18 months. No operative method seems to have been entirely satisfactory—operative measures having to be repeated in most cases. Numerous cases of spontaneous cure, that is, disappearance without actual removal of the papillomata themselves, have been reported.

The following case is illustrative with a history of increasing hoarseness and difficult breathing for the preceding six months. She was evidently suffering marked laryngeal obstruction. Laryngeal view was very difficult to obtain, but finally a granular mass which filled the entrance except for a very small chink posteriorly presented. The child was ordered taken to the hospital and the consent of the parents gotten to do a tracheotomy whenever I deemed it necessary. The next day, as her breathing was getting steadily worse, I did a low tracheotomy, a few whiffs of ether being used. Operation was without incident, although the neck was extremely short, the patient being very small for her age. At the end of one week I opened the larynx and thoroughly removed the masses of papilloma which practically filled the box of the larynx below the cords and extended also above them.

The patient was discharged at the end of the twenty-fifth day without the tube and with the laryngotomy wound healed. During the following five months she was perfectly well, with perfect comfort in breathing and with perfectly clear voice. During December, 1915, 6 months later, she suffered an attack of grippe, which seems to have been the starting point of a recurrence of her papillomata. which necessitated her readmission to the hospital on January 8. 1916, at 11:45 P. M. Immediate tracheotomy was done, followed one week later by laryngotomy. The following 152 days were spent in the hospital, the tube being worn continuously so that rest of the larynx for respiratory purposes would give the greatest chance of allowing the process to run its course without reinfection, if we may use such a term. After this the mother, who had become quite an expert in the care of the tube, looked after the patient at home and brought her to see me about once a week. I was confirmed in my idea of letting the patient wear the tube for an indefinite period by finding some three months after discharge from the hospital that there were small papillomatous masses on both posterior pillars of the pharynx, which later disappeared spontaneously. Phonation with the tube stopped, after removal of the inner tube, was clear but weak, but the child was afraid to have the inner tube out for more than a couple of minutes at a time. She wore the tube continuously for two years and one-half and I was about ready to dispense with it and close the tracheal opening, but did not have the opportunity, as she died of influenzapneumonia during an epidemic. The microscopist reported the masses removed as papilloma.

Notwithstanding the increasing facility and certainty with which laryngologists use the direct laryngoscope for the removal of growths in the larynx, and the numerous reports of its use in very young children. I am still quite firmly convinced that its use, without preliminary tracheotomy in children under four years of age, is not justified and that in very small children tracheotomy, followed by opening the larynx, is preferable, because this operation, when carefully done, permits absolutely perfect access to every portion of the organ and more perfect removal without undue traumatism of every particle of growth. As a matter of fact, I do not believe it is always possible to get a larynx perfectly cleared out by the direct method, even in adults, and with suspension. The various drugs applied locally by sprays, inhalation or otherwise in adult cases, with the idea of dehydration, limiting the blood supply of the growths or causing change in their structure, have in the main been unsuccessful, and to my mind are not applicable in small children. Radium and X-ray exposures have been used and a few good results therefrom have been reported.

Cases are reported of cure by removal followed by fulguration repeated at intervals.

I would make two classes of laryngeal papillomata in children. First. those in which no marked obstruction to breathing exists and in which the patients are in good general condition; and second, those in which there is progressive difficult respiration. In the first class, we may temporize in the hope of spontaneous cure, which has been reported by a number of observers, supplementing our waiting by such measures directed to the general health as may seem advisable. In the second class we must consider:

1. Removal of growths by the direct method without preliminary tracheotomy.

2. Simple tracheotomy, relying on laryngeal rests to bring about a cure.

3. Tracheotomy followed by direct laryngoscopic removal of the growths; and

4. Preliminary tracheotomy, followed later by laryngotomy.

If our knowledge of the causation of papilloma in the larynx were greater we would be in position to supplement our operative procedures by means to prevent the recurrence; but unfortunately every theory of causation seems to have been controverted by reported cases in which the assumed causative factors were lacking.

### DISCUSSION.

Dr. J. Payson Clark, Boston, Mass.: I still adhere to my position, which I have stated several times, in regard to the treatment of these cases; that no treatment should be undertaken that in any way will cause permanent injury to the larynx or leave a scar. Papillomata, as you all know, resemble histologically a dermal wart, the ordinary wart; and there is some activity of cellular growth at a certain period in the life of a child. which makes these growths very persistent. During that period removal by any method is not going to be successful. I believe in a preliminary tracheotomy in all cases in young children, owing to the size of the larynx, and owing to the danger of rapid growth and of obstruction of the larynx following. After doing a tracheotomy, I believe in giving the larynx a period of rest. Like an ordinary dermal wart, a laryngeal papilloma will often disappear.

Dr. George L. Richards, Fall River, Mass.: I had a patient, a girl of twelve, who came to see me because a physician had advised laryngotomy. She had difficulty in breathing and was absolutely hoarse. On both cords were masses of papilloma. After taking the time to train the child so that she would submit to having an applicator carried into the larynx, removed the papilloma. Then for a period of only a month the next year, I made applications of alcohol directly to the cords. I saw that child over a period of five years, from once to twice a year. She has now disappeared from view. When I last saw her, she was eighteen years old, and there never was any recurrence. She was saved any operation. She did not have a tracheotomy.

Dr. D. Crosby Greene, Jr., Boston, Mass.: I have had an experience with a patient with papilloma, upon whom I operated once or twice by the direct method, which I think has a bearing on the subject of this paper. After I had operated upon the child two or three times, his mother took him to another surgeon who operated upon him by thyrotomy and thoroughly cleaned out the larynx. Subsequently, within a year, I saw this patient with his larynx full of papilloma. Such an experience, it seems to me, is sufficient reason for not resorting to such a radical procedure as laryngotomy in these cases. If the growth tends to recur, even after radical operation, it seems to me that we are not justified in using the more radical procedure.

Dr. Henry L. Swain, New Haven, Conn.: I had a case that recurred, in an adult, and when I was just learning to do direct laryngoscopy. I took off the next two or three with the direct method, and had a return of four or five small papillomas in various parts of the larynx. The young woman became pregnant, and could not come to the office; and I suggested that a spray of alcohol in the larynx might be carried out by her family physician. It was done, and four or five papillomas in various parts of the larynx receded under this treatment, and had disappeared entirely by the time she was able to come to me again, with only the original growth remaining on the vocal cord. That I removed with direct laryngoscopy and followed this up with alcohol for some time with no recurrence.

Dr. Robert Clyde Lynch, New Orleans, La.: Just as much as I was in favor of the removal of papilloma by dissection some years ago, thinking that I had a cure for this condition, I am now opposed to it. The first fourteen cases that I had and operated on were relieved at the one sitting, and I have never been able to duplicate that result since. My experience covers ninety cases at the present time. I have reason to speak that way. I believe now that any cutting operation is likely to be followed by recurrence of the papilloma. That is almost certain in my experience; not only that; it seems to be followed by a type of papilloma that indurates below the level at which the tumor originally grew. Therefore, the deeper the tissue, the harder it is to combat it surgically ever afterwards. It is for that reason that thyrotomy or any type of operation except that described by Dr. Jackson this morning is not indicated. The best results that I had have been by drying the surface with alcohol and ether, and using either fulguration or the actual cautery. For a time, I thought that fulguration was the better of these two means; but now I am leaning towards the use of the actual cautery, applied practically in the same way as in laryngeal tuberculosis. The performance of a tracheotomy early in those cases, in which it is not absolutely essential for breathing, is to be looked on with fear and trembling; because the papilloma masses will automatically grasp themselves around the raw surfaces and at the distal end of the tube, and you will plant papilloma that did not exist into the trachea. You not only have laryngeal papilloma, but also tracheal papilloma to deal with, which increases the difficulty of the case. In practically every case of papilloma that I have seen there seemed to be the psychological moment for its disappearance. In other words, I have operated on cases any number of times. The greatest number of operations on any one patient was forty-two. We operated on one little patient forty-two times, which is an evidence of the inefficiency of type of surgery that we can use—and in some of these patients we had removed the papillomatous mass completely, apparently at the time, and expected the usual recurrence within a month or six weeks, and for some reason or other, there would be a cessation of the return of the growth. There apparently was no difference in the look of the tissue, from a pathologic or physiologic stand-point, at the time of operation; yet in some of the cases, there would be no recurrence; and I have never been able to tell, at the time of the sitting, whether this would be the last time to operate on the patient or not. That is one of the peculiar phases of the situation.

Dr. D. Bryson Delavan, New York City: In the small, well-defined, slowly growing, warty papillomata of the larynx, the use of alcohol, as suggested to me about twenty years ago by the late Dr. Charles H. Knight, will in many cases effect a cure. In certain other cases it will retard the progress of the growth, dimin-ish its size, and render its thorough removal more easy. But there are many papillomata of the more active type upon which this treatment has no effect. Also in the case of children, it has gen-erally been in my hands entirely impracticable. To be effective, the alcohol must be as pure as possible, at least 95%, and the applica-tions, in the form of spray, must be made at least once daily, the spray being driven well into the interior of the larynx. This the patient can be taught to do for himself, in order to secure the necessary frequency and regularity of treatment. In some cases a solution of sulphate of zinc, two or three grains to the ounce, makes an excellent substitute for the less agreeable spray of alcohol. In suitable cases the value of this method of treatment has been amply proved.

Dr. Oscar A. M. McKimmie, Washington, D. C. (closing): Since I recorded this case, I have not seen a case of papilloma in either a child or an adult. In so small a child, I should probably do again what I did in this case, because I believe that even the method suggested by Dr. Jackson this morning, of removing by forceps, offers as much chance of spreading the papilloma as laryngotomy. The latter, in the hands of the average laryngologist, I consider to be a safer operation. If I had a child over four years old, I should attempt removal by the indirect method, because I was brought up on that, and use it more skillfully than the direct method. If I had a smaller child, I should probably do a prelimi-nary tracheotomy, and remove the growth by subsequent laryn-gotomy.

### Presentation of Patients, Instruments and Reports.

Dr. Delavan, New York City: Presented a patient showing the splendid results following external applications of radium. Dr. Delavan then asked the patient to show the character of the voice as to the length of treatments.

Patient: I had two hours for the first time, and four and a half hours on each side. They were crossfired and the next time I had one hour and fifty minutes on each side. The third time I had two hours. My voice, as you hear, is coming back. I really think that it is getting better each day.

### DISCUSSION.

(Dr. Delavan's patient.)

Dr. Chevalier Jackson, Philadelphia, Pa.: I feel so enthusiastic over the results in this case, that I should like to say a word. After not so many weeks of perfectly painless treatment, she came in with all the enormous masses that had occupied the place of the ventricular bands simply melted away. It approached ideal medicine in a way which we practically never see. It looked as if that was one of those sad cases of inoperable malignancy. It is one of the most brilliant cures that I have ever seen, and I was so enthusiastic that I made these drawings.

Dr. Chevalier Jackson then presented a little girl who had masses of papillomatous growths removed with the crushing forceps. Her speech was clear and there had been no recurrence.

### General Measures in the Treatment of Laryngeal Tuberculosis.

By Lawrason Brown, M. D.,
Saranac Lake, N. Y.

While tuberculous laryngitis is rare in children and more often found at autopsy, it occurs in about 25% or more of adults with pulmonary tuberculosis, slightly more in men than in women, and next to tuberculosis, enteritis and colitis is the most frequent complication of pulmonary tuberculosis, due most likely to direct infection of the part by the sputum. Laryngeal tuberculosis is rarely, if ever, a primary disease, a statement with which I am sure many of you will agree.

One vital essential in the treatment of tuberculosis has become, if I may so express it, part of us. I refer to rest. We put the patient on silence and give the larynx absolute rest, except for such movement as occurs in breathing, swallowing and coughing. We forbid whispering, whistling and every other use of the larynx. The results from this absolute rest are just as striking as they are in the case of tuberculosis of the knee, of the hip, of the spine, or indeed of any other organ that can be given nearly 100% functional rest. Absolute rest of the larynx can probably be most nearly attained by performing tracheotomy and the use of the tube. Chevalier Jackson has reported three cases of laryngeal tuberculosis, supposed to be primary, who wore tracheotomy tubes and got better. In the vast majority of cases such radical measures are not necessary. How long such absolute rest should continue must depend upon how the lesion progresses. Lip whispering, then ordinary whispering, next an occasional sentence in speaking tones, is the method of progression, but singing, shouting, public speaking should be avoided for some months after recovery. Personally, I go further in the rest treatment and do not hesitate to put my patients to bed for six weeks, with wide open windows, or better still, upon a porch during the day and in a well ventilated room at night. I do this for the following reasons: Pulmonary tuberculosis is usually present and partial rest of the lung as much as is possible, is thus effected. Cough, which may injure the larynx when excessive, is better controlled by rest in bed than by any other means, for reduction of the number of respirations means lessened irritation of the irritable lungs, consequently lessened secretion, and in turn lessened cough, and so less sputum flowing over the larynx.

Recovery from laryngeal tuberculosis depends in most instances largely upon the condition of the pulmonary tuberculosis. With advancing pulmonary disease, fever and poor nutrition, it is diffi-

cult to promote healing in a tuberculous larynx, but I have seen it
done with the aid of the electrocautery. Few laryngologists still
seemed to hold to the idea that local treatment was the important
thing. In regard to local treatment, I feel that the laryngeal
dropper, devised by Dr. Yankauer of New York, is not yet widely
enough known and used, for I can now recall only one or two
patients who have come to me with laryngeal tuberculosis who
had ever previously employed it.

To produce rest and to facilitate swallowing, freedom from or
lessening of pain is necessary. I have tried injection of alcohol
into the superior laryngeal nerve with some success, but the respites have never been long. The insufflation of anethesin or
orthoform has been helpful. In these cases the laryngeal dropper
has proved a godsend. Before the application of drugs I have the
patient thoroughly rinse or wash out his larynx with physiologic
salt solution. Menthol (1%) in oil is an excellent application to
begin the method upon, for if the patient swallows it, no harm is
done. Then, stronger solutions of menthol, emulsions of anesthesin, or what I have found is best of all, Freudenthal's emulsion of
orthoform and menthol, can be applied as necessary. I have by
these methods been able to avoid largely cocaine, with its disagreeable after results. In a few cases I have not hesitated to
use morphin hypodermically when necessary. More recently I
have been interested in the use of a thin solution of gelatin suggested by Mr. Petroff from his studies in physical chemistry. He
afterwards placed in our hands a strongly immune serum (sheep
or goat). Spraying the larynx with these substances apparently
afforded a few patients marked relief, but in others was of little
avail.

In conclusion, I would like to say that about 100,000 persons die
from pulmonary tuberculosis in the United States every year. At
least 40 to 50 per cent of these have some laryngeal tuberculosis.
If patients live on the average about three years, there must be
about 300,000 or more patients in the United States, of whom 25 to
50 per cent have laryngeal tuberculosis, in all then, about 100,000
have laryngeal tuberculosis. Many of these are people with slight
or no means. Treatment of their throat condition must in large
part devolve upon the medical men doing tuberculosis work. They
feel their shortcomings and are eager to turn to you for help. But
when they see a patient with high fever dragged to a laryngologic
dispensary, which they know is wrong, they realize that they
or some one else has erred.

### Climate in the Treatment of Laryngeal Tuberculosis.

By Carroll E. Edson, M. D.,
Denver, Colo.
(By Invitation.)

Tuberculosis of the larynx is practically always secondary to an
active pulmonary tuberculosis. '

The extent and character of the primary lesions usually determine our choice of climate for the patient.

To discuss satisfactorily how the supervention of the laryngeal
infection may modify this selection, we must first have a clear

understanding of the part climate plays in the cure of tuberculosis of the lungs.

In my paper, as it will be printed, I have dealt at length with this portion of the subject.

How does climate especially help the patient with laryngeal tuberculosis, and what choice of meteorologic components is desirable in his case?

Tuberculosis of the larynx responds only in a general way and to a slight degree to the increased vitality induced by outdoor life and to general nutrition. The local laryngeal lesion is less directly affected by these factors than is pulmonary tubercle. Its arrest is more dependent on the third member of the physiologic triad, rest.

Under the establishment and maintenance of complete rest the prognosis of laryngeal tuberculosis is much better than commonly believed. This complete rest, incomparably the most important part of the treatment we can bring to bear, is curiously difficult to secure.

The first, the most effective means to this end, the hardest to obtain, is silence; the absolute avoidance of all phonation.

Next in value to silence in securing the fullest rest to the larynx is the abolition, reduction or control of cough from whatever source it arises.

The cough of infraglottic origin rising from the pulmonary disease will lessen with the improvement in that lesion. Climate, as I showed, is a valuable aid in securing that arrest and often gives surprisingly prompt results in diminishing the cough.

The local laryngeal irritation, most soothed by rest, may occasionally need local sedative applications. It is, however, to a considerable degree affected by atmospheric conditions presently to be mentioned, the control of which may greatly assuage the patient's discomfort.

The supralaryngeal cough caused by nasal and especially pharyngeal trouble is a factor of great importance in its wear upon the patient. From my observations it is not sufficiently appreciated or given enough detailed care. Even in purely pulmonary tuberculosis no small fraction of the most annoying cough is alleviated by proper and painstaking care of the catarrhal or obstructive congestion of the upper respiratory area.

In laryngeal tuberculosis the cough from these sources is especially harmful, for it remains always a nonproductive, unnecessary cough of purely mechanical violence.

Now it is in helping control and lessening the cough arising from the nose, pharynx and glottis that certain climatic factors play a definite and direct part. So important and so readily demonstrated is this role that the presence of a tubercular laryngeal lesion calls for especial consideration of them in the choice of climate. The later development of a laryngeal tuberculosis may for the first time make a change of climate advisable.

A patient with laryngeal tuberculosis does not endure well extremes of heat or cold. Such patients are prone to loss of appetite and poor nutritional balance, even before any pain or swallowing has occurred. This early loss of weight, and the frequently accompanying anemia is out of proportion to the added amount of tubercular disease. I believe it is the result of anxiety, discouragement and fear born of the knowledge and constant evidence of the new complication. Consequently any added cause for poor appetite and assimilation, such as heat or humid weather, is to be avoided.

Equally do such patients suffer from great cold, especially at night, and the irritation from breathing very cold air may excite so much cough as to prevent sleeping out. Thus one of the most valuable opportunities for combining fresh air and rest will be lost. Even though the daytime cold is modified by bright sunshine, very cold nights, or too wide a diurnal range in temperature, are to be avoided. For these reasons it may be advisable for a patient who can afford it to make a winter sojourn in a more southern, warmer station and change to a cooler, more bracing region in the summer months.

Abrupt or marked change in the temperature of the respired air readily induces cough as we well know. Climates characterized by such sudden or frequent changes are to be avoided.

Damp air, especially if at all cold or in motion, is an immediate excitant of cough to an inflamed larynx or sensitive rhinopharynx. Therefore, the patient will benefit most if sent to a mild, equable climate with a dry air, low relative humidity and long periods without wet weather.

Strong winds and dusty air are sedulously to be avoided. Frequently in the same region of generally similar climatic conditions one locality will have a topography giving shelter from the prevailing wind, it will be thus entirely suitable, while a station near at hand, not so protected is undesirable. Such local details are important to consider even after the general problem has been settled. Indeed, the whole success in the cure of laryngeal tuberculosis is a matter of appreciation of and attention to detail.

In this connection, may I add a word, even if it seem a criticism? Too often we see patients sent long distance from home at a sacrificing cost to gain the advantage of a better climate for living out of doors who, because of a laryngeal lesion, take frequent or even daily trips to the physician's office. There they sit in a crowded, often poorly ventilated room, waiting their turn for local applications. This travel and waiting is undertaken frequently when the exertion involved or the presence of fever should forbid such conduct. Any febrile patient with laryngeal lesions needing regular local treatment should be treated at his residence. If the laryngologist cannot give the time for such visits, the patient will be best placed in a sanatorium, where the means for local care are at hand and where he does not have to pass his waiting time indoors rereading a last year's copy of Outdoor Life.

These are briefly the principles underlying the use of climate in the cure of laryngeal tuberculosis,

There is no specific climate for tuberculosis.

The disease may heal in any climate.

Some climates, however, offer the patient an incomparably better opportunity to make use of the three requisites for cure: an outdoor life, increased nutrition, physiologic rest.

Laryngeal tuberculosis does not require a climate essentially different from that for pulmonary disease.

It does benefit, however, from a little more care in consideration of a few details. These are, equableness, without extremes of heat or cold, especially the latter; freedom from frequent, sudden changes in temperature; damp air, particularly in winter, high winds and dust.

A careful consideration of the balance between the patient's needs, his means and the reasonable advantage to be gained from a change in surroundings is necessary to avoid disappointment or disaster. To make a correct selection the physician must understand the climatic characteristics of both the home and the contemplated resort. He must have an accurate knowledge of and interest in meteorologic statistics and be able to interpret them properly in terms of physiologic effect upon the patient.

Further advance in the best utilization of climate will come with a greater appreciation of the fact that the physical modalities of temperature, humidity, sunlight, wind and barometric pressure, are real and definite in their action. The more complete our study and knowledge of this physiologic response, which they demand from a patient, the better use we shall be able to make of these climatic components in the environment we select for the invalids who seek our counsel or depend upon our care.

## The Treatment of Tuberculous Laryngitis by Suspension Laryngoscopy.

### By L. W. Dean, M. D.,
### Iowa City.

Using proper precautions, endolaryngeal operations may be performed upon the tuberculous larynx by suspension without detriment to a coexisting quiescent pulmonary condition.

It is quite impossible for me to do as accurate work by direct laryngoscopy as by suspension. I have done many more endolaryngeal operations by the direct method than by suspension. I cannot place my cautery or knife as accurately by the former as by the latter method, neither can I protect the larynx so well from the cautery point.

Unless there is some contraindication to its use, suspension laryngoscopy is to me the procedure of choice for endolaryngeal operations on the tuberculous larynx. The well illuminated larynx is thoroughly exposed. Both hands of the operator are free. He may have in one hand a spatula to expose better or to protect a certain area in the larynx, and in the other his galvanocautery ponit, punch or curette. He is at liberty to turn to his instrument table and select, if necessary, a different instrument without interfering with his work. He may take in his left hand a laryngeal speculum and expose the upper end of trachea, the anterior commissure or the interarytenoid space, leaving his right hand free for operative work on the part exposed. There is no hurry. The patient who is suspended the first time may feel that he is suffocating. The tuberculous case is particularly favorable for suspension. The emaciated neck makes the procedure a very easy one.

The work is done under local anesthesia. There is no excuse for loosening teeth. I frequently attach the tooth clips to a dental bridge, using a lead protector. There should not be the slightest danger of jaw fracture. The patient should be rapidly suspended, using every precaution for the patient's comfort. To get a good view it is not necessary to separate the jaws widely. Separating the jaws too widely may add to the patient's discomfort. It is not always necessary or advisable to bring the anterior commissure into view. It is never necessary to raise the patient's head from the table.

The anesthesia: Morphin, ¼ gr.; atrophin, 1/120 gr., is given twenty minutes preceding the operation. Ten per cent cocain is applied to the epiglottis and larynx, using a cotton swab. The swab is held in contact with the epiglottis and cords until all tendency to sagging disappears.

Suspension prevents hemorrhage and edema by permitting of exact incision and cauterization when operating in the larynx and so thoroughly expose bleeding points that they may be properly handled.

For amputating the epiglottis suspension laryngoscopy is the procedure of choice. Under local anesthesia, using the short Lynch tongue spatula, the epiglottis is distinctly exposed. It is grasped with a tenaculum forcep and using a Lynch knife, cleanly severed at its base. I have not noted any hemorrhage of importance following this procedure. It requires but a short time.

The decision as to whether the operation is to be performed by direct laryngoscopy. or suspension is made by the pulmonary expert. He approves of suspension for those cases who can have the endolaryngeal work done in this way without much risk of a reaction. The suspension in our hands gives the best results, and if it can be used without detriment to the patient, it is the method of choice. It is particularly desirable to suspend those cases needing cutting and curetting operations.

The frequency of suspension depends upon the needs of the larynx. Occasionally we have a case when galvanocautery is used under suspension every two weeks. These cases are usually ones that are discharged from the sanitarium whose larynges are scarred, the result of previous operations and the healing process, and who have returned for cauterization of suspicious small areas in the larynx.

The first essential thing in treating laryngeal tuberculosis by suspension laryngoscopy is to have the patient under the supervision of a pulmonary expert who has authority to say this patient shall or shall not be suspended.

Our tuberculous laryngitis cases are divided into four classes for treatment: First, those who remain in bed and receive only the simple medication; second, those who may sit up and have applied to the larynx mild astringents and antiseptics; third, those who receive endolaryngeal surgical procedures by direct laryngoscopy; and, lastly, those who are operated under suspension. The pulmonary expert, having before him the laryngologist's findings, decides in which class the case belongs.

While suspension laryngoscopy seems to me to be the ideal condition for the performance of endolaryngeal operations in cases with quiescent pulmonary conditions, it is particularly adapted to the treatment of superficial tuberculous ulcerations of the trachea. If these ulcerations are high up, using the laryngeal spatula these cases may be readily cauterized. If situated low down in the trachea a tracheoscope may be passed under suspension and proper treatment instituted.

## DISCUSSION.

Dr. Joseph B. Greene, Asheville, N. C.: Dr. Edison has told us what we have thought for a long time, that climate has no direct effect on the larynx itself, but only affected it directly through the general health of the patient. However, he has presented in a scientific way the influence of climate on the general condition of the patient.

To Dr. Lawrason Brown we are indebted for emphasizing to us the importance of rest to the voice in the treatment of laryngeal tuberculosis. It seems to me, however, that the general man who treats pulmonary tuberculosis is apt to pay too little attention to the laryngeal condition. The treatment of the larynx is different from that of the lung condition in that we are unable to use local measures in one case, while the larynx is easily accessible for local applications. It seems to me, further, that the treatment of laryngeal tuberculosis depends largely on the stage of the disease, and likewise upon the site of the lesion. It is obvious that silence which has been so well emphasized could have no effect on lesions of the epiglottis and could influence very slightly, if at all, chronic infiltrations in other situations of the larynx. In ulcerations of the epiglottis there is no treatment to my mind comparable to that of epiglottidectomy. In many cases of ulceration and infiltration I am in the habit of using applications of formalin with a great deal of benefit to the patient. There are certain cases, however, which require the use of electric cautery. For this treatment I am in the habit of using the indirect method, though Dr. Dean has told us of the advantages of suspension in these cases. In conclusion, I wish to emphasize the importance of alcohol injections into the superior laryngeal nerve for pain in laryngeal tuberculosis. The method of making this injection was presented so clearly by Dr. Fetterolf in a complete paper published in the Annals of Otology, Rhinology and Laryngology, March, 1912, that little difficulty is experienced in making a successful injection.

Dr. George B. Wood, Philadelphia. Pa.: The only method I have found that yields positive results in the treatment of tuberculosis is the application of the actual cautery. As far as the cure of the tuberculous process is concerned, I do not believe that lactic acid or any other drug has any influence in checking the progress of the disease except in so far as they cure and prevent secondary infections. The application of drugs, however, for the purpose of combating secondary infection and of protecting the larynx against further inoculation from the pulmonary sputum should be recognized as an important part of the treatment. I believe that the cautery should supplant all bloody operative procedures. There is a distinct danger in the use of the punch or other compressing instruments of forcing the tubercle bacilli from the local lesion into the neighboring lymphatics, and also the cut surface leaves an open channel for further infection from the pulmonary secretions. I have no hesitancy in asserting that the large majority of early cases of laryngeal tuberculosis can be cured by the use of the actual cautery, and I have frequently seen the laryngeal lesion healing while the lungs were rapidly breaking down. Of course, in extensive lesions of the larynx, especially where the disease is extrinsic, and in pharyngeal lesions, the prognosis is exceedingly bad, no matter what form of treatment is adopted; although I have seen large pharyngeal ulcers healed promptly after cauterization. The value of the cautery is not that it destroys the tuberculous lesion, but lies in the fact that it revitalizes an area which, because of the tubercle, has been deprived of its blood vessels. In a series of experiments on guinea pigs, I succeeded in producing cutaneous lesions of the abdomen by the use of an attenuated tubercle bacillus. The tubercles that were cauterized always healed promptly while the control was progressing. Histologic examination of the cauterized tubercle showed that within three days the eschar was surrounded by a network of capillaries and was thrown off by granulating tissue in about seven days, leaving a superficial ulcer which promptly healed. The rest of the tubercle, formerly free from any evidence of blood vessels, was now permeated with capillaries and the epithelioid cells were rapidly replaced by fibroblasts and in a comparatively short space of time no evidence of active tuberculosis could be detected in the region of the original lesion. From a clinical standpoint, a very important point in favor of the use of the cautery is its comparative ease of application by the indirect method. In a large majority of patients, laryngeal lesions can be cauterized during the ordinary office routine with no more discomfort to the patient than an ordinary laryngeal application.

Dr. Robert Clyde Lynch, New Orleans, La.: I should like to mention two cases that have yielded very nicely to the sun's rays, which were applied by the patients themselves, at a time during their convalescence when the pulmonary lesion was entirely quiet. Suspension certainly does facilitate the ease and accuracy of the application of the cautery. I think that the greatest number of cases of laryngeal tuberculosis that I have seen at any time were those of Dr. Dean; and in many of those cases it was almost impossible to tell that the patients had been the victims of previous tubercular ulceration. Healing, so far as my imagination went, was beyond expectation. These cases of laryngeal tuberculosis, as far as my experience in my own patients went, were remarkable. I do not think that Dr. Dean said enough about his routine treatment, as carried on in the institution that he has charge of. I saw fifty-five to sixty cases one afternoon, in all phases of ulceration of the larynx, and in all phases of activity and quiescence of the process in the lung; and I am sure that I saw fifteen that were as well as any larynx that I have looked into for some time. They were tubercular patients in whom the process had been active and the history records were there to show what had gone on.

Dr. Cornelius G. Coakley, New York City: I have divided the subject of laryngeal tuberculosis into two parts: First, the non-ulcerative form, and second, the ulcerative form. In the nonulcer-ative form, most of these patients were able to go away from their homes; and it is perfectly surprising the results that are obtained by the absolute silence that these patients are recommended to employ. They come back with larynges that are as clean as any normal larynx. Then they show on their vocal cords enormous thickening and infiltration, which in former years I was in the habit of letting go on to the ulcerative stage, involving the epi-glottis. I now have them treated in this manner; and you would not believe the degree of absorption that results. In a compara-tively short time, all these cases have improved so far as their pulmonary condition is concerned. They have come back with perfect respiration and voice. In the ulcerative type, you do not always get such good results, especially where the epiglottis and adenoid region are involved. All these patients have great diffi-culty in swallowing, and the greatest difficulty is in keeping up the nutrition of the patients. The thing which in my hands has given the patients the greatest relief from the difficulty and pain of swallowing, has been the application of orthoform, one grain; iodoform, one grain, and compound stearate of zinc, one grain. The patients can be readily taught to apply these themselves by taking the powder blower and making a blast and a pressure of the bulb with inspiration, at the same time. This will carry that mixture over all portions of the lower part of the pharynx, larynx and even down to the trachea. The first two or three applications are dis-agreeable to the patient from the cough produced; but in a short time the application can be made without producing any cough. I believe that the powder of compound stearate of zinc holds the orthoform and iodoform against these lesions, protects the ulcer from the streptococci that are present and limits their spread.

We have not had a chance to do very much treatment with sus-pension, because most of the patients that do come to us are able to be put on sanatorium treatment, where, I think, they do much better than at home. I object to home treatment, because it is difficult to carry out. The family will come in and interfere with the carrying out of the treatment. They cannot do this at the sanatorium.                                                     i

Dr. James E. Logan, Kansas City, Mo.: I have often taken these cases and put them into the old-fashioned prairie schooner and sent them across the plain, and in going across they have found the location in which they have improved most. Most of them have been improved. To my mind, the ideal treatment would be, if you could carry it out, to have a patient with tuberculous laryngeal ulceration go to the spot that benefits him, and there receive the suspension laryngoscopy after the lungs and other conditions have been improved sufficiently to accept that treatment. That, to my mind, would be the ideal method of treating those cases; but as far as my ability to benefit them at the altitude in which I live goes, I would say that I advise against their accepting treatment from me.

Dr. E. Ross Faulkner, New York City: I call this the irony of fate, that I have the privilege of saying a few words on the paper read by Dr. Lawrason Brown. I was his patient for a year, and I think that it is largely due to his treatment by rest that I am here today. I know that he believes in rest, for he kept me in bed for a year. I had a tuberculous larynx, and I had to rest it and not talk at all for three months. I am afraid that I was a sorry patient. Nevertheless, through the fact that Dr. Brown has the faculty of making his patients do what he wants them to, I would say I submitted to the treatment. I had numerous visitors, and it was difficult for me to keep quiet all the time. One thing he kept me from, and that is from any one's attempting to touch my larynx by means of suspension laryngoscopy. I do not know that I was weak enough to allow anyone to do that, anyway. Regarding rest, patients may be making progress and their balance may be upset by some slight thing. They may do something which in a person of ordinary activity would not be of importance, but will start them on a downhill course; whereas, otherwise they would have been taking a sure course towards recovery.

Last September a patient aged sixty-seven years came to the clinic with hoarseness, which she had had for four months. She had not lost weight. The only thing seen was an ulcer on the left vocal cord, with gradual infiltration spreading from the cord. I took it for an epithelioma. The other men there thought so, too, and demonstrated the case to the students. We had the Wasserman test done and the lungs examined, but did not have an X-ray made. I proceeded to do a thyrotomy. When I opened the larynx I found that it did not feel like an epithelioma. I removed the cord, and on examining the specimen, I thought it was an epithelioma, although the base did not appear indurated, but section proved it to be tuberculous. After removing it, I closed the wound, leaving a ridge of tissue, which afterwards made a very good cord. She got quite a fair voice, and the result was excellent. The old lady went on her way rejoicing, and is very well today.

Dr. Emil Mayer, New York City: In my clinic, it was our custom to give every patient one of the Yankauer droppers, so that he could make these applications. This, which is a simple apparatus, consists merely of an elongated dropper which is held in the patient's mouth. A little strip of adhesive is placed at the distal end, so that the patient may know just how far to introduce it. Then you can be sure that he always has it in far enough to reach the interior of the larynx. This invaluable little apparatus is particularly cheap, and we have to bear these things in mind. We cannot send all these patients away. They are not financially able to go any distance.

The value of the galvanocautery in these cases recalls a case treated by Dr. Fetterolf. The man made his residence in New York, and came to me because he has, in addition, a tuberculous ear. He had been treated by Dr. Fetterolf, who had applied (by the indirect method, of course) the galvanocautery. It was one of the most astounding things to see that man, the epiglottis, arytenoids and the interior of whose larynx, as the result of the condition that he had had before, were deeply involved, get a clear voice and reach a condition of restored health. On account of recurrent attacks of otitis, it became necessary for him to see me from time to time, so I have seen him for a matter of three years. Every once in a while I look at his larynx to see how things are; and if anyone wants a convincing proof of the value of galvano-cautery, all he needs to do is to see a case of this kind, on which I must compliment Dr. Fetterolf.

Dr. Lee Wallace Dean, Iowa City, Iowa (closing): Every case of laryngeal tuberculosis should be placed under the care of a tuberculosis expert before the therapeutic procedure is advised. The laryngologist should recommend to this expert on pulmonary tuberculosis what in his judgment would be the proper treatment of the larynx, basing his opinions on his findings. The pulmonary expert should be the one to advise whether the treatment suggested should be carried out or not.

### "Mucocele of the Nasal Accessory Sinuses; Two Cases of Pansinus Involvement With Recovery After Interval Operations."

By Virginius Dabney, M. D.,
Washington, D. C.

The various theories as to the eitology of this affection are presented: Injury, congenital showing of the duct, and a high deviation of the septum are given.

It is essentially an affection of the young, although the two cases presented by the writer were 25 and 62 years old, respectively.

It is not especially remarkable that the symptoms of mucocele should be so seldom seen or felt until late. While the affection is principally that of the frontal sinus, similar conditions exist in other sinuses. So slowly and insidiously do mucoceles develop that no symptoms are noticed by the patient before the tumor formation is advanced, or the retention of a large mass of mucus is established. There is absence of pain. Pressure symptoms are most marked.

In the early stages a diagnosis of mucocele is practically impossible. When further advanced, and there is loss of visual power with diminishing of the visual field, the diagnosis is more simple, especially when the radiograph is employed.

It is not always easy to differentiate these from malignant tumors, and often an examination of the contents becomes our only resource. Empyema is more difficult to differentiate than any other condition. The severity of the symptoms, pus in the nose, and the patient's distress are of help in differential diagnosis.

The prognosis of mucocele is uniformly good, and the treatment radical operation with drainage.

The writer presents the histories of two cases of this affection.

1. Female, 25; had asthma, nasal stoppage, burning, subject to colds, and of about six years' duration. Had had polyps removed. Pressure over the brow and antrum painful. Lids slightly swollen. Killian operation; later a double Luc-Caldwell operation was done and the same type of disease found in the antra as had existed in the frontal sinus. She had lost her asthma and her discomfort.

The second case was a woman 62 years old. During thirty years she has had numerous operations for the removal of polypi and ethmoid disease. She had asthma, numbness over the top of the head, fullness in the cheeks, constant severe headaches. Examination with the Roentgen rays confirmed the diagnosis of pansinusitis. Bilateral Killian operation showing many cysts and much thick, yellowish, bloodstreaked mucus. Four months later a bilateral Luc-Caldwell operation showed similar conditions in the antra.

These two cases present the classic symptoms and the extraordinary features that make mucocele of the nasal accessory sinus an interesting study. The nature of the growths, the type of secretion, the long duration and insidious development, the lack of insistent symptoms, distention of the cavities, were all present with an almost total absence of constitutional signs. In both radical operation effected cures.

## DISCUSSION.

Dr. Otto T. Freer, Chicago, Ill.: If the uncinate process is the subject of an inflammatory swelling, as it often is during antrum, ethmoidal or frontal sinus suppuration, it impinges upon the lower border of the middle turbinate, lying in contact with it, so that it completes the floor of the recessus frontalis, making of it a partly or completely closed cavity. Secretions are then more or less retained in the recessus, according to the amount of uncinate and associated swelling. My experience has not sustained the usual idea that antrum suppuration is secondary to the frontal sinus suppuration in these cases, the frontal sinus "draining into the antrum." Chronic antrum suppurations are in my experience nearly all of dental origin and the frontal sinus abscess follows that of the antrum. In aggravated cases of this sort the maxillary antrum, the recessus frontalis and the frontal sinus form one continuous lake of pus that drains under pressure through small fissures into the nasopharynx.

Should the uncinate process and middle turbinate for any reason become adherent, the recessus frontalis becomes a closed or nearly closed cavity and its bony walls and those of the frontal sinus and antrum are then subjected to chronic slight pressure from the fluid distending this cavity which escapes with difficulty, if at all, the result being a mucocele which is the most conspicuously evident where it affects the frontal sinus, because the floor of the frontal sinus, which is the roof of the orbit, being a thin, weak place, gives way, becoming absorbed with resulting displacement of the eye outward by the distended sac which takes the place of the firm frontal sinus floor. If the fluid distending the mucocele cavity becomes sterile, it contains merely mucus. I have observed two of these cases. In one of them the chronic pressure of the contents of the mucocele had led to absorption of the bone of the adherent uncinate process and middle turbinate, so that they formed a sac that depended from the middle meatus region and could be easily opened widely with a knife. A great deal of fluid gushed out. Exploration then showed disappearance of the orbital floor of the frontal sinus with enlargement of the natural opening into the antrum, so that it would admit a finger. The eye was displaced outward and downward to an extreme degree. While the broad drainage of the mucocele created caused it to disappear, the eye displacement remained permanent.

The second case was seen casually in the practice of another man and I do not know the result of drainage of the mucocele upon the eye displacement.

Dr. C. G. Coakley, New York City: Within the past fourteen years, I have had two cases that were diagnosed as mucocele. One was a patient on whom about ten or eleven years before I performed ethmoid exenteration for orbital cellulitis. The patient had been operated on a few days before by a confrere in New York. After a partial exenteration of the ethmoid, this orbital cellulitis developed very promptly, and demanded immediate operation. I cleaned out his ethmoid only. I exenterated the ethmoid only along the nose, like the second half of a Killian incision. The membrane in the frontal sinus was thickened, and there was some accumulation of pus. The patient had asked to have very little deformity caused. I was doing, as an experiment, that type of operation, hoping to get sufficient drainage from the frontal sinus to prevent having to do a complete Killian operation, or radical operation on the frontal sinus. The patient made a good recovery from both the frontal inflammation and the ethmoidal. For a long time one could pass a probe into the frontal sinus and wash it out, until all secretion had ceased. He disappeared from view, owing to residence in another country; but he returned at intervals for examination, and transillumation showed that all evidence of frontal sinus involvement on that side was absent. He returned again in June, a year ago, while I was away, and consulted a confrere in New York. He had a marked bulging in his forehead, and downward and outward displacement of the globe of the eye, which had been going on for several weeks.

The diagnosis of mucocele was made. The frontal sinus was opened, and the membrane only partially removed, giving temporary relief; but a permanent fistula discharging pus resulted. In November he came into my hands again; and I completed the operation, cleaning out the right frontal sinus. There had been a perforation of the interfrontal septum, so that the pus extended into the left frontal sinus. The patient made a good recovery. Considerable membrane remains in the right frontal. Nothing has been touched in the left frontal. There was an inflammatory process going on in the membrane.

If you want to call these conditions mucoceles, all right; but I think that the pathology is that of a chronic inflammation of the mucous membrane, without bacteria present, or with a low-grade bacterial content, which has become devitalized so that we cannot get a growth. For some reason—perhaps, owing to the explanation given by Dr. Freer, that of some previous injury—there has been an interference with the passage of the secretion of the nose. There has been an obliteration of the nasofrontal duct, and the result is a gradual accumulation of pus with bone absorption. If you look on it as a chronic lowgrade inflammatory process, you can understand better what is going on in these cases. In the first case, fibrous tissue had grown across the floor of the frontal sinus, so that no probe could be passed up into the frontal sinus. That I satisfied myself of three or four years before the present attack. The process had been that of chronic inflammation, where the outlet had been obstructed with some anatomic disturbance—possibly inflammation and possibly trauma.

Dr. Lewis A. Coffin, New York City: What I have understood as mucoceles are cavities confined to the ethmoidal tract, which contain a sort of oysterlike sterile masses. They may extend into and involve the frontals. The interesting thing is the absolute destruction of all the natural cell walls of the tract and the extension and enlargement of the limiting wall of the cavity. That is the real wonder to me. I suppose it is due to action of the osteoblasts and the osteoclasts, but how they work so as to preserve the even thickness of the retaining wall is altogether beyond me. I do not know how it differs from the cystic turbinate, which we find more frequently in the female than in the male; nor again do I know whether it is comparable to the cyst that we find in the jaw. We have seen cysts in the lower jaw as large as a robin's egg, which had evidently started from some diseased tooth. I was wondering whether, if, as Dr. Freer has suggested, the condition commences in the antrum and spreads upward, the infection may not come from the teeth. The antrum is so often infected from a diseased tooth that this origin seems possible. If so, this would mean that we have an aseptic cavity which had its origin in an infective process. The cases that I have seen generally presented a tumor between the nose and the inner canthus of the eye. Of course, this tumor was hard; because of the limiting bony wall. In one case the X-ray showed the existence of a mass as large as a hen's egg. When operated, it was found to be an osteoma. What is the chemistry that determines whether the growth shall be the one or the other, I do not know.

Dr. Hill Hastings, Los Angeles, Cal.: Dr. Dabney made the statement that the existence of sarcoma with the diagnosis of mucocele is not uncommon. Some years ago I reported before the American Laryngologic, Rhinologic and Otologic Society three cases of mucocele, in all three of which a diagnosis of sarcoma had been made. In two cases the mucocele had been shown up externally in the orbit, the third case was believed to be a mucocele of the antrum. It caused a bulging of the anterior wall of the maxillary sinus with rotation of the teeth. On operation the cyst filled the whole antrum except a very small area at the upper, outer angle. I have since doubted my original diagnosis of mucocele of the antrum and believe that it was a dentigerous cyst that almost filled the antrum. The orbital growth were, however, true mucoceles.

Dr. Joseph H. Bryan, Washington, D. C.: There is a condition known as mucocele. Just what the actual pathology is, I am not able to state; but undoubtedly it is an accumulation of pure mucus, due to a low-grade inflammation that has not gone on to suppuration. It is caused by a plugging of the cavity, and I believe is a pathologic condition.

Dr. Thomas J. Harris, New York City.: I should like to report a case of pneumocele. The man was a Russian, thirty-three years of age, who complained of crackling in the frontal region and vague pain over the head. There was a sense of fluctuation over the mass. The nose showed distinct ethmoiditis. There was a history of considerable time in the development of the disease. No swelling was seen beneath the orbit. The X-ray showed distinct frontal sinus disease. The diagnosis was not made. I thought that it was frontal disease, plus something else. Radical operation showed, first, a distinct air tumor with a very small opening into the frontal sinus, which was filled with pus, and a solitary sinus, not the left sinus at all; and an occluded nasofrontal canal. It would seem that the trouble had begun in the nose and proceeded up into the forehead.

Dr. Virginius Dabney, Washington, D. C. (closing): Dr. Freer's explanation of the condition is blocking of the natural outlet, which seems perfectly reasonable and is seen frequently. Dr. Coakley starts out by saying that there is really no such condition as mucocele, but he really doesn't mean this, as he later lays down a rule which covers the cases perfectly. He does mean that many of the cases so reported are not of this type; thus, the first case he refers to was certainly not a mucocele, and I doubt if the second one was. The sterility of the growths and the cavities of which he speaks is absolutely true and one one of the diseases's striking pecularities. A growth cannot be obtained from any attempted culture. Dr. Coffin speaks of finding very often a bony cyst filled with semisolid matter; this is interesting and falls within the domain of my subject. Likewise the enormous destruction of bone which he notes is similarly characteristic. Dr. Coffin's characterization of the contents as an "oyster-like" is especially graphic; nothing so well describes the growth. A cystic turbinate is one stage of a mucocele. Dr. Hastings speaks of sarcoma as one of the confused diagnoses, and he is entirely correct in his position. In the mass of literature through which I waded in preparing my paper, I found in the British Medical Journal an illustration under the heading, "Educational Mistakes." It was the picture of a man who looked like one of the gargoyles which peer down at you from Notre Dame; the most appalling deformity I've ever seen. This had been calmly accepted as a sarcoma for three years, being in reality a mucocele. I read Dr. Bryan's article, which was about 15 years in advance of its time. Hydrops antri is a term not to be tolerated. Pneumatocele referred to by Dr. Harris is spoken of more by the French than any others, and was not touched upon by me owing to its rarity and ease of differentiation, chiefly by the crepitation and lack of local and constitutional signs.

### Aspergillosis of the Maxillary Sinus.

By Ross Hall Skillern, M. D.,
Philadelphia, Pa.

James B., a large man about fifty years, presented himself with vague symptoms referred to the left maxiliary sinus. Some unilateral, apparently nonfetid, nasal discharge, a feeling of fullness over the left antrum, vague head pains, entirely atypical of sinusitis. No periods of congestion or depression and no postnasal discharge. Some cacosmia at times, but never marked.

Examination revealed a slightly congested, lateral nasal wall, otherwise normal. A needle puncture of the maxilliary sinus was made and considerable resistance was offered to the ingress of the normal saline solution. Being mindful of the fatalities reported by Gording following needle puncture in which there almost invariably was difficulty in forcing the irrigating solution into the sinus, I proceeded with the utmost caution, watching the patient closely for the appearance of any untoward symptom. Despite the continuation of gradual pressure, nothing developed, nor did any liquid escape from the nose, either anteriorly or through the choanae into the pharynx. As the resistance seemed to be lessening, another syringeful was tried and almost almost immediately some fluid returned from the nostril on that side. It appeared slightly turbid but no free pus was observed. After injection of at least sixteen ounces, there appeared in the washings small, white inspissated masses, which resembled cottage cheese. It immediately occurred to me that we were dealing with a case of cheesy metamorphosis of a sinus empyema, of a so-called "Verkäsung," which, of course, is a condition where the purulent secretion has been sterile and begins to organize into a semisolid mass. Continued lavage, which now was returning quite freely, brought forth considerable quantity of this cheesy material, some of which was set aside for pathologic investigation. Lavage was continued until the antrum was free, the injected fluid returning clear. The patient expressed himself as greatly relieved, saying his head felt lighter than it had for a long time.

He did not return for nearly a week, when further needle puncture and lavage were negative, the patient feeling quite well. He was to report should any of his old symptoms reappear, but as several months have now elapsed, we can consider the case as cured.

The pathologic examination by Dr. Case gave the following findings:

"The specimen was small, soft and possessed no characteristic appearance that might have suggested the diagnosis. It had been placed in formaldehyde solution, so that a cultural study was, unfortunately, not possible. Following the usual routine, it was imbedded in paraffin, stained with hematoxlyn and eosin and examined histologically.

As may be seen in the preparation under the microscope, it consists of a close myselial network with an occasional conidiaspore, surmounted by a fanlike arrangement of conidiaspores. The hyphae take a faint pink stain, but the fructifying bodies are yellowish in color, apparently resisting the penetration of the dye. Diagnosis: Aspergillus, probably of the species fumigatus."

Dr. Lee Maidment Hurd, New York City: I saw a woman fifty years of age, who came to me for some obstruction of breathing. She had a deflected septum and the usual signs of chronic nasal catarrh. Transillumination showed the left antrum to be dark. I washed out this antrum, and got slightly cloudy fluid with strips like cotton fibre. This fluid showed aspergillus with bacillus pyocyaneus. She gave no symptoms of this condition whatever. Being a nervous woman, she insisted on a cure. I washed the antrum out with saline, and later injected it with silver. Then I opened the antrum and instituted intranasal drainage—all with no effect. There was always turbid fluid looking like cotton fibre. I cannot remember all the different antiseptics I tried without success. At last, I inflated it every day with equal parts of boric acid and aristol; and within a week it cleared up. We could not quite identify the parasite, but it was present in every washing.

## Case of Intranasal Ethmoid Exenteration Accompanied by Uncontrollable Hemorrhage. Death.

By Dunbar Roy, M. D.,
Atlanta, Ga.

A male aged 18 had a suppurating ethmoiditis with numerous polypi. Operated on the left side with uneventful recovery. Four months later the right side was operated upon. Four days following this there was hemorrhage from that side readily checked. Two days later a severe hemorrhage occurred from both sides for which the nose was tightly packed. Ten days later free bleeding again from both nasal cavities. The blood always clotted freely. The greatest bleeding seemed to be from the left side, and the nose was packed. Blood still oozing, the left common carotid was tied under anesthesia.

Five days after this hemorrhage from the neck incision and again the following day.

It was decided to open the incision in the neck and tie the bleeding vessels. The patient took but a few whiffs of gas when he stopped breathing. No autopsy was allowed, but the incision in the neck was opened and all of the neck muscles and fascia were undermined and an immense cavity found filled with clotted blood. The suture on the carotid was firm and there was complete ligation.

No blood examination was made as the blood clotted freely and it was expected that the hemorrhage would be controlled.

Evidently a slow bacteremia had been progressing for some time due to the absorption for years of pus from the ethmoid cells, and this had undermined the coats of the blood vessels as well as the integrity of other body tissues.

While the immediate cause of death was the general anesthetic, this would not have produced death had there not been such an excessive loss of blood and the whole system in an abnormal state.

This unfortunate termination emphasizes the great danger of these extreme cases of necrosing ethmoiditis.

## Neuralgias of the Trigeminal Tract and Facial Neuralgias of Other Origin—Impressions Derived from a Survey of 555 Cases.

By Charles H. Frazier, M. D., Sc. D.,
Surgeon to the University Hospital, Philadelphia.

Major trigeminal neuralgia is the term that would be proposed as descriptive and distinctive; and in order that there may be no misunderstanding as to what is implied, the following brief sketch is its distinguishing and characteristic features.

Appearing suddenly and without any apparent exciting cause and with few exceptions after middle life, a sharp, shooting, stabbing, lancinating pain is experienced at first in one of the three divisions of the trigeminal nerve, usually the second or third.

The pain is likened by the patient to an electric shock, to a boring hot iron, to the tearing of flesh. The distribution of the pain has definite anatomic limitations, and without variation is referred to the terminal distribution of the nerve involved to the lips, gums, tongue, teeth, nose, forehead. The pain comes as a bolt from the sky and vanishes like a shooting star. "Attacks" indicate certain periods of time during which the patient is subject to paroxysmal seizures. The attacks are of varying duration, a week or two at first, and two or three in a year, but as time goes on the attacks are of longer duration and of greater frequency. The pain of renal and biliary colic is of great intensity, to be sure, but controlled at least in part by morphin  Not so the pain of trigeminal neuralgia. The habitual use of morphin is presumptive evidence that the patient is not a subject of the disease under discussion.

It would seem that peripheral infections, including sinus diseases, played no part in the etiology. These convictions have been forced upon me by a critical analysis of my clinical experiences. On my records there are only three instances in which either at the time of my first observation or previous thereto, had the patient been under treatment for sinus disease. For a hundred years and more the etiology has been a matter of speculation and we are as far today as ever from any clearcut conception or any convincing data as to the prevailing cause.

The following is a brief summary of observations upon types of neuralgia: We recognize, first of all, a definite clinical entity in what we prefer to call "major trigeminal neuralgia," the symptoms of which are so characteristic that a diagnosis can be made that should admit of no discussion. The etiology is still a matter of speculation. We recognize other neuralgias in the distribution of the trigeminal nerve that have a specific cause, some of them stimulating the major type, such as (1) the neuralgias due to tumors involving the sensory root, the ganglion or its several divisions; or (2) the neuralgia following herpes zoster. We recognize a third group of neuralgias, involving chiefly the ophthalmic division, that we believe to be of toxic origin; symptomatically they have nothing in common with the major type. We recognize a fourth or miscellaneous group in which the pain, though of great intensity but not paroxysmal, is referred chiefly to the orbit, temple and cheek, sometimes to the neck, associated frequently with general headache or hemicrania; a group in which our suspicion has been aroused as to the part the sympathetic system may play in its origin. Finally a group which we classify under the psychoneuroses or psychalgias.

In discussing the treatment of major trigeminal neuralgia, restricting the remarks chiefly to experience with the major operation, of these there have been 204 avulsions or sections of the sensory tract, 5 complete excisions of the ganglion and 5 partial excisions of the ganglion. The major operation has long since been robbed of its terrors; the mortality, once 5%, has been reduced to less than 1%, there having been but one operative fatality in the last 177 cases of my series. In the vast majority the patients, as one would anticipate, express complete satisfaction with the results.

At one time or another, I have introduced certain variations, to which I will refer in passing. For a while I have substituted section of the root for avulsion but to no advantage. In a few instances I have left intact the inner fasciculus of the sensory root, when the ophthamic division was not involved, in the hope that by so doing trophic keratitis might be avoided. I am now awaiting results; should in the course of time there be any recurrence in the series, this modification will have to be abandoned. Latterly I have been able to conserve the motor root and thus prevent the atrophy of the temporal muscles, which hitherto interfered with a perfect cosmetic result. This modification, furthermore, now makes it possible to operate on both sides in bilateral cases. All the technical difficulties have been mastered and the operation is now one of the most satisfactory the neurosurgeon is called upon to pertorm.

## DISCUSSION.

Dr. Greenfield Sluder, St. Louis, Mo.: In the course of Dr. Frazier's paper he spoke of the sinuses of the perinasal space, as, in all probability, not being the cause of trigeminal neuralgia. I have seen three such cases—at least, three that I thought were such cases. One was sent to me by Dr. Halsted, who can tell more of the story than I can of sphenoid suppuration, on which he operated and got relief for a year. Then the patient returned, and ultimately come to a Gasserian ganglion operation. I had a case of tic that was relieved by a simple operation on the sphenoid. This was only a short while ago, and may be considered as not finished. He may have further trouble. I have another case that was relieved some years ago, and has not returned; but my experience with trigeminal neuralgias, as described by Dr. Frazier is negligible. That is, my own experience. I have, however, repeatedly seen what I thought was major trigeminal neuralgia exhibit a sticking pain. There was a lowerhalf headache and pain, as a constriction about the eye, the upper jaw, the teeth, the ear, and the mastoid, almost more than back of the mastoid, with a point of tenderness attached. The shoulder blade, the arm, the forearm and the fingers were also involved. It was nearly a complete case, when it went down to his elbow. It repeatedly proved to be controllable by the nasal ganglion; by cocainization injection relieved it for a year and a half. Then an attack of coryza reestablished the pain, and it passed off in the wake of the coryza. Later, he developed another coryza, which reestablished the pain; and it did not pass off. It was injected a second time, and the patient has not yet had a recurrence. Pain of nasal ganglion origin can always be reestablished by virtue of the fact that the ganglion remains in the tissue superficial to the nose, and may be irritated again by inflammation in the nose. I think it is as well to put in here as elsewhere the question of a psychologic estimate of these cases. Dr. Cushing, last summer, gave three papers. In these articles he spoke of this lowerhalf headache and mentioned a case in which the pain was from the major neuralgia of the trigeminus. He expressed to me in conversation the opinion that these were all spilled over; and he put in the text the view that there is no reason to assume that the nasal ganglion is responsible for this symptom complex. He thought that it was more rational to assume that the second division of the fifth nerve was the origin of the pain and that it was spilled over. It is difficult or impossible for me to understand how these can be cases spilled over from the trigeminus, from my experience of Dr. Cushing's cases. He most kindly showed me some of these cases in the beginning of my observations, in 1909. I had seen enough to justify me in describing nasal ganglion cases, but my experience was that of a beginner and I did not understand his cases at the time; and I do not quite understand them now. A woman from whom he had removed the Gasserian ganglion at the distribution of the headache had a most violent headache, with sphenoiditis; and I opened the sphenoid, with instant relief from the frightful headache. I tried to open the sphenoid by a comprehensive opening, but could not get through by my customary technic; because the bone was so thick and hard. I used an eight-inch drill, and succeeded; but the hole closed up in a few days. I did not do any more comprehensive surgery. Some time later I heard that she was suffering about as much as before. That pain was not spilled over from the trigeminus, because the trigeminus was gone. Nor can these cases be explained by segmental overlapping, however, when the trigeminus was no longer there. I have done a dozen ophthalmoplegic migraines, in which the sphenoid was operated on with relief. To my mind, these cases are explicable by virtue of thin bone, which separates not merely the optic nerves, but also the third, fourth and sixth nerves. If these cases, then, be of sphenoidal origin, and explicable by the thin separation of the lining nerve trunks, that can readily recur for the same reason that established it in the beginning. You cannot change the thickness of the bone separating it or give more protection to the adjacent nerves.

Dr. Frazier spoke also of pain that was stopped by cocainization of the sphenopalatine or nasal ganglion. The fact of pain transmission then arose in my mind. The question of the sympathetic comes in; and it seems to me that, as no other nerve connection is available, it must then be assumed that the sympathetic, if not under normal conditions, at least under abnormal, becomes capable of afferent transmission. The literature on the subject of the possible sensory attributes of the sympathetic is very extensive.

Dr. Ross Faulkner, New York City: Dr. Frazier has established the surgical procedure, and has shown the world its great value in relieving suffering. Also, he has reduced the mortality from over 22% to less than 1%. Dana, some years ago, writing on tic douloureux, mentioned the fact that a case of two years standing can be cured by castor oil. I thought that there might be some truth in it; and in the cases that came to me, I tried it. To my surprise, some got rid of the pain for quite a long period. The method employed is almost as severe as operation. He gave it every night. It is, by all means, worth trying, and there is no doubt that some cases will get rid of the pain from that treatment.

The etiology of this thing has been very much of a mystery, and I have never been able to get any light on the solution of it. It occurs in all classes, the poor as well as the rich.

The method used by me for alcohol injection was practised for a long time by splitting the head of the cadaver and taking out the nerve. By using a good deal of cocaine, and employing a needle with an abrupt bevel to it, I was able to determine if the point of the needle was in the nerve. I used three or four drops of cocaine for anesthesia. Not more than ten drops of alcohol was used for that sort of injection. In a large number of cases there were permanent results. I have six cases, at least, that have never come back. The majority come back within a year, or even six months.

In the second division, I have not had satisfactory results. You cannot get into it, but must put the alcohol around the nerve. But in the third division, you can do so, and work easily into the substance of the nerve and get complete anesthesia with the injection of alcohol. The good results secured by this method justify its being tried in all cases in the third division. All cases should be treated with castor oil first; and then, if this fails and especially if they are confined to the third division, inject alcohol into the nerve. Continue to try a number of times, until you get in. With the first or second division, it is difficult to get a result, unless one injects the ganglion. I had one case in the first division alone which I did the ganglion injection with alcohol. I have had two such cases. I should not recommend it, however, because if the direction is not right, you might get into the cavernous sinus or the carotid artery.

Dr. Charles H. Frazier (closing): I should be disposed to agree with most of what has been said in the course of the discussion. To one remark I should, however, take exception. Dr. Sluder referred in his remarks to a case of "low grade tic." In my opinion there is no such thing. A correct diagnosis of tic douloureux presupposes a violent, excruciating pain—a pain of great intensity and severity. With regard to tic douloureux or the major trigeminal neuralgia there should be no conflict of opinion as to its recognition. It is quite distinct from that variety of neuralgia—sphenopalatine neuralgia, if you choose—to which the discussion this afternoon has been chiefly devoted. That the latter may be of sympathetic origin is not unlikely. Not until in suitable cases we have excised the sphenopalatine ganglion can we speak with any positiveness as to the part this ganglion, with its sympathetic connections, plays in the etiology. Alcohol injection of the sphenopalatine ganglion for obvious reasons is not comparable to injection of the Gasserian ganglion or its divisions.

In my address, I did not touch upon the subject of alcohol injection for the relief of trigeminal neuralgia. The subject is too big to discuss in a cursory way. In the management of patients I never urge one or the other method—alcohol injection or operation —but after laying the facts before the patient, leave the choice to him. In nine cases out of ten, if he has suffered for only a year or two, he will choose the injection; if for a longer time and he has had already several injections, he elects the operation.

I cannot agree with the statement of Dr. Faulkner as to variations in the period of relief following injections of the second and third divisions, nor do I agree with him in his prohibitive attitude towards injections of the ganglion. In very old people, in the exceptional case where there may be some contraindication to oper-ation, when the ophthalmic division is involved, and in cases of inoperable carcinoma of the face, I have not hesitated to recom-mend and practice ganglion injections. Particularly in the cancer group have I found these injections so welcome. By enabling the patient to eat without pain and to sleep without morphin, life for the time is quite transformed.

### Nasal Tuberculosis.
By William B. Chamberlin, M. D.,
Cleveland, Ohio.

Nasal tuberculosis is rare, but the primary form not as rare as ordinarily supposed. There is still some confusion in use of terms lupus and tuberculosis. Zarniko's classification into proliferative and ulcerative types is probably simplest and best. Zarniko thinks that the term lupus should be dropped, though Killian still clings to this term on account of the attenuated form of the infection and the chronicity of the involvement.

Symptoms are usually those due to nasal obstruction with in-creased secretion. Pain is rare. Bleeding and crust formation is occasionally present.

The place of predilection is usually the cartilaginous septum, inferior turbinal, nasal floor and lateral nasal wall being next in order. Bone involvement is secondary. Infection may be due to inhalation of infected air or to a direct lesion from the infected finger nail.

Tubercle bacilli are always rare and may not be found at all. Presence of giant cells in fields of epithelial and lymph cells estab-lish the diagnosis, even though typical tubercles and tubercle bacilli are not found. Typical miliary tubercles with centres of cheesy degeneration are pathognomonic.

Differential diagnosis from syphilis, malignancy and foreign body with granulation tissue is presented.

Treatment is surgical removal, with subsequent application of lactic acid or superheated air.

### DISCUSSION.

Dr. Emil Mayer, New York City: I am one of those who still feels that we should keep up with the term lupus, because there is a great big difference between tuberculosis and the attenuated form of tuberculosis that we call lupus. In the cases of lupus of the upper air passages that I have cited, and which I have watched patiently for eighteen or twenty years, I feel that I was justified in adhering to the original term. Why not consider the fingernail infection? These are cases in which the disease appears in the area that could easily be reached by the fingernail on entering the nose. There is another form that cannot be classed among the ulceratice or tubercular. In the cases cited Dr. Chamberlin spoke of either a destruction or a form of new growth. We have the lymph exudative forms, and I have seen cases of that kind of tuber-culosis of the nose in which the only symptom was that of repeated attacks of laryngeal spasm. Examination showed yellow exudate, which eventually showed miliary tuberculosis; and the patient went to pieces rapidly. In one case I made a diagnosis of tuberculosis in a young woman whose only evidence was a yellow exudate on the inferior and posterior portion of the uvula. Now the importance of making a differential diagnosis between lupus and tuberculosis, to my mind, is, in the first instance, the importance to the patient of the fact that you can tell him that he does not need a change of climate and will be just as well off at home as anywhere else; and, in the second, the importance to the patient of being relieved from any fear of the possibility of contagion, so far as his carrying the disease to anyone else is concerned. Why not treat them with the galvanocautery? That can be as safely done in the nose, and the conditions as thoroughly eradicated, as anywhere else, and with less danger from having an open wound in a tubercular patient and have a recurrence of his condition. 1 should like very much to have Dr. Chamberlin ultimately report what has happened to the second case. That patient, as I understood, had miliary tuberculosis; and I regard this as a most dangerous sort of condition to the patient, who may succumb in a very short time.

Dr. Lee Wallace Dean, Iowa City, Iowa: During the last two years we have been studying cases of chronic suppuration of the paranasal sinuses suffering from pulmonary tuberculosis. A similar investigation of chronic otorrhea in this class of patients showed that many of the mastoids were tuberculous. To our surprise we found that tuberculosis of the paranasal sinuses was a rare thing unless it was secondary to bone tuberculosis in the neighborhood of the diseased sinus. We have not found a single case where the sinus disease was tuberculosis unless it was secondary to bone tuberculosis. In one case of chronic maxillary sinus disease the purulent discharge contained acid fast bacilli and produced tuberculosis when injected into a guinea pig. Careful microscopic examination of the lining of the sinuses and the surrounding bone showed that there was no tuberculosis of the sinuses; that the bacillus tuberculosis was present as an accidental contamination.

Dr. B. Alex Randall, Philadelphia: I want to mention a case of tuberculosis, which more or less completely involved the nasal chambers themselves. Many of the teeth were loosened. These were all removed, and curettement of th alveolar processes carried out with the removal of much of the nasal mucosa by Harrison Allen, who had charge. The patient survived for twenty years or more.

Dr. Lee M. Hurd, New York City: I wish to report some cases of mistaken diagnosis. One of these was a case of socalled lupus—lupus of the lip and vestibule. Sections were found by one pathologist to be tubercular. Dr. Jonathan Wright doubted this, and said that granuloma from syphilis and from tuberculosis could not be told apart under the microscope. The case cleared up under mixed treatment. Other cases that were diagnosed as tubercular all cleared up under antisyphilitic treatment. They were all in the anterior part of the nose.

Dr. William B. Chamberlin, Cleveland (closing): With regard to Dr. Mayer's insistence on the term lupus, I personally cannot see any great justification for that term. Dr. Mayer did not hear my remark about the finger being the most probable cause of infection; airborne infection being the one most insisted on, and the fingernails being the most probable cause of infection. The type of cases he mentioned, I am glad to know of. I did not know anything of that type of case. His suggestion in regard to treatment is apropos. I think one should be careful in the use of galvanocautery, not to carry the cautery so deep that the cartilage becomes involved.

In many cases I made a probable diagnosis of tuberculosis, which was ultimately confirmed by the pathologist.

In regard to Dr. Dean's reference to tuberculosis in sinus cases, I would say that I have not found it in such cases.

## Some Observations on Localized Pulmonary Suppuration, Treated by Endobronchial Irrigation.

### By Charles J. Imperatori, M. D.,
### New York City.

Lung abscesses may be divided into three classes, those that are caused by aspiration, by embolism and another type, possibly a tubercular cavitation with a secreting lining of infecting organisms. Observations were conducted on seven cases, two being alive and still under treatment. Of the five deaths, one died from a carcinoma of the bronchus, one was operated elsewhere, that is, a pneumectomy was done, but the patient succumbed on the table and the other three cases died from an intercurrent pneumonia.

Of the five cases that died, four were autopsied and proven, beyond doubt, to be tubercular; one being a carcinoma with a tuberculosis. All of these cases were repeatedly examined, careful sputum analyses made, fluoroscoped, radiographed and decided that they were probably not tubercular and referred from either the medical, surgical or tubercular wards as cases for treatment. The remaining two cases, clinically, have the same characteristics that the other five had.

Simple bronchial irrigations, in the writer's opinion, in the control and treatment of lung abscesses of this type, are of little use. It is very possible, with the use of the spiral irrigating tubes of Lynah, better results may be obtained and this method shall be pursued in subsequent cases. Various medicaments were used in some of the early treatments of these cases, such as iodoform emulsion, iodin in olive oil, tincture iodin, weak Dakin solution—one and ten, and boric acid solution. All with negative results. Warm saline solution and the injection of olive oil, impregnated with the 5% bismuth, seemed to be as efficacious as anything.

Idiopathic lung abscess, and by that is meant that type of abscess other than that directly traceable to aspiration or trauma of some foreign substance, or the embolic abscess following some surgical procedure, is possibly a tubercular cavitation with a lining area of pyogenic organisms. This can not be given as a definite conclusion and is merely suggestive from these personal observations and must be proven by a larger series of cases.

## DISCUSSION.

Dr. Emil Mayer, New York: A patient with a purulent condition in his bronchus is a most unhappy individual, and anything that can be done to relieve these patients is of such value that it should receive every bit of recognition possible. As Dr. Imperatori says, not enough of this work has been done to enable one to state definitely what particular remedy is going to be of the greatest advantage. There is one thing, however, that I wish to call attention to, and have called attention to, in regard to this same subject, and that is the need of a certain amount of care in not doing irrigations too frequently. These patients receive, as a rule, a hypodermic injection of morphia, and require a fairly strong solution of cocaine to render the bronchus as free from cough and irritation as possible. It must be borne in mind that while we have a dreadful disease, yet we have no right to inflict on these poor individuals, in addition to their other suffering, either the morphin or the cocaine habit.

Dr. George Richards, Fall River, Mass.: I should like to ask what objection there would be to making a direct opening into the lung, resecting one or two ribs, and getting direct outward drainage? I had a case in which I was doubtul whether it was tubercular or not. The general surgeon, under general anesthesiu, resected the ribs and drained the abscess outwardly; and although the girl had suffered for two months, she slowly and continuously got well, and is at work at her occupation. Is there more risk from the surgical operation of making an opening directly into the lung? It is more or less disagreeable to the patient to make these irrigations. The technic must be of considerable difficulty on the part of the operator.

Dr. Henry L. Swain, New Haven, Conn.: Dr. Richards' question of an opening on the outside presupposes that you can readily discover where the abscess is and can get at it from the outside. I have run over a couple of cases in which that was not easy, even after the injection of bismuth. That couldn't always be done with any degree of safety or accuracy.

I should like to ask Dr. Imperatori how much trouble he has in getting his patients accustomed to the dosage? He spoke of it as though he always operates on the recumbent patient? I have sometimes thought that if I could get the patient to sit up so that the stuff would stay in better than when lying down, it would be a good thing.

Dr. Henry L. Lynah, New York City: I believe that most of the lung abscesses are due to aspiration, because all of the surgeons agree that embolic cases die rather early. The patients which I have had the good fortune to bronchoscope are all still alive. In washing out the abscess cavities, as advised by Yankauer, I never have been able to recover any of the solution by suction, for it is always coughed out through the bronchoscopic tube mouth as fast as it is injected. Personally I believe that the dilatation of bronchial stenoses and the establishment of proper lung drainage is what improves the cases. I only use suction after bronchoscopic dilatation, and seem to have obtained some results. Bleeding, edematous and fungating granulations are always touched with 10 to 20% nitrate of silver. As to the injections of bismuth sub-carbonate in olive oil, that was not done with any idea of curing the cases, but was purely for purposes of definite localization of the abscess cavity. All of the patients, however, improved. Dr. Wm. H. Stewart attributed the improvement to the secondary action of the X-ray on the metallic substance in the lung. We have had bismuth remain in the lung for ten months after injection, but often when the bismuth disappears the abscess is healed.

In cases following tonsillectomy early bronchoscopic examination is always indicated while the process is in the pneumonic stage, and before definite cavitation has taken place. We have had some startling recoveries in these early cases after removal of sloughs from the edematous bronchus and bronchial dilatation and aspiration.

Dr. William B. Chamberlin, Cleveland, Ohio: Dr. Lynah's remarks illustrate a case of mine in which removing granulation tissue and plugging one branch proved beneficial. This boy, 18 years of age, had given a history of purulent expectoration since he was six years old, probably produced by a foreign body. We could find no evidence of it. If it was a foreign body, it gave no shadow on the plate. Subsequent to the injection, the purulent discharge decreased decidedly, and the odor almost entirely disappeared. There was marked improvement after such treatment, no bismuth being used. He had gained ten pounds in weight, and the odor had entirely disappeared.

Dr. R. B. Canfield, Ann Arbor, Mich.: I would like to add a case of pulmonary abscess similar to the last described by Dr. Imperatori. It occurred in a child of 11 years who had a pulmonary abscess of two years' standing of unknown etiology, from which she expectorated about six ounces of foul pus at intervals of five or six days. The abscess was located in the lower left lobe. It was plainly seen through the bronchoscope, communicated with the bronchus through a small opening, and was lined by foul smelling granulation. Bronchosopy, aspiration and the use of compound tincture of benzoin secured a satisfactory recovery after several treatments. The satisfactory result of the treatment was confirmed by the X-ray, which showed a steady diminution in the size of the abscess and its ultimate obliteration.

Dr. Harmon Smith, New York City: I should like to ask whether, if in tuberculous, there is danger of hemorrhage; and whether the use of iodine and olive oil would not enable the patient to retain it?

Dr. Charles J. Imperatori, New York City (closing): The point is to find out whether I am correct in my assertion that these lung abscesses may be caused by any other means than by straight aspiration and embolism. All these cases were seen in the wards of Bellevue Hospital. They were not cases that came directly to the otolaryngologic service, but were transferred to it. They were surgical, medical or tubercular cases. They were assumed not to be tuberculous; although several, from the radiographic plate, had been diagnosed as such, and then the diagnosis was changed. I have not had any cases following tonsillectomy. I have not had any embolic cases. In the four autopsies, there were found distinct tubercles, from the size of a pea to that of a hazel nut, within a centimeter or so of the abscess cavity.

Answering Dr. Meyer, I would say that the patient never gets more than a quarter of a grain of morphin. That is measured in minims. Usually, the patients get six or seven minims of Magendie solution. The amount of cocaine is never more than a dram. The method of cocainization is with a Cohen applicator. Make an application to the base of the tongue, and then the cushion of the epiglottis. With an applicator syringe at the same time, you touch the larynx and inject a drop of cocaine. Then wait five minutes and do it again. Use an atomizer and spray the trachea with three or four sprays of a ten per cent cocaine. Then, as the bronchoscope is passed, make one application to the carina.

Answering the questions, I would say that I know of one case in which outside drainage was done, and several cases in which olive oil and iodin were used by the general surgeon. I always bronchoscope the patient in the reclining position, and usually employ a 7 m. m. tube. I expect to have a 5 m. m. tube to get into the smaller bronchi. I do not believe that any of the solution stays there, but the reason for injecting the saline solution is to soften up and liquify the pus that I did not seem to be able to suck out with our aspiration apparatus. Following Yankauer's technic, I injected eight ounces and sucked it out. Knowing that Dr. Lynah was injecting these lung abscesses and radiographing them, and hearing that he was curing them, I decided to use bismuth. At first I used bismuth subnitrate; but later I changed it to bismuth subcarbonate. I have never used iodin. In regard to the danger of hemorrhage in tuberculous cases, when I was working at the Riverside Hospital, I irrigated a number of abscesses, with negative results. If any cases showed a tendency to bleeding, I discontinued the use of the bronchoscope indefinitely.

### Group Head Surgery.
By B. R. Shurly, M. D.,
Detroit, Mich.

This system will win or fail if guiding hands steer it safely from the shoals of commercialism and fee splitting. If efficiency and humanitarianism are not sacrificed by greed, disloyalty, lack of harmony and cooperation, the group system is sure to win.

The advantages to the patient are self-evident. He realizes fully the necessity of laboratory, X-ray and dental examinations and hospital observation at a fair fee.

The group system adds the danger of machine diagnosis and repair shop methods. It is said that one of our automobile hospitals is so highly specialized that the operating room similizes the assembling plant to such an extent that one man prepares the field, a second makes the incision, a third operates, a fourth sews up the wounds, and a fifth puts on the dressing, while the sixth, the anesthetist, moves the patient to his room, and a seventh brings in another patient. Humanitarianism is so far removed that the eighth who takes the history is the only one who can recognize the patient on the street some weeks later, if the patient is lucky enough to get there.

Group head surgery must be affiliated with, or control a head hospital and teaching opportunities to be scientifically progressive and efficient.

In our own specialty, at the beginning of the war, regular medical officers were assigned to duty as eye, ear, nose and throat specialists, who were usually without interest or training in the work. Your committee changed this immediately. Group head surgical units were organized and successfully performed enormous labor in this country and abroad. The original estimate of 200 beds in a 1000-bed hospital devoted to Army Hospital work was approximately correct.

## ADVANTAGES OF GROUP PRACTICE.

The advantages of group practice are, first, better diagnosis and scientific work, cooperation, mutual interest, conservation of effort, quick service to the profession and the public, the division of labor, specialization along lines particularly interesting to the individual, the pleasure of working among the sick where no man thinks he owns the case, co-operative system in buying of instruments and general equipment, conservation of office space, the use of team work at all times of the day or night, the practical value of an office and hospital together that can be operated by the same staff for the mutual advantage of the patient and the practitioner.

If state and industrial medicine with health insurance are to absorb private practice, it will be necessary to adopt a feudal group system to protect the practitioner and the public who demand private service. It will be of advantage in case state medicine and state hospitals increase to combine with other groups for their personal protection and existence. The success of the group is in relation to the ordinary attributes of industry, intelligence, harmony and a spirit of co-operation, all of which characteristics ultmately receive their full reward.

## DISADVANTAGES OF GROUP PRACTICE.

The personal equation is lost between the physician and the patient; the machine and dispensary methods prevail, unless carefully guarded. It is difficult to obtain a group of men who are temperamentally fitted to associate in harmonious endeavor. It is difficult to find practitioners who will always operate under the Golden Rule, but as this is difficult in almost any walk of life, it may not be considered as a disadvantage. It is difficult to obtain men who do not overestimate their personal value and who entertain sufficient broad and humanitarian views to handle patients properly.

### Report of Cases of Cancer of the Esophagus Treated by Radium.
#### By D. C. Greene, M. D.,
#### Boston, Mass.

It is remarkable that cancer in the esophagus is in the majority of cases well advanced before the patients begin to be troubled by difficulty in swallowing. This accounts in part for the signally unsuccessful results of treatment in a curative way. Pain has been frequently absent, especially when the middle and lower thirds of the esophagus have been the regions involved. The most favorable location for early recognition is in the upper end of the esophagus, because here as a rule dysphagia and pain occur relatively early.

In the treatment of cancer of the esophagus with radium we are confronted with serious obstacles. Esophagoscopy has rendered the diagnosis of the site and nature of the lesion a relatively simple matter, but it is usually impossible to determine accurately its size and extent. The surface application of radium by means of bougies loaded with radium tubes, has in our hands been productive of only discomfort and aggravation of symptoms without any beneficial results. This method was at best inaccurate and apt to cause burns of the normal epithelium on account of the dislodgement of the applicator from the original position in which it was placed. The method of permanent implantation of small tubes of the emanation seemed to be worth trial and during the past year I have treated a series of eighteen cases by this method. Radium seeds of a value from one to three millicuries have been shown to have an area of effective radiation of about one centimeter. The destruction of the radium is an element of danger which must be reckoned with in placing the seeds, since perforation of the wall of the esophagus into the aorta or into a bronchus may result from an implantation too close to the outer wall.

The technic of the method employed has been as follows: Under ether a medium sized Mosher esophagoscope is passed down to the growth, the field is cleared by suction, and a seed inserted into the most prominent portion of the growth to a depth of about a centimeter. The trocar used for this purpose is made of sufficient length to be passed through a 17-inch esophagoscope and sufficiently heavy and rigid not to bend enough to interfere with accurate placing and insertion of the point when the instrument is held at its proximal end. The usual dosage has been about 5 m. c. in single tubes or distributed in two or three tubes.

The following history is presented as typical: A woman 55 years, consulted me on December 9, 1920, on account of difficulty in swallowing, first noticed six months previously. For the past two months she had been able to take nothing but liquids and these with increasing difficulty. There had been marked loss of weight and she presented a decidedly emaciated appearance. X-rays taken before I saw her showed a constriction of the esophagus just below the arch of the aorta, extending about four inches downward. On December 16th esophagoscopic examination showed a red granular tumor mass obstructing the lumen at ten and three-quarters inches from the teeth. This mass appeared to be growing from the right side, from about three-quarters of the circumference. A very small lumen could be seen in the left anterior quadrant. A specimen was removed for examination and one seed, 7 m. c., was inserted into the center of the presenting mass. A No. 26 French bougie was passed into the stomach. Histologic examination of the specimen was made by Dr. J. H. Wright, who reported squamous cell carcinoma. This patient had two subsequent treatments at three and four-week intervals. The esophagoscopic examinations showed some sloughing and ulceration of the region of the insertion of the seed, but no noticeable change in the size of the lumen. The patient got along fairly comfortable for three months and had no difficulty in swallowing liquids during this time, and the weight remained almost stationary. During the latter part of March she began to be troubled by cough on taking nourishment. This became so severe that a gastrostomy was advised and performed on March 30th. Five days later she had a severe hemoptysis and died. The autopsy showed an annular carcinomatous mass involving the wall of the esophagus for about five inches from the level of the bifurcation downward. There was a posterior fistula into the aorta and an anterior one into the left primary bronchus. The latter lesion undoubtedly was responsible for the onset of cough.

In only one case was a definite view of the whole tumor obtained, and an opportunity given to insert the radium effectively. The tumor in this case was situated on the anterior wall back of the cricoid.

In general, it may be stated that patients can be given a moderate degree of relief for two or three months by this method. It has been possible to accomplish this degree of palliation with relatively little discomfort from the treatment. Of the eighteen cases treated by this method, fifteen were males and three were females. The tumor was located in the upper third of the esophagus in six, in the middle third in three, and in the lower third in nine cases. The youngest was 45 and the oldest 65 years of age. The average age was 57 years. The average duration of life after beginning treatment was three and a half months. Four patients are under treatment. Only one of these is showing definite improvement in the local condition and in general health. Another, who has been under treatment for five months, is gaining in weight and swallowing better, but the local process as shown by the esophagoscope is still active. The remaining two are rapidly failing. One of these has been under treatment seven months and the other five months. In nearly every instance the patient was able to swallow liquids up to the end and gastrostomy was advised only twice.

### Report of a Case of Carcinoma of the Larynx, and One of Sarcoma of the Nasopharynx Treated With Radium.

By John R. Winslow, M. D.,

Baltimore, Md.

The first was a male aged 56. Dysphagia and dyspnea: fairly clear voice; rapid loss of flesh. Sputum and Wasserman negative. Duration of symptoms, nine months.

There was a large lobulated intralaryngeal tumor. smooth, red and without ulceration. It was apparently attached to the left arty-cartilage, with a tongue-like projection into the hypopharynx.

Although the larynx was almost completely filled by the growth. the dyspnoea was not striking. Removal of specimen diagnosed to be carcinoma.

Preliminary tracheotomy followed by seven hours of radiation, externally screened by three millimeters of lead, and held at a distance of one centimeter from the skin.

This was succeeded by immediate dysphagia and a bad skin burn with ulceration of the neck. This took one year to heal.

In about two weeks all symptoms relative to breathing or swallowing disappeared and within a month all trace of the growth had vanished.

The second case was that of a white boy, aged 19, who had difficulty of breathing through the left nostril. He was a mouth breather, speech thick and nasal.

A voluminous tumor was found in the epipharynx, with smooth surface and firm to touch. Specimen showed sarcoma.

Tracheotomy, with subsequent removal of the growth. Recurrence in about two months. This was treated by radium, partly by direct contact, but mainly by needles inserted into the growth. Because of unavoidable interruptions, treatment was extended over more than two years. Patient has been free from symptoms of growth for about a year.

### Radium Emanation; Its Advantages Over Radium for Use in the Upper Air Passages. A New Way of Applying It.

By Otto T. Freer, M. D.,
Chicago, Ill.

The limited distance to which the radium rays are therapeutically effective is in part due to their divergence in all directions in the matter of light rays so that only moderately far from their source they become too far apart to influence materially morbid states. The greater the amount of radium or its emanation placed at the source, however, the greater will be the distance to which rays sufficiently close together to give the required therapeutic effect will be projected.

Radium applications to the larynx and laryngopharynx are the most difficult regions for exact and prolonged applications of radium emanation. The applicator is passed into the larynx with the aid of the laryngeal mirror, as in ordinary swabbing of the larynx. Only for the papillomas of childhood are suspension laryngoscopy and a straight applicator needed. The larynx is anesthetized with a 5% spray of cocaine, followed soon by swabbing the laryngeal interior with pure cocaine flakes upon a moist swab. The clamp is then put on with the help of an assistant. Anesthesin powder is then puffed into the pharynx and larynx to heighten the local insensibility. It intensifies the action of the cocaine and quiets the retching caused at times by cocaine in certain throats. The applicator is now introduced, the screen being placed exactly upon the spot in the glottis, upper larynx or fossapyriformis, where it is wanted, while the assistant guides the vertical stem of the applicator into the open jaws of the clamp. He instanely closes upon it when the screen is in the right place, where it stays until the clamp is opened. The saliva pump is then started and the patient left to himself in the assistant's care. Should retching occur after a time, anesthesin powder or a little cocaine spraying will usually stop it without the removal of the applicator, but if it becomes violent, the applicator is taken out, cocaine sprayed into the throat and the applicator replaced. Retching may often be prevented if the patient retain his napkin hold upon the tongue during the session. Some patients quietly endure the presence of the applicator for an hour or more; others need it taken out once or twice in an hourly session.

For applications to the tonsil and faucial regions, an applicator is used that lacks the laryngeal bend.

For nasal applications a headband is used, upon whose forehead four small clamps are fastened. They consist merely of a piece of brass tubing opened widely enough on one side to admit length-wise a stem of copper wire with a capsular screen soldered to its end. A set screw penetrates the wall of the tube and fixes the stem at any point desired. The small clamps are affixed to the forehead plate upon their unopened sides. By proper bending of the wire stem the screen may be made to fit into the desired place in the nasal cavity, or pernasally, in the nasopharynx, where it is held in place by closing the clamp.

Six laryngeal carcinomas and four pharyngeal ones were treated with the applicators and emanation. Mention of previous cases treated with radium needling is omitted. Three of the laryngeal carcinomas were intrinsic, involving the arytenoids, the aryepiglottic folds and fossaepyriformes. Three were intrinsic, involving the right vocal cord in each instance. In the extrinsic cases the appearance of the larynx became normal in from four to eight weeks after the last treatment, inspection showing no trace of the growth. So far, no patient has shown a local relapse, but in one the larynx has been invaded from without by rapidly growing glandular tumors. The intrinsic case patients permitted the use of large three and four-case screen in the glottis as long as needed, for a full hour in several instances. In the most extensive of the intrinsic when first seen the carcinomatous mass buried both the right vocal cord and ventricular band, the right side of the larynx being immobile. There was no ulceration. Three weeks after the last of four intralaryngeal treatments of 100 millicurie hours each, the patient recovered his voice, which had been a hoarse whisper for half a year. The right vocal cord regained some of its motion and became clearly outlined, all trace of the carcinoma disappeared. This condition has become stationary, cicatricial retraction binding the right cord partly down. While the disappearance of a carcinoma takes the number of weeks mentioned, almost immediate improvement in the symptoms, preceding the disturbance of the reaction, has been repeatedly seen, as for instance, the melting away of the verrucous excrescenses of a papillary carcinoma of the pharynx lying just above the left arytenoid body inside of a week after the first raying.

The treatment of malignant laryngeal disease with radium rays requires a comparatively large dose of emanation, from 100 to 200 millicuries applied at each sitting, in order to reduce the time of the raying to a minimum in the irritable laryngeal region and to flood the territory under treatment to its utmost pathologic limits with rays sufficiently close together to destroy all microscopic carcinomatous implants. Small radium doses can not do this.

## Radium in the Treatment of Laryngeal Carcinoma, With a Review of the Literature.

### By Fielding O. Lewis, M. D.,
### Philadelphia, Pa.

The writer treated sixteen cases of carcinoma of the larynx with radium since January, 1917, with the following results:

One case in which total laryngectomy had been performed, which had recurrence in the thyroid gland, died six months after operation. Another, in whom a complete laryngectomy was performed two weeks ago, has had large doses of radium within the larynx, and radium plaques applied externally for the past year. While doing nicely, it is too early to record accurate results. Another, in which thyrotomy had been performed, with recurrence of the disease in the external·wound, was treated by radium needles and died eight months after the thyrotomy. One with early involvement on the right side of the larynx was treated by radium needles inserted directly into the growth, had early retrogression, later showed signs of beginning activity, was thyrotomized. The patient is still living and there is no evidence of recurrence after four months.

The remaining twelve cases, which were considered inoperable were tracheotomized and treated vigorously by introducing needles into the growth and radium applied externally.

In two of these remaining twelve cases there was marked retrogression of the growth, so much so that the site of the lesion was hardly perceptible, and the patient's condition remained so for many months. Recurrence developed, and in spite of the use of radium, they died in about a year after their first treatment.

Out of 109 cases above recorded, ten were living at the time the reports were published, showing a mortality of about 91 per cent.

The method of applying radium in the cases which came under our observation was as follows: The first three or four cases were treated by introducing the capsule, properly screened, into the larynx, after the patient has been thoroughly cocainized, using a 20 per cent cocaine solution within the larynx, preceded by a hypodermic of ¼ grain of morphin sulphate. The radium was held in position after the manner described by Jackson and Janeway. Later, 8⅓ to 12½ m. g. needles, to which strings were securely tied, were introduced into the growth, the number depending upon the size of the lesion. These were left in position in some instances for seven to twelve hours. In addition to the needles, external applications were also used.

From reports, the writer is of the opinion that more recent, improved technic in the use of radium emanations, as practiced at the Memorial Hospital in New York, offers more encouraging results.

From the writer's experience and from published reports, it would seem that radium is only indicated in the socalled inoperable cases of carcinoma of the larynx, meaning those cases in which there is marked involvement of the cervical glands, epiglottis, base of the tongue, and the esophageal wall. Its analgesic effect in the cases, in moderate doses, constitutes one of the most important benefits. It is valuable for those patients who refuse operation. It perhaps exercises a beneficial effect in blocking the lymphatics before a radical operation upon the larynx. Such brilliant results have been obtained in early intrinsic malignancy of the larynx by thyrotomy that in these cases radium should not be thought of except possibly as a postoperative measure. In the more advanced type of intrinsic cancer of the larynx, laryngectomy has prolonged the lives of many by surgeons in all parts of the world. Here, again, radium should not be considered a means of treatment except before or after operations.

## DISCUSSION.

Dr. Henry L. Swain, New Haven, Conn.: I should like to know whether radium emanations should be used in laryngeal fibromata, and whether these growths will yield to that treatment.

Dr. Henry L. Lynah, New York: I should like to know whether Dr. Freer has made pathologic sections of any of these cases.

Dr. Norval H. Pierce, Chicago: I should say, without equivocation, that the last case that Dr. Freer reported was one of carcinoma. The only possible way to substantiate the diagnosis was by histologic study. Here was a man within the danger zone as to age, who had hoarseness, increasing since January last. There was distinct lagging of the cord, fusiform growth, with more ulceration, I think, than Dr. Freer tells us. If this case recovers, my enthusiasm for radium treatment will be greatly increased. I wish to accentuate that, because I believe that it is a case of carcinoma.

Dr. Cornelius G. Coakley, New York: I have clinically seen similar lesions which had all the appearance to me of being carcinoma; and in all these cases, I feel that it is unwise to regard the condition as carcinoma. One should remove a section, and I have been surprised how often I have been mistaken in the clinical phases when compared with the pathologist's report. Tuberculosis simulates the signs in the chest, and I think it would be unwise to consider it carcinoma.

Dr. Robert Clyde Lynch, New Orleans, La.: I should like to ask whether there was any effect on the top of the cord in the case which Dr. Pierce spoke of, and what Dr. Freer thinks necessary in order to screen the normal half of the larynx while exposing the diseased side?

Dr. Henry L. Swain: I should like to ask whether the flat container can be made to screen one side more than the other?

Dr. Freer (closing): In respect to the various questions, I would say regarding sarcoma that I spoke, perhaps, a little too optimistically about these growths; but my experience has been that they yield readily to radium, and this is confirmed by the literature. Most men speak of nasal sarcomata as singularly good-natured under radium treatment. Many will disappear after simple surgical work. Their good nature is pretty well substantiated. I had similar success with radium in the old days, even when the sarcoma had got back into the nasopharynx and eustachian tube. Of course, there are some that will not do it; but these growths are better natured than are sarcomata elsewhere. With regard to nasopharyngeal sarcoma, I have not had much experience, except when it complicated nasal sarcoma. It disappeared then, with the nasal sarcoma; but I cannot speak authoritatively on the subject.

Even when Sir Felix Semon was writing about laryngology and took such deep interest in carcinoma of the larynx, it was regarded as a dangerous thing to cut a piece off from a carcinoma in the larynx. The danger of squeezing cancer cells into the larynx was, too, regarded as risky. When a thing appears to be carcinoma, I do not like to cut a piece out, unless I intend to take the whole thing away. larynx and all, if it proves to be such. If I intend to treat it with radium, to cut into the growth may spoil my purpose because the cells travel fast.

Regarding Dr. Coakley's thought that the cord was intact, I would say that I cut a piece out of the center of the cord, with the elastic fibers, where there was a chance of its getting better; and leaving the fibres was a bad thing. It looked like carcinoma, and there was no reason to think that it was tubercular. It is hard to mistake tuberculosis of the larynx. The symptoms indicated carcinoma, and I think that I am justified in considering it highly probable that it is carcinoma.

As to screening, we do not want to screen anything in the neighborhood of carcinoma. We want to illuminate everything in the large area about carcinoma. The carcinoma is simply an evidence of widespread infection. Half the neck may be involved. You want to effect all that you can.

Dr. D. Bryson Delavan, New York City: Much time will be required to establish our knowledge of the efficacy of radium treatment in these cases. Meanwhile. more must be learned regarding the effects of the treatment. Many cases must be treated and they must be kept under careful observation long enough to determine the ultimate actual results. This will require a period of years, rather than months. Again, the uses of radium itself and the possibilities of its action must be better understood. For that reason it is most desirable that the work of Madame Curie, the most brilliant investigator in this department, should be continued by her. At the present time our watchword should be "Patience." No doubt it may require several years to establish much regarding it, but in the meantime, it would be well to refrain from opposition based upon theoretical speculation and to study the subject judiciously and with open minds.

Dr. Harmon Smith, New York City: Radium has more effect on sarcomata than on carcinomata, and particularly lymphosarcomata. Those in the nasopharynx yield more readily and quickly than do carcinomata in that region. The question arises as to the application of radium before or after operation. In view of the fact that radium shuts off the channels by which the growth is disseminated, I think it should be done before. A low order of carcinoma of the larynx that disappears with the application of radium is likely to make us draw the wrong inference. Unless we have some more definite evidence than the clinical observation, we cannot yet determine the effect of radium on these growths.

Dr. Cornelius G. Coakley, New York: I wonder whether the method, as employed by the Institute in New York, is not more generally known. They use a pharyngeal tube, of which the proximal end is just external to the lip. The distal end passes over the epiglottis and over the arytenoid, and the whole pharynx is packed with gauze. . This does just what Dr. Winslow's technic does, but it

saves the patent from tracheotomy and is just as easy to work
with; and I am surprised that this method is not known and employed more in the reports in the literature. The whole tube can
be easily taken out at any time, if there is respiratory obstruction;
but I have never seen any during even a long anesthesia, when
given in that way. It seems to me that the great advantage in
the application of radium has been by the seed method, the use of
radium emanations being preferable to that of radium salts. The
burns that were so frequently obtained in the earlier methods are
avoided. I wonder how necessary it is to have such an apparatus
as was exhibited to us by Dr. Freer. Dr. Janeway was the first
one that I knew of to employ radium within the larynx, and devised
a method by which it could be kept there for at least two hours.
The statement, as he made it to me, made it seem possible that by
simply cocainizing the larynx. one could give the patient a suitable curved applicator that he could hold in his larynx for two
hours. That was demonstrated to me, however; and I wonder
whether such an apparatus could not be done away with. It did
not seem possible to me that the patient himself could hold it in
contact with the exact site of application for the required length
of time. but this is so.

Dr. Henry L. Swain, New Haven:  I wish to refer to an experience that I had, thanks to Dr. Ingersoll, with a case of apparent
lymphosarcoma in the neck. The growth had originally been in
the tonsils. and he had been subjected to massive doses of radium
within and X-ray without. An impovement had resulted and absolute cure had apparently occurred. The patient was sent to me,
to see whether, later on, the man might not need more X-ray—he
living near me. I had the feeling that he did not. At the Boston
meeting we had him come on; and we saw him and concluded that
he was well. He has since died of metastasis, and numerous metastases were found in the abdominal glands. the liver and the lung.

The question arises: Did the massive dosage locally given have
anything to do with driving the thing in, as the laity would put
it, and as his family think? Or had the case progressed so far
that metastasis had started before the radium was applied? That
is the probable solution; but we must consider whether the absorption of the products, when so much living tissue is devitalized, and
the svstem disposes of that being formed at the time of devitaliza-
tion, has anything to do with the future life of the patient.. These
cases seem like acute Hodgkin's disease in the way that they come
up so quickly. The tumor came quickly to its full growth, and
then disappeared again; and it seems unlikely that it led to the
metastasis that occurred.

Dr. Coakley objected to calling the growth carcinoma which Dr.
Freer had treated. It does not make so much difference what it
was. It seemed to be carcinoma, and was treated and got well.

Dr. Lewis said something about making radium application to
the severer cases. I presume he meant the inoperable ones. I
should prefer to hope that very early use of radium might cut the
epithelial changes and render operation unnecessary.

Dr. Arthur W. Watson, Philadelphia: It may be of interest to
the Association to know that the patient I reported a few years
ago as having been treated with radium, a case of carcinoma of

the larynx. is still living and perfectly well. I have examined him quite recently.

In regard to the case reported by Dr. Winslow, a fibrosarcoma of the nasopharynx, it has seemed curious to me that in nearly all cases of fibroma of the nasopharynx that I have seen, and I have seen quite a number, the pathologist's report on a portion removed was sarcoma or fibrosarcoma.

Dr. James E. Logan, Kansas City, Mo.: The description Dr. Freer has just given of his method of applying radium emanations to the interior of the larynx in the treatment of malignant diseases of that organ is very interesting and instructive. With increased experience in this method of procedure he will undoubtedly be able to give to the profession a more comprehensive plan from which we can accomplish more good than has been our experience of the past.

Dr. Winslow's report of the case treated by extralaryngeal application of radium in which a very severe burn followed and a subsequent marked improvement resulted, may open the way to external application of radium or its equivalent, is the method to be employed because of its ease of application, but we have a great deal yet to learn before we can determine what method is best.

It is interesting to note the difference of opinion between pathologists in the diagnosis of intranasal tumors. In one of my cases (Dr. Freer will remember the patient) I removed what my pathologist diagnosed as a spindlecelled sarcoma of the nasopharynx. Recurrence took place six months later, at which time I refused to perform the second operation. The patient went to the Cook County Hospital, Chicago, and the pathologist there diagnosticated a simple fibroid tumor. A second operation was attempted and the patient died on the table. We are never certain of recovery in these cases.

Many years ago I reported a case of round celled sarcoma, recovery after eight years of no recurrence after operation. The patient finally died of a sarcoma of the pancreas. Of course, we have all removed nasal growths with the electrolytic needle and also by galvanocautery without recurrence, so I take it that we are at least progressing. Recurrences have been prevented by the use of radium on tumors located in other parts of the body, suggesting, as I believe, that surgical interference in the first place should be followed by the use of radium, or as suggested by Dr. Smith, we might use the X-ray first, then surgery, and then radium.

Dr Norval H. Pierce, Chicago: I rather antagonize the view that Dr. Coakley put forward in regard to always substantiating the laryngoscopic diagnosis of cancer of the larynx by microscopic examination. Of course, this is a very old and much discussed question; and I believe that it is a dangerous formula to have such extensive credence among laryngologists. I have been rather extensively criticised in Chicago, by some of my colleagues, for holding the viewpoint that whenever we can escape cutting into a carcinoma of the larynx for microscopic examination, we should. Regarding the case that Dr. Freer reported today, which I saw: Here was a fusiform infiltration of the vocal cords in a man sixty odd years of age. The card lagged. He was hoarse from January until May. There had been some hoarseness preceding this. Ulceration was very marked when the tumor was touched with peroxide of hydrogen. What could this have been?

First, we think of carcinoma; then tuberculosis, syphilis and ordinary lowgrade inflammation, socalled. Against the latter was the fact that this man's larynx was entirely healthy, with the exception of this growth on the vocal cord. There were no other infiltrations; no other thickenings.

He had never shown any evidences of tuberculosis. There were no tubercle bacilli in his sputum. It could not have been tuberculosis.

It could not have been syphilis. He had three or four Wassermanns made. He never had had a history of syphilis. He was rather a moderate gentleman in his habits. His spinal fluid had been examined and was negative to Wassermann.

Now, suppose we had cut into this man, and instead of being impure scientists, we had become pure scientists and destroyed this man's vocal cord. That would have been the only way that we could have done it, because it was an intramural affair. You could not have done it from the surface. It would have been necessary to take a large piece for diagnosis; not a small piece. Then, such enough, we have a carcinoma of the larynx. Then the picture or prognosis is entirely changed. At best. he would have had an area of ulceration under radium, with a destroyed voice. At is it, so far, Freer tells me, his voice is good and the tumor has disappeared. I would rather be an impure scientist and have an impure scientist handle the case under these conditions.

Dr. C. J. Coakley, New York: Two or three times a year it happens that cases are referred to me for an opinion, in which other men whose opinions I regard as most valuable, have made a diagnosis of carcinoma of the larynx. I invariably, in these cases, remove a section, if I am not frankly able to confirm that diagnosis. If I find the pathologic report not satisfactory, as it may not be, I take a second piece before I am willing to submit that patient to the operative procedure advised by previous surgeons. If you are going to carry out Dr. Pierce's idea, you must not put anything in the larynx. such as a swab, which is going to bruise it. I do not believe that Dr. Freer has a technic by which he can remove the larynx without bruising it and squeezing the epithelial cells. Nor must we put radium in, because we are bruising the larynx also by this procedure. I do feel that it is not wise to subject a patient to a serious operation without being sure of your diagnosis. No man should have a section taken unless he is willing to go on with the surgical means necessary in the case.

Dr. H. H. Forbes, New York City: Emanations are not new to us. We have followed out, in the radium work in the hospital, a combined system. In other words, while I feel competent to put in either the needles or emanation, I do not feel now that, with our limited experience in simply the growths of the pharynx. esophagus and larynx, I am in quite a position to judge the quality and quantity or the type of material to be used in these new growths. All the men who are interested in the Endoscopic Association realize that. with our technic, we are able. not only to view the parts, but also to make the examination. With Dr. Coakley, I feel that if it is possible, we should remove sections. We are then able to treat the cases and watch them.

There are two or three points that occur to me. One is that we have discarded entirely the socalled tubes or capsules in our esophageal and laryngeal work. We are using the needle. We have not the facilities for preparing the seeds of the emanation element, where the gas is formed. Whether we shall have to come to that, and give up the needles, I do not know. To be candid, it seems to me that those who are using the emanations are getting better results than we who are using simply the needles. If there is an objection to using the needle and there is a possibility of infection from their use, the same possibility would apply to the seeds. To avoid that, we have used a thoroughly aseptic method of preparing the patient, with alcohol or iodin used over the surface of the growth before using the needles. However, I do not believe that it is entirely the fault of our method of treatment.

In regard to the question of screening, I do not feel that the gentlemen have emphasized it sufficiently; and while I have only an opinion to offer, I do not think that, with an element as active as radium, we should expose normal tissues to it yet. I cannot feel, in my own mind that radium is going in there to destroy simply the abnormal tissue and not to destroy a certain amount of normal tissue. I think that the reaction is going to be on the normal tissue also. Unfortunately, the cases that we have had have not been of the type Dr. Freer spoke of in reporting his case of apparent cure in the larynx. I do feel, from the advanced cases that have come to us, among which we have had a number of deaths, that if I were to see these cases over again, I would not expose them to the radium treatment.

Dr. Henry L. Lynah, New York City: I believe that most of the lung abscesses are due to aspiration, because all of the surgeons agree that embolic cases die rather early. The patients which I have had the good fortune to bronchoscope are all still alive. In washing out the abscess cavities as advised by Yankauer, I never have been able to recover any of the solution by suction, for it is always coughed out through the bronchoscopic tubemouth as fast as it is injected. Personally, I believe that the dilatation of bronchial stenoses and the establishment of proper lung drainage is what improves the cases. I only use suction after bronchoscopic dilatation, and seem to have obtained some results. Bleeding, edematous and fungating granulations are always touched with ten to twenty percent nitrate of silver. As to the injections of bismuth subcarbonate in olive oil, that was not done with any idea of curing the cases, but was purely for purposes of definite localization of the abscess cavity. All of the patients, however, improved. Dr. Wm. H. Stewart attributed the improvement to the secondary action of the X-ray on the metallic substance in the lung. We have had bismuth remain in the lung for ten months after injection, but often when the bismuth disappears the abscess is healed.

In cases following tonsillectomy early bronchoscopic examination is always indicated while the process is in the pneumonic stage and before definite cavitation has taken place. We have had some startling recoveries in these early cases after removal of the sloughs from the edematous bronchus and bronchial dilatation and aspiration.

Dr. Robert Clyde Lynch, New Orleans:  I have had seven cases of which four have died.  They were treated by the use of needles. I have used only twenty-five milligrams of radium.  The needles were planted right into the growth and left for four, six, eight and twelve hours at a time.  We made the patients more uncomfortable by this procedure, instead of giving them analgesia.  They suffered more intensely than if they had been left alone; and I believe that they died sooner than they otherwise would have.

Talking about Dr. Smith's remark concerning a case that he reported, two or three years ago, in which he did laryngectomy after a previous application of radium, the cuts show what looks like cartilaginous tissue.  There was tremendous sloughing of the parts, and the man died from the sloughing process.

If operation is decided on, the time for the application of radium is after the operation, rather than before, on that account.

I want to ask Dr. Freer whether the radium seeds that he used contain four hundred millicuries of radium.  Dr. Freer's results were so different from those that I have been able to see in the cases of the men who have been using radium in my section of the country and in the reports from other sections, that I was wondering whether the tremendous difference in the content of the element used accounted for his results as compared with ours.  In my section of the country, we are disposed to be a little pessimistic about the results of radium around the mouth and upper esophagus. Our results, not only in my own hands, but also in those of Matas and Miller, and those who had considerable experience in operative work in the mouth and throat, are poor, and, in a general way. we are disposed to be pessimistic about the results obtained in the mouth, pharynx and upper esophagus.

Dr. D. Crosby Greene, Boston, Mass. (closing):  I wish to call attention to the fact that I did not claim in my paper to have cured any patients, but that they had been relieved.  The method has been palliative in the majority of cases.  With seed implantations one gets necrosis of the part of the tumor which presents in the lumen.  The patients have reported as being more comfortable and swallowing better.  The end results have, however, been bad in all but one case.  Nevertheless, I think that the method gives some promise of accomplishing more, so I intend to continue its use, hoping to gain increasing effectiveness by combining its use with that of Dr. Duane's new X-ray apparatus. which promises to be more effective than anything yet produced in that line.  With regard to Dr. Freer's apparatus, I feel that in the face of the results that he has reported, if he continues to get such results, we must acknowledge that he has made a great advance in the application of radiation within the larynx.  Our experience at the Huntington Hospital has not been like his.  We have had some good results from radiation and I expect to show next week in Boston two cases of apparent cure of cancer of the larynx by radiation.  In one case one and a half years, and in the other two years, have elapsed since the procedure was undertaken.  Our results following the method of surface application of the radium to the larynx have not been so successful as Dr. Freer's.  We have not had such an ingenious method of application as he has produced and I wish to pay tribute to his ingenuity and skill in administrating radium in this way. I have found almost always a considerable amount of inflammatory reaction following the application of radium in the larynx; so much so that I have performed as a routine, preliminary tracheotomy. This does no harm and is the only way to forestall sevede dyspnea which is apt to come on during the period of reaction, so that the cure can be attributed to the radium only. But our records of surface application to the larynx have not been as successful as Dr. Freer's. We have not had such an ingenious method of application as he has produced, and I wish to pay tribute to his remarkable ingenuity and skill in administeding the radium emanations in this way. I have found, almost invariably, a considerable amount of reaction after the application of radium in the larynx; so much so, that I do a tracheootomy beforehand. It does not do harm in these cases, particularly if there is sufficient infiltration to nadrow the space so that breathing is difficult. Anyway, I think that it does good in itself, and avoids the danger of acute stenosis of the larynx in the bad cases.

Dr. John R. Wilson, Baltimore (closing): The important point in these cases is diagnosis. For that, unless exceptionally, we are dependent upon the pathologist. To make sure, I resorted to three pathologists, and none of them agreed. The last examination was made of an alcoholic specimen, some two years after the operation. It is possible that, by maceration. the appearances were altered in some way; so that what was originally a roundcelled sarcoma gave the appearance of a spindlecelled sacroma or fibrosarcoma. I do not know whether that is possible or not. The laryngeal case that I reported could have been treated by any method. It happened that at that time the more recent methods were not known. The skin burn was due to inexperience, as it was one of the first cases of laryngeal tumor treated in this institution. It seems to me that Dr. Freer's doses are enormous. I am not responsible for the physical side of the treatment. The tubes given me were represented as emanations of pure gamma rays. How they get the gamma rays isolated, I do not know. They were handed to me as pure gamma rays, and were certainly active.

Dr. Fielding O. Lewis, Philadelphia (closing): Relative to the length of time that the patients are able to retain these applications in the larynx, I might say that we used preliminary tracheotomy in our cases, because we found that the reaction was so severe that tracheotomy had to be done later. There was also an added advantage in putting the larynx at rest. Dr. Swain stated that he would prefer to use radium in early cases of carcinoma of the larynx. I feel differently, because in cases treated by radium there are so few cured; whereas, in thyroidotomy, about 75 or 80 per cent of cures are obtained when the cases are seen early.

Regarding biopsy, I feel that there are borderline cases in which it is necessary to remove a specimen. In the case of an old man that I saw six months ago, in which I asked Dr. Jackson to cooperate, there was a small ulcerated growth of a few months' duration on the vocal cord. His Wassermann and other examinations were negative by direct larynogoscopy. I removed the growth in toto; and histologic examination of the growth showed it to be simply a papilloma with an ulcerated surface.

# INDEX OF THE LITERATURE.

## SECTION 1.—LARYNGOLOGY AND OTOLOGY—GENERAL AND HISTORICAL.

**Baldenweck, L.** Otorhinolaryngology in France in 1920.
Méd., Paris, 1921—II—290.

**Boot, G. W.** Ear as source of focal infection.
Illinois M. J., Oak Park, 1921—XXXIX—549.

**Brown, R. G.** Recent advances in ear, nose and throat specialty from point of view of general practitioner.
Med. J., Australia, Sidney, 1921—I—437.

**Canuyt, G.** Importance of blood pressure in ear, nose and throat disease.
J. de méd. de Bordeaux, 1921—LXXXXII—271.

**Gutmann, A.** Interrelationship of eye and dental disease.
Deutsche med. Wchnschr., Berl., 1921—XXXXVII—565.

**McBride, P.** Some discarded theories and methods.
J. Laryngol., Lond., 1921—XXXVI—269.

**Menetrier, P., and Coyon, A.** Lesions in the air passages of the gassed.
Ann. de méd., Par., 1921—IX—409.

**Morton, J. B.** Relation of eye, ear, nose and throat to general medicine.
Illinois M. J., 1921—XL—97.

**Nobécourt, M.** Overlapping infections of air passage.
Presse méd., Par., 1921—XXIX—513.

**Palmer, G. T.** Ventilation, weather and common cold.
J. Lab. & Clin. M., St. Louis, 1921—VI—602.

**Rovinsky, A.** Sea bathing and the ear.
Med. Rec., N. Y., 1921—C—12.

**Sluder, G.** The borderland of rhinology, neurology and ophthalmology.
J. Am. M. Ass., Chicago, 1921—LXXVII—688.

**Wiener, M., and Loeb, H. W.** Eye in relation to ear, nose and throat.
South M. J., Birmingham, 1921—XIV—491.

## SECTION 2.—RESPIRATORY SYSTEM, EXCLUSIVE OF THE EAR, NOSE AND THROAT.

**Haberkamp.** Paralysis of respiratory organs in infancy.
Monatschr. f. Kinderh., Berl., 1921—XXI—163.

**Menetrier, P., and Coyon, A.** Lesions in the air passages of the gassed.
Ann. de méd., Par., 1921—IX—409.

**Mullin, W. V.** The accessory sinuses as an etiologic factor in bronchiectasis.
Ann. Otol., Rhinol. & Laryngol., St. Louis, 1921—XXX—683.

Nobécourt, M. Overlapping infections of air passage.
Presse méd., Par., 1921—XXIX—513.

## SECTION 3.—ACUTE GENERAL INFECTIONS, INCLUDING DIPHTHERIA, SCARLET FEVER AND MEASLES. THE EAR, NOSE AND THROAT.

Achard, C. Diphtheritic paralysis.
Bull. méd., Par., 1921—XXXV—567.

Arnold-Larsen, A. Influenza statistics.
Ngesk. f. Laeger. Kjobenh., 1921—LXXXIII—903.

Bullowa, J. G. M. Tonsils and scarlet fever.
Am. J. Dis. Child., Chicago, 1921—XXII—29.

Busacchi, P. Nervous manifestations after diphtheria.
Riv. di clin. pediat., Firenze, 1921—XIX—180.

Carey, B. W. Diphtheria control.
J. Am. M. Ass., Chicago, 1921—LXXVII—668.

Chesney, A. M. Immunologic study of bacillus influenzae.
J. Infect. Dis., Chicago. 1921—XXIX—132.

Crouzon and Marceron. Influenza as factor in tuberculosis.
Bull. Soc. méd. d. hop., Par., 1921—XXXXV—965.

Curtis, L. Diphtheria.
Med. Rec., N. Y., 1921—IC—1098.

Ekvall, S. Immunity to diphtheria and the Schick reaction.
Upsala Läkaref. Förh., 1921—XXVI—219.

Frothingham, C. Influenza.
Am. J. M. Sc., Phila., 1921—CLXI—528.

Glenny, A. T., Allen, K., and O'Brien, R. A. Schick reaction and
diphtheria prophylactic immunization with toxin-antitoxin
mixture.
Lancet, Lond., 1921—I—1236.

Haguenan, J. Meningeal reaction in diphtheritic paralysis.
Bull. soc. méd. d. hop. de Par., 1921—XLV—996.

Hall, M. W. Etiology of influenza.
Mil. Surgeon, 1921—XXXXIX—300.

Hannah, B. Schick reaction in control of diphtheria.
Pub. Health J., Toronto, 1921—XII—250.

Hartmann, H. W. Diphtheroid bacilli.
Schweiz. med. Wchnschr., Basel, 1921—LI—657.

Hogan, J. F. Laryngeal diphtheria.
J. Am. M. Ass., Chicago, 1921—LXXII—662.

Imperatori, C. J. Some observations on localized pulmonary suppuration, treated by endobronchial irrigation.
Ann. Otol., Rhinol. & Laryngol., St. Louis, 1921—XXX—665.

Kay, M. B. Subcutaneous emphysema due to ruptured larynx in
untreated case of diphtheria.
J. Mich. M. Soc., Grand Rapids, 1921—XX—240.

Lenoble et al. Pulmonary tuberculosis involving esophagus.
Bull. soc. méd. d. hop., Par., 1921—XLV—890.

**Lietz, F. H.** Diphtheria in the newborn.
Monatschr. f. Geburtsh. u. Gynaek., Berl., 1920—LII—340.

**Lippman, H.** Diphtheria bacilli in sputum.
München. med. Wchnschr., 1921—LXVIII—772.

**Lo Presti-Seminerio, F.** The Schick reaction.
Pediatria, Florence, 1921—XXIX—503.

**Martinez, Vargas.** Treatment of diphtheria.
Siglo méd., Madrid, 1921—LXVIII—648.

**Merklen, P., Weiss, M., de Gennes, L.** Meningeal reaction in diphtheritic paralysis.
Bull. soc. méd. d. hop. de Par., 1921—XLV—990.

**Mixsell, H. R., and Giddings, E.** Certain aspects of postdiphtheritic diaphragmatic paralysis: Report of eight fatal cases in four thousand two hundred and fifty-nine cases of diphtheria.
J. Am. M. Ass., Chicago, 1921—LXXVII—590.

**Morgnio, L.** Treatment of diphtheria.
Rev. med. d. Uruguay, Montevideo, 1921—XXIV—293.

**Munoyerro and Acosta, R.** Shick reaction in diphtheria.
Arch. Espanol. d. Pediat., Madrid, 1921—V—193.

**Olitsky, P. K., and Gates, F. L.** Experimental studies of nasopharyngeal secretions from influenza patients.
J. Exper. M., N. Y., 1921—XXX—713.

**Opitz, H.** Diphtheria bacilli in nose in childhood.
Monatschr. f. Kinderh., Berl., 1921—XXI—170.

**Opitz, H.** Paradoxic reaction to diphtheria vaccine.
Jahrb. f. Kinderh., Berl., 1921—XCV—139.

**Park. W. H.** Degree of immunity to diphtheria insured by a negative Shick test.
Am. J. Dis. Child., Chicago, 1921—XXII—1.

**Pfaundler, M.** Serotherapy in diphtheria.
München. med. Wchnschr., 1921—LXVIII—781.

**Pilot, I.** Bacteriologic studies of upper respiratory passages: diphtheria bacilli and diphtheroids of adenoids and tonsils.
J. Infect. Dis., Chicago, 1921—XXIX—62.

**Poulard.** Diphtheritic paralysis of accommodation.
Paris méd., 1921—XI—57.

**Rivers, T. M., and Poole, A. K.** Growth requirements of influenza bacilli.
Johns Hopkins Hosp. Bull., Balt., 1921—XXXII—202.

**Roello, G.** Joint complications of influenza in children.
Riforma med., 1921—XXIX—654.

**Schick, B.** Predisposing factor in diphtheria.
N. York M. J., 1921—CXIV—197.

**Smith, S. Calvin.** Observations on the heart in diphtheria.
J. Am. M. Ass., Chicago, 1921—LXXVII—765.

**Stark, H. H.** Retrobulbar neuritis, secondary to disease of the nasal sinuses.
J. Am. M. Ass., Chicago, 1921—LXXVII—678.

**Taylor, J. A.** Lingual application of iodin as prophylactic in cerebrospinal meningitis and influenza.
Brit. M. J., Lond., 1921—II—776:

**Treupel and Stoffel.** Chronic influenza.
München. med. Wchnschr., 1921—LXVIII—763.

**Tso, E.** Diagnosis and treatment of diphtheria.
Nat. M. J. China, Shanghai, 1921—VII—55.

**Vaglio, R.** Immunization against diphtheria.
Pediatria, Napoli, 1921—XXIX—463.

**Walker, T. D.** Free diphtheria antitoxin.
J. Med. Ass. Georgia, Atlanta, 1921—X—554. ....

**Ward, G.** Shick reaction.
Brit. M. J., London, 1921—I—928.

**Wildegans.** Surgical complications of influenza.
Mitt. a. d. Greuzgeb. d. med. u. chir., Jena, 1921—XXXIII—429.

**Zingher, Abraham.** Diphtheria prevention work in the public schools of New York City.
J. Am. M. Ass., Chicago, 1921—LXXVII—835.

## SECTION 4.—SYPHILIS.

**Maybaum, J. L.** Nonsuppurative neurolabyrinthitis, with special reference to focal infection and syphilis as causative factors.
Ann. Otol., Rhinol. & Layngol., St. Louis, 1921—XXX—719.

**Ramadier, J.** Ear test for inherited syphilis.
Presse méd., Par., 1921—XXIX—624.

**Stimson, P. M.** Syphilis of trachea and bronchi: Résumé of diagnostic features; three case reports.
Am. J. M. Sc., Phila., 1921—CLXI—740.

## SECTION 5.—TUBERCULOSIS.

**Barajas y de Vilches, J. M.** Pharyngeal tuberculosis.
Siglo méd., Madrid, 1921—LXVIII—413.

**Bourgeois, H.** Tuberculosis of the tonsil.
Méd., Paris, 1921—II—302.

**Broca, A.** Treatment of tuberculous adenitis.
Progrés méd., Par., 1921—XXXVI—227.

**Clairmont, A., and Suchanek, E.** Progressive pulmonary tuberculosis after goiter operations.
Arch. f. klin. chir., Berl., 1921—CXV—995.

**Crouzon and Marceron.** Influenza as factor in tuberculosis.
Bull. Soc. méd. d. hop., Par., 1921—XXXXV—965.

**Kurzak, H.** Tuberculosis of the sphenoid bone.
Ztsch. f. Tuberk., Leipz., 1921—XXXIV—433.

**Leegaard, F.** Tuberculosis of middle ear.
Laryngoscope, St. Louis, 1921—XXXI—374.

**Nather, K.** Tuberculosis of the thyroid.
Mitt. a. d. Greuzgeb. d. Med. u. Chir., Jena, 1921—XXXIII—375.

**Stafford, F. B.** Laryngeal tuberculosis with special reference to sunlight treatment.
Virginia M. Month., Richmond, 1921—XXXXVIII—239.

**Steck, H.** Relations between exophthalmic goiter and tuberculosis.
Schweiz. med. Wchnschr., Basel, 1921—LI—535.

**Weller, C. V.** Incidence and histopathology of tuberculosis of tonsils.
Arch. Int. Med., Chicago, 1921—XXVII—631.

## SECTION 6.—ANATOMY, PHYSIOLOGY AND PATHOLOGY.

**Gill, E. G., and Graves, K. D.** Tonsils from clinical and pathologic standpoint.
South. M. J., Birmingham, 1921—XIV—498.

**Goldman, A., Mudd, S., Grant, S. B.** Reactions of nasal cavity and postnasal space to chilling of body surface. II. Concurrent study of bacteriology of nose and throat.
J. Infect. Dis., Chicago, 1921—XXIX—151.

**Meyer, J., Pilot, T., Pearlman, S. J.** Bacteriologic studies of upper respiratory passages; incidence of pneumococci, hemolytic streptococci and influenza bacilli (Pfeiffer) in nasopharynx of tonsillectomized and nontonsillectomized children.
J. Infect. Dis., Chicago, 1921—XXIX—59.

**Mudd, S., Goldman, A., and Grant, S. B.** Reactions of nasal cavity and postnasal space to chilling of body surface.
J. Exper. M., Baltimore, 1921—XXXIV—11.

**Pilot, I.** Bacteriologic studies of upper respiratory passages: diphtheria bacilli and diphtheroids of adenoids and tonsils.
J. Infect. Dis., Chicago, 1921—XXIX—62.

**Pilot, I., and Pearlman, S. J.** Bacteriologic studies of upper respiratory passages: hemolytic streptococci of adenoids.
J. Infect. Dis., Chicago, 1921—XXIX—47.

**Pilot, I., and Pearlman, S. J.** Bacteriologic studies of upper respiratory passages: Influenza bacilli (Pfeiffer) of adenoids and tonsils.
J. Infect. Dis., Chicago, 1921—XXIX—55.

**Pilot, I., and Pearlman, S. J.** Bacteriologic studies of upper respiratory passages: Pneumococci and nonhemolytic streptococci of adenoids and tonsils.
J. Infect. Dis., Chicago, 1921—XXIX—51.

**Schaeffer, J. P.** Aberrant vessels in surgery of the palatine and pharyngeal tonsils; the sigmoid or tortuous cervical internal carotid artery and the visible pulsating arteries in the wall of the pharynx.
J. Am. M. Ass., Chicago, 1921—LXXVII—14.

**Scott, S.** Effect produced by obscuring the vision of pigeons previously deprived of the otic labyrinth.
Brain, Lond., 1921—XXXIV—71.

## SECTION 7.—EXTERNAL NOSE.

**Aboulker, H.** Correction of deformed nose.
Méd., Paris, 1921—II—313.

**Esser, J. F. S.** Opertion on nose without incising skin.
Deutsche. Ztschr. f. Chir., Leipz., 1921—CLXIV—211.

**Frank, I., and Strauss, J. F.** An invisible scar method in cosmetic nasal surgery.
Ann. Otol., Rhinol. & Laryngol., St. Louis, 1921—XXX—670.

**Metzenbaum, M.** Nasal deformities of developmental type.
Ohio M. J., Columbus, 1921—XVII—382.

**Selfridge, G.** Cosmetic surgery of nose.
Laryngoscope, St. Louis, 1921—XXXI—337.

**Stotter, J., and Stotter, A. L.** Correction of nasal deformities with autogenous transplants.
Ohio M. J., Columbus, 1921—XVII—384.

## SECTION 8.—NASAL CAVITIES.

**Bickel, A.** Present status of knowledge of colds.
Deutsche. med. Wchnschr., Berl., 1921—XXXXVII—780.

**Bilancioni, G.** Sarcoma in nasal fossa.
Tumori, Roma, 1921—VIII—22.

**Chamberlin, W. B.** The endonasal operation of the lacrimal sac.
Ann. Otol., Rhinol. & Laryngol., St. Louis, 1921—XXX—643.

**Cohen, L.** The management of recent fractures of the nose.
Am. Otol., Rhinol. & Laryngol., St. Louis, 1921—XXX—690.

**Good, R. H.** Simplified intranasal operation for obstruction of nasolacrimal duct.
Am. J. Ophth., Chicago, 1921—IV—597.

**Gradle, H.** Congenital atresia of puncta lacrimalia of one side.
Arch. Ophth., N. Y., 1921—I—349.

**Griessmann, B.** Treatment of ozena.
München. med. Wchnschr., 1921—LXVIII—849.

**Griscom, J. M.** Relation of intranasal pressure to heterophoria.
Penn. M. J., 1921—XXIV—804.

**Lermoyez, J.** Spasmodic coryza from chilling.
Bull. soc. méd. d. hop., Par., 1921—XXXXV—1183.

**Lyons, H. R.** Radium in treatment of myxomatous nasal polyps.
Am. J. Roentgenol., New York, 1921—VIII—407.

**Mosher, H. P.** Mosher-Toti operation on lacrimal sac.
Laryngoscope, St. Louis, 1921—XXXI—284.

**Mudd, S., Goldman, A., and Grant, S. B.** Reactions of nasal cavity and postnasal space to chilling of body surface.
J. Exper. M., Baltimore, 1921—XXXIV—11.

**Opitz, H.** Diphtheria bacilli in nose in childhood.
Monatschr. f. Kinderh., Berl., 1921—XXI—170.

**Palmer, G. T.** Ventilation, weather and common cold.
J. Lab. & Clin. M., St. Louis, 1921—VI—602.

1130 INDEX OF THE LITERATURE.

Patterson, J. A. Ocular diseases of nasal origin.
Am. J. Ophth., Chicago, 1921—IV—513.

Post, M. H. Glaucoma and nasal (sphenopalatine, Meckel's) ganglion.
Arch. Ophth., N. Y., 1921—I—317.

Reynaud, G. L. Hay fever: Report on successful detoxication method of treatment.
N. York M. J., 1921—CXIII—875.

Rosenblatt, S. Removal of tooth from nares.
Illinois M. J., 1921—XL—96.

Roy, D. Case of intranasal epithelioma cured by excision and radium. Literature.
Ann. Otol., Rhinol. & Laryngol., St. Louis, 1921—XXX—748.

Scheppegrell, W. The intensive treatment of hay fever.
Med. Rec., N. Y., 1921—C—191.

Tarneaud, J. Treatment of ozena.
Méd., Paris, 1921—II—328.

Walker, I. C. Frequent causes and treatment of seasonal hay fever.
Arch. Int. Med., Chicago, 1921—XXVIII—71.

Woods, E. A. Causes and results of deflection of nasal septum.
Northwest. Med., Seattle, 1921—XX—210.

Woods, R. Malignant granuloma of nose.
Brit. M. J., Lond., 1921—I—65.

## SECTION 9.—ACCESSORY SINUSES.

Ballenger, H. C. Diagnosis of nasal accessory disease.
Illinois M. J., Oak Park, 1921—XXXIX—525.

Dean, L. W., and Armstrong, M. Some indications for operation on nasal sinuses in children.
Laryngoscope, St. Louis, 1921—XXXI—273.

Dutrow, H. V. Diagnosis and treatment of maxillary sinusitis.
Laryngoscope, St. Louis, 1921—XXXI—296.

Emerson, F. P. Polypoid degeneration of lining of antrum of Highmore.
Laryngoscope, St. Louis, 1921—XXXI—292.

Hautant, A. Cancer of the maxillary sinus.
Med., Paris, 1921—II—309.

Kurzak, H. Tuberculosis of the sphenoid bone.
Ztsch. f. Tuberk., Leipz., 1921—XXXIV—433.

Lyons, H. R. Puncture of antrum of Highmore.
Minnesota Med., St. Paul, 1921—IV—319.

Mullin, W. V. The accessory sinuses as an etiologic factor in bronchiectasis.
Ann. Otol., Rhinol. & Laryngol., St. Louis, 1921—XXX—683.

Patterson, J. A. Ocular diseases of nasal origin.
Am. J. Ophth., Chicago, 1921—IV—513.

Pollock, H. Pulsating sphenoiditis.
Ann. Otol., Rhinol. & Laryngol., St. Louis, 1921—XXX—744.

**Robinson, C. A.** Case of long-lasting suppuration of nasal sinuses successfully treated by galvanic current.
Arch. Radiol. & Electroth., Lond., 1921—XXV—386.

**Swan, C. J.** Treatment of paranasal sinus diseases in relataion to secondary infections from this source.
Illinois M. J., Oak Park., 1921—XXXIX—527.

**Thomson, E. S.** Some clinical phases of ocular involvement in sinus disease.
Am. J. Ophth., Chicago, 1921—IV—507.

## SECTION 10.—PHARYNX, INCLUDING TONSILS AND ADENOIDS.

**Barajas y de Vilches, J. M.** Pharyngeal tuberculosis.
Siglo méd., Madrid, 1921—LXVIII—413.

**Bourgeois, H.** Tuberculosis of the tonsil.
Méd., Paris, 1921—II—302.

**Bullowa, J. G. M.** Tonsils and scarlet fever.
Am. J. Dis. Child., Chicago, 1921—XXII—29.

**Clark, J. G.** Death following operation of tonsillectomy with reference to motor driven apparatus for anesthesia.
Ohio M. J., Columbus, 1921—XVII—631.

**Cowley, R. H.** Local versus general anesthesia in tonsillectomy.
Kentucky M. J., Bowling Green, 1921—XIX—468.

**de Angelis, F.** Vincent's angina in children.
Pediatria, Napoli, 1921—XXVIIII—339.

**Elmendorf, D. F.** Vincent's angina.
Mil. Surgeon, 1921—XXXXIX—287.

**Flanary, D. L.** A new instrument for the enucleation of tonsils in capsule.
J. Am. M. Ass., Chicago, 1921—LXXVII—201.

**Fort, A. G.** Tonsils, with special references to local anesthesia.
J. Med. Ass., Georgia, Atlanta, 1921—X—618.

**Frank, I.** Retropharyngeal abscess.
J. Am. M. Ass., Chicago, 1921—LXXVII—517.

**Freer, O. T.** Radium emanation in upper air passages as compared to radium: A method of applying it with especial reference to laryngeal carcinoma.
Illinois M. J., 1921—XXXX—85.

**Gill, E. G., and Graves, K. D.** Tonsils from clinical and pathologic standpoint.
South. M. J., Birmingham, 1921—XIV—498.

**Goldman, A., Mudd, S., Grant, S. B.** Reactions of nasal cavity and postnasal space to chilling of body surface. II. Concurrent study of bacteriology of nose and throat.
J. Infect. Dis., Chicago, 1921—XXIX—151.

**Goodall, J. B.** Vincent's infection of gums and buccal membranes.
W. States Nav. M. Bull., Wash., 1921—XV—542.

**Goodyear, H. M.** New tonsil instrument.
J. Am. M. Ass., Chicago, 1921—LXXVII—201.

**Greene, J. B.**  A palate-tonsil retractor.
J. Am. M. Ass., Chicago, 1921—LXXVII—39.

**Hug, T.**  Foreign bodies in air and food passages.
Beitr. z. klin. Chir., Tübing., 1921—CXXII—153.

**Jackson, C.**  Symptomatology and diagnosis of foreign bodies in air and food passages, based on study of 789 cases.
Am. J. M. Sc., Phila., 1921—CLXI—625.

**Kay, M. B.**  Subcutaneous emphysema due to ruptured larynx in untreated case of diphtheria.
J. Mich. M. Soc., Grand Rapids, 1921—XX—240.

**Kynaston, J.**  Cause and treatment of adenoids.
Practitioner, Lond., 1921—CVI—407.

**Lapage, C. P.**  Chronic nasopharyngeal infection, chronic toxemia and distressed heart in children.
Brit. M. J., Lond., 1921—II—4.

**Mangabeira Albernaz, P.**  Chemical cauterization of tonsils.
Brazil méd., Rio de Jan., 1921—II—4.

**Meyer, J., Pilot, T., Pearlman, S. J.**  Bacteriologic studies of upper respiratory passages; incidence of pneumococci, hemolytic streptococci and influenza bacilli (Pfeiffer) in nasopharynx of tonsillectomized and nontonsillectomized children.
J. Infect. Dis., Chicago, 1921—XXIX—59.

**Milligan, W.**  Diathermy in inoperable pharyngeal and epilaryngeal malignancy.
Laryngol., etc., Edinburgh, 1921—XXXVI—369.

**New, G. B., and Hansel, F. K.**  Melanoepithelioma of the palate.
J. Am. M. Ass., Chicago, 1921—LXXVII—19.

**Olitsky, P. K., and Gates, F. L.**  Experimental studies of nasopharyngeal secretions from influenza patients.
J. Exper. M., N. Y., 1921—XXX—713.

**Pilot, I.**  Bacteriologic studies of upper respiratory passages: diphtheria bacilli and diphtheroids of adenoids and tonsils.
J. Infect. Dis., Chicago, 1921—XXIX—62.

**Pilot, I., and Pearlman, S. J.**  Bacteriologic studies of upper respiratory passages: hemolytic streptococci of adenoids.
J. Infect. Dis., Chicago, 1921—XXIX—47.

**Pilot, I., and Pearlman, S. J.**  Bacteriologic studies of upper respiratory passages: Influenza bacilli (Pfeiffer) of adenoids and tonsils.
J. Infect. Dis., Chicago, 1921—XXIX—55.

**Pilot, I., and Pearlman, S. J.**  Bacteriologic studies of upper respiratory passages: Pneumococci and nonhemolytic streptococci of adenoids and tonsils.
J. Infect. Dis., Chicago, 1921—XXIX—51.

**Poppi, A.**  Pathology of nasopharyngeal cavity.
Monograph. Oto.-Rhino.-Laryngol. Internat., Paris, 1921—II—117.

**Pybus, F. C.**  Retropharyngeal abscess: Five cases.
Practitioner, Lond., 1921—CVI—403.

**Ramadier, J.** Total tonsillectomy.
Méd., Paris, 1921—II—325.

**Robb, J. M.** Local tonsillectomy technic.
J. Mich. M. Soc., Grand Rapids, 1921—XX—303.

**Rouget, J.** Adhesion of the palate and pharynx.
. Méd., Paris, 1921—II—327.

**Schaeffer, J. P.** Aberrant vessels in surgery of the palatine and
pharyngeal tonsils; the sigmoid or tortuous cervical internal carotid artery and the visible pulsating arteries in the
wall of the pharynx.
J. Am. M. Ass., Chicago, 1921—LXXVII—14.

**Searcy, H. B.** Searcy tonsillectome.
South. M. J., Birmingham, 1921—XIV—639.

**Shambaugh, G. E.** Tonsils as foci for systemic infection.
Illinois M. J., Oak Park, 1921—XXXIX—531.

**Thomasson, W. J.** Two cases of hemorrhage following peritonsillar abscess.
Kentucky M. J., Bowling Green, 1921—XIX—611.

**Wall, G. A.** Juvenile nasopharyngeal fibroma. Report of case treated by Kocher's osteoplastic method.
Laryngoscope, St. Louis, 1921—XXXI—287.

**Warren, L. P.** New tonsil forceps.
J. Am. M. Ass., Chicago, 1921—LXXVII—285.

**Watkins, S. S.** Primary scleroma of larynx in negro born in Maryland.
Surg., Gynec. & Obst., Chicago, 1921—XXIII—47.

**Weller, C. V.** Incidence and histopathology of tuberculosis of tonsils.
Arch. Int. Med., Chicago, 1921—XXVII—631.

**Witherbee, W. D.** Principles involved in Roentgen ray treatment of tonsils.
Laryngoscope, St. Louis, 1921—XXXI—305.

## SECTION 11.—LARYNX.

**Canavan, M. M.** Edema of glottis in obscure deaths.
Am. J. M. Sc., Phila., 1921—CLXII—273.

**Carson, N. B.** Cancer of the larynx.
Ann. Otol., Rhinol. & Laryngol., St. Louis, 1921—XXX—761.

**Castilho Marcondes, F.** Suspension laryngoscopy.
Brazil méd., Rio de Jan., 1921—XXXV—271.

**Fein, J.** Cadaver position of the vocal cords.
Deutsche. med. Wchnschr., Berl., 1921—XXXXVII—591.

**Franz, L.** Topography of recurrent nerve.
Beitr. z. klin. Chir., Tübing., 1921—CXXII—366.

**Freer, O. T.** Radium emanation in upper air passages as compared
to radium: A method of applying it with especial reference to laryngeal carcinoma.
Illinois M. J., 1921—XL—85.

**Friedman, J., and Greenfield, S. D.** Cases of foreign body in larynx and esophagus.
N. York M. J., 1921—CXIII—818.

**Hill, F. T.** Dislocation of epiglottis.
Laryngoscope, St. Louis, 1921—XXXI—320.

**Hogan, J. F.** Laryngeal diphtheria.
J. Am. M. Ass., Chicago, 1921—LXXII—662.

**Hug, T.** Foreign bodies in air and food passages.
Beitr. z. klin. Chir., Tübing., 1921—CXXII—153.

**Jackson, C.** Symptomatology and diagnosis of foreign bodies in air and food passages, based on study of 789 cases.
Am. J. M. Sc., Phila., 1921—CLXI—625.

**Jonas.** Apparatus for heliotherapy of larynx.
Wien. klin. Wchnschr., 1921—XXXIV—280.

**Landivar, R., and Bogliano, H.** Suture of the larynx.
Semana Méd., Buenos Aires, 1921—XXVIII—549.

**Lannois, M.** The larynx in tabes.
Méd., Paris, 1921—II—297.

**Moure, E. J., and Portmann, G.** Total laryngectomy.
Presse méd., Par., 1921—XXIX—561.

**New, G. B.** Treatment of multiple papillomás of the larynx in children.
Ann. Otol., Rhinol. & Laryngol., St. Louis, 1921—XXX—631.

**Pfeiffer.** Plastic correction of defects in larynx and trachea.
Zentralbl. f. Chir., Leipz., 1921—XXXXVIII—965.

**Stafford, F. B.** Laryngeal tuberculosis with special reference to sunlight treatment.
Virginia M. Month., Richmond, 1921—XXXXVIII—239.

**Taylor, J. M.** Endoscopic removal of sand spurs from larynx and tracheobronchial tree.
J. Am. M. Ass., Chicago, 1921—LXXVII—685.

**Thomson, St. C.** Intrinsic cancer of larynx.
Brit. M. J., London, 1921—I—921.

**Tompkins, G. J.** Acute obstructive laryngitis in children.
Virginia M. Month., Richmond, 1921—XLVIII—193.

**Turner, A. L.** Paralysis of vocal cords, secondary to malignant tumor of mamma.
J. Laryngol., etc., Edinburgh, 1921—XXXVI—373.

**Uchermann, V., and Harbitz, F.** Amyloid tumor in larynx.
Norsk. mag. f. laegevidensk., Kristiania, 1921—LXXXII—497.

## SECTION 12.—TRACHEA AND BRONCHI.

**Carman, R. D., and Sutherland, C. G.** Aneurysm of aorta and abscess of the tracheobronchial lymph glands.
Am. J. Roentgenol., New York, 1921—VIII—269.

**Gerhartz, H.** Tuberculosis of bronchial and cervical glands.
Med. Klin., Berl., 1921—XVII—806.

**Hall, G. C.** Esophagoscopy and bronchoscopy in diagnosis and treatment. Safe rules to follow in emergency cases.
Kentucky M. J., Bowling Green, 1921—XIX—482.

**Hawes, J. B.** Bronchoesophageal fistula and traction diverticulum.
  Am. J. M. Sc., Phila., 1921—CLXI—791.

**Hug, T.** Foreign bodies in air and food passages.
  Beitr. z. klin. Chir., Tübing., 1921—CXXII—153.

**Jackson, C.** Symptomatology and diagnosis of foreign bodies in
  air and food passages, based on study of 789 cases.
  Am. J. M. Sc., Phila., 1921—CLXI—625.

**Kästner, H.** Roentgen findings in the trachea.
  Beitr. z. klin. Chir., Tübing., 1921—CXXII—455.

**Mullin, W. V.** The accessory sinuses as an etiologic factor in
  bronchiectasis.
  Ann. Otol., Rhinol. & Laryngol., St. Louis, 1921—XXX—683.

**Peltason, F.** Perforations of esophagus into air passages.
  Deutsche med. Wchnschr., Berl., 1921—XLVII—709.

**Pfeiffer.** Plastic correction of defects in larynx and trachea.
  Zentralbl. f. Chir., Leipz., 1921—XLVIII—965.

**Picard, E.** Fistula between esophagus and trachea.
  Arch. f. klin. chir., Berl., 1921—CXV—744.

**Sgalitzer, M.** Varieties in shape of trachea.
  Arch. f. klin. chir., Berl., 1921—CXV—967.

**Stimson, P. M.** Syphilis of trachea and bronchi: Résumé of diagnostic features; three case reports.
  Am. J. M. Sc., Phila., 1921—CLXI—740.

**Taylor, J. M.** Endoscopic removal of sand spurs from larynx and
  tracheobronchial tree.
  J. Am. M. Ass., Chicago, 1921—LXXVII—685.

## SECTION 13.—VOICE AND SPEECH.

**Blanton, S.** The medical significance of the disorders of speech.
  J. Am. M. Ass., Chicago, 1921—LXXVII—373.

**Ellison, E. M.** Sensory aphasia.
  N. York M. J., 1921—CXIII—796.

## SECTION 14.—ESOPHAGUS.

**Bensande, E., and Gueiraux, G.** Idiopathic dilatation of the esophagus.
  Rev. de méd., Par., 1921—XXXVIII—65.

**Besande, R., and Lelong, M.** Esophagoscopy.
  Presse méd., Par., 1921—XXVIIII—413.

**Carroll, C. H.** Open safety brooch in esophagus for nine months.
  Lancet, Lond., 1921—I—1300.

**Dufourmentel, L.** Radium treatment of cancer of the esophagus.
  Méd., Paris, 1921—II—321.

**Friedman, J., and Greenfield, S. D.** Cases of foreign body in
  larynx and esophagus.
  N. York M. J., 1921—CXIII—818.

**Greig, D. M.** "Cardiospasm," congenital narrowing of esophagus
  and esophagectasia.
  Edinb. M. J., 1921—XXVII—89.

**Hall, G. C.** Esophagoscopy and bronchoscopy in diagnosis and treatment. Safe rules to follow in emergency cases.
Kentucky M. J., Bowling Green, 1921—XIX—482.

**Hawes, J. B.** Bronchoesophageal fistula and traction diverticulum.
Am. J. M. Sc., Phila., 1921—CLXI—791.

**Hotz, G.** Radium treatment of cancer of the esophagus.
Schweiz. med. Wchnschr., Basel, 1921—LI—460.

**Hug, T.** Foreign bodies in air and food passages.
Beitr. z. klin. Chir., Tübing., 1921—CXXII—153.

**Jackson, C.** Esophageal stenosis following the swallowing of caustic alkalis.
J. Am. M. Ass., Chicago, 1921—LXXVII—22.

**Jackson, C.** Symptomatology and diagnosis of foreign bodies in air and food passages, based on study of 789 cases.
Am. J. M. Sc., Phila., 1921—CLXI—625.

**Lavergne De.** Ulcer of the esophagus.
Bull. soc. méd. de hop., Paris, 1921—XLV—681.

**Lenoble et al.** Pulmonary tuberculosis involving esophagus.
Bull. soc. méd. d. hop., Par., 1921—XLV—890.

**Lotheissen, G.** Esophageal stricture.
Wien. klin. Wchnschr., 1921—XXXIV—342.

**Lüpke, H.** Operative treatment of diverticulum of the esophagus.
Beitr. z. klin. chir., Tübing., 1921—CXXI—612.

**Madlener, M.** Antethoracal artificial esophagus.
Beitr. z. klin. Chir., Tübing., 1921—CXXII—299.

**Neff, F. C.** Congenital absence of middle portion of esophagus.
Am. J. Dis. Child., Chicago, 1921—XXII—57.

**Peltason, F.** Perforations of esophagus into air passages.
Deutsche med. Wchnschr., Berl., 1921—XLVII—709.

**Picard, E.** Fistula between esophagus and trachea.
Arch. f. klin. chir., Berl., 1921—CXV—744.

**Rockey, A. E.** Radium treatment of cancer of the esophagus.
J. Am. M. Ass., Chicago, 1921—LXXVII—30.

**Skinner, E. H.** Congenital atresia of esophagus.
Am. J. Roentgenol., N. Y., 1921—VIII—319.

**Sternberg, S.** Corrosion of esophagus in the gassed.
Wien. klin. Wchnschr., 1921—XXXIV—265.

**Tenckhoff, B.** Operation on trachea by using tracheoscope.
München. med. Wchnschr., 1921—LXVIII—676.

**Vogel, R.** Foreign bodies in esophagus.
Arch. f. klin. chir., Berl., 1921—CXV—910.

**Von Fink, F.** Deep seated foreign bodies in esophagus.
Zentralbl. f. Chir., Leipz., 1921—XLVIII—623.

**Watkins, S. S.** Fifty-cent piece in esophagus for three months; removal through mouth.
Kentucky M. J., Bowling Green, 1921—XIX—523.

## SECTION 15.—ENDOSCOPY.

**Besande, R., and Lelong, M.** Esophagoscopy.
Presse méd., Par., 1921—XXVIIII—413.

**Carroll, C. H.** Open safety brooch in esophagus for nine months.
Lancet, Lond., 1921—I—1300.

**Castilho Marcondes, F.** Suspension laryngoscopy.
Brazil méd., Rio de Jan., 1921—XXXV—271.

**Friedman, J., and Greenfield, S. D.** Cases of foreign body in
larynx and esophagus.
N. York M. J., 1921—CXIII—818.

**Hall, G. C.** Esophagoscopy and bronchoscopy in diagnosis and
treatment. Safe rules to follow in emergency cases.
Kentucky M. J., Bowling Green, 1921—XIX—482.

**Hug, T.** Foreign bodies in air and food passages.
Beitr. z. klin. Chir., Tübing., 1921—CXXII—153.

**Taylor, J. M.** Endoscopic removal of sand spurs from larynx and
tracheobronchial tree.
J. Am. M. Ass., Chicago, 1921—LXXVII—685.

**Tenckhoff, B.** Operation on trachea by using tracheoscope.
München. med. Wchnschr., 1921—LXVIII—676.

**Vogel, R.** Foreign bodies in esophagus.
Arch. f. klin. chir., Berl., 1921—CXV—910.

## SECTION 16.—EXTERNAL EAR AND CANAL.

**Arbuckle, M. F.** Earache in its clinical significance.
Illinois M. J., Oak Park, 1921—XXXIX—547.

**Colledge, L.** Injuries to the ear in modern warfare.
J. Laryngol., Lond., 1921—XXXVI—283.

**Day, H. F.** Reconstruction of ears.
Boston M. & S. J., 1921—CLXXXV—146.

**Faulder, T. J.** Injuries to the ear in modern warfare.
J. Laryngol., Lond., 1921—XXXVI—277.

**Friedman, J., and Greenfield, S. D.** Foreign bodies in external
auditory canal.
Med. Rec., N. Y., 1921—C—365.

**Liébault, G.** Foreign bodies in the ear.
Méd., Paris, 1921—II—319.

**Putelli, F.** Fibroma of external ear.
Tumori, Roma, 1921—VIII—42.

## SECTION 17.—MIDDLE EAR, INCLUDING TYMPANIC MEMBRANE AND EUSTACHIAN TUBE.

**Arbuckle, M. F.** Earache in its clinical significance.
Illinois M. J., Oak Park, 1921—XXXIX—547.

**Boot, G. W.** Otitic brain abscess.
Illinois M. J., 1921—XL—122.

**Colledge, L.** Injuries to the ear in modern warfare.
J. Laryngol., Lond., 1921—XXXVI—283.

**Faulder, T. J.**  Injuries to the ear in modern warfare.
J. Laryngol., Lond., 1921—XXXVI—277.

**Fernández Seco, J.**  Grave complications of otitis media.
Siglo med., Madrid, 1921—LXVIII—552.

**Ivins, H. M.**  Treatment of eustachian tube and middle ear.
Iowa M. J., Des Moines, 1921—XI—201.

**Lampe, H. F.**  Chronic mastoiditis with extensive cholesteatoma.
Laryngoscope, St. Louis, 1921—XXXI—307.

**Leegaard, F.**  Tuberculosis of middle ear.
Laryngoscope, St. Louis, 1921—XXXI—374.

**Liébault, G.**  Foreign bodies in the ear.
Méd., Paris, 1921—II—319.

**Sallender, F. W.**  How are we treating the eustachian tube?
Iowa M. J., Des Moines, 1921—XI—199.

**Schwartz, A. A.**  Chronic purulent otitis media.
Laryngoscope, St. Louis, 1921—XXXI—311.

**Texier, V.**  Mastoid operations with chronic otitis.
Méd., Paris, 1921—II—307.

**Wrigley, F. G.**  An intracranial complication of chronic middle ear
suppuration.
J. Laryngol., etc., Edinburgh, 1921—XXXVI—381.

## SECTION 18.—MASTOID PROCESS.

**Brooks, E. H.**  When to operate on mastoid in children.
Wisconsin M. J., Milwaukee.

**Callison, J. G.**  Double mastoid operation; acute thyrorenal exhaustion.
Laryngoscope, St. Louis, 1921—XXXI—359.

**Colledge, L.**  Injuries to the ear in modern warfare.
J. Laryngol., Lond., 1921—XXXVI—283.

**Faulder, T. J.**  Injuries to the ear in modern warfare.
J. Laryngol., Lond., 1921—XXXVI—277.

**Gill, E.**  Atypical mastoiditis with report of three cases.
Virginia M. Month., Richmond, 1921—XLVIII—156.

**Glogau, O.**  Primary mastoiditis with perisinus and extradural abscess. Operation. Recovery.
Laryngoscope, St. Louis, 1921—XXXI—318.

**Goodyear, H. M.**  Case of extensive lateral sinus thrombosis, with
special reference to low resection.
Laryngoscope, St. Louis, 1921—XXXI—365.

**Hays, H. M.**  Acute bilateral mastoiditis; meningitis; aseptic operation; recovery.
Laryngoscope, St. Louis, 1921—XXXI—302.

**Lampe, H. F.**  Chronic mastoiditis with extensive cholesteatoma.
Laryngoscope, St. Louis, 1921—XXXI—307.

**Perkins, C. E.**  Two cases of advanced suppurative disease of lateral sinus and jugular vein.
Med. Rec., N. Y., 1921—C—195.

**Spencer, F. R.** Roentgenology of the mastoids with conclusions based on one hundred cases.
Ann. Otol., Rhinol. & Laryngol., St. Louis, 1921—XXX—770.

**Texier, V.** Mastoid operations with chronic otitis.
Méd., Paris, 1921—II—307.

## SECTION 19.—INTERNAL EAR.

**Arganaraz, R.** Physiologic nystagmus.
Semana méd., Buenos Aires, 1921—XXVIII—666.

**Colledge, L.** Injuries to the ear in modern warfare.
J. Laryngol., Lond., 1921—XXXVI—283.

**Faulder, T. J.** Injuries to the ear in modern warfare.
J. Laryngol., Lond., 1921—XXXVI—277.

**Lafon, C.** Nystagmus and nystagiform movements.
J. de méd. de Bordeaux, 1921—XCII—374.

**Lewitt, F. C.** Equilibrium and vertigo.
Laryngoscope, St. Louis, 1921—XXXI—347.

**Maybaum, J. L.** Nonsuppurative neurolabyrinthitis, with special reference to focal infection and syphilis as causative factors.
Ann. Otol., Rhinol. & Layngol., St. Louis, 1921—XXX—719.

**Pentimalli, F.** Nystagmus from protein intoxication.
Riforma med., 1921—XXXVII—578.

**Perkins, C. E.** A case of labyrinthitis and cerebellar abscess.
Ann. Otol., Rhinol. & Laryngol., St. Louis, 1921—XXX—742.

**Robertson, C. M.** A review of the medical aspect of aviation.
Ann. Otol., Rhinol. & Laryngol., St. Louis, 1921—XXX—776.

**Scott, S.** Effect produced by obscuring the vision of pigeons previously deprived of the otic labyrinth.
Brain, Lond., 1921—XLIV—71.

**Sears, W. H.** Practical use of Barany tests away from medical centers.
Penn. M. J., 1921—XXIV—798.

**Wells, W. A.** Vertigo from point of view of otologist.
N. York M. J., 1921—CXIII—859.

## SECTION 20.—DEAFNESS AND DEAFMUTISM, AND TESTS FOR HEARING.

**Callison, J. G.** Progressive systemic deafness as an endocrine syndrome.
N. York M. J., 1921—CXIV—48.

**Hays, H. M.** Needed measures for the prevention of deafness during early life.
J. Am. M. Ass., Chicago, 1921—LXXVII—263.

**Peck, A. W.** Social alleviation of adventitious deafness.
J. Am. M. Ass., Chicago, 1921--LXXVII—267.

**Ramadier, J.** Ear test for inherited syphilis.
Presse méd., Par., 1921—XXIX—624.

**Sonnenschein, R.**  Resonators as possible aid in tuning fork tests. A preliminary report.
Ann. Otol., Rhinol. & Laryngol., St. Louis, 1921—XXX—703.

## SECTION 21.—FOREIGN BODIES IN THE NOSE, THROAT AND EAR.

**Carroll, C. H.**  Open safety brooch in esophagus for nine months.
Lancet, Lond., 1921—I—1300.

**Friedman, J., and Greenfield, S. D.**  Cases of foreign body in larynx and esophagus.
N. York M. J., 1921—CXIII—818.

**Friedman, J., and Greenfield, S. D.**  Foreign bodies in external auditory canal.
Med. Rec., N. Y., 1921—C—365.

**Hall, G. C.**  Esophagoscopy and bronchoscopy in diagnosis and treatment.  Safe rules to follow in emergency cases.
Kentucky M. J., Bowling Green, 1921—XIX—482.

**Hug, T.**  Foreign bodies in air and food passages.
Beitr. z. klin. Chir., Tübing., 1921—CXXII—153.

**Jackson, C.**  Symptomatology and diagnosis of foreign bodies in air and food passages, based on study of 789 cases.
Am. J. M. Sc., Phila., 1921—CLXI—625.

**Liébault, G.**  Foreign bodies in the ear.
Méd., Paris, 1921—II—319.

**Taylor, J. M.**  Endoscopic removal of sand spurs from larynx and tracheobronchial tree.
J. Am. M. Ass., Chicago, 1921—LXXVII—685.

**Watkins, S. S.**  Fifty-cent piece in esophagus for three months; removal through mouth.
Kentucky M. J., Bowling Green, 1921—XIX—523.

**Vogel, R.**  Foreign bodies in esophagus.
Arch. f. klin. chir., Berl., 1921—CXV—910.

**Von Fink, F.**  Deep seated foreign bodies in esophagus.
Zentralbl. f. chir., Leipz., 1921—XLVIII—623.

## SECTION 22.—ORAL CAVITY, INCLUDING TONGUE, PALATE AND INFERIOR MAXILLARY.

**Ansaldi, C.**  Tumor in accessory salivary gland.
Policlin., Roma, 1921—XXVIII—277.

**Ashhurst, A. P. C.**  Recurrent unilateral subluxation of mandible excision of interarticular cartilage in cases of snapping jaw.
Ann. Surg., Phila., 1921—LXXIII—712.

**Babonnier and Hubac.**  Fatal epidemic encephalitis with parotitis.
Bull. Soc. méd. de hop., Paris, 1921—XLV—732.

**Brémond, L.**  Treatment of paradental cysts.
Méd., Paris, 1921—II—315.

**Brophy, T. W.**  Cleft palate and harelip procedures.
Minnesota Med., St. Paul, 1921—IV—283.

**Shearer, W. L.** Cleft palate and harelip.
Minnesota Med., St. Paul, 1921—IV—293.

**Walton, L., and Aimes, A.** Importance of oral infection.
Progrés. méd., Par., 1921—XXXVI—253.

**Vean, V., and Ruppe, C.** Median upper harelip.
Arch. de méd. d. enf., Par., 1921—XXIV—241.

## SECTION 23.—FACE.

**Babonnier and Hubac.** Fatal epidemic encephalitis with parotitis.
Bull. Soc. méd. hop., Paris, 1921—XLV—732.

**Blumer, G.** Case of extensive cavernous angioma of head, face
and neck, with attacks of fever and somnolence.
Boston M. & S. J., 1921—CLXXXV—58.

**Fort, J. T.** Malignancy of face and jaws.
Kentucky M. J., Bowling Green, 1921—XIX—456.

**Kennon, R.** Tumors of salivary glands, with their after-history.
Brit. J. Surg., Bristol, 1921—IX—76.

**König, F.** Plastic operations on lips.
Beitr. z. klin. Chir., Tübing., 1921—CXXII—288.

**Netter, Césari, and Durand, H.** The salivary glands in epidemic
encephalitis.
Bull. soc. méd. d. hop., Paris, 1921—XLV—721.

**Plewka, W.** Suppurative parotitis in the newborn.
Arch. f. Kinderh., Stuttg., 1921—LXIX—279.

**Schwartz, E.** Actinomycosis of the salivary gland.
Beitr. z. klin. chir., Tübing., 1921—CXXI—629.

**Vean, V., and Ruppe, C.** Median upper harelip.
Arch. de méd. d. enf., Par., 1921—XXIV—241.

## SECTION 24.—CERVICAL GLANDS AND DEEPER NECK STRUCTURES.

**Blumer, G.** Case of extensive cavernous angioma of head, face
and neck, with attacks of fever and somnolence.
Boston M. & S. J., 1921—CLXXXV—58.

**Broca, A.** Treatment of tuberculous adenitis.
Progrés méd., Par., 1921—XXXVI—227.

**Carp, Louis.** Ranula of branchial origin.
Surg., Gynec. & Obst., Chicago, 1921—XXXIII—182.

**Gerhartz, H.** Tuberculosis of bronchial and cervical glands.
Med. Klin., Berl., 1921—XVII—806.

**Gilman, P. J.** Branchial cysts and fistulas.
J. Am. M. Ass., Chicago, 1921—LXXVII—26.

**Gödde, H.** Deep lymphangioma in the neck.
Deutsche. Ztschr. f. Chir., Leipz., 1921—CLXIII—135.

**Quick, D.** The conservative treatment of cervical lymphatics in
intraoral carcinoma.
J. Am. M. Ass., Chicago, 1921—LXXVII—436.

**Speer, E.** Treatment of torticollis.
München. med. Wchnschr., 1921—LXVIII—672.

## SECTION 25.—THYROID AND THYMUS.

**Baker, A. E.**  Nohyperplastic toxic goiter.
J. South. Car. M. Ass., Greenville, 1921—XVII—108.

**Bär, E.**  Operative treatment of exophthalmic goiter.
Beitr. z. klin. chir., Tübing., 1921—CXXII—87.

**Barr, J.**  Hyperthyroidism and hypothyroidism.
Practitioner, Lond., 1921—CVI—381.

**Bartlett, W.**  Importance of goiter being recognized by general
public.
Ohio M. J., Columbus, 1921—XVII—461.

**Bartlett, W.**  Various operative procedures indicated for different
kinds of goiter.
J. Missouri M. Ass., St. Louis, 1921—XVIII—275.

**Berblinger, W.**  The pituitary with thyroid deficiency.
Mitt. a. d. Grenzgeb. d. Med. u. Chir., Jena, 1921—XXXIII—92.

**Bircher, E.**  Pathology of the thymus.
Schweiz. Arch. f. Neurol. u. Psychiat., Zurich, 1921—VIII—208.

**Boothby, Walter M.**  The basal metabolic rate in hyperthyroidism.
J. Am. M. Ass., Chicago, 1921—LXXVII—252.

**Bram, I.**  The psychic factor in exophthalmic goiter.
J. Am. M. Ass., Chicago, 1921—LXXVII—282.

**Brunner, H. C.**  Accessory intrathoracic goiter.
Beitr. z. klin. Chir., Tübing., 1921—CXXII—114.

**Callison, J. G.**  Double mastoid operation; acute thyrorenal exhaustion.
Laryngoscope, St. Louis, 1921—XXXI—359.

**Clairmont, A., and Suchanek, E.**  Progressive pulmonary tuberculosis after goiter operations.
Arch. f. klin. Chir., Berl., 1921—CXV—995.

**Dubs, J.**  Technic for goiter operations.
Deutsche Ztschr. f. Chir., Leipz., 1921—CLXIII—257.

**Frazier, C. H., and Adler, F. H.**  Basal metabolism estimations in
goiter.
Am. J. M. Sc., Phila., 1921—CLXII—10.

**Garner, M., and Block, S.**  The epinephrin thyroid test.
Bull. Soc. med. d. hop. de Paris, 1921—XLV—1137.

**Gerstenberger, H. J.**  Factor of position of diaphragm in Roentgen
ray diagnosis of enlarged thymus.
Am. J. Dis. Child., Chicago, 1921—XXI—534.

**Gilman, P. K.**  Acute suppurative thyroiditis.
Calif. State J. M., San Francisco, 1921—XVIIII—294.

**Grunenberg, K.**  Vegetative nervous system in exophthalmic goiter.
Deutsche med. Wchnschr., Leipz., 1921—XLVII—648.

**Hagenbuch, Mary.**  Strumitis.
Mitt. a. d. Greuzgeb. d. Med. u. Chir., Jena, 1921—XXXIII—181.

**Hammett, F. S.**  Studies of thyroid apparatus.  Action of thyroxin
on isolated intestinal segment.
Am. J. Physiol., Balt., 1921—LVI—386.

**Hammett, F. S.** Studies of thyroid apparatus. I. stability of nervous system as factor in resistance of albino rat to loss of parathyroid secretion.
Am. J. Physiol., Baltimore, 1921—LVI—196.

**Hammet, F. S., and Tokuda, K.** Studies of thyroid apparatus; changes in amount of intestine; contracting substances of thyroid of albino rat according to age.
Am. J. Physiol., Balt., 1921—LVI—380.

**Holst, J.** Glycosuria and diabetes in exophthalmic goiter.
Acta Med., Scandinavia, Stockholm, 1921—LV—662.

**Judd, E. S.** Consideration of treatment of lesions of thyroid gland.
Minnesota Med., St. Paul, 1921—IV—315.

**Labbé, M., and Stévensin, H.** Action of thyroid and parathyroids on respiratory interchanges.
Ann. de méd., Par., 1921—IX—264.

**Mayo, C. H.** Thyroid and its diseases.
Iowa M. J., Des Moines, 1921—II—297.

**Mayo, C. H.** The thyroid.
Med. Rec., N. Y., 1921—C—177.

**Mosenthal, H. O.** Clinical value of basal metabolism determinations in diseases of thyroid gland.
N. York M. J., 1921—CXIV—41.

**Nather, K.** Tuberculosis of the thyroid.
Mitt. a. d. Greuzgeb. d. Med. u. Chir., Jena, 1921—XXXIII—375.

**Peabody, F. W., Sturgis, C. C., Tompkins, E. M., and Wearn, J. T.** Epinephrin hypersensitiveness and its relation to hyperthyroidism.
Am. J. M. Sc., Phila., 1921—CLXI—508.

**Plummer, Henry S.** Interrelationship of function of the thyroid gland and of its acive agent, thyroxin, in the tissues of the body.
J. Am. M. Ass., Chicago, 1921—LXXVII—243.

**Rogoff, J. M., and Goldblatt, H.** Attempt to detect thyroid secretion in blood obtained from glands of individuals with exophthalmic goiter and other conditions involving thyroid.
J. Pharmacol. & Exper. Therap., Balt., 1921—XVII—473.

**Rubeli, H.** Lingual goiter and pregnancy.
Monatschr. f. Geburtsh. u. Gynaek., Berl., 1920—LII—295.

**Ryser, H.** Explanation of sudden thymic death.
Schweiz. med. Wchnschr., Basel, 1921—LI—554.

**Schmidt, E. O.** Exophthalmic goiter.
Mitt. a. d. Grenzgeb. d. Med. u. Chir., Jena, 1921—XXXIII—512.

**Seymour, M.** Myxedema following treatment of Grave's disease with Roentgen ray.
Boston M. & S. J., 1921—CLXXXV—261.

**Simpson, C. A.** Radium and Roentgen ray treatment of hyperthyroidism.
N. York M. J., 1921—CXIV—36.

**Stanton, J.** Goiter.
Boston M. & S. J., 1921—CLXXXIV—693.

Sträuli, A. Retrogression of goiter after shifting.
Beitr. z. klin. Chir., Tübing., 1921—CXXII—44.

Steck, H. Relations between exophthalmic goiter and tuberculosis.
Schweiz. med. Wchnschr., Basel, 1921—LI—535.

Tixier, L., and Duval, H. Exophthalmic goiter with thyroid tumor and metastases.
Bull. soc. méd. d. hop., Par., 1921—XLV—874.

Tsuji, K. Effect of diet on thyroid functioning.
Acta scholae med. univ. imp. Kioto, 1920—III—713.

Yamanoi, S. The persisting thymus.
Schweiz. med. Wchnschr., Basel, 1921—LI—557.

Yamanoi, S. Thymus lipomas.
Zentralbl. f. Chir., Leipz., 1921—XLVIII—785.

Wilson, L. B. Malignant tumors of thyroid.
Ann. Surg., Phila., 1921—LXXIV—129.

Wolff, G. Malignant goiter.
Beitr. z. klin. Chir., Tübing, 1921—CXXI—56.

## SECTION 26.—PITUITARY.

Berblinger, W. The pituitary with thyroid deficiency.
Mitt. a. d. Grenzgeb. d. Med. u. Chir., Jena, 1921—XXXIII—92.

Fabris, S. Pituitary test in children.
Pediatria, Napoli, 1921—XXVIIII—548.

Friedman, E. D. Unusual hypophysial syndrome.
N. York M. J., 1921—CXIV—113.

Monakow, P. v. Pathology of the pituitary.
Schweiz. arch. f. Neurol. u. Psychiat., Zurich, 1921—VIII—200.

Schulmann, E. Clinical features of pituitary polyuria.
Médicine, Paris, 1921—II—799.

Walton, A. J. Surgery of pituitary gland.
Lancet, Lond., 1921—I—1168.

## SECTION 27.—ENDOCRANIAL AFFECTIONS AND LUM-BAR PUNCTURE.

Boot, G. W. Otitic brain abscess.
Illinois M. J., 1921—XL—122.

Coburn, R. C. New pharyngeal tube for anesthesia in oral and head surgery.
Med. Rec., New York, 1921—C—155.

Fenton, R. A. Case of bilateral thrombosis of lateral sinuses not originating from otitis.
Northwest. Med., Seattle, 1921—XX—155.

Glogau, O. Primary mastoiditis with perisinus and extradural abscess. Operation. Recovery.
Laryngoscope, St. Louis, 1921—XXXI—318.

Goodyear, H. M. Case of extensive lateral sinus thrombosis, with special reference to low resection.
Laryngoscope, St. Louis, 1921—XXXI—365.

**Haguenan, J.** Meningeal reaction in diphtheritic paralysis.
  Bull. soc. méd. d. hop. de Par., 1921—XLV—996.

**Hays, H. M.** Acute bilateral mastoiditis; meningitis; aseptic operation; recovery.
  Laryngoscope, St. Louis, 1921—XXXI—302.

**Merklen, P., Weiss, M., de Gennes, L.** Meningeal reaction in diphtheritic paralysis.
  Bull. soc. méd. d. hop. de Par., 1921—XLV—990.

**Perkins, C. E.** Two cases of advanced suppurative disease of lateral sinus and jugular vein.
  Med. Rec., N. Y., 1921—C—195.

**Shelden, W. D.** Tumors involving the Gasserian ganglion.
  J. Am. M. Ass., Chicago, 1921—LXXVII—700.

**Symonds, C. P.** Case of bilateral eighth nerve tumors associated with multiple neurofibromas and multiple endotheliomas of meninges.
  J. Neurol. & Psychopathol., Bristol, 1921—II—142.

**Taylor, J. A.** Lingual application of iodin as prophylactic in cerebrospinal meningitis and influenza.
  Brit. M. J., Lond., 1921—II—776.

## SECTION 28.—CRANIAL NERVES.

**Achard, C.** Diphtheritic paralysis.
  Bull. méd., Par., 1921—XXXV—567.

**Burrows, H.** Bilateral hypoglossal palsy due to gunshot wounds.
  Brit. M. J., Lond., 1921—II—776.

**De Schweinitz, G. E.** Ocular interpretations of disorders of pituitary body and their nonsurgical treatment.
  Virginia M. Month., Richmond, 1921—XXXXVIII—179.

**Frank, L. W.** Trifacial neuralgia; symptomatology and treatment.
  Kentucky M. J., Bowling Green, 1921—XVIIII—229.

**Franz, L.** Topography of recurrent nerve.
  Beitr. z. klin. Chir., Tübing., 1921—CXXII—366.

**Landon, L. H.** Surgical neuralgia of fifth cranial nerve.
  Ohio M. J., Columbus, 1921—XVII—452.

**Magnus, V.** Trigeminal neuralgia.
  Norsk. Mag. f. Laegevidensk., Kristiania, 1921—LXXXII—420.

**Maybaum, J. L.** Nonsuppurative neurolabyrinthitis, with special reference to focal infection and syphilis as causative factors.
  Ann. Otol., Rhinol. & Layngol., St. Louis, 1921—XXX—719.

**Norman, N. P., and Johnston, H. M.** Neuralgias of superior and inferior maxillary branches of fifth nerve caused by dental pulp nodules.
  N. York M. J., 1921—CXIV—88.

**Ombrédanne, L.** Correction of facial paralysis.
  Presse méd., Par., 1921—XXIX—636.

**Perkins, C. E.** A case of labyrinthitis and cerebellar abscess.
  Ann. Otol., Rhinol. & Laryngol., St. Louis, 1921—XXX—742.

**Post, M. H.** Glaucoma and nasal (sphenopalatine, Meckel's) ganglion.
Arch. Ophth., N. Y., 1921—I—317.

**Poulard.** Diphtheritic paralysis of accommodation.
Paris méd., 1921—XI—57.

**Rooker, A. M.** Case of facial paralysis.
Laryngoscope, St. Louis, 1921—XXXI—363.

**Sachs, E., and Alvis, B. Y.** Anatomic and physiologic studies of eighth nerve.
Arch. Neurol. & Psychiat., Chicago, 1921—VI—119.

**Shelden, W. D.** Tumors involving the Gasserian ganglion.
J. Am. M. Ass., Chicago, 1921—LXXVII—700.

**Symonds, C. P.** Case of bilateral eighth nerve tumors associated with multiple neurofibromas and multiple endotheliomas of meninges.
J. Neurol. & Psychopathol., Bristol, 1921—II—142.

**Wrigley, F. G.** An intracranial complication of chronic middle ear suppuration.
J. Laryngol., etc., Edinburgh, 1921—XXXVI—381.

## SECTION 29.—PLASTIC SURGERY.

**Aboulker, H.** Correction of deformed nose.
Méd., Paris, 1921—II—313.

**Brophy, T. W.** Cleft palate and harelip procedures.
Minnesota Med., St. Paul, 1921—IV—283.

**Day, H. F.** Reconstruction of ears.
Boston M. & S. J., 1921—CLXXXV—146.

**Frank, I., and Strauss, J. F.** An invisible scar method in cosmetic nasal surgery.
Ann. Otol., Rhinol. & Laryngol., St. Louis, 1921—XXX—670.

**Pfeiffer.** Plastic correction of defects in larynx and trachea.
Zentralbl. f. Chir., Leipz., 1921—XLVIII—965.

**Selfridge, G.** Cosmetic surgery of nose.
Laryngoscope, St. Louis, 1921—XXXI—337.

**Shearer, W. L.** Cleft palate and harelip.
Minnesota Med., St. Paul, 1921—IV—293.

**Stotter, J., and Stotter, A. L.** Correction of nasal deformities with autogenous transplants.
Ohio M. J., Columbus, 1921—XVII—384.

## SECTION 30.—INSTRUMENTS.

**Coburn, R. C.** New pharyngeal tube for anesthesia in oral and head surgery.
Med. Rec., New York, 1921—C—155.

**Flanary, D. L.** A new instrument for the enucleation of tonsils in capsule.
J. Am. M. Ass., Chicago, 1921—LXXVII—201.

**Goodyear, H. M.** New tonsil instrument.
J. Am. M. Ass., Chicago, 1921—LXXVII—201.

**Greene, J. B.** A palate-tonsil retractor.
J. Am. M. Ass., Chicago, 1921—LXXVII—39.

**Perthes, G., and Jüngling, O.** Radium applicator for mouth.
Zentralbl. f. Chir., Leipz., 1921—XLVIII—958.

**Searcy, H. B.** Searcy tonsillectome.
South. M. J., Birmingham, 1921—XIV—639.

**Warren, L. P.** New tonsil forceps.
J. Am. M. Ass., Chicago, 1921—LXXVII—285.

## SECTION 31.—RADIOLOGY.

**Dufourmentel, L.** Radium treatment of cancer of the esophagus.
Méd., Paris, 1921—II—321.

**Freer, O. T.** Radium emanation in upper air passages as compared
to radium: A method of applying it with especial reference to laryngeal carcinoma.
Illinois M. J., 1921—XL—85.

**Hotz, G.** Radium treatment of cancer of the esophagus.
Schweiz. med. Wchnschr., Basel, 1921—LI—460.

**Kästner, H.** Roentgen findings in the trachea.
Beitr. z. klin. Chir., Tübing., 1921—CXXII—455.

**Lyons, H. R.** Radium in treatment of myxomatous nasal polyps.
Am. J. Roentgenol., New York, 1921—VIII—407.

**Perthes, G., and Jüngling, O.** Radium applicator for mouth.
Zentralbl. f. Chir., Leipz., 1921—XLVIII—958.

**Rockey, A. E.** Radium treatment of cancer of the esophagus.
J. Am. M. Ass., Chicago, 1921—LXXVII—30.

**Roy, D.** Case of intranasal epithelioma cured by excision and radium. Literature.
Ann. Otol., Rhinol. & Laryngol., St. Louis, 1921—XXX—748.

**Seymour, M.** Myxedema following treatment of Grave's disease
with Roentgen ray.
Boston M. & S. J., 1921—CLXXXV—261.

**Simpson, C. A.** Radium and Roentgen ray treatment of hyperthyroidism.
N. York M. J., 1921—CXIV—36.

**Spencer, F. R.** Roentgenology of the mastoids with conclusions
based on one hundred cases.
Ann. Otol., Rhinol. & Laryngol., St. Louis, 1921—XXX—770.

**Witherbee, W. D.** Principles involved in Roentgen ray treatment of
tonsils.
Laryngoscope, St. Louis, 1921—XXXI—305.

## SECTION 34.—EYE.

**Ball, J. M.** Proper treatment of acute suppurative dacryocystitis.
Am. J. Ophth., Chicago, 1921—IV—447.

**Bär, E.** Operative treatment of exophthalmic goiter.
Beitr. z. klin. chir., Tübing., 1921—CXXII—87.

**Bram, I.** The psychic factor in exophthalmic goiter.
J. Am. M. Ass., Chicago, 1921—LXXVII—282.

**Chamberlin, W. B.** The endonasal operation of the lacrimal sac.
Ann. Otol., Rhinol. & Laryngol., St. Louis, 1921—XXX—643.

**De Schweinitz, G. E.** Ocular interpretations of disorders of pituitary body and their nonsurgical treatment.
Virginia M. Month., Richmond, 1921—XLVIII—179.

**Good, R. H.** Simplified intranasal operation for obstruction of nasolacrimal duct.
Am. J. Ophth., Chicago, 1921—IV—597.

**Gradle, H.** Congenital atresia of puncta lacrimalia of one side.
Arch. Ophth., N. Y., 1921—I—349.

**Griscom, J. M.** Relation of intranasal pressure to heterophoria.
Penn. M. J., 1921—XXIV—804.

**Grunenberg, K.** Vegetative nervous system in exophthalmic goiter.
Deutsche med. Wchnschr., Leipz., 1921—XLVII—648.

**Gutmann, A.** Interrelationship of eye and dental disease.
Deutsche med. Wchnschr., Berl., 1921—XLVII—565.

**Holst, J.** Glycosuria and diabetes in exophthalmic goiter.
Acta Med., Scandinavia, Stockholm, 1921—LV—302.

**MacMillan, J. A.** New operation for treatment of lacrimal obstruction.
Am. J. Ophth., Chicago, 1921—IV—448.

**Morton, J. B.** Relation of eye, ear, nose and throat to general medicine.
Illinois M. J., 1921—XL—97.

**Mosher, H. P.** Mosher-Toti operation on lacrimal sac.
Laryngoscope, St. Louis, 1921—XXXI—284.

**Patterson, J. A.** Ocular diseases of nasal origin.
Am. J. Ophth., Chicago, 1921—IV—513.

**Post, M. H.** Glaucoma and nasal (sphenopalatine, Meckel's) ganglion.
Arch. Ophth., N. Y., 1921—I—317.

**Schmidt, E. O.** Exophthalmic goiter.
Mitt. a. d. Greuzgeb. d. med. u. chir., Jena, 1921—XXXIII—512.

**Sluder, G.** The borderland of rhinology, neurology and ophthalmology.
J. Am. M. Ass., Chicago, 1921—LXXVII—688.

**Stark, H. H.** Retrobulbar neuritis, secondary to disease of the nasal sinuses.
J. Am. M. Ass., Chicago, 1921—LXXVII—678.

**Thomson, E. S.** Some clinical phases of ocular involvement in sinus disease.
Am. J. Ophth., Chicago, 1921—IV—507.

**Tixier, L., and Duval, H.** Exophthalmic goiter with thyroid tumor and metastases.
Bull. soc. méd. d. hop., Par., 1921—XLV—874.

**Wiener, M., and Loeb, H. W.** Eye in relation to ear, nose and throat.
South M. J., Birmingham, 1921—XIV—491.

# INDEX OF AUTHORS.

# INDEX OF TITLES.

19.
746 -4

·

RF
1
A64
v. 30
Biological
& Medical
Serials

Annals of otology, rhinology
and laryngology

PLEASE DO NOT REMOVE
CARDS OR SLIPS FROM THIS POCKET

UNIVERSITY OF TORONTO LIBRARY

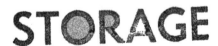

STORAGE

Lightning Source UK Ltd.
Milton Keynes UK
UKHW012033121218
333853UK00008B/569/P